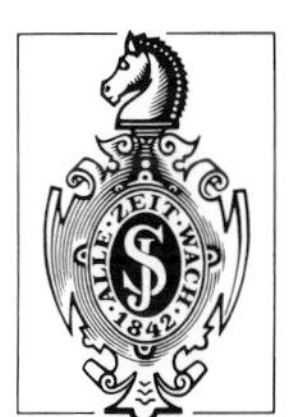
ALLE ZEIT WACH
1842

Coordinating Editor	Chapter Authors	Contributors
M. Allgöwer	M. Aebi	M. Allgöwer
	F. Behrens	F. Baumgart
	Ch. Colton	J.R. Border
	R. Ganz	M. Bühler
	S.T. Hansen	W. Dick
	U. Heim	A. Fernandez
	D. Höntsch	R. Frigg
	R.K. Marti	S. Gertzbein
	J. Mast	G. Hierholzer
	J.M. Matta	F. Magerl
	P. Matter	P. Matter
	S.M. Perren	E. Morscher
	W.W. Rittmann	M.E. Müller
	H. Rosen	S.M. Perren
	Th. Rüedi	P. Regazzoni
	J. Schatzker	Th. Rüedi
	L. Schweiberer	
	R. Szyszkowitz	
	M. Tile	
	H. Tscherne	
	J.K. Webb	
	B.G. Weber	
	S. Weller	
	H. Willenegger	

M. E. Müller · M. Allgöwer
R. Schneider · H. Willenegger

Manual of INTERNAL FIXATION

Techniques Recommended by the AO-ASIF Group

Contribution on Biomechanics by S.M. Perren

Coordinating Editor
M. Allgöwer

Third Edition, Expanded and Completely Revised
With 500 Illustrations, Mostly in Color

Springer-Verlag
Berlin Heidelberg NewYork
London Paris Tokyo
Hong Kong Barcelona

Foreign language editions of the 1st edition

German edition

Springer-Verlag
Berlin Heidelberg New York 1969

French edition

Masson et Cie., Éditeurs
Paris 1970, 1974

Italian Edition

Aulo Gaggi, Editore
Bologna 1970

Japanese Edition

Igaku Shoin
Tokyo 1971

Spanish Edition

Editorial Científico-Médica
Barcelona 1971, 1972, 1975, 1977

Foreign language editions of the 2nd edition

German Edition

Springer-Verlag
Berlin Heidelberg New York 1977

Spanish Edition

Springer-Verlag
Berlin Heidelberg New York 1979

French Edition

Springer-Verlag
Berlin Heidelberg New York 1979

Italian Edition

Piccin Editore
Padova 1981

Chinese Edition

Springer-Verlag
Berlin Heidelberg New York Tokyo 1983

Japanese Edition

Springer-Verlag
Tokyo 1988

3rd Edition 1991
Corrected 3rd printing 1995

ISBN 3-540-52523-8 3rd Edition Springer-Verlag Berlin Heidelberg New York Tokyo
ISBN 0-387-52523-8 3rd Edition Springer-Verlag New York Berlin Heidelberg Tokyo
ISBN 4-431-52523-8 3rd Edition Springer-Verlag Tokyo Berlin Heidelberg New York

ISBN 3-540-09227-7 2nd Edition Springer-Verlag Berlin Heidelberg New York
ISBN 0-387-09227-7 2nd Edition Springer-Verlag New York Heidelberg Berlin

Library of Congress Cataloging-in-Publication Data. Manual of internal fixation: techniques recommended by the AO-ASIF Group / M.E. Müller ... [et al.]; coordinating editor, M. Allgöwer. – 3rd ed., expanded and complete rev. p. cm. Includes bibliographical references and index. ISBN 3-540-52523-8 (alk. paper): ISBN 0-387-52523-8 (alk. paper). 1. Internal fixation in fractures. I. Müller, M.E. (Maurice Edmond), 1918. II. Allgöwer, Martin. III. Arbeitsgemeinschaft für Osteosynthesefragen. [DNLM: 1. Fracture Fixation, Internal. WE 185 M294]. RD103.I5M8313 1990 617.1'5--dc20 DNLM/DLC for Library of Congress 90-10386 CIP

Reproduction of the figures: Gustav Dreher GmbH, Stuttgart

Typesetting, printing and bookbinding: Universitätsdruckerei H. Stürtz AG, Würzburg

2124/3111-54 – Printed on acid-free paper

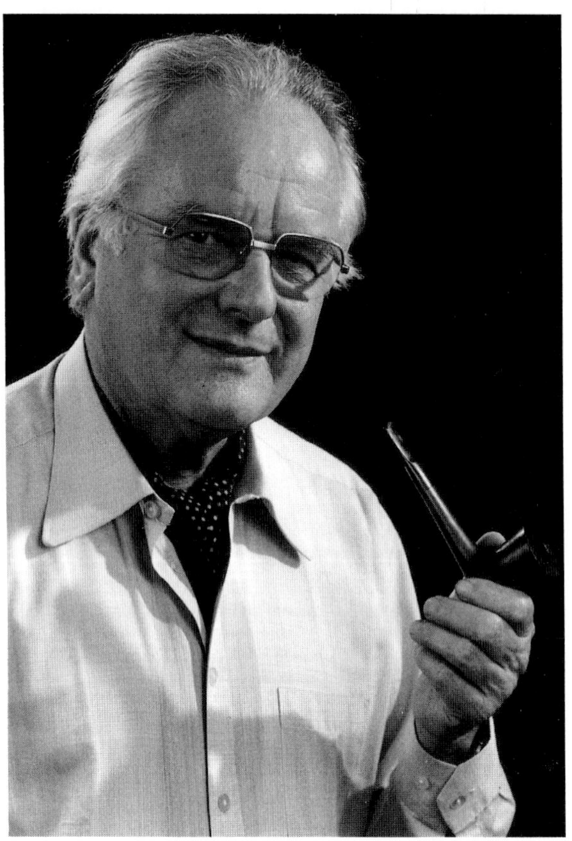

In Memoriam

Professor
ROBERT SCHNEIDER, MD
1912–1990

For twenty years (1958–1978) Robert Schneider was the chairman of the Swiss AO group. Under his leadership it achieved pre-eminence in the field of operative care of fractures and brought about a global revolution in the treatment of fractures and trauma. This achievement bears witness to the greatness of this sincere and honest man and self-critical scientist more than any words.

Robert Schneider was the head of a small county hospital in Grosshöchstetten. His isolation from the academic atmosphere of a university did not, however, stifle his productivity. His leadership talents, his abilities as an organizer, his immediate grasp of and insight into the most complex problems, his abilities as an orthopedic surgeon and healer and his personal warmth brought him the friendship and admiration of patients and colleagues alike.

A close friend and colleague of the founders of the AO, he was a wise choice as chairman of the Swiss AO group. The valuable discoveries and developments he made in AO techniques, implants, and instruments were numerous. He was meticulous in his preoperative planning and assiduous in documenting every operative procedure.

Robert Schneider published some forty scientific papers and in 1981 a much admired monograph on total hip replacement, a revised edition of which was translated into English in 1989. He also chronicled the first twenty-five years of the Swiss AO in the book *25 Jahre AO – Schweiz*.

Of the four AO Manual editors, he is the first to leave us. The trusted advisor to his Swiss colleagues and father figure of the Spanish and German AO groups, he will be remembered by many friends. For future students of the AO philosophy and methods, his achievement and scholarship will live on.

PREFACE TO THE THIRD EDITION

In the early 1950s, the pioneering work of Robert Danis on operative treatment of fractures was in danger of falling into oblivion. Maurice E. Müller, impressed and intrigued by his contacts with Danis, first critically applied internal fixation and immediate mobilization to some 80 patients and found the basic concept confirmed, but in need of further development with regard to technology, clinical application, and scientific analysis. In 1958 he assembled a group of friends, general and orthopedic surgeons, willing to invest time and effort in helping to create the necessary armamentarium and to form a study group for clinical trials. This group was set up in the same year under the name Arbeitsgemeinschaft für Osteosynthesefragen (AO), later on to be known in English-speaking countries as the Association for the Study of Internal Fixation (ASIF).

The first report on operative treatment of fractures by Müller, Allgöwer, and Willenegger, published in 1963, stressed the advantages of early open reduction and internal fixation. This book, first published in German, amusingly lost an important part when translated into English. At the suggestion of worried American and English partners, a picture series showing the healing pattern of 188 tibial fractures operated on in Chur between December 20, 1961 and April 26, 1962 was left out. Operating on fresh tibial fractures was considered by many to be a policy that might discredit the whole AO effort in the United States as well as in the United Kingdom!

The technical solutions embodied in various operative fixation methods for fractures, osteotomies, and arthrodeses accepted and used by the Swiss AO group were discussed and demonstrated in detail in 1969 in the first edition and in 1979 in the second edition of the *Manual of Internal Fixation*. Both editions were reprinted many times.

These reprintings in themselves would not have justified an entirely revised edition only to illustrate small changes. It had, however, become obvious that the extensive research carried out at the Davos institute deserved a more prominent position within the manual. By the same token, successful basic and clinical contributions from many countries outside of Switzerland were rightly felt to merit recognition.

To pay tribute to the international support in achieving the worldwide impact of the "AO philosophy," the AO/ASIF foundation was created in 1984, calling on 80 trustees from 15 different countries.

It was thought inappropriate to delegate the task of rewriting the manual again to the relatively small "Swiss team" – many of our courses actually have a remarkably international faculty. At the second general assembly of the foundation, the need for such a third edition was generally recognized and all 80 trustees agreed to be assigned to one of the 20 working groups charged with reediting the 20 chapters of the previous manuals. These group members met two to three times, the conceptional input being extremely valuable. The chairman of each group was given the onerous task of acting as the chapter author. In several chapters certain surgeons and/or basic researchers have made particularly significant contributions and they therefore figure as "contributors." The table of contents not only indicates the chapter authors and the contributors but also the group members in recognition of their efforts at the onset of this four-year endeavor!

It was decided that the third edition should preserve the general layout as well as the system of instructive drawings with only very few X-rays. Ample room had to be provided for new implants and techniques, and the technical section had to be preceded by a detailed report on "state-of-the-art biomechanics." The AO classification of fractures, as well as a classification of soft tissue injuries, also had to be included. This considerable increase in scope more than doubled the number of pages but it still was possible to keep the book to one volume.

We would not wish to conclude this preface without a general remark concerning modern trauma care in general. In the course of the past decade, evidence accumulated that early total care not only improves the outcome of localized lesions, but also reduces the incidence of ARDS (adult respiratory distress syndrome) and MOF (multiple organ failure). It became obvious that these complications of the period after injury depend not only on the initial severity of the trauma, but also on treatment methods, particularly early total care in the first few hours. The successful early neutralization of the traumatic lesions and prevention of the secondary spread of pathophysiological disorders has formed the basis of the remarkable progress in understanding and treating trauma reactions of the human body. Many years later, this led to a comprehensive report by John Border and collaborators on the pathophysiology and treatment of blunt multiple trauma, published in 1990.

We would like to express our sincere appreciation for the excellent work by the staff of Springer-Verlag, for the invaluable help of Sarah Nevill in streamlining and typing the various manuscripts, and last but not least to Klaus Oberli and the late Julius Pupp for their careful illustrations.

October 1990 The Editors

PREFACE TO THE SECOND EDITION

The goal of the Association for the Study of the Problems of Internal Fixation (AO/ASIF) is not just the propagation of internal fixation. The name of the Association implies its activity; it concerns itself with the problems of internal fixation. It has two main spheres of activity. The one deals with the question of indications for internal fixation in fracture treatment. The other deals with biomechanical improvements of internal fixation for fractures, osteotomies and non-unions.

The difficulties and failures which over the decades plagued internal fixation were, apart from wound infection, largely the result of lack of knowledge of basic scientific facts. Bone healing in the presence of internal fixation was poorly understood. The Association (AO) began its studies by focusing on this problem. These efforts led to the foundation of the Laboratory for Experimental Surgery in Davos. A research programme was developed which encompassed the fields of biology, biomechanics and metallurgy. Research in these fields was pursued at Davos as well as in the associated hospitals and institutions. New bone instruments and implants were developed and constantly modified in accordance with the new biomechanical discoveries made in the basic laboratory and associated hospitals. The evaluation of the newly developed methods was greatly enhanced by careful clinical documentation of the patients during their initial treatment and follow-up. Another important source of suggestions and advice have been the AO basic and advanced courses which have been held regularly both in Switzerland and in other countries. They represent an international effort of considerable magnitude: by the end of 1976, 55 basic courses had been held with almost 20,000 general and orthopaedic surgeons having participated.

The manual, as its name implies, is designed chiefly to convey technical details. The technical recommendations, however, are based upon fundamental research, as well as upon the vast clinical experience of over 50,000 operatively treated fractures, osteotomies and non-unions. Simply because in the manual we dwell on the operative methods of stabilization of most of the skeleton, one should not assume that we wish to minimize the issue of indications for operative intervention. Although in this second edition we discuss the indications in greater detail than we did in the first, they still remain the personal responsibility of the surgeon. Operative fracture treatment is a most worthwhile but a very difficult and demanding therapeutic method. We must reiterate what we stated in 1963 in our book *The Technique of Internal Fixation of Fractures* and in the first edition of this manual in 1969. Internal fixation should not be carried out by an inadequately trained surgeon, nor without the necessary equipment and adequate sterile operating room conditions. Advocates of internal fixation who lack self-criticism are much more dangerous than sceptics or outright opponents. We hope that our readers will understand our efforts in this direction and pass on to us any constructive criticism.

We wish to express our gratitude to all the members of the AO who took part in the revision of this manual as well as to our marvellous artist Mr. K. Oberli and to our dear and dependable collaborator Miss E. Moosberger.

The Editors

CONTENTS

3 SCREWS AND PLATES AND THEIR APPLICATION

Chapter Author: J. Schatzker

Group Members: Initial input by A. Alho and J. Sheehan is gratefully acknowledged

With 58 Figures

8 FOREARM AND HAND/MINI-IMPLANTS

Chapter Author: U. Heim
Group Members: J.M. Ortega, A. Pannike, and B. Spiessl
With 22 Figures

11 PROXIMAL FEMUR

Chapter Author: R. Ganz
Group Members: N.J. Canha, F. Gonzalo-Vivar, and E. Trojan
With 16 Figures

12 FEMORAL SHAFT AND DISTAL FEMUR

Chapter Author: H. Tscherne
Group Members: E. Beck and B. Mallin
With 12 Figures

13 PATELLA AND TIBIA

Chapter Author: R. Szyszkowitz
Group Members: M. Allgöwer, H.P. Burch, R. Teitge, and H. Vasey
With 30 Figures

15 FOOT

Chapter Author: S.T. Hansen
Group Members: H. Bèzes, G. Friedebold and M. Landolt
With 7 Figures

16 THE SPINE

Chapter Authors: M. Aebi and J.K. Webb
Contributors: W. Dick, S. Gertzbein, F. Magerl, and E. Morscher
Group Members: H. Cotta, F. Magerl, E. Morscher, S. Olerud, and J.K. Webb
With 41 Figures

17 COMPOUND FRACTURES

Chapter Authors: W.W. Rittmann and J.K. Webb
Group Members: A. Appley and E. Zerbi

18 FRACTURES IN CHILDREN

Chapter Authors: Ch. Colton and R.K. Marti
Group Members: P. Optecam, E. Sander, and Ph. Spiegel
With 26 Figures

20 INFECTIONS

Chapter Author: H. Willenegger
Group Members: F. Brussatis, H. Grove, and K. Korzinek

LIST OF ADDRESSES

Aebi, Max, P.D. Dr., Klinik und Poliklinik für Orthopädische Chirurgie, Inselspital, CH-3010 Bern

Allgöwer, Martin, Prof. Dr., International Society of Surgery (ISS) / Société Internationale de Chirurgie (SIC), Hauptstr. 63, CH-4153 Reinach BL 1

Baumgart, Frank, Prof. Dr. Ing., Schweizerisches Forschungsinstitut, Laboratorium für Experimentelle Chirurgie, CH-7220 Davos

Behrens, Fred, M.D., F.R.C.S., Orthopaedic Department, Case Western Reserve University, Metro Health Systems, 3395 Scranton Road, Cleveland, OH 44109, USA

Border, John R., M.D., University of Buffalo, Department of Surgery, School of Medicine and Biomedical Sciences, Eric County Medical Center, 462 Grider Street, Buffalo, NY 14215, USA

Bühler, Markus, AO Dokumentation, Belpstr. 24, CH-3014 Bern

Colton, Christopher, M.D., F.R.C.S., Consultant Orthopedic Surgeon, University Hospital, Queen's Medical Centre, GB-Nottingham NG7 2UH

Dick, Walter, P.D. Dr., Leitender Arzt, Orthopädische Universitätsklinik, Felix-Platter-Spital, CH 4055 Basel

Fernandez, Alberto, Dr., Hospital Britanico, Av. Italia 2424, Montevideo, Uruguay

Frigg, Robert, Schweizerisches Forschungsinstitut, Laboratorium für Experimentelle Chirurgie, CH-7220 Davos

Ganz, Reinhold, Prof. Dr., Universität Bern, Klinik und Poliklinik für Orthopädische Chirurgie, Inselspital, CH-3010 Bern

Gertzbein, Stanley D., M.D., F.R.C.S. (C), 2075 Bayview Avenue, Toronto, Ontario M4N 3M5, Canada

Hansen, Sigvard T., Prof. Dr., Harborview Medical Centre, 325 Ninth Avenue, Seattle, WA 98104, USA

Heim, Urs, P.D. Dr., Mattenstr. 17a, CH-3073 Gümligen-Bern

Hierholzer, Günther, Prof. Dr., Ärztlicher Direktor der Berufsgenossenschaftlichen Unfallklinik, Großenbaumer Allee 250, W-4100 Duisburg, FRG

Höntsch, Dankwart, Dr., Berufsgenossenschaftliche Unfallklinik, Rosenauerweg 95, W-7400 Tübingen, FRG

Magerl, Fritz, P.D. Dr., Klinik für Orthopädische Chirurgie, Kantonsspital St. Gallen, CH-9007 St. Gallen

Marti, René K., Prof. Dr., Academisch Medisch Centrum, Meibergdreef 9, NL-1105 AZ Amsterdam Z.O.

Mast, Jeffrey, M.D., Department of Orthopaedic Surgery, Wayne State University, Hutzel Hospital, 4707 St. Antoine Blvd., Detroit, MI 48201, USA

Matta, Joel M., M.D., USC Orthopedic Medical Group, 2300 South Flower Street, Suite 2000, Los Angeles, CA 90007, USA

Matter, Peter, Prof. Dr., Chirurgische Abteilung, Spital Davos, CH-7220 Davos

Morscher, Erwin, Prof. Dr., Orthopädische Universitätsklinik, Felix-Platter-Spital, CH-4055 Basel

Müller, Maurice E., Prof. Dr., Fondation Maurice E. Müller, Murtenstr. 35, CH-3008 Bern

Perren, Stephan M., Prof. Dr., Schweizerisches Forschungsinstitut, Laboratorium für Experimentelle Chirurgie, CH-7220 Davos

Regazzoni, Pietro, P.D. Dr., Departement für Chirurgie, Kantonsspital Basel, CH-4031 Basel

Rittmann, Willy-Werner, Prof. Dr., Kantonsspital St. Gallen, Chirurgische Abteilung, CH-9007 St. Gallen

Rosen, Howard, M.D., Stewart House, 70 East 10th Street, New York, NY 10003, USA

Rüedi, Thomas, Prof. Dr., Rätisches Kantons- und Regionalspital Chur, Chirurgische Klinik, CH-7000 Chur

Schatzker, Joseph, Dr., M.D., B.Sc. (Med.), F.R.C.S. (C), Sunnybrook Medical Centre, 2075 Bayview Avenue, Toronto, Ontario M4N 3M5, Canada

Schneider, Robert (†), Prof. Dr. med., Alpenstr. 15, CH-2500 Biel

Schweiberer, Leonhard, Prof. Dr., Direktor der Chirurgischen Universitätsklinik, Innenstadt, Nußbaumstr. 20, W-8000 München 2, FRG

Szyszkowitz, Rudolf, Prof. Dr., Departement für Unfallchirurgie, Universitätsklinik für Chirurgie, Auenbruggerplatz, A-8036 Graz

Tile, Marvin, M.D., B.Sc. (Med.), F.R.C.S. (C), Surgeon-in-Chief, Sunnybrook Medical Centre, 2075 Bayview Avenue, Toronto, Ontario M4N 3M5, Canada

Tscherne, Harald, Prof. Dr., Unfallchirurgische Klinik der Medizinischen Hochschule, Konstanty-Gutschow-Str. 8, W-3000 Hannover 61, FRG

Webb, John K., M.D., F.R.C.S., Queen's Medical Centre, GB-Nottingham, NG7 2UH

Weber, Bernhard G., Prof. Dr., Rorschachstr. 150, Silberturm, CH-9007 St. Gallen

Weller, Siegfried, Prof. Dr., Berufsgenossenschaftliche Klinik, Rosenauer Weg 95, W-7400 Tübingen, FRG

Willenegger, Hans, Prof. Dr., AO-International, Balderstr. 30, CH-3007 Bern

1 BASIC ASPECTS OF INTERNAL FIXATION

1.1 Aims and Principles

1.1.1 Introduction

Every fracture leads to a complex tissue injury involving bone and surrounding soft parts. Immediately after the fracture and during the repair phase, we see local circulatory disturbances and manifestations of local inflammation, as well as pain and reflex immobilization. These three factors, circulatory disturbance, inflammation, and pain, a result of dysfunction of joints and muscles, lead to the so-called fracture disease (Lucas-Championniere 1907).

Fracture disease is caused by two main pathogenic factors: pain and lack of physiological challenge to the bone-muscle complex by movement and changing mechanical load. In the lower limb, this means lack of weight-bearing, in the upper limb, lack of normal muscle work. Fracture disease is therefore a clinical state manifested by chronic edema, soft tissue atrophy and patchy osteoporosis. Edema, as such, induces intermuscular fibrosis and muscular atrophy. These fibrotic processes cause muscles to develop unphysiological adhesions to bone and fascia and therefore lead to stiffness of adjacent joints.

These sequelae, if fully developed, are very often not completely corrected by long-term physiotherapy. At best they keep the patient out of work for weeks or months, and all too often they lead to partial or even total invalidity. In 1945, the rate of permanent partial invalidity compensated by the Swiss National Insurance Company was 35% following tibia fractures and some 70% after femur fractures. Thus, permanent impairment is more often due to the sequelae of fracture disease than to defective bone healing in malalignment or non-union.

1.1.2 Life Is Movement, Movement Is Life

This should be the guiding principle of fracture care! Full, active, pain-free mobilization results in a rapid return of normal blood supply to both the bone and the soft tissues. It also enhances articular cartilage nutrition by the synovial fluid, and when combined with partial weight-bearing, it greatly decreases post-traumatic osteoporosis by restoring an equilibrium between bone resorption and bone formation. A satisfactory internal fixation is achieved only when external immobilization is superfluous and when full, active, pain-free mobilization of muscles and joints is possible. This is the AO's main objective and is best achieved by stable internal fixation during the bone healing process.

Major fractures, particularly of long bones, the pelvis, and the spine, have repercussions on the homeostasis of the accident victim as a whole but primarily on the cardiorespiratory system. This new edition of the *AO Manual* is directed at dealing with the local lesions involving fractures. A detailed study supported by the AO group of the general reaction to, and the treatment of, severe trauma is being published by Border et al. (1990).

At the outset in 1958, the AO formulated four treatment principles which were expected to improve the results of fracture treatment in general and of internal fixation in particular (Müller et al. 1984). Some 30 years later it appears timely to evaluate the extent to which these four principles have stood the test of time. They were:

- *Anatomical reduction* of the fracture fragments, particularly in joint fractures.
- *Stable internal fixation* designed to fulfill the local biomechanical demands.
- *Preservation of the blood supply* to the bone fragments and the soft tissue by means of atraumatic surgical technique.
- *Early active pain-free mobilization* of muscles and joints adjacent to the fracture, preventing the development of fracture disease

The first of these principles, *anatomical reduction*, has kept all its importance in the reconstituting of full function in all joint fractures and is also valuable with regard to length, rotation, and axes of meta- and diaphysis. In diaphyseal fractures it has received certain corrections with regard to reduction of cortical fragments, where it has become related to the method of operative treatment employed. It is of primary importance in fixation by lag screws with or without protection by neutralization (protection) plates. To achieve optimal mechanical strength, the cortical circumference must be fully reconstructed and placed under interfragmental, as well as axial, compression.

However, there is a precarious balance to be struck between early mechanical perfection and devascularization of the detachment fragments. The idea of the "biological fixation" has branched off in two directions. The first relates to the application of flexible plates and the second concerns the application of conventional plates bridging a complex fracture zone with only three or four screws anchored proximally and distally in the intact parts of the fractured bone.

So-called flexible plates have been devised in an endeavor to avoid the "stress protection" formerly believed to be instrumental in plate-induced cortical osteoporosis. This has clearly been demonstrated to be a misconception. Plate osteoporosis after "flexible plating," rather than being decreased, is increased because of the more marked vascular disturbance caused by the tightly fitting plate. In contrast to conventional plates, the LC-DCP (limited-contact DCP) preserves periosteal blood supply (see pp. 62, 74), causes less osteoporosis than the DCP with a flat undersurface, and furthermore allows the cortical bone underlaying the plate to develop a thin callus bridge. Clinically this is probably of limited importance because thanks to rapid remodeling, cortical healing following application of a normal DCP is successful in a large majority of cases. However, the possibility of avoiding cortical osteoporosis underlying the plate is of considerable scientific and even clinical interest.

The second very successful line of thought led to the idea of the bridge plate (Müller and Witzel 1984; Heitemeyer and Hierholzer 1985) and the wave plate (Brunner and Weber 1981). The basic idea is to leave the fracture zone and its fragments undisturbed by fixing the plate to the intact part of the bone distal and proximal to the fragment area. When a multifragmentary fracture area is bridged using a wave plate two advantageous mechanisms come into play: (1) when the plate spans an extended fracture area the inner part of the plate, not fixed to the bone, undergoes more distributed deformation, so that sites of excessive deformation prone to fatigue failure are avoided, and (2) the plate applied at a distance to the bone permits better vascular access to the repair tissue and benefits more from the mechanical support provided by the repair tissue due to better leverage.

Similar considerations apply to the second principle, *stable fixation*. All methods of operative fixation must provide adequate stability to maintain length, axes and rotation. Lag screw fixation, with or without neutralization plates, depends on "absolute stability" for optimal healing, which occurs by direct angiogenic (haversian) bridging of the precisely reduced fracture. In these cases, visible "cloudy callus" is indicative of lost stability, for which nature has tried to compensate. It shows the need for a reduced challenge to the fracture area by decreased weight-bearing.

The bone healing pattern is completely different from that of direct angiogenic union when plates are applied in a bridging mode or when medullary nailing or external fixation is used. With these latter methods, a certain amount of interfragmentary movement is inevitable, even desirable, and nature has to supplement stabilization by producing callus to solidify the "welding" of the fragments.

In summary, callus-free healing is not an aim in itself. It is a fascinating biological property of living cortical bone under conditions of absolute stability and good vascularity. It is clinically only relevant in interfragmentary compression by means of lag screws with or without neutralization plates.

Emphasis on the third principle of *atraumatic surgical technique* has, if anything, increased. It concerns not only the soft tissues but also the bony fragments and, in particular, their vascularity (Mast et al. 1989)!

The fourth principle, *early pain-free mobilization*, has certainly stood the test of time, and proof is at hand that after most fractures permanent impairment has significantly decreased with the advent of immediate postoperative mobilization. A new dimension has been added and abundantly documented in the last two decases – the merit of early total care of the severely traumatized patient in the hours following the accident. A good number of pathophysiological events, earlier thought to be caused by trauma, have now been shown to be related to treatment modalities. In particular, if the human body lies for an extended period of time in the unphysiological supine position, this can lead to long-lasting cardiorespiratory disturbance, which often ends in multiple organ failure. These problems are discussed in Chap. 6 and are detailed in a separate book entitled *Blunt Multiple Trauma: Comprehensive Pathophysiology and Care* by Border et al. (1990).

In summary, the initial working hypothesis expressed in the four treatment principles has seen certain changes in emphasis but, all in all, has stood the test of time!

1.2 Basic Aspects

A review of bone as a material, its fracture and spontaneous healing should help to understand the problems and basic goals of fracture treatment.

1.2.1 Bone as a Material

The strength of bone (Fig. 1.1) *is about 1/10 that of steel.* The apatite structure of bone is at the basis of its excellent compressive strength. The tensile elements of bone, i.e., the collagen fibers, are generally thought to be weaker. The tensile strength of the tibia, for instance, is about 20% less than its compressive strength. That of the radius, on the other hand, is higher by 20% (Knets 1980). The strength of cancellous bone is very variable and usually less than 1/10 of that of cortical bone (Yamada and Evans 1970).[1] Compression applied to bone using so-called rigid implants is maintained due to the elastic deformability of the bone. A comparably small loss (about 10%–20%) is explained by the time-dependent deformation under load ("creep" or, vice versa, "stress relaxation"). This phenomenon was earlier attributed to "visco-elasticity of bone". A dominant quality of bone is its *brittleness*: bone behaves more like glass than like rubber. When bone is deformed (e.g., elongated) only about 2% of its length, it breaks.

The anisotropy of bone, i.e., its different mechanical properties along different axes, does not play a major role in internal fixation and will therefore be disregarded here.

Bone serves as a framework for soft organs and allows for locomotion. (It furthermore stores minerals, primarily calcium, a function which will not be discussed here.) To function as a skeleton, the bones must be stiff. As we shall see on p. 50, this stiffness is the main reason why the stability achieved using internal fixation may be jeopardized by minimal bone fracture surface resorption.[2] During normal activity, and much more so during sports activity, bone must resist large forces.

[1] The ultimate tensile or compressive strength of bone is about 1 MPa. A segment of the tibia may therefore be loaded with the weight of a small car without risk of failure (see Fig. 1.1a). For practical purposes one should keep in mind that a standard 4.5-mm screw anchored, for example, in one femoral cortex, is able to resist 400 N per millimeter of cortical thickness. Such a screw could therefore carry the weight of three persons.

[2] The Young's modulus of axial stiffness of cortical bone amounts to 20 GPa. As a practical example, a tibia loaded by body weight shortens about 60 μm or six cell layers only. The stiffness of a plated and compressed diaphyseal bone segment is such that only 10 μm shortening results from a load of 1000 N being applied axially. Bone, therefore, corresponds to a very stiff spring, a fact which is of importance in internal fixation. The stiffness of cancellous bone as a material is 1/5–1/10 that of cortical bone in axial compression. In bending and torque the geometry plays a more important role, compensating for the difference in material properties.

Fig. 1.1 Strength of bone.

Bone is a comparatively strong material. Its strength exceeds by far the requirements of heavy physical activity.

a Compressive strength. A short segment of the tibia diaphysis is able to carry the weight of a small car.

b Holding strength of a screw within cortical bone. A standard 4.5-mm cortex screw, anchored in only one cortex, can withstand 2500 N (the weight of three persons).

Fig. 1.1

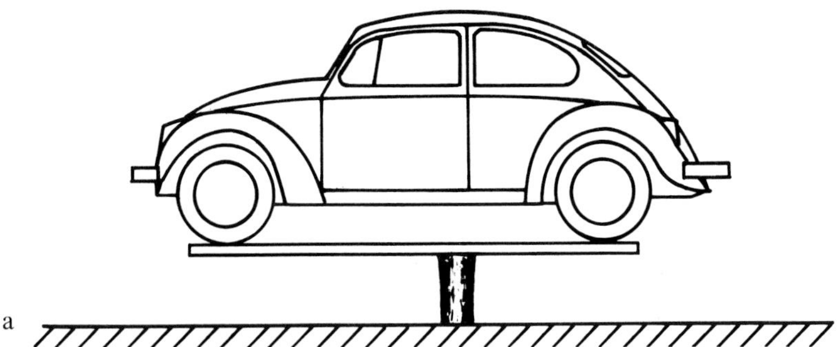
a

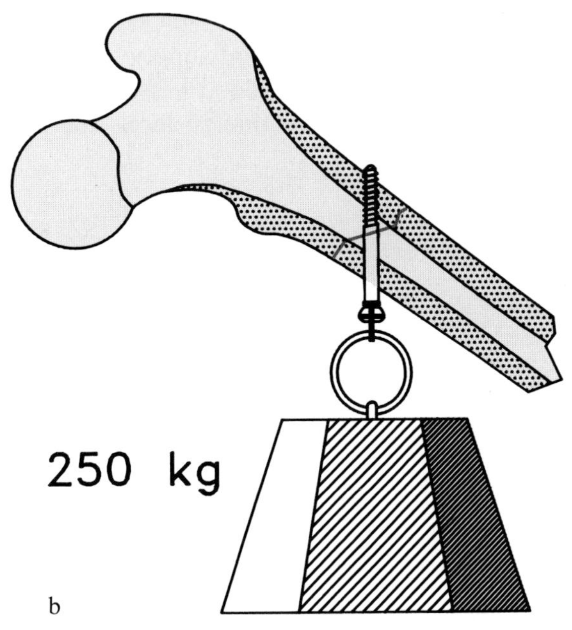

b

1.2.2 The Bone Fracture

The skeleton provides a rigid frame for physical activity and for the protection of the soft organs. The basic requirement for optimal locomotor function is adequate anatomic shape and stiffness (i.e., resistance to deformation under load).

Bone fractures as a result of mechanical overload. The fracture interrupts, within fractions of a millisecond, the structural integrity and with this the stiffness of the bone (Fig. 1.2; Moor et al. 1989). The shape of the fracture depends mainly upon the type of load exerted and upon the energy released. Torque results in spiral fractures, avulsion in transverse fractures, bending in short oblique fractures, while axial compression (especially in metaphyses) results in impaction (fractures without contact between the main fragments after restoration of original length of the bone). The degree of fragmentation depends upon the energy stored prior to the process of fracturing; thus wedge fractures and multifragmentary ones are associated with a high energy release. In this context the rate of loading plays a certain role.

A special phenomenon is the implosion which occurs immediately after disruption. As Moor and coworkers have shown, such implosion (and with it marked soft tissue damage due to cavitation in a similar way as in gunshot wounds) is observed using high-speed cinematography.

In addition to the diminished blood supply brought about by the soft tissue damage, the disruption of the intracortical blood vessels running along the bone axis results in a necrotic deeper layer of the fracture surface. The immediate surface is supported by diffusion.

Fig. 1.2 The bone fracture.

The sequence of events resulting in a spiral fracture with additional (butterfly) fragment analyzed using high-speed cinematography. A human cadaver tibia was fractured using axial torque. The process resulting in a butterfly fracture was recorded at 10000 frames per second (Moor et al. 1989).

a Tissue trauma. When the applied torque reaches the limit of the strength of the bone, the disruption results in an abrupt opening of a fracture gap. A temporary vacuum is created. An implosion succeeds which can be compared in its effect to the process of cavitation in high-velocity gunshot wounds. Marked tissue trauma in the areas of cavitation results.

b Sequence of events and timing. The schematic diagram visualizes the sequence of events in the process of fracturing. Within 400 μs the fracture is fully developed. The sequence leading to the dissolution of the butterfly fragment is also shown.

Fig. 1.2

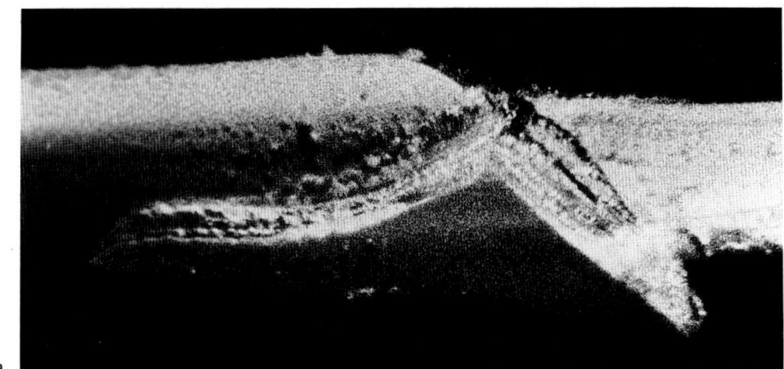

a

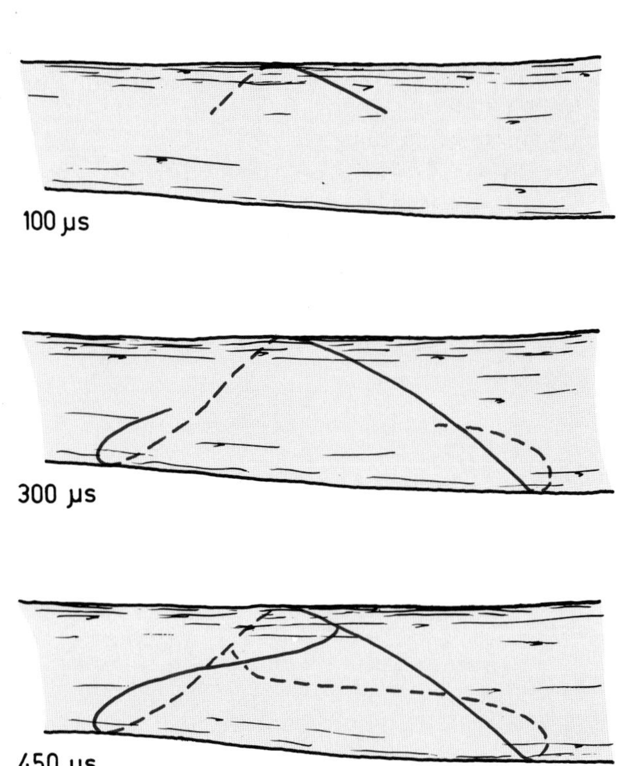

b

1.2.3 Spontaneous Bone Repair: Healing Without Treatment

Nature is able to unite untreated fractures (Fig. 1.3). In the absence of treatment, however, significant malalignment frequently results with consequent impaired function of the skeleton.

1.2.4 Basic Aims of Fracture Treatment

Fracture treatment in general strives for complete and early recovery of limb function. Therefore solid union in *proper anatomic shape* is the basic goal. In respect to diaphyseal fractures, this means at least correct relative positioning of the bone segments which carry the articulations (i.e. restoration of overall length, and reduction of flexural and torsional malalignment). In intra-articular fractures, precise reconstruction of the articular surfaces is a goal in its own right. The reconstruction of the anatomy generally offers the best chance for optimal recovery of function and is preferred to "tolerable malalignment".

Fig. 1.3 Fracture healing without treatment.

The fractured femur of a dog united solidly without treatment; however, marked malalignment resulted. The fracture had been neither reduced nor splinted. (Courtesy of G. Sumner-Smith).

Fig. 1.3

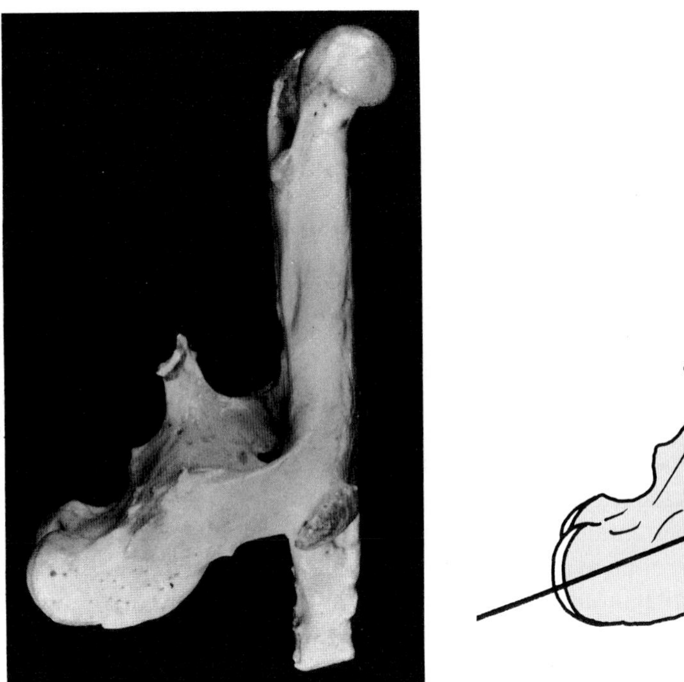

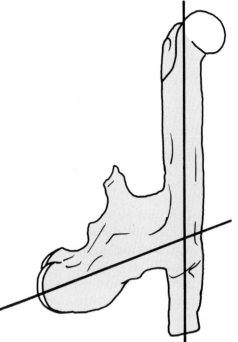

1.2.5 Aims of Operative Fracture Treatment

Three indications for internal fixation stand out:

1. Long-lasting immobilization of soft tissues, especially around the joints, may result in *fracture disease* (see p. 1).
2. In the case of a fracture involving the load-bearing *articular surfaces*, precise reconstruction of these surfaces is of paramount importance. Any incongruity (Fig. 1.4) of the articulating surfaces gives rise to areas of high stress and thus promotes post-traumatic arthrosis.
3. Recovery of function after some fractures of long bones is particularly dependent upon early exact and stable reconstruction, as well as upon immediate mobilization to prevent permanent impairment. *Double forearm fractures* and supracondylar femur fractures are examples.

It should be re-emphasized that the goal of fracture treatment is not only solid union but, equally important, early and full recovery of limb function (see Schatzker and Tile 1987), which includes bone *and* soft tissue integrity.

The surgical treatment of a reactive (hypertrophic) non-union aims at restoring the mechanical environment so that even without direct surgical modification of the interfragmental fibrocartilaginous tissue, uneventful solid healing in anatomically correct position results (Fig. 1.5). Here again the stable fixation allows immediate recovery of pain-free (at least partial) limb function. The solid union following appropriate stable internal fixation is extremely reliable: nearly a 100% union rate in noninfected non-unions of the tibia is reported by Weber and Cech (1973). "Of 127 noninfected non-unions of the tibia 126 achieved sound union; one was radiologically persistent without symptoms. Of 122 infected non-unions of the tibia 117 resulted in sound union and two were radiologically persistent with drainage. Three non-unions had neural and vascular intolerable symptoms in the foot, for which amputation was performed" (Weber and Brunner 1981). The rate of union, the correction of malalignment as well as retaining of joint function lead to optimal results unmatched by nonsurgical treatment such as electrical stimulation. According to the same authors, "Most non-unions are more than simply an ununited fracture of a bone: shortening, angulation, joint stiffness, muscle atrophy, neural and vascular disorders, drainage and infection are additional problems needing treatment. . . . Electrical stimulation may heal the bone gap, but it is unable to produce a positive

---

Fig. 1.4 Precise anatomical reduction is required.

Fractures which compromise articulating surfaces of joints result in post-traumatic arthrosis due to overload following the loss of even stress distribution.

Fig. 1.5 Surgical treatment of a non-union after unsuccessful conservative management.

In a pet Appenzeller dog many attempts to treat the non-union failed; simple correction of malalignment and stabilization led to prompt healing.

a Fully developed non-union. Malalignment has led to an increased bending load which does not allow the repair tissues to stabilize the fracture sufficiently, which is a prerequisite of solid union.

b Operative treatment. The surgical treatment consisted in correcting the angulation by the application of a tension band plate to the convex surface of the malalignment. When the plate was put under tension, the fracture straightened out. The interfragmentary tissue was not touched.

c Prompt solid union after correction of the biomechanical situation. Once the angulation was corrected and the non-union stabilized, prompt and solid healing resulted within 3 months.

Fig. 1.4

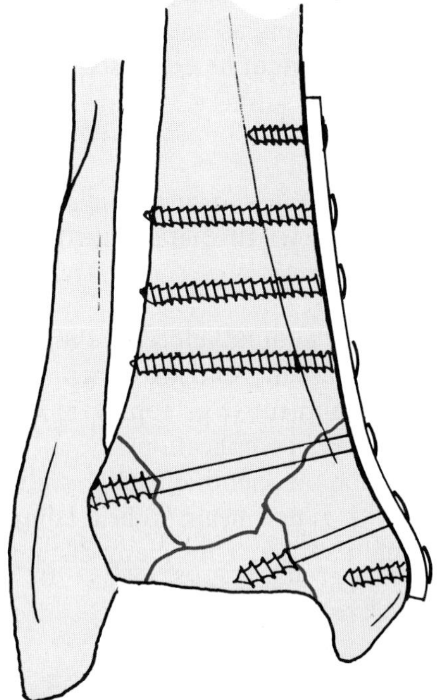

Fig. 1.5

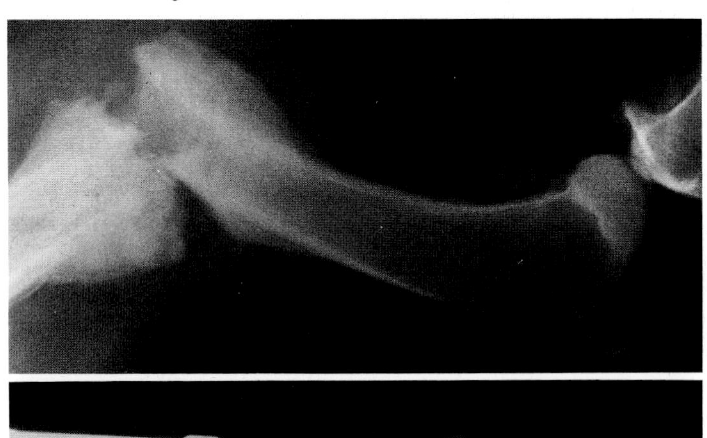

a

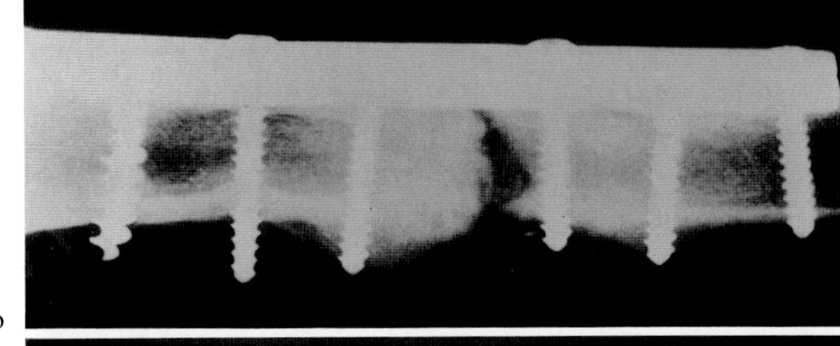

b

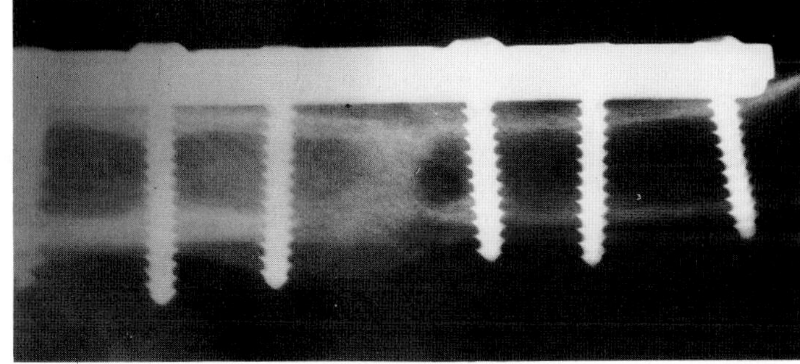

c

effect on the other negative phenomena. It is therefore important to consider a non-union as an injured limb, not simply as an ununited broken bone; e.g. the quality of a certain treatment for non-union cannot be expressed by the rate of ossification only, disregarding angulation, shortening and stiffness."

1.3 Scientific Background to Internal Fixation*

Internal fixation requires a sound understanding of the principles and techniques involved for adequate use of the implants and instruments. The understanding of biological reaction to changes in the environment (e.g., forces, blood supply, etc.) is basic to achieving the desired result and avoiding complications.

The following section on scientific background is intended to convey an understanding of fracture treatment; it is not meant to be a complete overview of the science underlying today's art of internal fixation. Thus many distinguished contributions in this field could not be considered.

1.3.1 Technical Background

In fracture healing, a close relationship exists between mechanical input and biological reaction. Internal fixation requires a good knowledge of the mechanical factors, which provide the optimal environment for reliable and undisturbed fracture healing and for functional restitution of the injured limb as a whole.

1.3.1.1 Stability

The stability of a fracture (spontaneous or after fixation) determines most of the biological reactions during the process of healing. If the blood supply is adequate, the type of healing and the occurrence of delayed or non-union depend mainly upon mechanical conditions related to stability (see p. 16). Stable reconstruction of the fractured bone (e.g., by exact adaptation and compression) minimizes the load to be carried by the implant. Stability of fixation is therefore a critical parameter with respect to implant fatigue and corrosion. The term *stability of fixation* and the factors determining the degree of stability will therefore be discussed.

The use of the term "stability" differs in medical and technical sciences. Stability in internal fixation is used to describe the degree of immobility of the fracture fragments. Stable fixation means a fixation with little displacement under load. A special condition is described by the term *absolute stability*. This defines complete absence of relative dis-

* The efforts of Martin Allgöwer and Chris Colton to transform the rough manuscript into hopefully readable shape are gratefully acknowledged. Joe Schatzker's and Emanuel Gautier's comments on improvement of the logical outline were invaluable. The scientific work was largely performed by the collaborators of the Laboratory for Experimental Surgery, Davos, a competent and outstandingly committed team. The reviews of Frank Baumgart, Frederick Baumgärtel, Jacques Cordey, Richard Meinig, Berton Rahn, Adam Schatzker, and Slobodan Tepic, the artwork of Piet Imken and the late Julius Pupp, and the photography of Emir Omerbegovic and Claudia Güntensperger, and the management by Vreni Geret have contributed to a large extent. I would like to thank my family for friendship and patience.

placement between (compressed) fracture surfaces. Within the same fracture surface, areas of absolute and of relative stability may be present simultaneously (see Fig. 1.8).

Stability, Strain and Fracture Healing

The degree of instability is best expressed as magnitude of strain[3] (deformation of the repair tissues):

Relative motion between bone fragments is compatible with initial fracture healing, provided that the resulting strain remains below the critical level for the formation of that repair tissue (Perren and Cordey 1977, 1980). It goes without saying that if strain is too low, mechanical induction of tissue differentiation (by irritation) fails. In stably fixed fractures with low strain, internal remodeling of bone seems to be induced by necrotic areas.

The critical parameter determining the effect of instability upon cellular elements is the resulting strain. Strain characterizes the condition of deformation of the tissue elements, taking into account the degree of displacement *and* the gap width (relative deformation $\delta L/L$).

Analyzing fracture healing in terms of strain of the repair tissues is more appropriate than judging it merely by the displacement (instability), because strain expresses the deformation of the tissue element (e.g., cell) and allows the surgeon to determine the amount of critical deformation by considering relative displacement (fracture instability) *and* fracture gap width.

The analysis of mechanical conditions using the concept of strain allows one to understand why fractures with a single, narrow gap are very intolerant of even minute amounts of displacement (such displacement may not be detected by vision but must be "*detected by intellect*"). Instability is better tolerated by multifragmentary (comminuted) fractures because the overall displacement is shared between many fracture gaps. Therefore, at any single gap the relative displacement is greatly reduced. If the reduction is not precise the situation is furthermore tolerant to displacement as the strain is reduced due to the larger gap width (see p. 16).

The importance of close adaptation and increased stability achieved by means of compression will be discussed (see p. 30) in the light of the fact that close but insufficient adapation lacking compression may be dangerous. This is due to problems of tissue differentiation under high strain conditions and large implant load resulting in more corrosion.

Fractures may be inherently stable or may stabilize spontaneously through the biological process of tissue formation, with subsequent differentiation into tissues with increasing stiffness, from granulation tissue to bone. The simultaneous increase in the diameter of the callus provides the repair tissues with improved leverage for stabilization. Motion-induced fracture surface resorption results in widening of the gap and a consequent further reduction of relative tissue deformation (strain).

If the resulting strain within the repair tissues (in and around the fracture) exceeds a critical limit, further differentiation and thus healing may be prevented. The expression of instability in terms of strain within the repair tissues allows for a logical understanding of the bone healing process (biology of strain, see p. 60). It explains why some fixation methods without total abolition of interfragmentary mobility, may allow healing (e.g., in non-unions fixed using intramedullary nailing), while other methods leaving only very small gaps do not tolerate even macroscopically invisible displacement.

---

[3] For definition of strain see p. 16

Living bone reacts to high strain conditions at a bone-bone or bone-implant interface by surface resorption (Fig. 1.31) (Perren et al. 1975). Thus in healing under conditions of relative instability, the distance between the surfaces is widened, meaning that for a given amount of displacement, the resulting strain of the individual tissue element (cell) is reduced (see also Figs. 1.9, 1.10).

Stability and Implant Loading

The degree of stability achieved has a determining effect upon the amount of load borne by the implants used for fixation (Fig. 1.6). The load carried by the implant is critical with respect to possible fatigue failures and/or to (fretting) corrosion.

Fatigue

Stable fixation of adapted fragments restores the "structural continuity" by the recovery of the load-bearing capacity of the fractured bone. It therefore reduces the load placed upon the implants. "The bone must protect the implant" (Weber, pers. comm.). The relative increase in load resulting from incorrect use of an implant is much larger than the relative increase in strength provided by metallurgical improvements of the implant. *A bad surgeon will by far outweigh a good metallurgist* – the surgeon changes the loading of the implant by a factor of two to four times while the metallurgist may only improve the strength of the metal by up to 30%. The latter is often achieved at the expense of give (ductility) or of tissue tolerance of the material.

The measurement of bending load placed upon an internal fixation plate, as carried out by Klaue et al. (1985), shows an important effect of stability in protecting implants from overload.

Corrosion

As we will outline later (see p. 95), the most important type of corrosion (practically the only one remaining) for implant materials conforming to today's international standards (ISO)[4] is fretting corrosion. Fretting is produced by a changing load applied across and displacing an interface between two metal components of an implant, such as a screw and a nail. The more dynamic the load carried by the implant, the more likely is fretting to cause repeated disruption of the protective "passive layer." Stable fixation helps to reduce corrosion.

[4] ISO = International Standards Organization, Technical Committees TC 150: "Surgical Implants", TC 164 "Biocompatibility Testing".

Fig. 1.6 The effect of stability of fixation upon implant loading. Short oblique osteotomies of sheep tibial diaphyses bridged by plates (Klaue et al. 1985).

a In one group only a plate is used to merely bridge the fracture (splinting plate); no lag screw is used to produce interfragmental compression.

b In another group a lag screw – here applied through the plate – provides additional stability.

c The initial *bending load* of the plate (*ordinate*, microstrain) is markedly larger without lag screw. Eventually bone union reduces the load (*abscissa*, days after surgery).

d The bending load of the plate is continuously smaller when a lag screw is applied. This explains why the technique of application rather than metallurgy determines fatigue failure.

Fig. 1.6

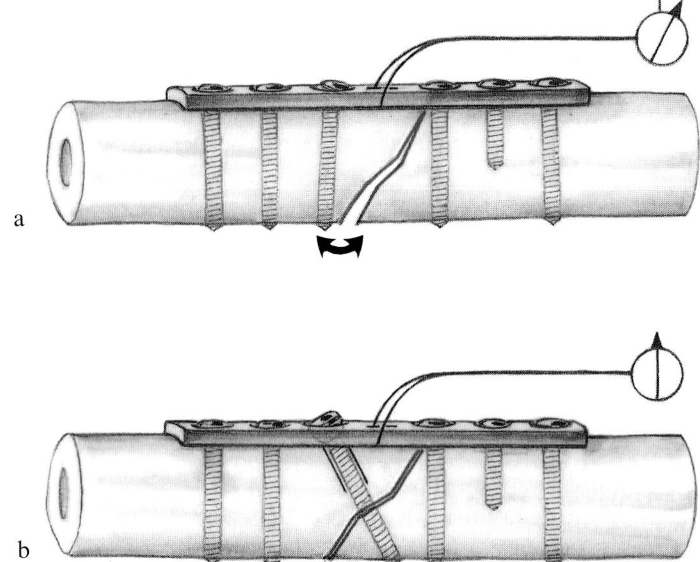
a
b

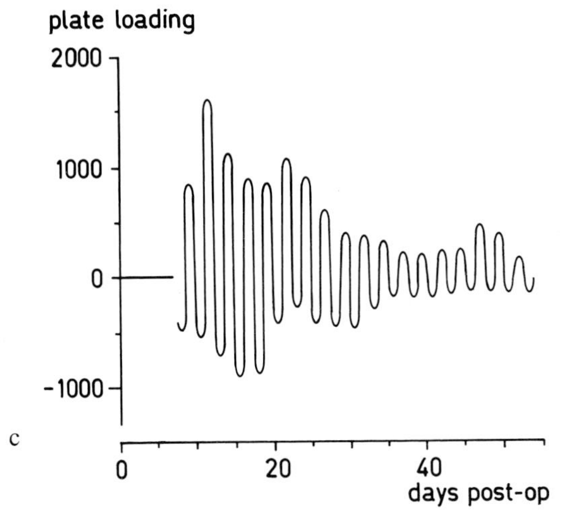
plate loading
2000
1000
0
-1000
c
0
20
40
days post-op

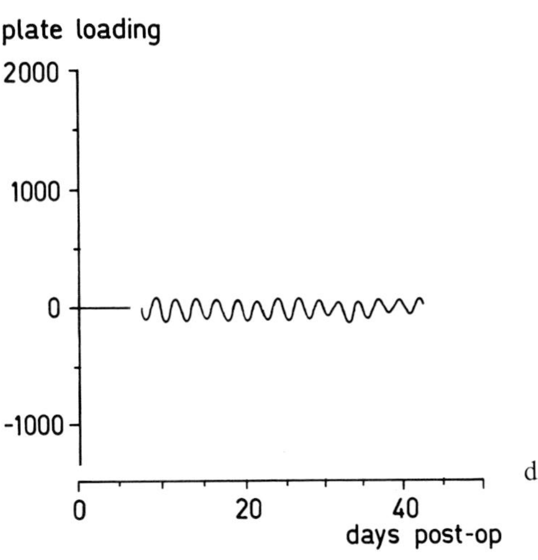
plate loading
2000
1000
0
-1000
d
0
20
40
days post-op

Besides the influence of stability upon the pattern of fracture healing and solid implant-to-bone contact which avoids biological loosening (see pp. 46, 47 and 56), stability of fixation exerts an influence upon the mechanical performance of the implant and upon corrosion. The latter determines the biological tolerance of the implant.

1.3.1.2 Force, Stress, Strain, Stiffness

Force (N)[5] acting upon a material results in a state of internal *stress*. The unit of stress (σ), force/area, is N/m^2. Force deforms a material. The deformation ratio, *strain* ($\varepsilon = \delta L/L$) is unitless and may be reported as percent change of the original dimension (Fig. 1.7). The relationship between the acting force and the resulting deformation is called *stiffness*: the less the stiffness the larger the deformation. The term *rigidity* is often used synonymously with stiffness in the medical literature.

All three elements – force, stress and strain – may be split into static (constant) and dynamic (changing over time) components[6] (Fig. 1.7c).

1.3.1.3 General Aspects of Load

Load may consist of up to three components of forces and three components of moment; load acts upon a material or a device.

Types of Mechanical Load

Load may or may not change (appreciably) with *time*. A load which does not change with time is called static,[8] while periodically or intermittently changing load is dynamic in nature. The compression exerted by an implant applied under tension is static. The forces generated by the function of the limb (e.g., locomotion) are dynamic or functional forces.

---

[5] Forces are expressed in newtons: 10 N ~1 kp ~2.2 lbf. Moments are expressed in newton meters: 1 Nm ~10 kp·cm ~ft·lb/1.37.

[6] In technical sciences the terms static and dynamic are used to define the equilibrium of a situation.

[7] The state of stress can be "visualized" by applying an imaginary cut. To re-establish the previous balance of forces a force must be applied to the cut surface. The amount of force per unit area of the cut surface corresponds to the amount of previous internal stress (σ).

[8] A more appropriate term would be "stationary".

Fig. 1.7 Force, stress, and strain.

a An externally applied force (F) results in a deformation (δL) of a body and in an internal state of stress F/A (σ=force/area). The limit of failure can be described by strength as well as by strain (ε) (elongation at rupture).[7]

b The mechanical behavior of a given material can be characterized by a stress-strain diagram. The stress and strain interdependence is plotted. The limit of failure can be described by the strength (a limit of stress σ_{max}) as well as by maximal deformation (ε_{max}=strain at rupture).

c The three components of forces and three components of moments which describe the loading of a device.

Fig. 1.7

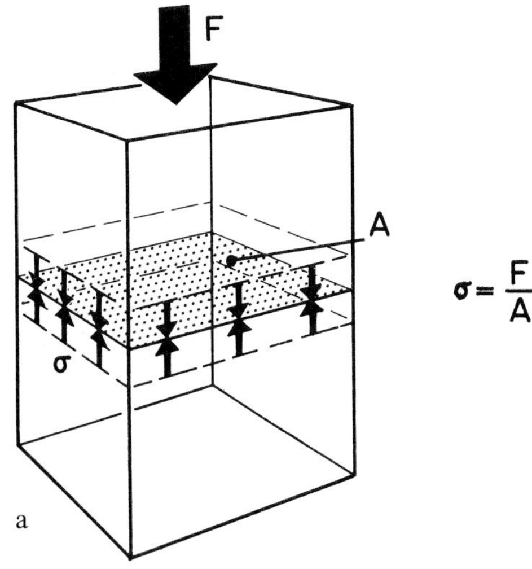

a

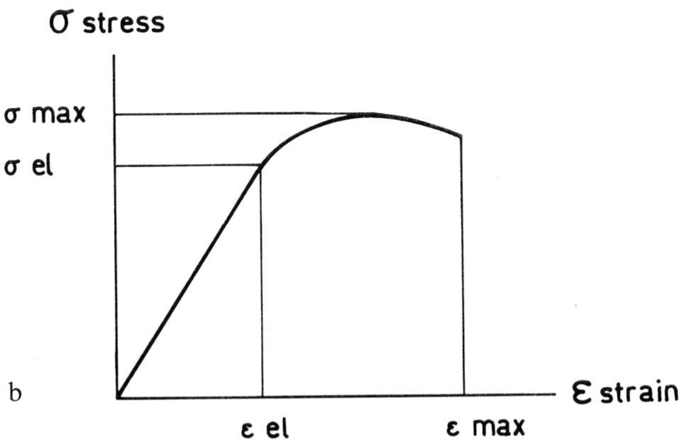

b

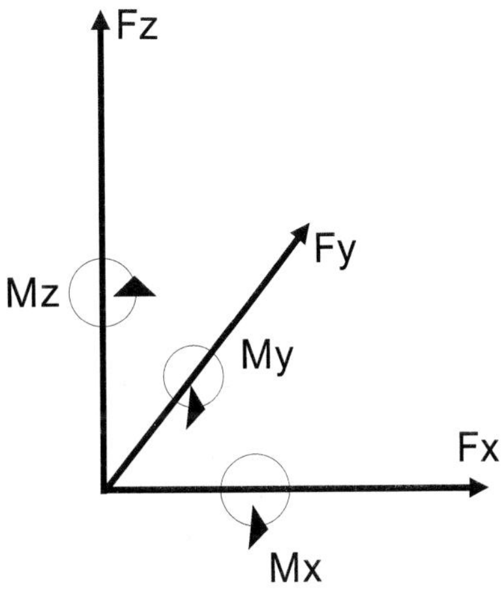

c

No component under consideration is evenly distributed over the fracture area:

1. The static force generated by the implant.
2. The dynamic force resulting from function of the limb (which tends to destabilize the fracture).
3. The amount of contact surface upon which the forces act.

Therefore at different sites different mechanical conditions may exist (Fig. 1.8a, b). According to the different mechanical conditions locally dissimilar types of fracture healing are observed (Fig. 1.8c) within the same fracture area.

A simple mechanical analysis shows that the tension band wiring (Fig. 1.8a) as described by Pauwels (1954) and the tension band plating as outlined by Müller et al. (1963), if performed without lag screw application, result in conditions which vary with time and location.

The different *mechanical conditions* are:

1. A site immediately adjacent to a compression plate may experience a high compressive load (which could eventually exceed the strength of the bone cortex, leading to irreversible deformation such as localized microfractures; Rahn et al. 1971). A minimal dynamic component may be superimposed.
2. A site a little farther from the plate may experience a high static load but within the limits of strength of the bone and with a small component of dynamic load superimposed (stable condition).
3. A site even farther from the plate may exhibit a balance, with lesser stabilizing and greater destabilizing forces resulting in intermittent contact.
4. At the opposite cortex the fracture gap may remain open continuously, with a changing gap width as the varying (dynamic) tensile forces continuously exceed the compressive stabilizing forces.

The mechanical conditions which prevail within the fracture surface cannot be described with one term only, as at different places (or at different times at the same place) a multitude of changing conditions may exist simultaneously.

The *bone reaction* may vary accordingly within the same fracture (Fig. 1.8c). The different types of healing are:

1. Internal remodeling or "contact healing" of overloaded contact areas. It is especially interesting to note that areas which have undergone local overload, but which remain

---

Fig. 1.8 Different mechanical conditions and types of healing within the same fracture surface.

a Different conditions within a fracture surface at different times of observation (tension band wiring of the olecranon, see p. 16 and 44). The preload exerted by the wire is shown by *black triangles* (static compression); the changing load due to function (pull of the triceps muscle and related articular compression producing additional compression of the fracture surface) is shown by *open arrows*.

b Different conditions within a fracture surface at different times of observation: tension band plating of shaft fracture without interfragmental compression (either by prebending of the plate or by interfragmentary lag screw) bears an inherent risk of delayed union. The use of plates only, without lag screw or prebending, should therefore be avoided.

c Different types of healing within the same fracture. This histological section (courtesy of J. Craig) demonstrates within the same fracture area all stages from direct healing to delayed healing. In *area A* direct bone healing is seen, in *area B* indirect bone healing, and in *area C* delayed healing.

Fig. 1.8

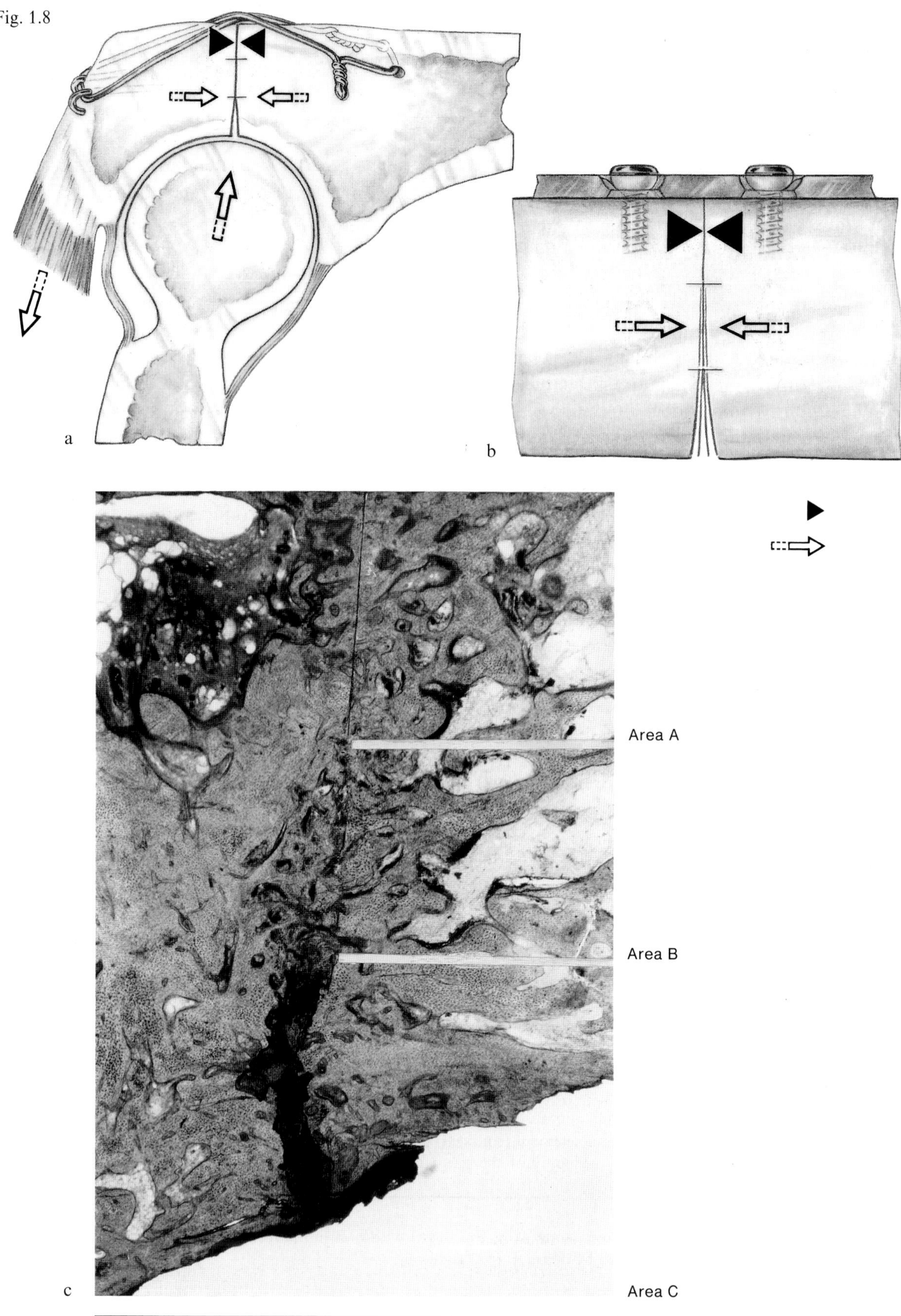

stably fixed by adjacent contact areas, exhibit direct internal remodeling as demonstrated by Rahn (see above).

2. Internal remodeling or "contact healing" of intact contact areas (see p. 70).
3. Fracture surface resorption and indirect healing (see p. 68).
4. Delayed healing. The non-united gap will eventually fill by indirect bone formation (see p. 70).

The *effect* of load consists of deformation[9] of an intact bone, and/or of providing varying degrees of stability of a fracture. Static compression generally stabilizes, while dynamically applied tension or shear tends to result in instability of the interface. The effect of combined forces depends upon their relative values at a given time and place as outlined above. The surgeon will aim to apply enough static compression to maintain stability in the presence of any opposing dynamic tensile forces which may act upon the fractured bone. Small areas of local overload are not of basic concern, as the bone as a whole is able to resist high loads. Generalized overload exerted prior to onset of bone union, though, results in the mechanical breakdown of the internally fixed fracture. (The French term "debricolage" (see Glossary p. 109) seems to be appropriate to describe a condition where the fragments of a fracture, which were previously fixed together, simply fall apart. This describes a condition where no biological reaction plays a role. Two possible causes can come into play: the construction may be too weak or the load excessively large.)

Load applied to bone or implant (e.g., axial tension) produces an internal state of *stress* within the material. Stress increases with load, but it decreases with increasing load-bearing surface.[10] Increasing stress may reach a critical level of strength of the material and the material may fracture. Here the critical condition of the fracture is described in terms of *strength* (e.g., ultimate tensile strength).

Load applied to a material produces stress within the material and thus invariably results in deformation (strain) of the material. Strain (Figs. 1.9, 1.10) is expressed as

---

[9] The other effect of force, acceleration, is not considered here.

[10] Stress is expressed as force per unit area N/m^2 ($\sim 1\ kp/mm^2 = 10 \times 10^6\ N/m^2 = 10\ MPa$).

Fig. 1.9 Large strain in small gaps.

The deformation of the cells or tissues is critical. It depends not only upon the degree of displacement (δL) of the fragments (instability), but also (and more importantly) upon the initial width of the fracture gap (L). For very small gaps (e.g., smaller than 0.1 mm) an imperceptible displacement (0.1 mm) may result in very high strain (> 100%) of any one individual tissue element, for example, the cell.

a A small displacement (5 μm) in a small gap between the fragments (here about one cell layer thickness, ~10 μm) results in a strain of 50%.

b A somewhat larger displacement (10 μm) in a small gap reaches the limit of strain tolerance of the cell. The change of the gap width from 10 to 20 μm is not visible to the naked eye (i.e., the surgeon does not see such instability).

Fig. 1.10 Small strain in large gaps.

Strain of the individual tissue element (e.g., cell) of the repair tissue within the fracture gap (and adjacent to it) may be reduced by widening of the gap (from 10 μm in Fig. 1.9a to 40 μm in Fig. 1.10 by bone surface resorption) and/or by shearing the overall displacement by multiple serial gaps. Both conditions are usually seen in multifragmentary fractures.

a A small displacement (5 μm, same as in Fig. 1.9a) within an initially wide gap (40 μm) results in strain (~12%) which is tolerated by dense fibrous tissue.

b A somewhat larger displacement (10 μm, same as in Fig. 1.9b) within an initially wide gap (40 μm) results in strain (~25%) which is tolerated by granulation tissue.

Fig. 1.9

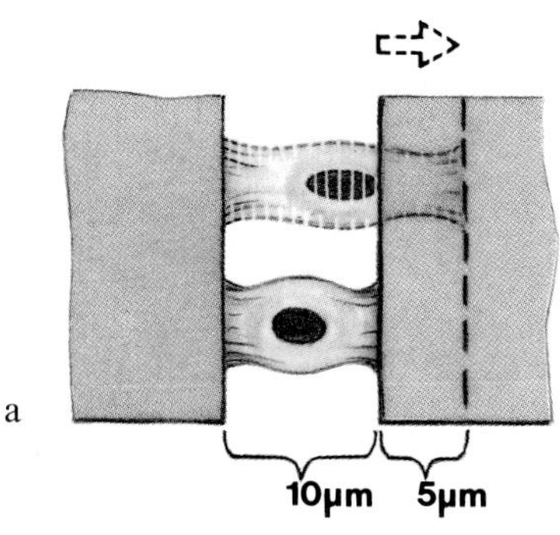

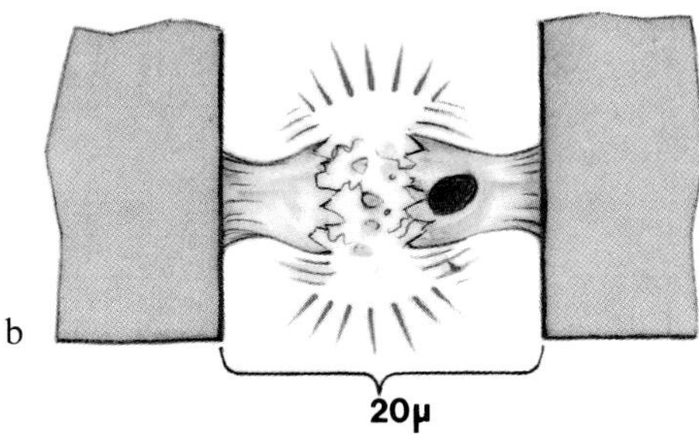

Fig. 1.10

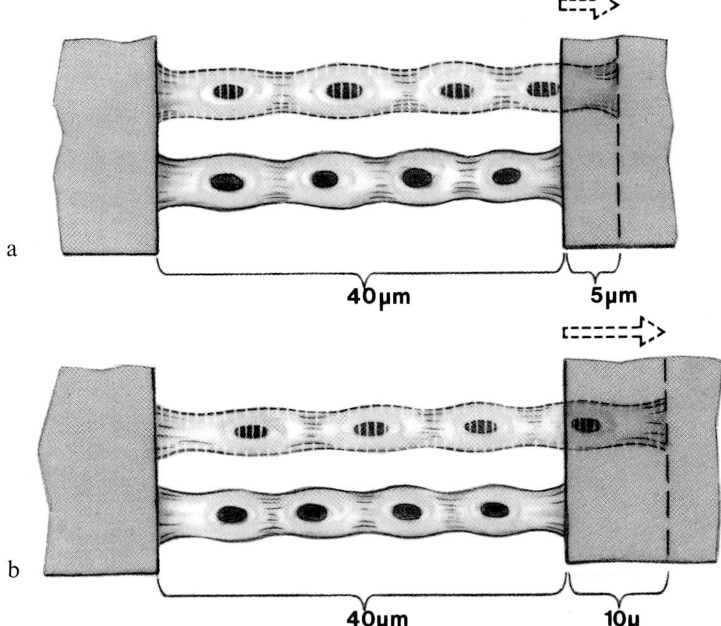

relative (e.g., percentage) increase or decrease in length in relation to original length (see p. 16, 17). Increasing load (stress) may reach the critical level of strength. Deformation may also reach the critical level of *elongation at rupture* (or strain at rupture) and the material may fracture. In the initial stages of fracture healing, when strength and stiffness of the repair tissues do not play a relevant role, it is more appropriate to specify the critical condition of the tissues involved in fracture healing in terms of *tolerated strain* (see Table 1.1) than in terms of stress.

Table 1.1. Critical strain levels of repair tissues

Elongation at rupture of different tissues	
Granulation tissue	100%
Dense fibrous tissue	20%
Cartilage	10%
Cancellous bone	2%
Lamellar bone	2%

The values taken from Yamada and Evans 1970 show that critical elongation (at rupture) of lamellar bone is small. The value of parenchyma has been taken to replace the missing data for granulation tissue.

When the load-bearing surface is large, the critical limit of load at fracture is best expressed as stress (stress equal to or smaller than strength). When the load-bearing surface is small, and with this the contribution of the tissue to stabilization minimal, the critical limit is best expressed in terms of strain (limit of strain tolerance). The former condition is defined by load, the latter is defined by deformation. Though the two characteristics represent two aspects of the same condition, critical mechanical conditions of tissue differentiation in fracture healing and non-unions are more easily understood using a clear concept of strain.

Bone Failure

Fractures of previously intact diaphyseal bone occur as a rule due to a single state of excessive stress. Failures of initial small bone bridges in fracture healing are best understood to be the result of an episode of excessive strain because the force potentially acting by far exceeds the strength of the tissue. The only critical parameter then is the deformation allowed by the width of the gap between the fracture surfaces nearby.

Implant Failure

With respect to the implant, two conditions exist which may lead to failure: a single massive overload or multiple smaller overloads ("fatigue") Why under certain conditions does a thicker plate seem to break more readily?

When an implant bridging a long defect is increasingly loaded (e.g., by increasing weight-bearing), the stress generated may eventually reach the limit of strength and the implant fails. This commonly understood behavior may be called "load-driven failure."

Another condition exists in a highly loaded fracture area: when surface resorption with gap widening occurs, then eventually the strain of the implant reaches the critical limit – "deformation-driven failure." Given sufficient load, the failure of, for example, a plate depends upon gap width and thickness of the plate. The thicker plate fails at a smaller angle of bending because the surface of the thicker plate experience a higher strain for the same angle of bending. This analysis is of importance concerning implant failure, because in internal fixation "deformation-driven" conditions often prevail.

1.3.1.4 Physiological Load

Physiological activity of a limb consists of movements by muscle forces and weight-bearing. Both result in bone loads with complex patterns of static and dynamic components of torque, bending, and axial load. The effect of physiological load may again be analyzed as consisting of three components of forces and/or three components of moments (see p. 18). Loading of a fracture surface statically by the implant and dynamically by functional load results in a complex pattern whereby areas of overload, areas of reversible deformation, areas of intermittently open gaps, and areas of constantly open gaps of changing size can exist simultaneously. An example of such a complex loading situation is the condition produced by a tension band wiring of a fractured olecranon or patella (Fig. 1.8a, see p. 19 and p. 44). Hertel (1984) has demonstrated that the stress generated within a conventional plate is increased 14 times if a plate hole is placed on top of an open defect (open fracture gap). If in addition a screw hole near the fracture is left open, i.e., not fixed to bone, the plate experiences 0.3 times higher stress at this site. Plate holes with and without screws did not show relevant differences in measured loading when the bone was perfectly adapted and thus was able to carry load.

1.3.1.5 Principles of Surgical Stabilization

There are two basically different mechanisms of fracture fixation: *splinting* and *compression*. The two differ in the mechanism of stabilization and in the degree of stability achieved.

Splinting

The fixation by splinting (Fig. 1.11) consists in connecting a (more or less) stiff device to the fractured bone. This device reduces the mobility of the fracture in proportion to its stiffness. Splinting is achieved using a great variety of methods, ranging from external splints, i.e., plaster fixation, to internal fixation by plates and medullary nails and also includes the transcutaneous splints: the external fixators. *The effect of splinting is to reduce (not abolish) fracture mobility.* Thus pain is reduced and the limb is protected from excessive deformation. Some people advocate the use of plates made of a material of stiffness similar to that of bone. As fracture mobility depends proportionally upon the stiffness of the splint, however, there is no point in using such a plate.

A special type of splinting is *buttressing*, where a stiff splint serves to maintain the shape of a bone after a complex fracture or in the presence of a defect. The implant bridges the segment of the bone which cannot carry the load. The implant is then subjected to full functional load until the bone resumes the load. In this case, special precautions have to be taken to avoid failure of the unprotected implant.

Table 1.2. The relative stiffness of bone, plate and nail

	Bending	Torque
Tibia	1	1
Plate	1/25	1/20
Nail	1/3	1/150

The stiffness of so-called rigid internal fixation implants made of steel may be similar to that of bone under axial loading, but a plate is 25 times less stiff than a corresponding bone in bending, or 20 times less in torque.

Coupling of Splints

As mentioned above, the splint must be connected (coupled) to the fractured bone. The effectiveness of a splint fixed to bone depends to a great extent upon the stiffness of the softest element within the chain: bone/coupling by soft tissues/splint. Plaster as such is very rigid due to its large dimensions. However, it provides very limited stabilization of the fracture, due to the flexible coupling between plaster and bone by soft tissues. While a plaster cast is very effective in nonoperative treatment (Böhler 1938; Latta et al. 1980; Sarmiento 1984), it will hardly ever unload a stable internal fixation, because it allows significant angulation of the bone fragments and, in addition, increases inertial loading. When a fracture which is fixed by lag screw and plate is deformed by an applied bending load, the screws pull out at a very small overall deformation. A plaster cast does not, therefore, reliably prevent screws from pulling out, nor does it prevent a plate from failing in fatigue, should the surgeon fail to reduce external loading. Stripping of threads occurs at bending angles which are smaller than the angulation allowed for by the plaster.

Coupling of the noninterlocked intramedullary nail in respect to bending is good; in respect to axial load and torsion it depends upon friction (whereby, in the case of torsion, the friction is not only small but its leverage is minimal). Coupling in stable external fixators depends mainly upon the stiffness of the pin. Here the thread offers much less stiffness than the shaft of the pin, the flexural and torsional stiffness changing with the fourth power of the critical diameter. The critical diameter is the core diameter of the thread or the outer diameter of the shaft.

Fig. 1.11 Basic tools in internal fixation. 1: Splinting.

a External splinting by plaster cast relies upon the same basic mechanisms as does splinting for emergency care: A splint is fixed to the bone. Because of its stiffness it reduces (but does not abolish completely) the mobility of the fracture fragments. A splint by necessity carries part or all of the load, particularly if contact is missing between the fracture fragments. Coupling between plaster cast and bone is comparatively loose due to the interposition of the soft tissues.

b The plate used as a splint: The plate may theoretically be used to keep the fracture fragments apart. The plate carries a full functional load until solid union occurs. Coupling between the plate and bone is very tight; plate fixation of simple fractures (in relation to achieving the goal of reliable and undisturbed fracture healing) does not well tolerate fracture surface resorption (locking splint).

c The nail used as a splint: A splint always deforms when loaded. The splint therefore reduces but does not abolish instability (relative stability). The nail is comparatively strong, and splinting using intramedullary nails (once again in relation to achieving the goal of reliable and undisturbed fracture healing) tolerates fracture surface resorption well (gliding splint).

Fig. 1.11

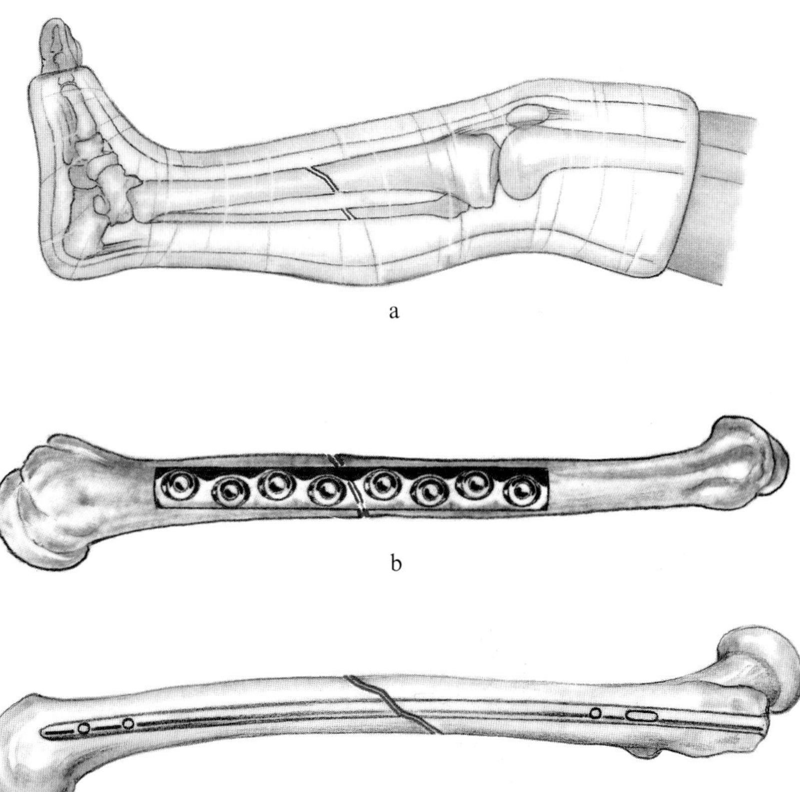

Enhancement of Splints

A plate is known to be flexible and due to its asymmetric positioning not strong enough to carry the full load of limb function. Müller and Witzel (1984) and Mast et al. (1988) have proposed supplementing a minimal internal fixation with a temporary external fixator (Fig. 1.12a, b). The large lever arm of the external fixator allows for efficient unloading of the internal fixation until bone has "taken" and can take over its function of contributing stiffness and strength.

Unloading of Bone by Implanted Splints

Classical splints are the nail and the external fixator. Special consideration is given here to the plate as splint. As we will see, plate splinting is used to reduce the physiological load placed upon, for example, a screw fixation. Unloading of the plated bone segment is a prerequisite of the function of the protection plate and the buttress plate. Most other implants act in a similar way and unload, or protect, fractured bone from excessive physiological forces so as to permit undisturbed fracture healing during early functional treatment and to prevent mechanical breakdown of the incompletely healed fracture. On the other hand, a mechanically reconstructed bone, because of its "structural integrity," protects the implant, for example, from repeated bending and thus from fatigue failure.

Fig. 1.12 Enhancement of the splint.

a A multifragmentary fracture is splinted using a plate with a minimum of surgical exposure and screws. The procedure does not demand exact reduction. The plate fixation alone would not be strong enough, therefore it is protected using an external fixator.

b The callus bridge provides solid support of the far cortex. The external fixator can therefore be removed at 6 weeks. (Courtesy of F. Baumgärtel).

c As soon as the callus provides support the external frame is removed. Thus the time of transcutaneous connection is minimized and the internal fixation adapted to the healing process.

Fig. 1.12

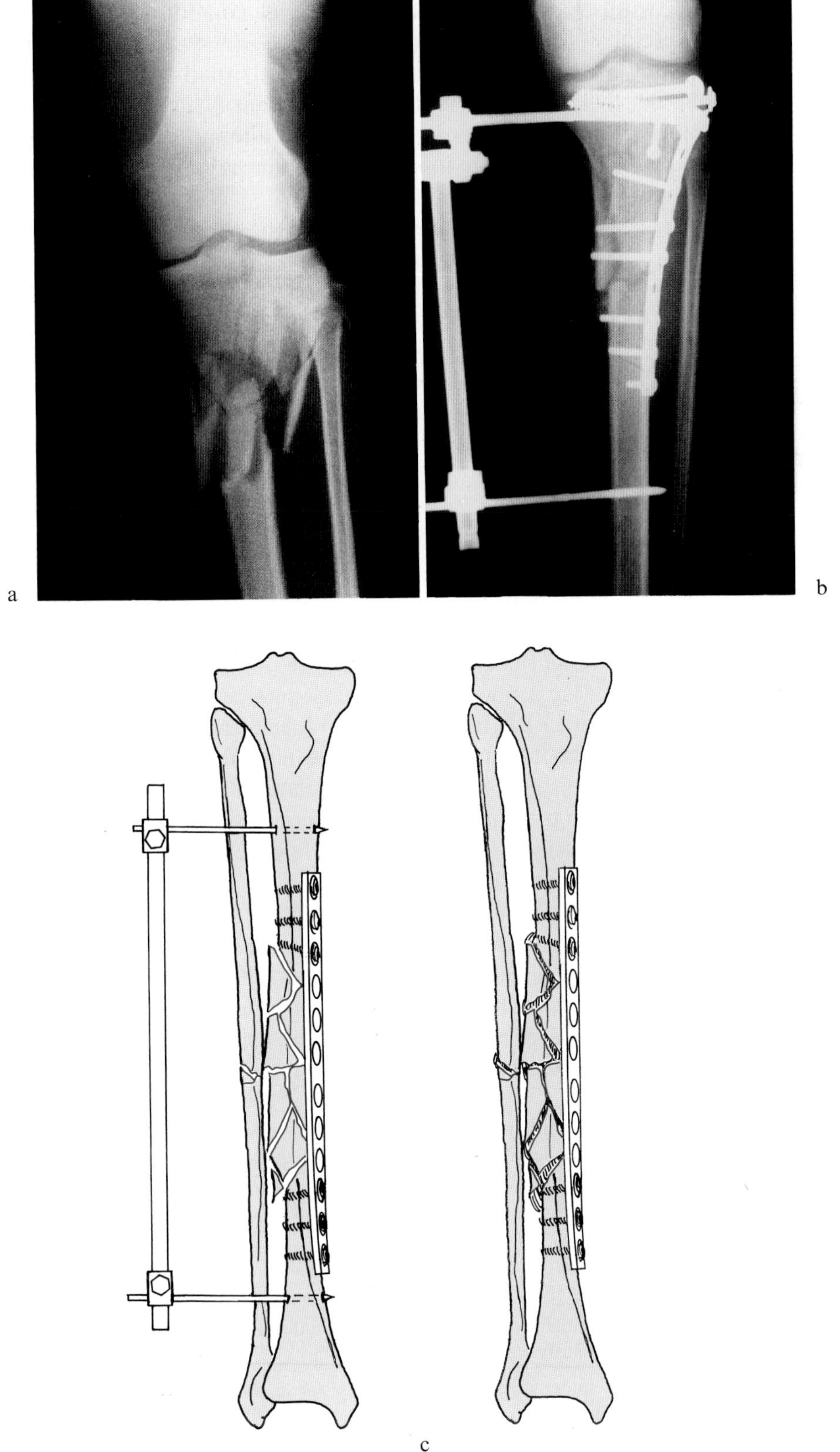

a b c

Gliding and Nongliding Splints

There are two basic splinting principles: one which allows gliding of the fragments along the implant, the other which prevents it (Fig. 1.13). A conventional nonlocked intramedullary nail allows for gliding of the bone along the nail because the friction between nail and bone is generally small, as the radial expansion forces of the nail "in reality" are comparably small. A plate, as a rule, does not allow gliding because the friction resulting from the plate screws is large (each screw produces compression between plate undersurface and bone in the range of up to 3000 N).[11]

The intramedullary nail is an efficient tool for treating a fracture without any additional fixation. The small displacement at the fracture, allowed for by the (noninterlocked) nail, may result in shortening of the fragment ends due to resorption. The possibility for gliding along the nail allows (should resorption occur) coaptation of the fracture and restabilization.

A plate applied to a simple fracture, without additional measures (such as interfragmental compression), would not provide sufficient stability to prevent fragment and resorption induced by micromotion between the fragment ends. When such shortening occurs, the high friction between plate underside and bone surface does not allow for coaptation. The plate then bears all the load placed upon the bone and is prone to fatigue failure. Plate fixation therefore requires the use of interfragmental compression by screws and/or axial compression by the plate with or without prebending of the plate (or contact brought about by functional load) to ensure bony contact able to carry load without intermittent displacement. As a rule the plate should not be used to stabilize a fracture of a weight-bearing bone, but to unload (protect) a fracture stabilized by other means (e.g., lag screws): a fracture is splinted to be partially unloaded (protected), provided bone contact has been restored. When a fracture gap beneath the splint remains open, the bone at the fracture area is completely unloaded by the splint.

It is an important goal of the use of a plate to at least partially unload the fractured bone which has been previously fixed using screws. Stress shielding is, therefore, a prerequisite, and not primarily a disadvantageous side effect, of the treatment. This fact has often been misunderstood in recent years.

A further fact to be mentioned here is that, with respect to axial loading, the stiffness of a so-called "rigid internal fixation plate" made of steel is equal to that of, for example, the tibia. However, the plate is many times less stiff than the bone in bending and torque. The nail is "soft" under torsional loading. Torque coupling between the nonlocked nail and the bone is, as a rule, not tight. Locked nails provide tight torque coupling, once the initial "play" of the bolts or screws within the holes in the nail has been overcome.

[11] If a frictional coefficient (metal to bone) of 0.4 is assumed and if three screws are applied in each fragment, the surface undergoing a normal force of up to 3000 N per screw is able to resist more than 3600 N of tangentially applied force (on each side of the fracture) without sliding.

Fig. 1.13 Gliding and nongliding splints.

a Gliding splint: a medullary nail applied without interlocking allows the fragments to close a fracture gap which underwent surface resorption.

b Non-gliding splint: under conditions similar to those shown in a, a plate (especially the round hole plate) does not allow gliding. In this case of a technically incorrect plate fixation (wrong position and function of lag screw, bad leverage of plate screws) a small gap was left open. The relative motion of the fragments (due to incomplete loosening of the implant) produced a high strain condition (see p. 16). A delayed union developed. *Left*, immediately after operation; *right*, 8 months after operation. (From Perren and Boitzy 1978).

Fig. 1.13

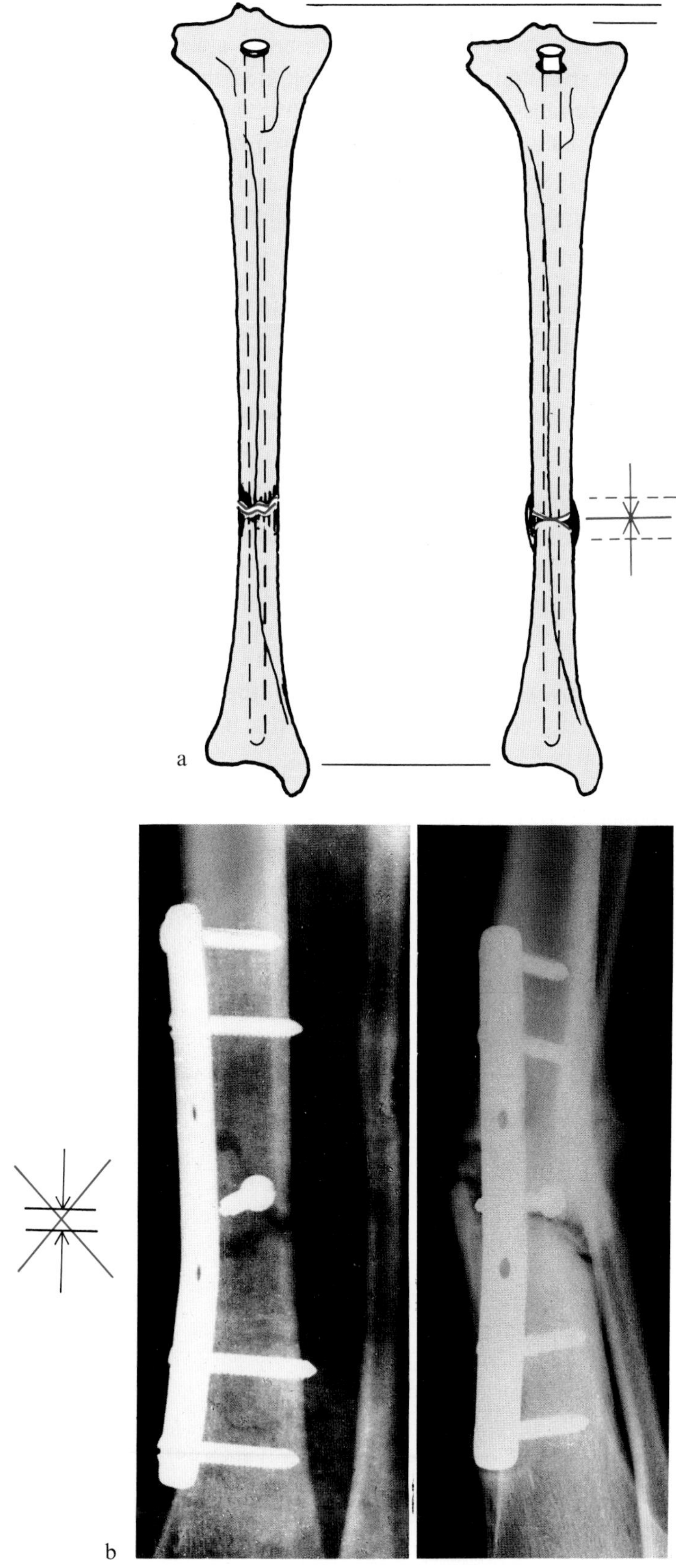

Compression

Compression is a very elegant tool to stabilize a fracture because efficient stabilization is achieved with minimal amounts of implanted material. Compression fixation consists in pressing two surfaces (bone-to-bone or implant-to-bone) together.

According to its alteration with time, two different types of compression are distinguished:

1. Static compression, i.e., compression which does "not" change with time. Once applied, static compression remains virtually unaltered.
2. Dynamic compression: limb function, for instance, results in periodic partial loading and unloading of the contacting surfaces due to dynamic forces resulting from function. The wire or plate applied as tension band transforms the functional tension into compression. A fixation results which allows some load-induced movement.

The *effect of compression* is twofold:

1. Compression produces preloading, i.e., the surfaces remain in close contact as long as the compression applied remains larger than any opposite-acting force (e.g., tension from physiological load which results in bending; Fig. 1.14a).
2. Compression produces friction, i.e., the compressed surfaces resist sliding displacement as long as the friction produced by compression remains larger than the shearing force applied (Fig. 1.14b, c). Local shear at a transverse fracture results mostly from torque applied around the long axis of the bone, while inclined surfaces such as oblique fractures undergo shear when the bone is loaded along its long axis, e.g., by weight-bearing.

Different *methods* are used to produce compression. They differ not only in the implant used but also in the mechanism by which compression is applied and in the efficiency of the compression.

Fig. 1.14 Basic tools in internal fixation. 2: Compression.

a Stabilization by compressive preload. Preload is effective whenever the compression which stabilizes the interface exceeds the tension induced by bending (Perren 1971).

b Compression stabilization by sufficient friction. Compression of an interface produces friction, which opposes displacement by shear. This mechanism is most important in stabilization of interfaces of a structure placed under torque load. No displacement occurs.

c Loss of compression stabilization by insufficient friction. If the friction generated is too small and/or the torsional (shear) load placed upon the fracture too large, the surfaces slide along each other: instability.

Fig. 1.14

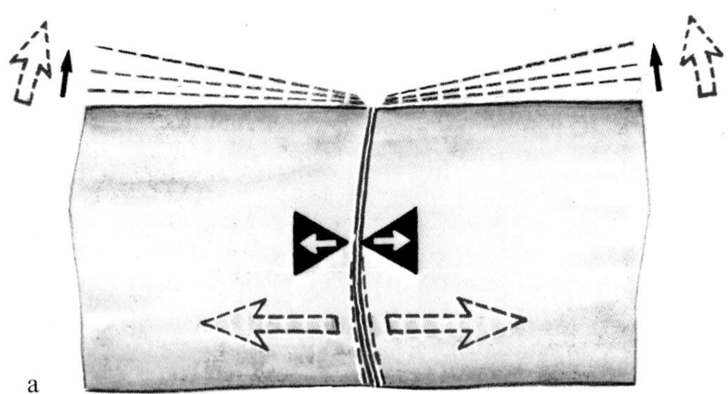

a

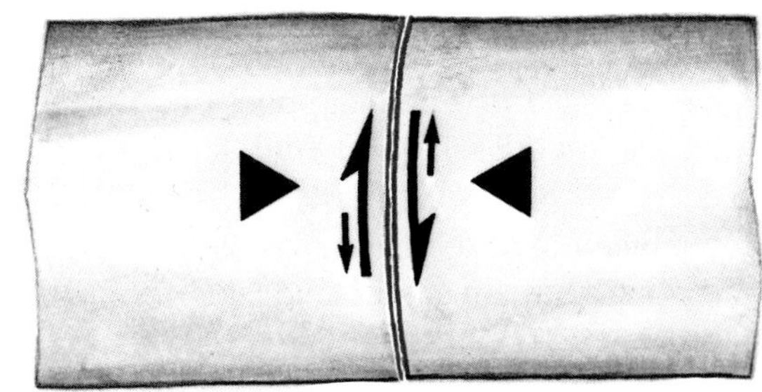

b

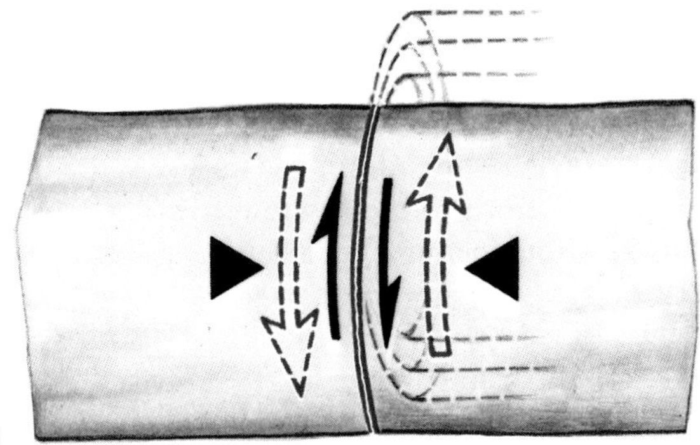

c

Interfragmentary Compression Applied by Lag Screw

A fracture may be compressed by application of a screw across the fracture (Fig. 1.15), whereby the screw thread is anchored within the fragment near the tip of the screw. Thus when the screw is tightened this fragment will be pressed against the fragment retained by the head of the screw (Fig. 1.15b). The prerequisite of the function of the lag screw is that the bone fragment near the head of the screw is not coupled to the thread of the screw. This may be achieved by using a screw with a partial thread or by removing the thread within the bone fragment near the head of the screw by overdrilling (gliding hole). For a gliding hole to function properly, the screw must be positioned in the axis of the drill hole (i.e., forces acting perpendicular to the long axis of the screw will lead to engagement of the screw thread with the wall of the gliding hole and thus to loss of lag screw effect).

The compression exerted by a lag screw is very efficient because (among other reasons) it is relatively large. Brennwald et al. (1975) and von Arx (1975) have determined that the force applied by expert surgeons using a plate screw amounts to 2000–4000 N. It is important to note that the force exerted by the lag screw acts from within the fracture surface (Fig. 1.15d) in contrast to the compression exerted by the plate (see below).

It is noteworthy that the direction along which the compression acts (inclination of lag screw) must coincide fairly well with a perpendicular to the fracture surface. As Johner et al. (1983) have shown, sliding occurs if the compression applied to a smooth osteotomy is inclined only 20° in relation to an axis perpendicular to the fracture surface.

The theory of the bisecting angle applies only to the special case of the spiral fracture, where a spiral surface and a longitudinal surface connecting the two ends of the spiral are – on average – perpendicularly compressed. Here an inclination corresponding to the bisecting angle in relation to the visible fracture line of the spiral is chosen.

The presumption that an axial load acts along the long axis of the bone shaft is only correct for short stretches within a complex loading pattern. It is therefore safest to select an inclination of a lag screw such that it is perpendicular in respect to the "average" inclination of the fracture surface.

A further important aspect of lag screw fixation consists in the comparably limited range of action of the lag screw: the stress generated across the fracture tapers off quite quickly with the distance to the screw axis. A single lag screw therefore does not offer good stabilization in respect to torque acting within the fracture plane.

Lag screw fixation provides motionless fixation ("absolute stability"), but the strength offered is often considered to be inadequate, i.e., functional loads applied may result in displacement. Single overload applied to lag screw fixation results in irreversible loss of compression. Therefore, the lag screw fixation is often protected by a plate with a so-called neutralization (better: "protection") function. The combination of lag screw

---

Fig. 1.15 Principles of lag screw technique.

a In order to find the best location and inclination, forceps compressing the fracture temporarily substitute for the function of the lag screw. They are also adjusted to prevent shear of the fracture.

b The lag screw replaces the forceps in location and position (inclination) for best stabilization.

c The lag screw is best positioned at right angles to the fracture plane. The use of the bisecting angle is only correct for fixing osteotomies with less than 40° inclination according to Johner et al. (1983). If the inclination of the osteotomy corresponds, for instance, to 60°, the osteotomy will be displaced due to insufficient inclination of the lag screw.

d The photoelastic analysis shows that the range within which compression acts is relatively small. This explains why rotation cannot be countered by a single lag screw.

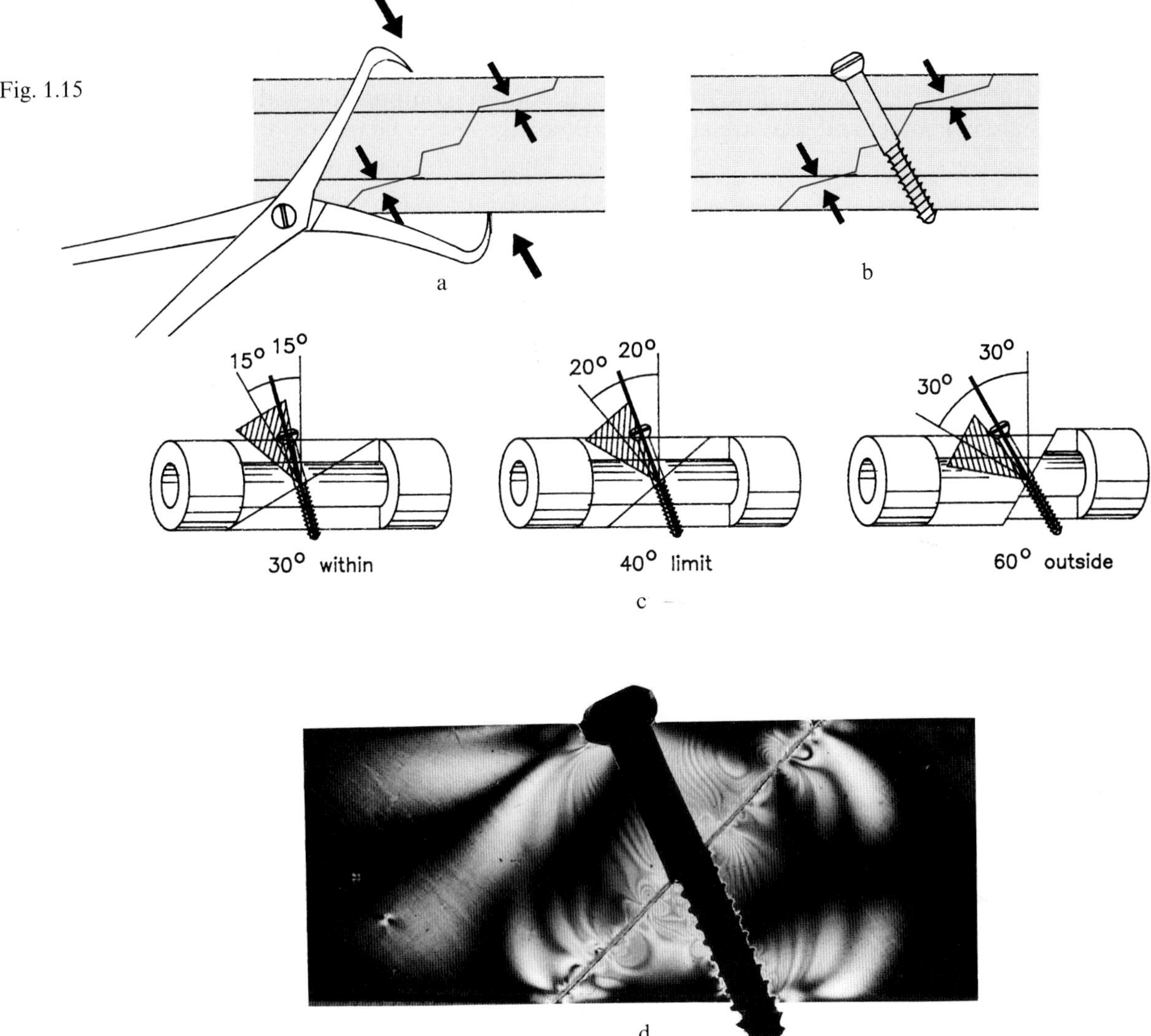
a
b
15° 15°
30° within
20° 20°
40° limit
30°
30°
60° outside
c
d

Fig. 1.15

and protection plate fixation has been studied by Barraud (1982) and Eisner et al. (1985). Diehl (1976) analyzed stability and strength of different types of internal fixation of femur and tibia in respect to early rehabilitation.

Axial Compression Exerted by the (Compression) Plate

Compression using a plate (Fig. 1.16) is produced by applying a pretensioned plate to the bone. The prerequisite for this application of compression is that the bone fragments are in contact and thus are able to carry load.

Fig. 1.16 Compression exerted by the plate. A plate provides stable fixation only under very special conditions.

a Method of test: First the stiffness of the plated intact bone is determined. Then stiffness is determined with the plate fixed to the tension side and finally with the plate fixed to the compression (bending) side.

b Method of evaluation: The deformation produced by the bending moment applied is plotted. The slope of the curve for the plated intact bone is taken as reference for maximal stability, the one for a plate bridging a defect is taken as reference for minimal stability.

c A plate placed at the tension side provides good stability of fixation.

d A plate placed at the compression (bending) side provides minimal stability.

e See p. 36.

Fig. 1.16

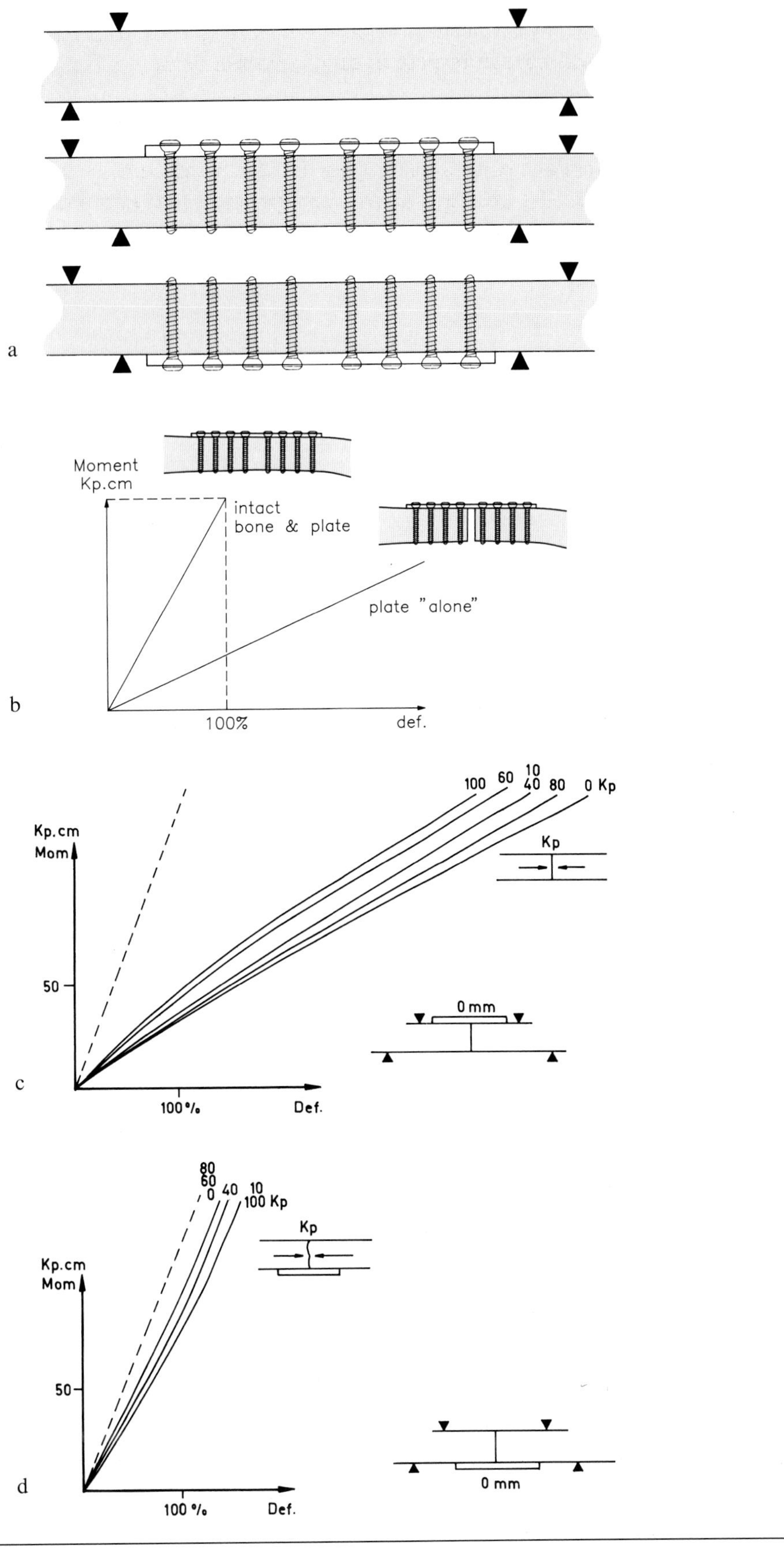
a
Moment
Kp.cm
intact
bone & plate
plate "alone"
100%
def.
b
100
60
10
40
80
0 Kp
Kp
Kp.cm
Mom
50
0 mm
100%
Def.
c
80
60
0
40
10
100 Kp
Kp
Kp.cm
Mom
50
0 mm
100 %
Def.
d

Fig. 1.16 Compression exerted by the plate (continued).

e Axial compression without prebending (*top*) results in compression near the plate only. Prebending without axial compression (*center*) results in adaptation of the far cortex only. The combination of axial compression and prebending (*bottom*) results in compression of the whole cross section.

Fig. 1.16

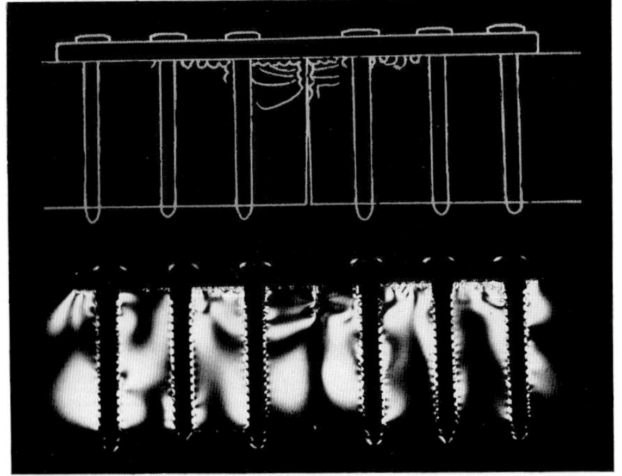

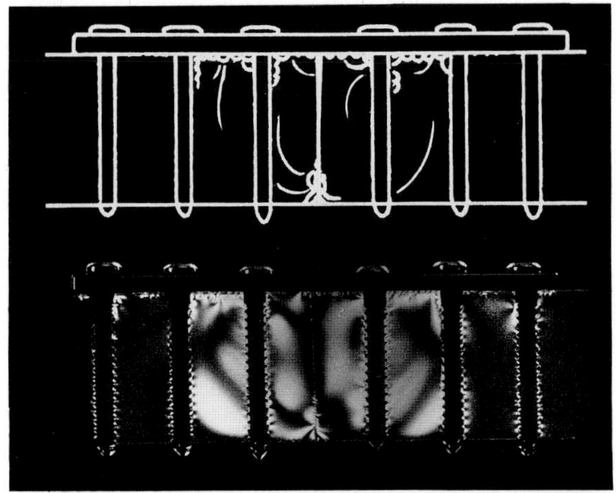

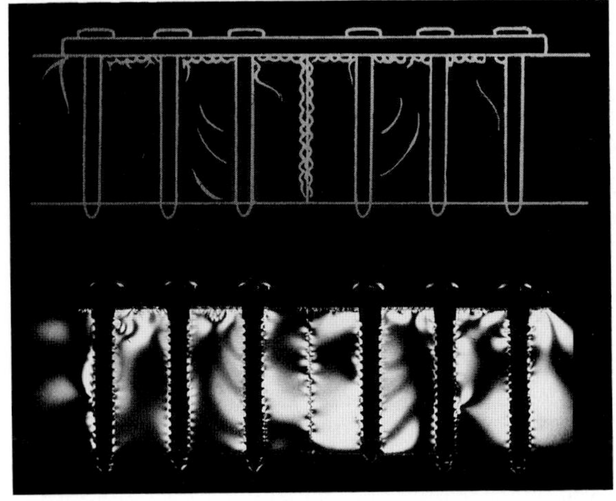

e

Compression by Prebending of the Plate

When a plate which is exactly contoured to the bone exerts axial compression, then only the near cortex is compressed. To achieve compression of the far cortex the plate may be bent so as to elevate its midsection from the bone surface.

When a prebent plate is fixed to the bone, the bend is straightened out. Due to its elastic recoil, the plate has a tendency to recover the bend which was applied by plastic (irreversible) deformation. It therefore exerts a bending moment which tends to close and to compress the far fracture gap (i.e., the one away from the plate). While in earlier days smooth bending was advocated (Fig. 1.18a), it has become evident that only the part of the bend spanning the distance between the inner screws is active (Fig. 1.18b). Therefore a comparably sharp bend between these plate holes should be applied. The angle of bend should be such that an eight-hole, 4.5-mm small DCP be elevated about 2 mm from the bone surface. The effect of this method depends upon the balance of the prebend and axial compression applied (Fig. 1.18). It should be noted that compression which is equal in both cortices is not an aim in itself. Good stability only requires that the far cortex be compressed enough to maintain contact under physiological loading without being overloaded. The compression of the far cortex is important in respect to stabilizing against torque and shear resulting from it. The displacement of a plated transverse osteotomy under torque load occurs around an axis near or within the plate. In this context the lever arm of the far cortex is many times larger then the one of the near cortex.

The advantage of prebending over the lag screw is that single overload, which opens the fracture gap, usually does not result in plastic deformation of the plate. Once the load has subsided the fracture is again stabilized due to the elastic recoil of the plate.

Prebending increases stability and it may be combined with the interfragmentary lag screw. It is especially efficient in bones of small diameter and/or in soft bone. The disadvantage of prebending is that of the elastic recoil of a prebent plate may disturb the reduction achieved.

The effect of prebending a plate on compression of the fracture surface and stability has been determined by Hayes and Perren (1971), Perren et al. (1974), and Aeberhardt (1973). Gotzen et al. (1981) analyzed extensively the prebending of plates, while Gotzen et al. (1980) and Haas et al. (1985) included different aspects of positioning of plate screws as well.

When comparing the effects of prebending and lag screws, Claudi et al. (1979) and Regazzoni (1982) observed that prebending is superior for small bones and for porous bones, while lag screw compression is superior in large and dense bones. A further advantage of prebending is that it tolerates incidences of overload. After overload the prebent plate returns to normal function, whereas the screw threads are irreversibly stripped.

Fig. 1.17 The effect of axial compression superimposed on that of prebending.

a The plate placed on the tension side: Initial stable conditions for all degrees of load and compression.

b The plate placed on the compression (bending) side: No compression, no stability. Increasing range of stable conditions with increasing compression.

Fig. 1.18 The effect of shallow versus sharp bending.

a A shallow bend has a minimal effect as only the bend enclosed within the inner screws is active.

b A sharp bend is effective.

Fig. 1.17

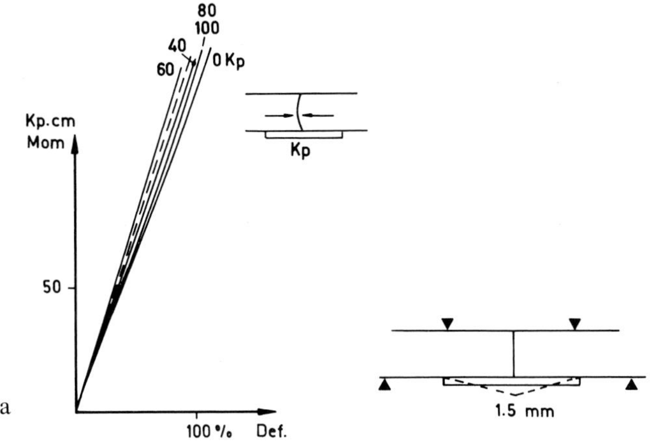

a

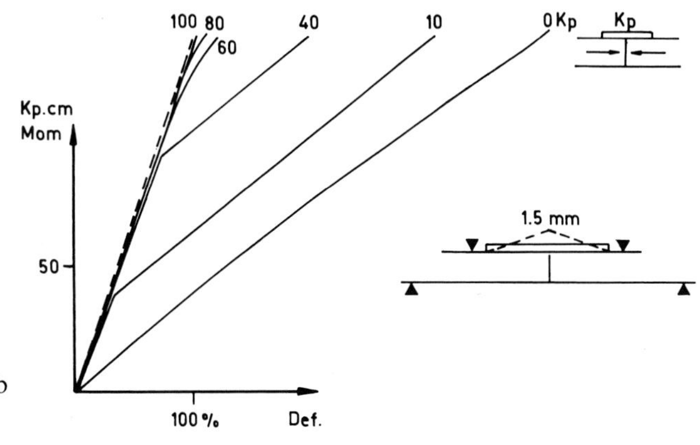

b

Fig. 1.18

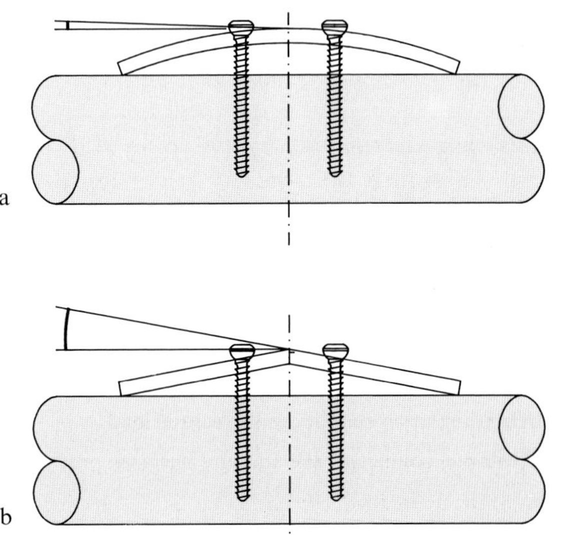

a

b

Fig. 1.19 The effect of prebending upon stability under torque load.

a Torque applied without contact at the fracture surfaces produces shear. The axis of rotation is within the plate.

b Pure axial compression is ineffective in respect to torque load. The friction produced by axial compression is located near the plate and has a small lever arm.

c Prebending produces friction far from the plate, i.e., with good leverage.

Fig. 1.20 Practial application of prebending. The plate should first be contoured to fit the bone surface snugly (a). A comparably sharp bend should then be applied (b); the midsection is therefore elevated (c) and when fixed to the bone, the plate compresses the far cortex as well (d).

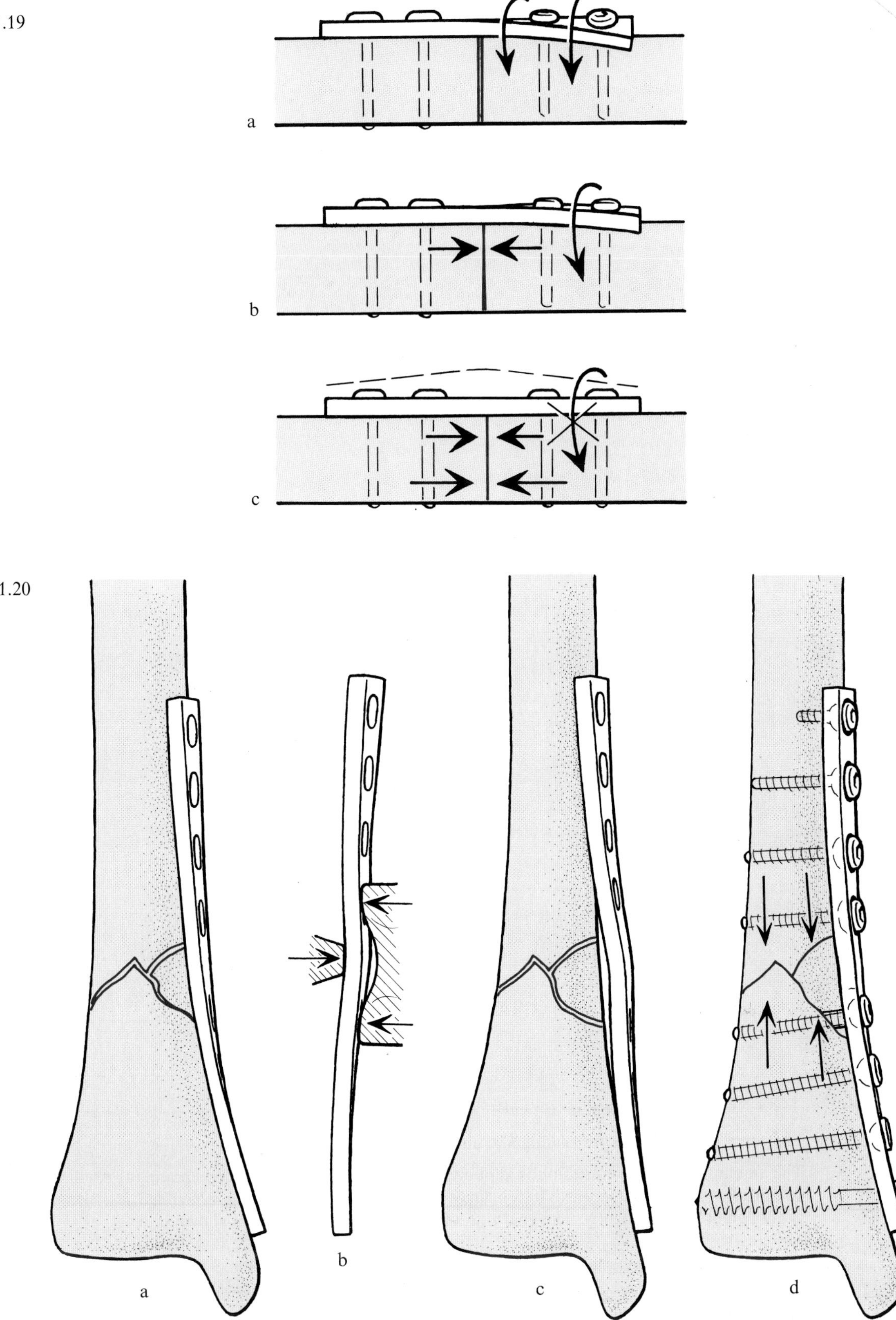
Fig. 1.19
a
b
c
Fig. 1.20
a
b
c
d

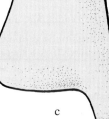

Fig. 1.21 The correlation between prebending and amount of axial compression.

The amount of axial compression is kept constant. A small amount of prebending (a) results in minimal compression of the far cortex. If too large an amount of prebending is applied (c), the near cortex is not compressed efficiently. The goal is to balance the two principles as shown in b.

Fig. 1.22 The appropriate sequence of application of the screws in a prebent plate.

To fix a prebent plate to the bone, the inner screws should be applied first and the outer thereafter (a). If the outer screws are applied first, the near cortex opens because the plate is too long in relation to the bone spanned between the outer screw holes (b).

Fig. 1.21

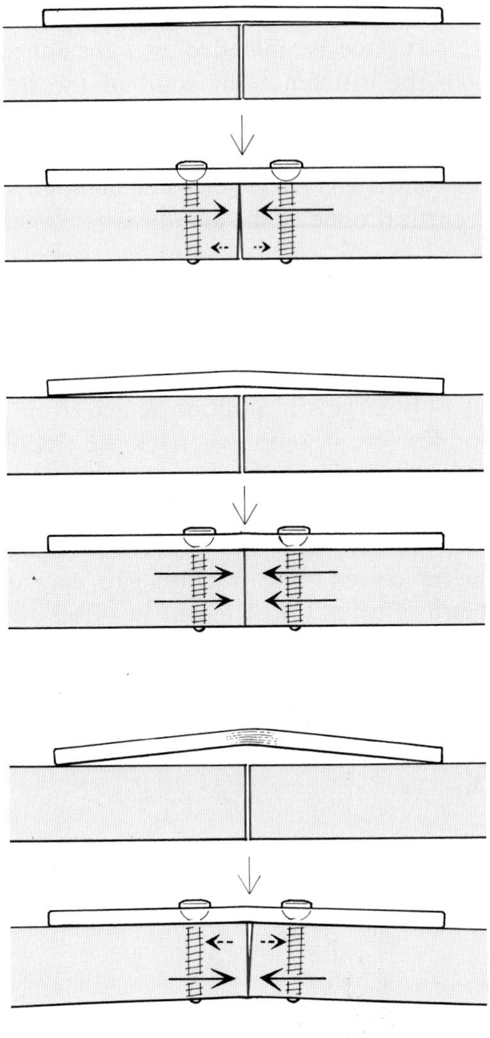

a

b

c

Fig. 1.22

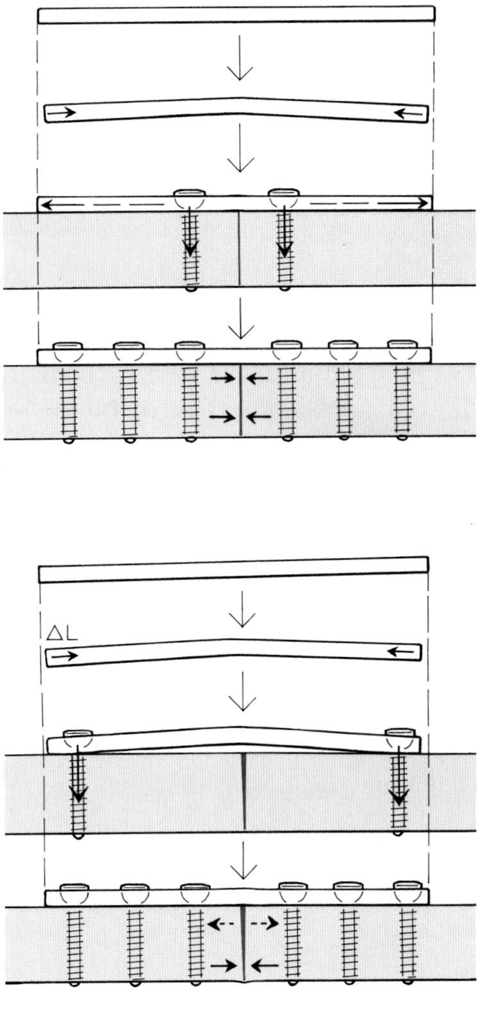

ΔL

a

b

Tension Band Fixation

Tension band fixation (Fig. 1.23) relies upon compression produced by the dynamic component of the functional load. The classic example of a tension band consists of a wire applied to the outer surface of a transversely fractured patella. This wire, together with the supporting condyles, transforms the tension applied by the quadriceps muscle into dynamic compression acting at the inner surface of the patella. The often discussed question of the magnitude and direction of the forces acting at different places of the patella fracture has a simple answer: the outer surface is unloaded and the inner surface is loaded. The remaining force is equal to the difference (or sum) of the static preload and the dynamic component of the force.

The tension band allows for some load-induced movement. Such fixation is often used at the metaphyses, where cancellous bone is less affected by small amounts of instability and reacts faster than is the case for cortical bone of the diaphysis.

Comparison of Compression by Screw and Plate

A cortical bone screw tightened by the "average surgeon" produces around 3 kN of compressive force. A plate used for axial compression results in about 0.6 kN. The compression produced by the screw is not only large; in addition it acts from within the fracture surface and results in more or less even compression of the fracture surface. The compression exerted by a straight plate contoured to fit the bone surface in turn acts asymmetrically from outside the fracture surface. The resulting compression is high near the plate (where it may even exceed the strength of bone; Rahn et al. 1971) and low within the fracture surface in the far cortex. The fracture gap may open in the cortex opposite to the plate. The asymmetric effect of the plate may be offset by prebending it (Bagby and Janes 1957). Prebending, though, is only efficient if the plate is not too soft.

Fig. 1.23 Tension band: Dynamic compression used for stabilization.

The wire placed at the anterior surface of the patella compresses the anterior part of the transverse fracture (a). Together with the pull of the muscle and the resistance of the patellar ligament a balanced compression is produced (b). The balance is of temporary nature and the inner fracture surface displaces somewhat intermittently, a situation which is well tolerated by the cancellous bone.

Fig. 1.23

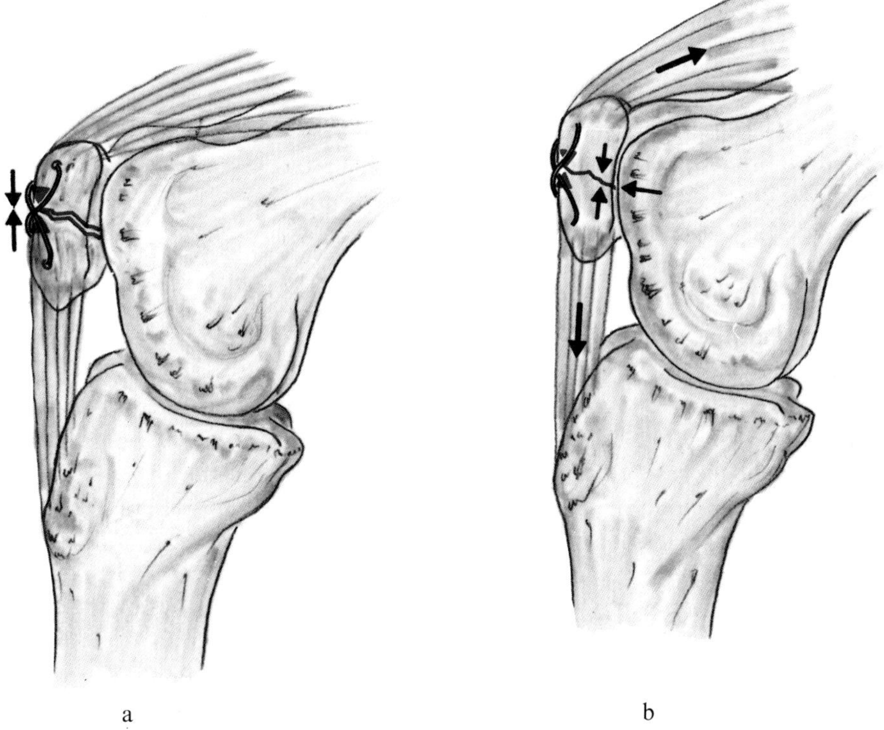

1.3.1.6 Mechanics of Interfaces

In fracture treatment by internal fixation, contact zones are established between bone and bone and between bone and implants. The bone reaction at these interfaces depends upon mechanical conditions which therefore play a determining role in the outcome of the healing process. The mechanical condition of the interface has two facets: one is the load transmitted, the other is deformation of the tissue between the bone fragments.

The deformation of repair tissues results in a relatively large displacement of the fracture fragments if the tissues between the fragments are soft. To describe the mechanical condition of relative displacement at the fracture gap, the term "stability" is used. More or less stability is synonymous with less or more relative displacement, which describes different grades of relative stability. When the fracture surfaces are adapted and compressed, the immediate contact surfaces do not displace. This is "absolute stability".

Unstable Interface

A bone placed under (repeated) dynamic load deforms cyclically, a behavior which is explained by the spring-like characteristic of the bone (Fig. 1.24). This deformation has been used experimentally in vivo to produce displacement between a plate and bone so that the effect of instability can be studied. A screw (or bolt) inserted at the free plate end is subjected to periodic unloading, while the other end of the plate is rigidly fixed to the bone by two screws under high common preload. This results in intermittent minimal displacements at the contact surface between the unloaded screw (or bolt) and the bone cortex.

Two observations appear to be noteworthy:

Investigating the hypothesis that interface instability induces bone resorption, Ganz et al. (1975) produced conditions of minute amounts of instability between a screw and the threaded hole within the bone. Their method consisted of the fixation of an instrumented plate to a functionally loaded bone, whereby only one end of the plate was fixed by inserting screws tightly. The other plate end was left "free" by inserting the experimental screw only with a small amount of torque in order to maintain the correct position rather than to use it for fixation of the plate to the bone. Functional compressive loading

---

Fig. 1.24 Method of producing instability in the experiment.

To study the effect of controlled instability upon implant loosening by bone surface resorption, advantage was taken of the fact that bone shortens cyclically under weight-bearing during walking. Comparing bone with a stiff spring demonstrates how one can bring about relative displacement between the free end of a plate and the underlying bone. The displacement amounts only to a few micrometers. The plate is solidly fixed at the other end by two screws under high common preload.

a, b Schematic diagrams of the nonloaded and loaded situations of a plate fixed only at one end to the bone. Bone shortens under axial compression, and a relative displacement between the free end of the plate and the underlying bone results.

c Initial situation without functional load: The unloaded bone has its original length. A small amount of compression preloads the inner surface of the cylinder to produce bone contact.

d Situation with functional load: The loaded bone is now shorter. The small initial compression is unloaded, the inner surface opens temporarily, and the outer experiences intermittent contact.

e Biological reaction to intermittent unloading and instability: In spite of the fact that the above-mentioned displacement amounts to only a few micrometers, bone surface resorption is initiated. Thus, a small initial instability results in gross loosening due to the biological reaction.

Fig. 1.24

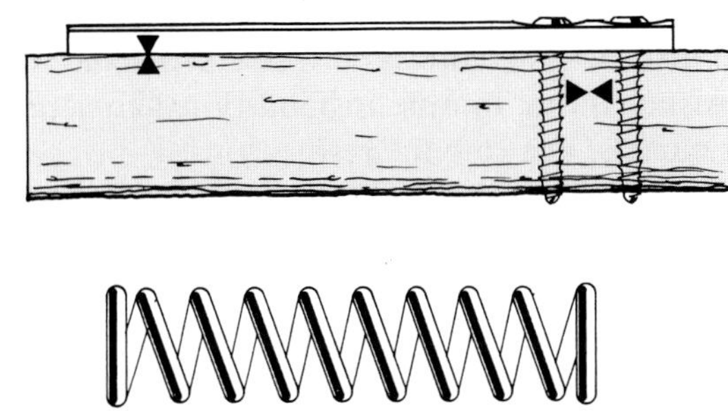

a

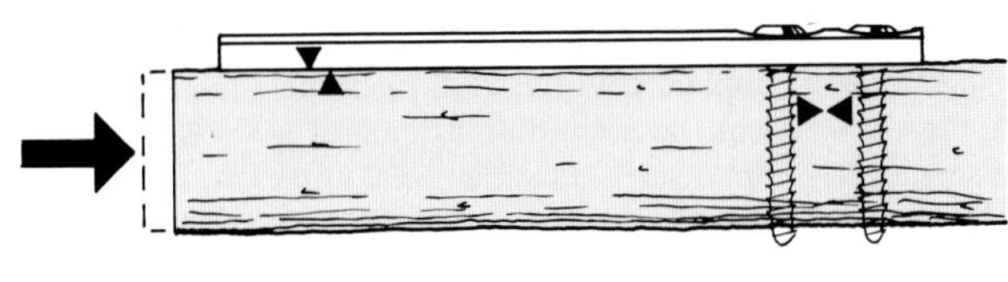

b

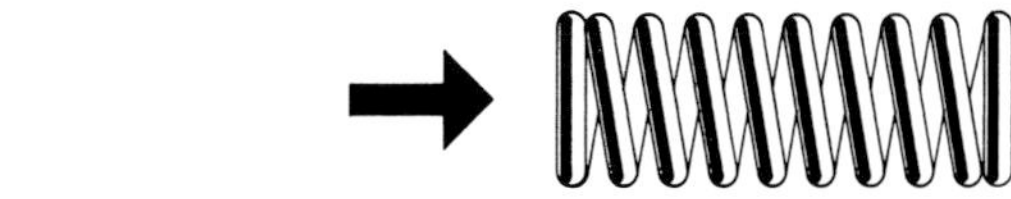

c

d

e

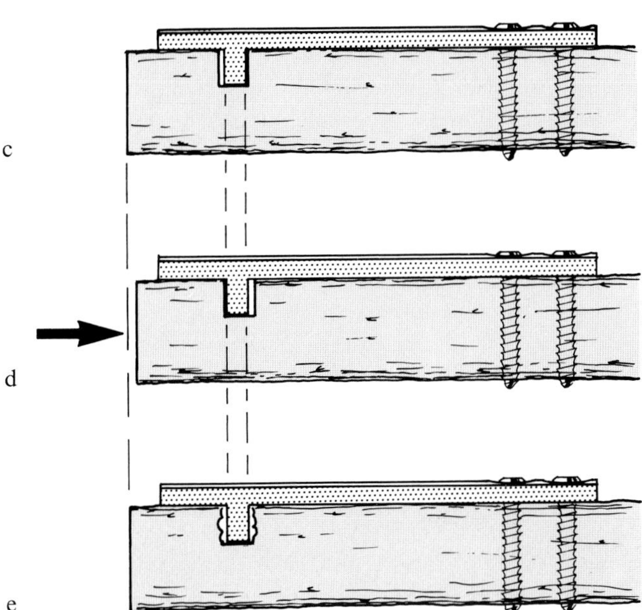

shortens the plated bone segment by less than 10 μm. This displacement results in inclination of a screw which is not tightly driven into bone. Figure 1.24 illustrates a simplified version of the same experiment (Brennwald pers. comm. 1976) in which a short fixed bolt was used instead of the tilting screw. The displacement and the resulting bone resorption are displayed. Initial minute instability led to secondary massive instability, in both experimental models, due to bone resorption.

Stadler et al. (1982) used a hydraulically operated plunger to study bone surface reaction to high interface strain (Fig. 1.25). High interface strain produced by the plunger hitting the bone surface intermittently led to bone surface resorption, while low strain conditioned in which the plunger displaced the same amount but at a distance to the bone surface, did not.

Thus, initially small instability will, by the process of micromotion-induced bone surface resorption, lead to secondary gross instability.[12]

---

[12] The relationship between applied compression, resulting shortening, and effect of minimal resorption is visualized in Fig. 1.17. It can be seen that a load of 1000 N results in about 10 μm shortening of the compressed segment. Minimal surface resorption completely abolished the compression.

Fig. 1.25 Experimental method used to study bone reaction at unstable interfaces (Stadler et al. 1982).

a Hydraulically operated bellows with plunger mounted within a U-shaped jig.

b X-ray showing the apparatus applied to the proximal metaphysis of the tibia.

c Cross section of the tibia: the histological section shows the marked bone surface resorption in the vicinity of an intermittently contacting plunger surface.

d Cross section of the tibia: no resorption in the case of a plunger which cycled at a distance from the bone surface.

Fig. 1.25

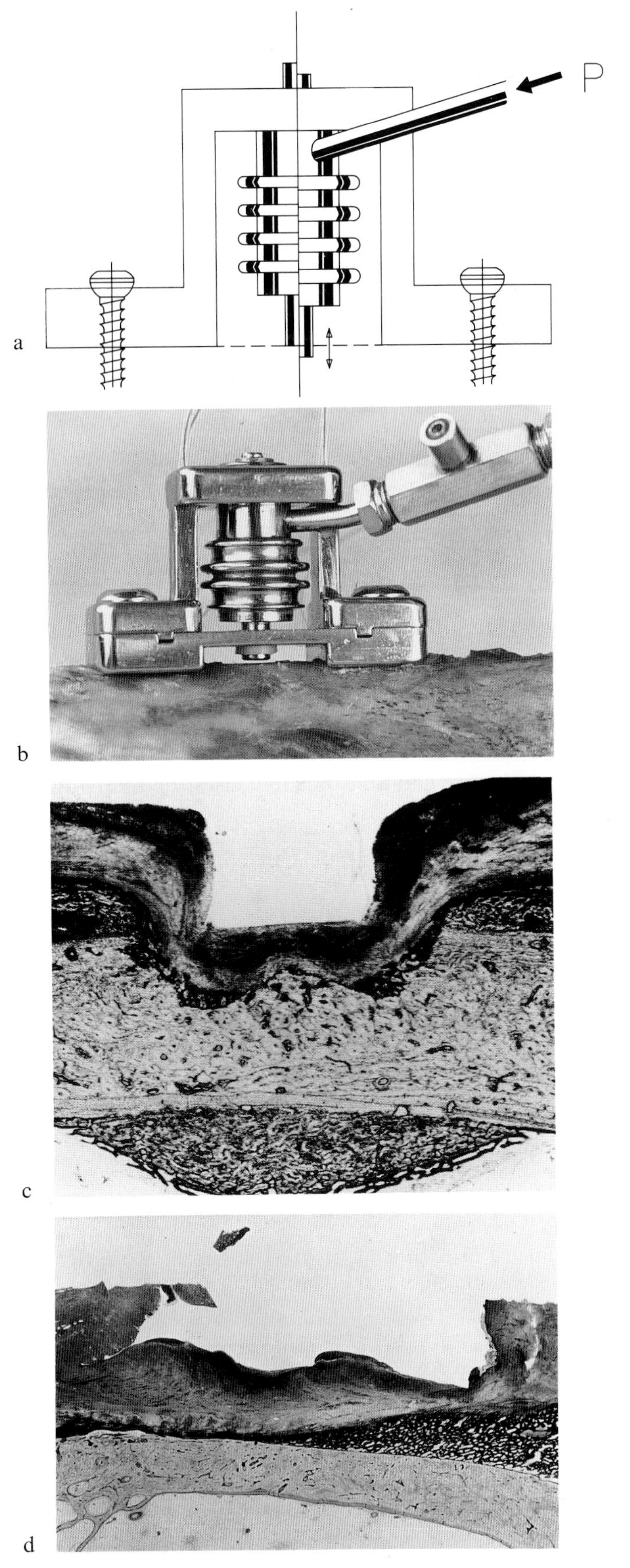

Mechanically Induced Pin Loosening in External Fixation

The pins used with external fixators often loosen at the pin-bone interface. Huiskes et al. (1985) felt that this was due to mechanical failure of bone due to local overload. While this may occur in metaphyseal bone, there is now good evidence that in cortical bone surface resorption induced by micromotion is much more common (see p. 56). Two methods to decrease micromotion have been used empirically in the past: (1) the pins were prebent before they were fastened to the longitudinal rods (bending preload), or (2) the size of the pin shaft was selected so that its diameter was larger than the drill hole (radial preload) (Behrens 1982, 1989).

Experiments carried out by Hyldahl et al. (1988) (Figs. 1.26, 1.27) have cast doubts on the effectiveness of bending preload, but they have clearly demonstrated that radial preload can significantly reduce surface resorption compared to pins inserted without preload. They showed that the range of possible misfit between the borehole and pin diameter was much smaller than hitherto assumed (see p. 62).

In external fixation utilizing a frame – particularly in fusions and in osteotomies – micromotion of the parallel Steinmann pins can be reduced by bending the pins against each other.

Mechanically Induced Non-union

Unstable interfaces between bone fragment ends may result in a mechanically induced non-union even in the presence of intact biological reactions (reactive or hypertrophic non-union) (Weber and Cech 1973). In this case the tissue differentiation from soft to more stiff tissues and the increase in cross section are unable to reduce the mobility of the fragments. The bone formation at the fragment ends results in reduction of the width of the fracture gap and thus increases the interfragmental strain.

Fig. 1.26 The effect of bending versus radial preload in pins of external fixators.

a Pneumatically operated external fixator rod, which allows application of a cyclical bending load to the single pin at the right. In b–d, a cross section of the near cortex is illustrated schematically.

b Without additional load, bending produces a tight fit at the right side of the pin, while radial preload results in an equal amount of preload around the pin.

c With an additional load pushing the pin to the right, the bent pin increases the gap on the left, the radially preloaded one decreases somewhat the preload at the left without displacement.

d With an additional load pushing to the left, the gap with the bent pin becomes smaller and the radially preloaded pin does not show displacement.

Fig. 1.27 Effect of radial preload of external fixator pins to prevent pin loosening: *Abscissa*: The three groups from left to right: no preload, radial preload, bending preload. *Ordinate*: Loss of bone contact surface in percent. The effect of different conditions of radial preload: *left*, the exactly fitting pin with marked resorption of the contact surface. *Middle*, the slightly oversized pin with minimal resorption. *Right*, bending preload was applied. It reduced somewhat but did not prevent the resorption and loosening.

Fig. 1.26

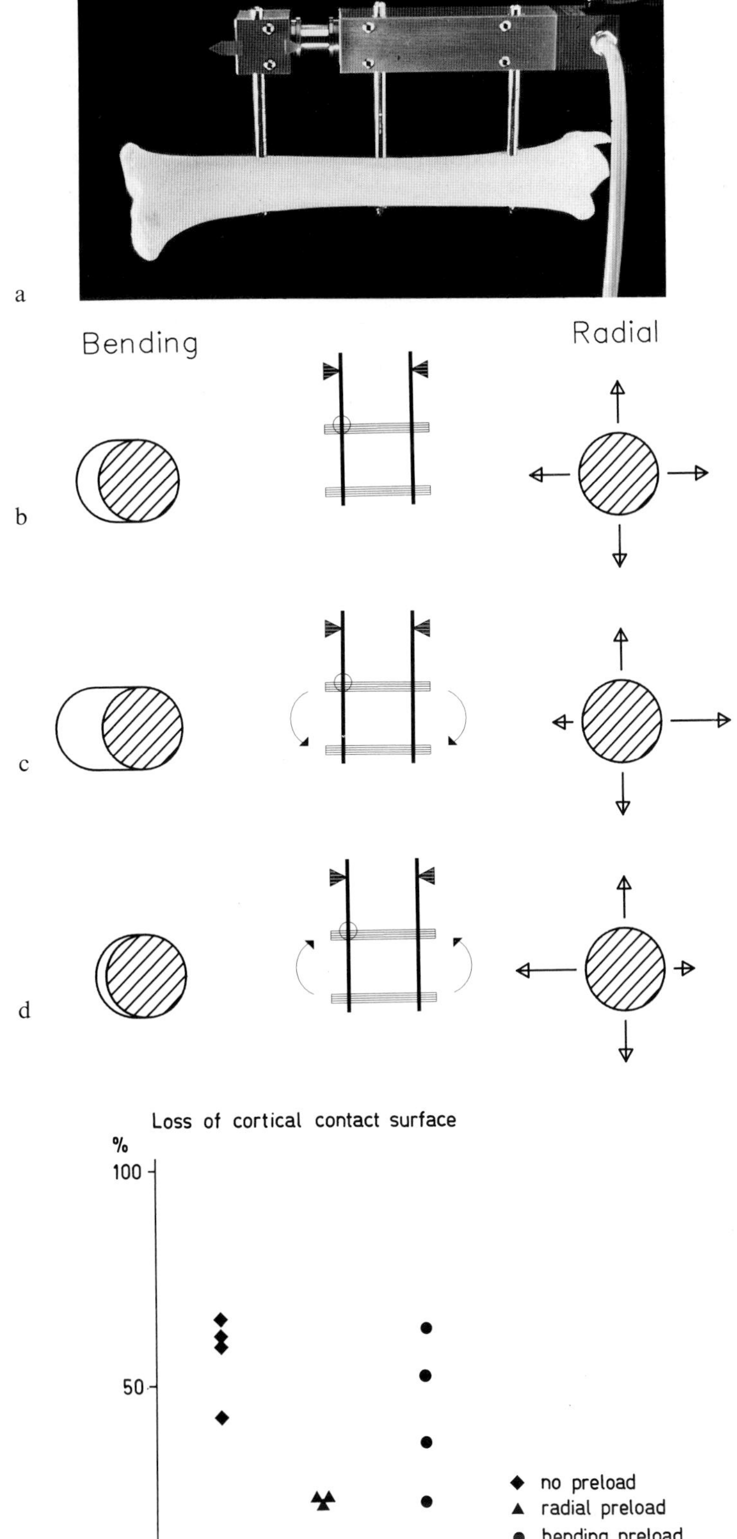

Fig. 1.27

Stable (Compressed) Interface

Screws submitted to bending and thus stabilized by compression (at the interface) were studied in the same experiment in which unstable interfaces were examined. Less bone surface resorption was observed. It is important to note that in this experiment, in spite of very high internal compressive stresses, the bone did not show resorption in the stable areas of contacting interface. Figure 1.28 explains the relationship between compression applied and fracture surface resorption: maintenance of compression proves the absence of such resorption.

Figure 1.29 shows why the blood supply of bone is not disturbed by compressive load. Consider the behavior of a brick wall with a drill hole through its thickness. A rubber hose carrying water through the hole will for practical purposes exhibit the same flow whether the brick wall is heavily loaded or not. The flow will change markedly when the brick wall collapses, but not before. The same holds true for blood vessels within the stable framework of hydroxyapatite.

1.3.2 Biological Reactions

Cellular function determines the reliability and quality of fracture healing. In fracture healing with preserved vascularity this cellular function is primarily controlled by the mechanical environment. The elements of biological reaction to the mechanical environment are outlined in this section.

The mechanical environment is mainly determined by the forces acting on and the resulting deformation leading to displacement of fracture fragments. Two biomechanical events play a role:

1. Cellular function, which results in tissue formation, destruction, and differentiation, is controlled by mechanical input. Tissue deformation (strain) due to instability induces both callus formation and bone resorption at contacting interfaces (i.e., between bone fragments as well as between bone and implant). This resorption in turn results in increased instability of the fracture site. Intense staining of soft repair tissues may necessitate several stages of tissue differentiation, whereby soft tissues which tolerate deformation (e.g., granulation tissues) are replaced by a series of tissues (e.g., connective tissues) which are progressively stiffer and which tolerate less strain. This process is called indirect healing.

If on the other hand small gaps are stabilized by contact surfaces nearby, and if such contact surfaces are maintained in close apposition by interfragmental compression, the gap and the contact surface provide low strain conditions. Under these conditions direct bone formation is possible and bone surface resorption, as well as callus formation,

---

Fig. 1.28 The effect of resorption at the compressed interface upon the amount of compression.

a A bone segment within a C-clamp of original length L, no compression.

b Deformation (shortening) of 10 μm results in a compression of 1000 N.

c When the bone segment undergoes shortening of 10 μm due to fragment end resorption at the "fracture site," the compression is abolished.

Fig. 1.29 The effect of compression upon blood flow within cortical bone.

Large amounts of compression within the bone are well tolerated. However, even minimal compression of the soft tissues at the bone surface results in complete obliteration of periosteal blood supply.

Fig. 1.28

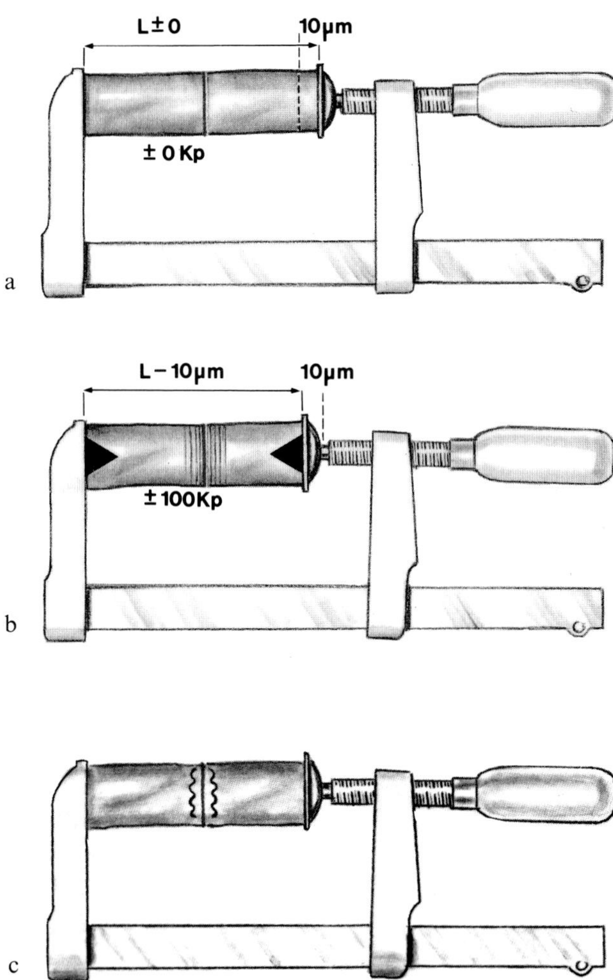

Fig. 1.29

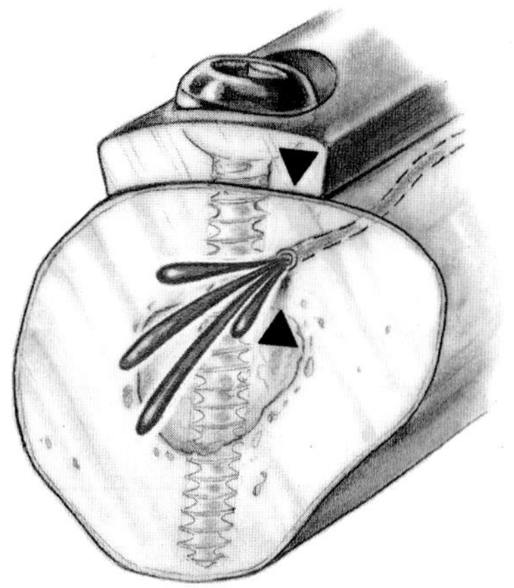

is absent. This type of healing is called direct healing (contact healing and gap healing). The surface of the contact zones is very small and corresponds to the compression applied times the strength of bone. Therefore the contact zone of a fracture amounts to only a small fraction (a few percent) of the cross-sectional area.

2. Cellular function results in changes in the material properties, in the geometry of the fracture fragments, and the (soft and hard) tissues connecting the fragments.[13]

1.3.2.1 Stability and Compression

Compression, Behavior and Effects

For decades the clinical observation that soft tissues undergo pressure necrosis (pressure sores) when continually compressed led to the belief that bone also underwent pressure necrosis. The observed resorption of the vertebrae near a pulsating aortic aneurysm had been incorrectly explained as resulting from "pressure-induced necrosis". Instead of undergoing pressure necrosis, bone as a tissue is exceptionally well suited to function under mechanical load; its cells and blood vessels are protected by a stiff framework.

Compression by Plate

Using instrumented compression plates, Perren et al. (1969a, b) demonstrated that the static compression applied decreased only gradually over a period of several months (Fig. 1.30).

Compression by Screws

The forces exerted by screws, as measured in simulated internal fixation by von Arx (1973), are larger (2–4 kN by screw compared to 0.6–1 kN by plate) and more efficient than the ones produced by "compression" plates. The use of instrumented washers implanted for an extended period of time (Blümlein et al. 1977) demonstrated the maintenance of very high forces applied to a relatively small area of living bone in the sheep (Fig. 1.33).

[13] The changes in material properties affect the stiffness of the fracture linearly, while the changes in geometry may affect torsional and flexural stiffness in proportion to the cube of the diameter.

Fig. 1.30 Flexible fixation using plates (Hutzschenreuter et al. 1969).

a A thin, flexible plate results in callus formation.

b A thicker, more rigid plate results in smaller, better structured callus and no resorption of the fragment ends.

Fig. 1.30

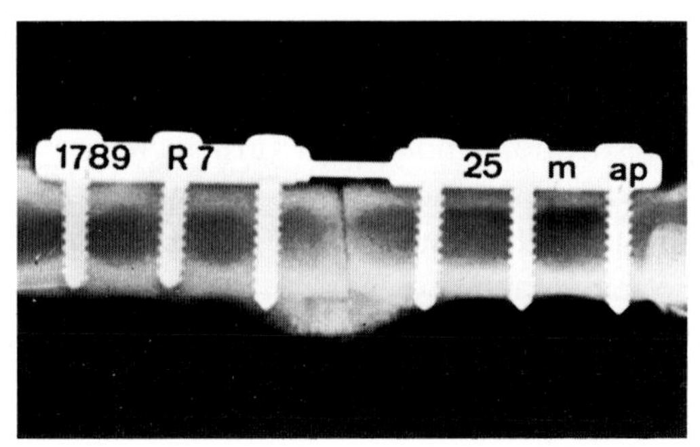

a

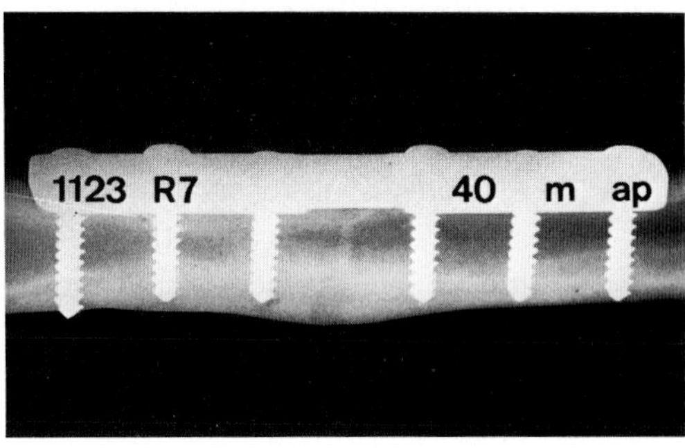

b

"Pressure Necrosis"?

In the experiments using instrumented plates and instrumented screws, the conditions were very sensitive to minute amounts of bone resorption at the compressed interfaces. Thus resorption of a one cell layer thickness of bone ($\sim 10\ \mu m$) would have resulted in a prompt, noticeable loss of compression (Fig. 1.28). The absence of such reaction demonstrated the absence of induction of bone resorption even by excessive compressive forces. Still, the incidence of implant loosening, under conditions suggestive of initial instability, led to further studies of "pressure necrosis."

1.3.2.2 Biomechanics of Instability

The effect of instability on bone biology is apparent, especially at the bone surfaces (Fig. 1.31). Instability induces bone resorption and this in turn increases the instability of fixation, either by plates or screws. Bone resorption induced by even minimal instability at the interfaces may therefore compromise the results of an internal fixation when techniques are applied which require the maintenance of absolute stability of fixation. Such techniques would include screws and plates used for the treatment of simple diaphyseal fractures. In a rigid system, applied forces will result in minimal deformation; conversely, a minimal change of geometry (for example, due to bone surface resorption) results in loss of applied compression.[14]

Induction of Bone Surface Resorption

Using the model of a plate bridging intact and functionally loaded living bone (Fig. 1.24), Perren et al. (1975) demonstrated the effect of relative and intermittent displacement between contacting surfaces of living cortical bone (Fig. 1.31). The induction of bone surface resorption was apparent with displacements in the range of less than one cell diameter (1–3 μm). Using hydraulically activated experimental implants in the sheep tibia, Stadler et al. (1982) induced surface resorption with a plunger intermittently contacting the bone surface, even with small forces.

Induction of Callus Formation

It is well known that mechanical irritation of living bone induces "callus" formation (as do other "irritating" factors). In the experiments of Stadler et al. (1982), callus formation was induced when the plunger cycled at a distance from the bone surface. Küntscher

[14] The terms rigidity and stability are often confused. Stability is used here to define a state of absence of relative displacement between contacting surfaces ("bone to bone" or "bone to implant"). Stiffness or rigidity defines the relation between force applied and resulting deformation or displacement. The latter definition correctly implies that there always results some degree of deformation or displacement under load in stiff or rigid internal fixation. The term "stable internal fixation" should therefore be used to express the absence of load-dependent displacement at the interface between fragment ends or between bone and implant.

Fig. 1.31 Induction of bone resorption in the experiment.
a Model according to Fig. 1.24.
b Stable interface: no resorption.
c Unstable interface: biological loosening.

Fig. 1.31

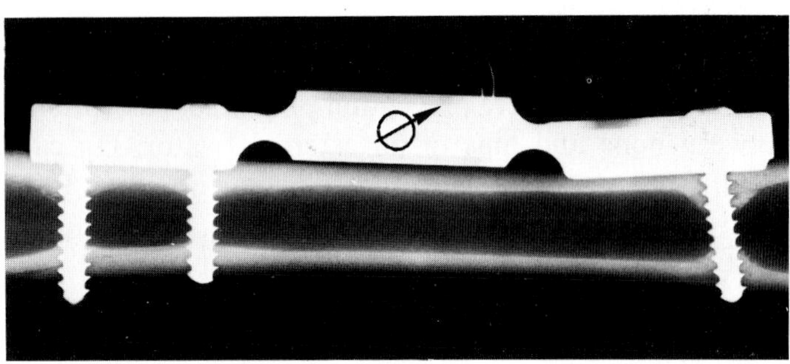

a

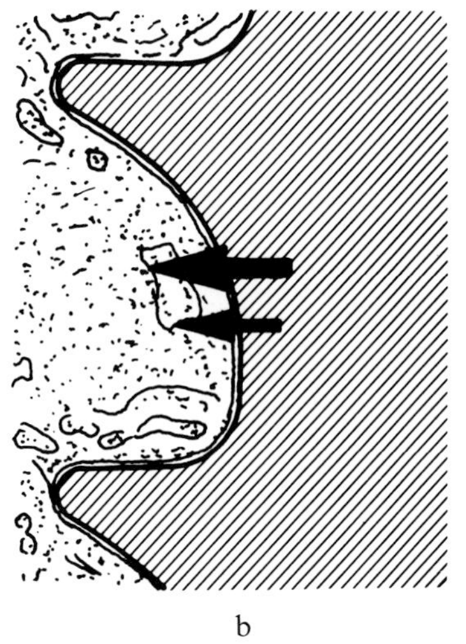

b

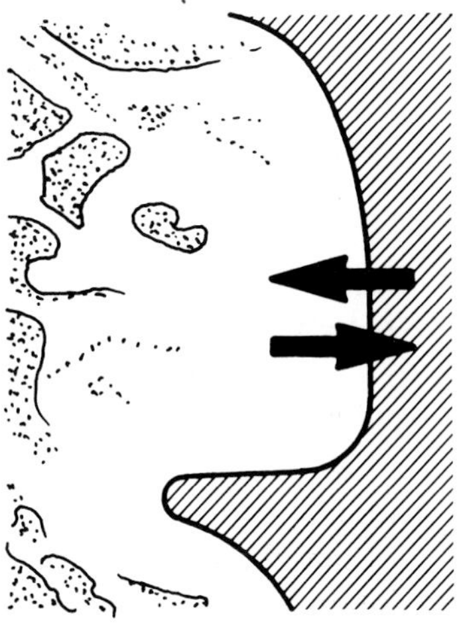

c

(1970) and later Danckwardt et al. (1971) demonstrated induction of periosteal callus formation when a corroding metal or plastic was inserted into the bone marrow cavity. Infection is also known to induce the formation of a "cloudy callus" under certain circumstances.

1.3.2.3 Biomechanics of Stability

As we will see when discussing direct or primary healing, compressed bone surfaces do not undergo surface resorption of the fragment ends (see p. 70). Avoidance of such surface resorption is of importance in preventing a "nongliding" implant such as plate and screw from keeping fracture fragments apart and preventing spontaneous stabilization by interdigitation. The latter could occur if the fragments could slide together.

Another situation where prevention of contact resorption is of importance is the interface between bone and pins of an external fixator. On careful scrutiny, pin loosening in external fixation is detected in 60% of pins in situ a 3–5 months. However, one does not readily detect pin loosening using X-rays: as Hente (1988) has shown, a 4.5-mm pin inserted into a 48-mm drill hole does not appear radiologically loose in spite of a 0.3-mm gap which could have occurred due to resorption. The effects of pin loosening may be:

1. Loss of stability, an effect which, in elastic fixation using external fixators, is not too important.
2. Pin track infection. This relation is evident though not yet clearly proven.
3. Loss of sealing between the skin surface and the medullary cavity. This may be the reason for the problems encountered when an external fixator is replaced by an intramedullary nail.

1.3.2.4 Reaction to Changes of Physiological Loading

The theory that bone structure reacts mainly to changes in functional loading is one of the most widely accepted and unfortunately most often misused theories. Bone adaptation to changes in load according to Wolff's law (Wolff 1893, 1986) applies primarily to cancellous bone: adaptation is slow and less important in cortical bone. In conventional internal fixation using plates, which transmit forces by friction, the unloading of the bone due to the implant is of temporary nature.

The biological reactions of bone and of hard and soft repair tissues to mechanical influences have recently been studied by Goodship and Kenwright (1985) and Lanyon and Rubin (1985). In fracture healing the reaction of the cortical bone to mechanical load probably plays a lesser role.

Fig. 1.32 Measurement of plate compression in vivo (Perren et al. 1969a, b).

a Instrumented plate. An internal fixation plate (DCP) fitted with strain gauges and a wire connection. This plate allowed precise determination of the amount of compression applied to living bone as well as the changes in vivo.

b Compression measurement in sheep tibia. A transverse osteotomy of a sheep tibia has been fixed using two DCPs applied at right angles. (Here only one of the two plates is illustrated).

c Compression applied to cortical bone in vivo. The initial value of compression of 1800 N force decreases very slowly. This pattern of change in compression proved that pressure necrosis with surface resorption in the compressed area did not occur.

Fig. 1.32

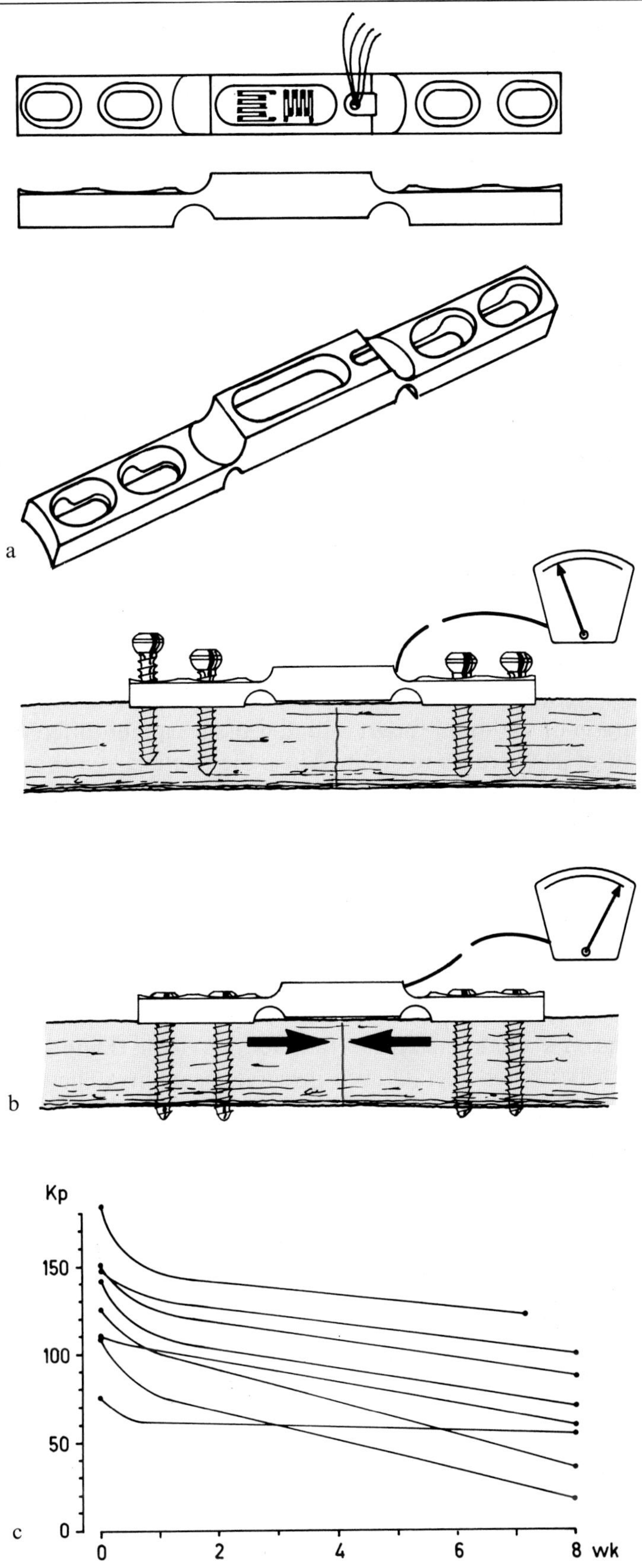

Reaction to Unloading by Implants

Many authors have studied the reaction of cortical bone to unloading by implants, and the mechanical effects of stress shielding are impressive. The cortical bone near a plate, for example, is unloaded. Depending upon the type of load applied, the opposite cortical bone is loaded either less or more than normal (Cochran 1969; Woo et al. 1976; Claes et al. 1982; Cordey et al. 1987; Gautier 1988).

While mechanical unloading has been indisputably demonstrated, and while bone changes are observed after internal fixation, the question remains of which structural changes are due exclusively to the change in mechanical load. After prosthetic replacement, after arthrodesis, and after long-term implantation of angle blade plates structural changes of the cancellous bone have been observed. Nonetheless, to validate the hypothesis that the changes in bone structure seen after internal fixation using straight plates in cortical bone are irrefutably linked to unloading, a close relationship between the mechanical challenge and the structural changes would have to be demonstrated. The apparent paradox is explained by the fact that plates transmitting force mainly by friction based upon compression of the plate to the bone (e.g., the straight plates) lose their close coupling, and therefore their ability to contribute to general unloading, around half a year after implantation (though they may still protect against peak load).

Reaction to Strain

Strain is defined as relative deformation (by a given stress or vice versa). The basic assumption of the strain theory is that a tissue cannot differentiate when strained beyond the limit of its tolerance to strain. Thus, the relation of *momentary strain* to *tissue-specific strain tolerance* determines the potential for its differentiation. As Pauwels (1965, 1980) has pointed out, the differentiation in failed healing of a fracture does not take a new direction, it is simply haltered at a certain level. There is obviously a lower limit of strain (*strain induction level*) below which no differentiation is initiated though the strain level would be tolerated.

Strain Controlling Fracture Healing

The surgeon is often amazed by the fact that some fractures heal under gross instability while others do not tolerate even invisible instability. The concept of strain (Perren and Cordey 1977, 1980) considers the deformation sustained by the individual cell. If the deformation present within the repair tissue exceeds the elongation which would lead to tissue (cell) disruption (elongation at rupture) of the next tissue to be developed, then the differentiation comes to a halt. A tissue cannot exist under conditions of strain exceeding the elongation at which rupture occurs.

With a grasp of this concept of strain, that is deformation which is expressed independently of geometry (see p. 16), the surgeon can now understand why in some situations (e.g., spontaneous healing of complex fractures) marked instability is compatible with the development of solid union, while under other conditions (closely adapted but not

---

Fig. 1.33 Measurement of screw compression in vivo (Blümlein et al. 1977).

a Instrumented washer for in vivo measurement of screw compression. A washer is fitted with strain gauges and a transcutaneous wire connection.

b Recording compression exerted by screws in vivo. Three different groups of initial compression and their changes in vivo are plotted. Over a period of 16 weeks the compression regressed very slowly.

Fig. 1.33

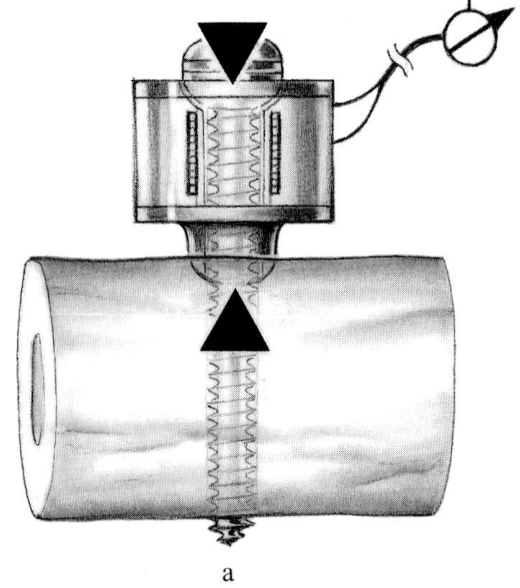

a

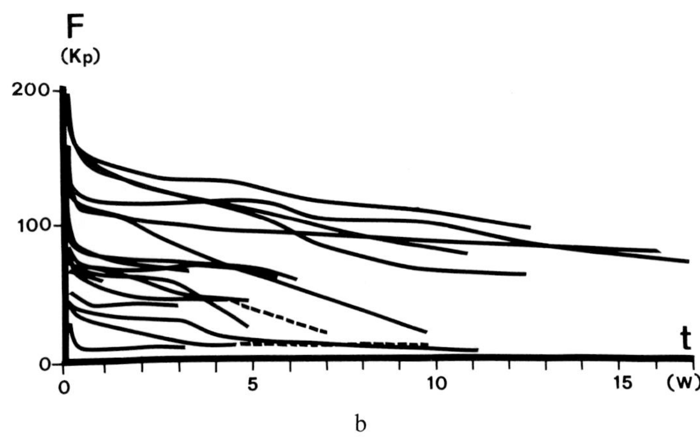

b

compressed fractures) even minute amounts of instability may not be compatible with solid union.

Reaction to Interface Conditions Grossly Exceeding the Strain Within the Bone

We have shown that radial preload is a very efficient tool in preventing intermittent displacement at the pin-bone interface. How much misfit can be tolerated mechanically? Here again strain is the critical parameter which allows one to determine the mechanically optimal misfit, i.e., the most favorable relation between the size of the drill hole and the diameter of the pin.

Biliouris et al. (1989) have recently studied this question and have come up with the statement that when using a 4.5-mm pin, a misfit of 0.1–0.2 mm is optimal; a misfit of more than 0.2 mm results in local mechanical breakdown of the bone at the interface. Instability and surface resorption and/or sequestration of a ring (ring sequestrum) may result. Both processes result in loss of optimal stability at the interface.

1.3.2.5 Disturbance of Blood Supply to Bone

Due to the Fracture

A fracture induces several different circulatory changes. It disrupts the longitudinal blood vessels, and the open ends of these blood vessels undergo thrombosis. Bone just deep to the fragment ends is no longer nourished and will become necrotic. The ensuing remodeling may lead to demarcation and formation of a sequestrum. Cavitation (see p. 6) at the time of fracture and displacement of the fracture fragments also add to the vascular trauma. In any case the fracture results in disruption of the longitudinal blood supply within bone. A thin surface layer of bone nourished by diffusion is superimposed on a deeper band of non-perfused and hence necrotic bone.

Due to the Soft Tissue Trauma

Stripping of the periosteum results in damage to the periosteal blood supply but particularly in damage to the nutrient artery. The latter is detrimental to the overall blood supply of bone. Stripping of the periosteum may occur from displacement of the fracture fragments and/or as a result of inappropriate surgical procedures.

Due to the Implant Contact

Implant-to-bone contact invariably results in damage of the radial perfusion of bone (Fig. 1.34) (Rhinelander and Wilson 1982). Gunst et al. (1979) demonstrated a correlation between the implant contact and the damage to blood supply using the method of Luethi et al. (1982) which had been developed to determine the implant (plate) to bone contact area.

Fig. 1.34 Blood supply, remodeling, and porosis beneath plate.

a Disturbed blood supply.

b Remodeling of the necrotic area, progressing towards the plate.

c Areas of normal bone and remodeled, temporary porotic bone: early temporary porosis.

Fig. 1.34

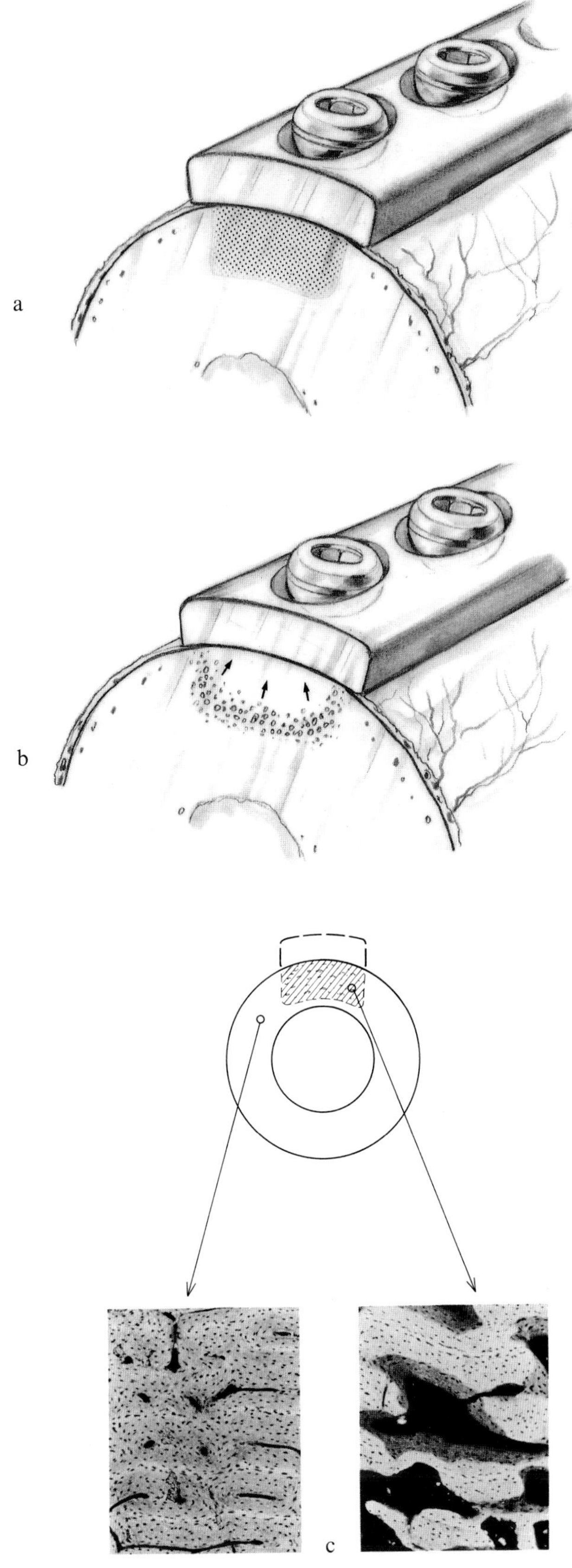

1.3.2.6 Reaction to Disturbance of the Blood Supply

There are two consecutive effects of damage to the cortical bone blood supply: first, necrosis occurs, and second, remodeling follows (Fig. 1.34). The remodeling starts within the adjacent living bone and moves toward the necrotic bone, eventually leading to removal and replacement of the necrotic area.

The blood supply is first disrupted by the displacement of the fracture fragments. It is also damaged by the cavitation phenomenon during fracture (see Fig. 1.2). Conservative treatment or open reduction may further compromise the blood supply. External splints may impede the blood supply because the soft tissues are not exercised. Internal splints (e.g., plates or nails) may hinder blood supply by their contact with bone, where they compress the blood vessels which enter or exit from bone (Fig. 1.34). From the experiments by Rhinelander (1978) and Ganz and Brennwald (1975), we know that if the fracture is stabilized, the medullary circulation may recover within 1–2 weeks. With regard to the blood supply, the surgeon must weigh the negative (surgical trauma) against the positive (faster recovery of blood supply) effects of different types of treatment.

Early Temporary Bone Loss near Implants

Uhthoff et al. (1971), Coutts et al. (1976), Moyen et al. (1978), and Matter et al. (1974) reported changes in the structure of long bones in the vicinity of the plate. The bone loss was explained on the basis of "Wolff's law" (Wolff 1893, 1986), which states that bone adapts its structure to mechanical loading conditions. The work of Woo et al. (1976) and Claes et al. (1980) seems to support the theory of "stress protection" of bone loss in plated bone. Tonino et al. (1976) and Tayton et al. (1982) proposed the use of soft plastic or carbon plates in order to minimize stress shielding.

Possible effects of static compression and tension applied to living cortical bone have been studied by Matter et al. (1974). They found no statistical difference in the remodeling rate regardless of the comparatively large amounts of static forces applied to the bone.

Based on recent experiments three findings emerge:

1. Early temporary bone loss is seen in the vicinity of literally all implants, including intramedullary nails (Fig. 1.35), fixator externe pins (Pfister et al. 1983) etc.
2. Early temporary bone loss exhibits a close relationship to the vascular damage brought about by implantation and by the presence of the implant (i.e., implant to bone contact). The pattern of early temporary porosis does not show a correlation with any conceivable type of unloading (Gautier et al. 1986).
3. Plastic plates, which were softer than standard metal plates, showed more porosis, contrary to expectations based on the mechanical theory of stress protection (Gautier

---

Fig. 1.35 Blood supply, remodeling, and porosis around a nail.

a Disturbed blood supply: circular area around nail.

b Initial remodeling in the demarcation area between necrotic and live bone. Cross section with disulfine intravital staining of blood supply at higher magnification. Within the demarcation zone enlarged canals of the osteons are seen. These represent osteons in remodeling with temporary porosis.

c Remodeling of the necrotic area progressing towards the nail.

d The rate and direction of the remodeling process were determined using the "polychrome sequential labeling method" (Rahn et al. 1980).

Fig. 1.35

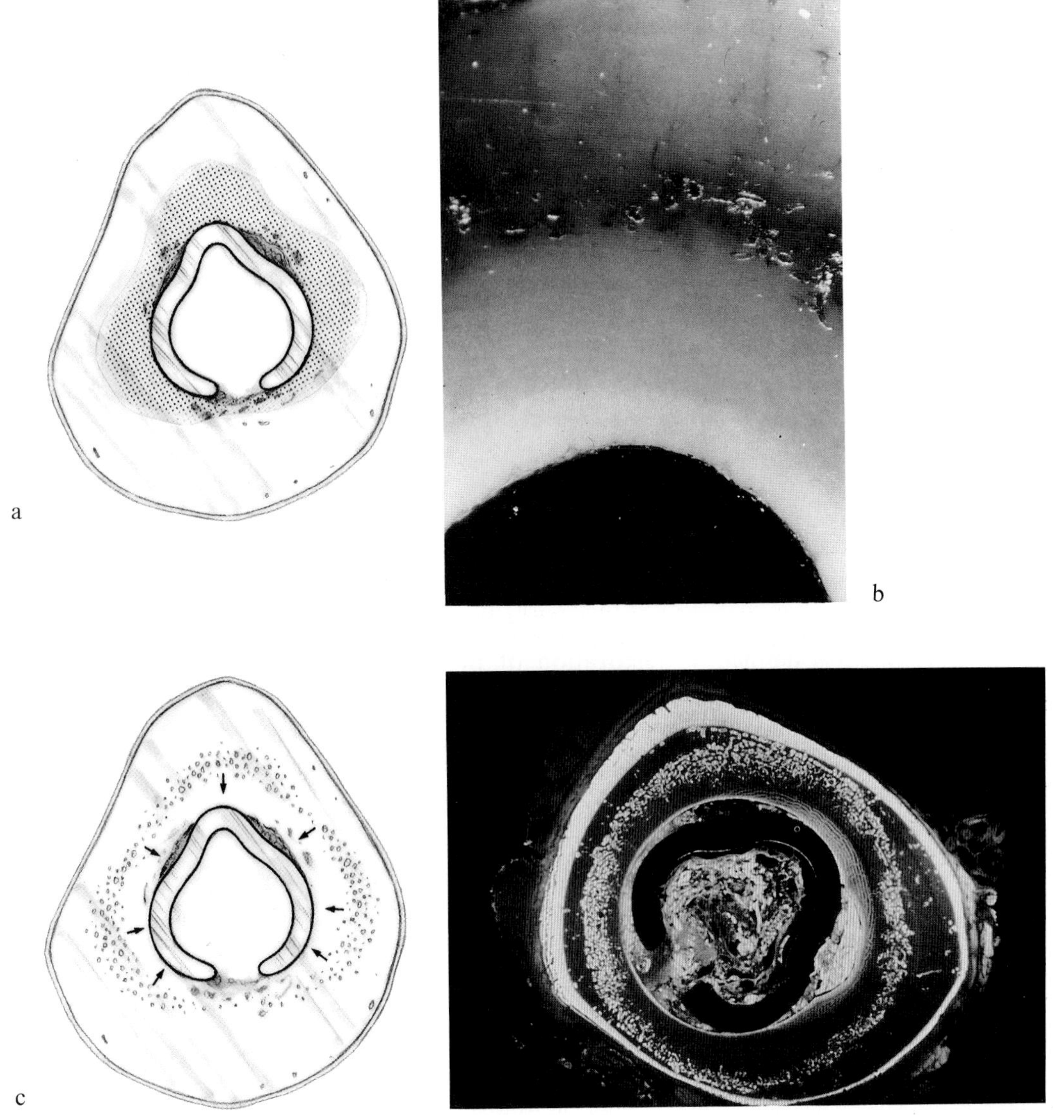

et al. 1986). The softer plate may adapt more snugly to the bone and result in increased vascular damage.

The early temporary bone loss disappears 3 months following surgery, and at 1 year the cross section of the bone appears to be nonporous. Some authors have stated that the late changes in bone structure due to unloading by the implant may result in refractures (Kessler et al. 1988; Leu et al. 1989). Using quantitative computer tomography, Cordey et al. (1985) studied the bone structure of the tibia after plate removal in a series of 70 patients. They observed only small changes in bone structure (less than 20%) when density and geometry were used to calculate expected strength. At the time of plate removal the plate is no longer rigidly pressed to the bone. Thus, force transmission between bone and plate via friction is lost and the plate induces unloading only at peak load.

Working on the hypothesis that implant-to-bone contact and the subsequent damage to blood supply is the cause of early bone loss, Jörger et al. (1987) and Vattolo et al. (1986) studied the immediate changes in blood supply (Fig. 1.36) and the bone loss under normal and special undercut plates 3 months following surgery (Fig. 1.37). The grooves reduced vascular damage and, as a corollary, also mitigated bone porosis which accompanies haversian remodeling.

1.3.3 Bone Healing

Healing is defined as restoration of the original integrity. To the surgeon this means regaining the stiffness of the bone structure. For the biologist, the microscopic restoration of the original structure may take years of internal remodeling.

A prerequisite for healing is an adequate biological capacity to react. Biomechanical conditions control the activity of the cells, with the mediators being of either a chemical or an electrical nature.

Fig. 1.36 Vascular damage produced by different plates.

a Plates with smooth undersurface and with grooves as used by Jörger and Vattolo in their investigation designed to compare the changes in blood flow and in haversian remodeling. The grooves are located between the plate holes, where the conventional plate is excessively strong.

b Using disulfine blue as a vital marker of blood supply, the cross sections of the sheep tibias displayed a markedly better blood supply beneath a grooved plate.

Fig. 1.37 Vascular damage and consequent haversian remodeling.

a At 12 weeks a distinct difference in remodeling is seen. The bone is porotic beneath a conventional smooth plate. The porotic area, which in cases of high rates of remodeling may sequestrate, reaches the periosteal surface of the bone, where plate contact retards the revascularization.

b With grooved plates the porosis is much less pronounced and does not reach the surface of the bone plated.

c There is literally no porosis if, under similar circumstances, a plate is applied as an internal fixator, i.e., at a distance from the bone surface (Tepic and Predieri 1989).

Fig. 1.36

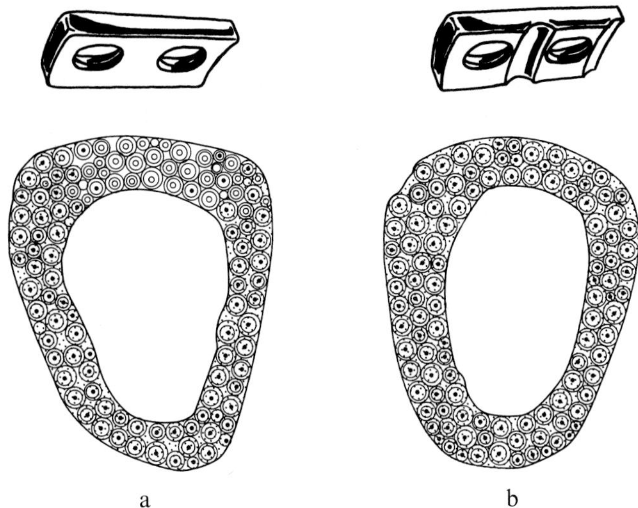

Fig. 1.37

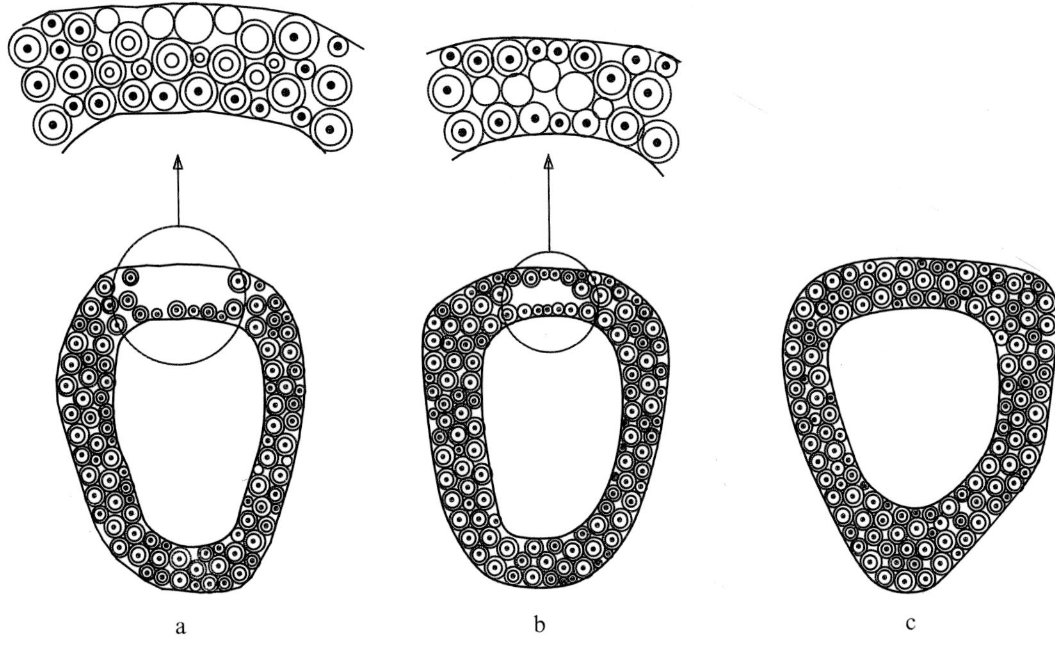

1.3.3.1 Basic Requirements

Fracture healing cannot proceed without adequate biological activity; living pluripotent cells must be available locally. These cells require a blood supply for nutrition and most likely for cellular support. One can safely assume that, given biological integrity, the *cells* surrounding a fracture are pluripotent and able to form bone. The critical parameter, therefore, is whether or not these cells are stimulated to repair the fragment ends with living, solid bone. Adequate *blood supply* to the repair tissues is crucial.

1.3.3.2 Type of Healing

With the onset of stable internal fixation a new type of healing was observed. First "healing by primary intention" (Lane 1913) and "soudure autogène" (Danis 1947, 1949) were observed radiologically and then "primary bone healing" was observed histologically (Schenk and Willenegger 1963). The term primary bone healing is replaced in this paper with the term "direct bone healing" to avoid confusion and to avoid an implicit qualification. The direct healing is based upon the process of angiogenic bone formation (Krompecher 1967). Different types of healing are outlined here because they have direct implications upon the rationale for various treatment modes.

1.3.3.3 Spontaneous (Indirect) Healing of Bone

This consists of three elements (Fig. 1.38):

1. Granulation tissue forms first around the fragments and later between the fragments as well. This is the callus precursor.
2. The fracture gap then widens due to surface resorption of the fragment ends, i.e., when plates and screws are used for stabilization.
3. Bone formation progresses through a series of different steps from granulation tissue to cortical bone (indirect bone formation).

Radiologically the process of indirect bone healing is characterized by the appearance of callus, by the widening of the fracture gap, and then by the filling of the fracture gap with newly formed bone, which is first patchy in appearance and then gradually acquires a more distinct and dense structure. The latter is achieved through a process of internal remodeling of the haversian system which may last several years.

Fig. 1.38 Healing pattern.

a Spontaneous healing, (indirect healing). Radiography of cortical bone following a transverse fracture without fixation. Abundant callus formation, bridging starts at the lower periosteal side in this picture (Rahn 1987).

b Direct (or primary) healing.
An oblique fracture fixed stably using a lag screw and plate healed by internal remodeling alone. The radiological picture and the histological section of such healing showed neither relevant periosteal nor endosteal callus formation specific to the fracture area. As can be seen in this histological picture, direct healing proceeds without resorption of the fragment end surfaces: i.e. contact healing. This figure shows an extremely precise adaptation achieved under experimental conditions (Tepic and Predieri 1989). In reality contact zones are comparably infrequent and do, therefore, contribute only little to the strength of healing.

Fig. 1.38

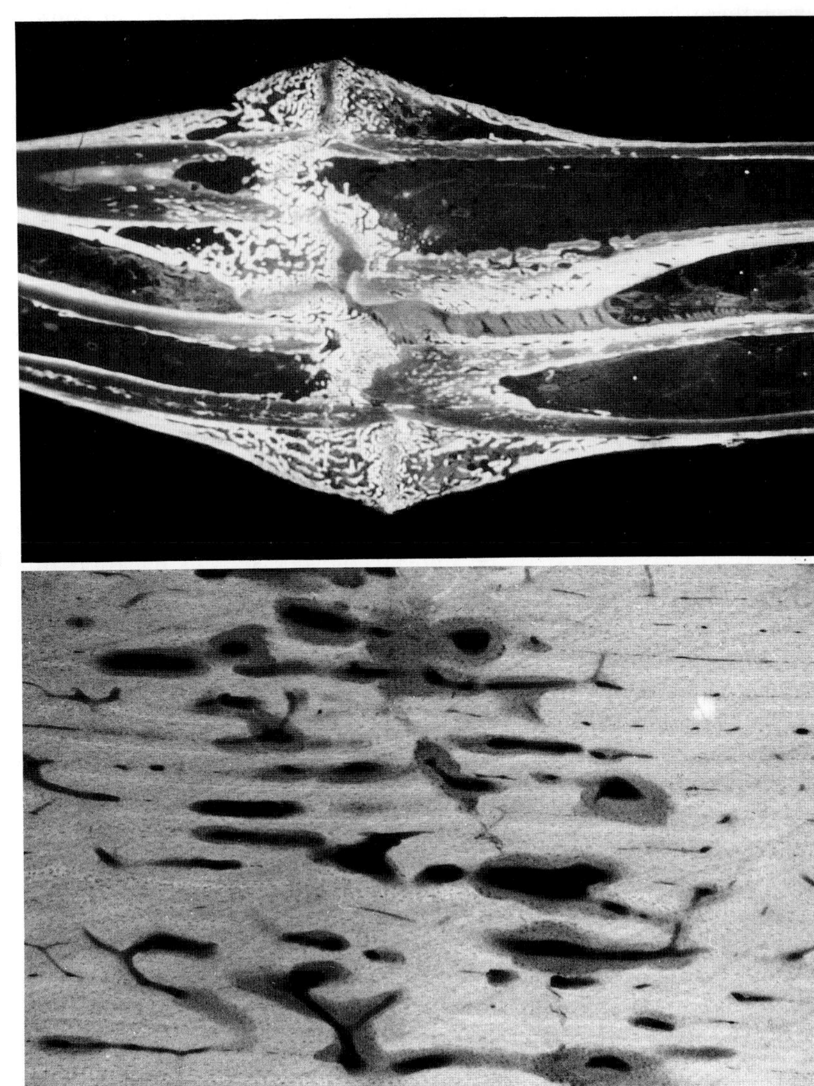

1.3.3.4 Direct (or Primary) Bone Healing

Direct bone healing bypasses the different steps outlined for indirect healing and skips directly to internal remodeling (Fig. 1.39) in contact zones (contact healing) (Fig. 1.39a) or to filling of stable gaps with lamellar bone and consequent remodeling or plugging (gap healing, Fig. 1.39b). The surface of immediate contact within a fracture is directly related to the compression applied (Ashhurst 1986). It amounts in reality to only a small fraction (a few percent) of the total cross section.

In direct healing no relevant amount of *callus*, especially of callus which specifically bridges the fracture line, becomes visible radiologically. *Fragment end resorption* does not occur. The process of internal remodeling of the haversian system, uniting the fragment ends, is the only process resulting in solid union. Direct healing does not lead to faster union. The absence of fragment end resorption may be of utmost importance when non-gliding splints are used. The radiological appearance of direct fracture healing is characterized by virtual absence of callus formation. The fracture gap does not truly widen, but may appear to do so due to intense remodeling near the fracture surface. Therefore the surgeon is guided mainly by the absence of signs of complications, such as callus formation, which would indicate instability and fragment end resorption (shortening). Callus is not considered to be undesirable per se, but its appearance under conditions which require absence of fragment end shortening is a sign of a critical instability.

1.3.3.5 Non-union

Bone healing may come to a stop (Fig. 1.5) when one or both of two elements are disturbed:

1. The mechanical conditions of strain.
2. The capacity for biological reaction.

In the first case a hypertrophic non-union is seen (Fig. 1.5a). The treatment (Fig. 1.5b) then must aim to correct the mechanical instability by using an internal splint. In the second case a nonreactive or atrophic non-union is present. The treatment here consists in inducing bone formation by applying a living bone graft as well as providing mechanical stability.

Fig. 1.39 The elements of direct or primary bone healing.

a Contact healing: The initial direct bone healing and final healing in all cases consist of remodeling of the haversian system. In the case of contact healing, this remodeling is essentially the only element upon which healing relies. The histological section depicts the "cutter head" with osteoclasts and osteoblasts at a distance producing a new vascularized osteon (Perren and Cordey 1980).

b Osteon: Histological appearance of an osteon tunneling the bone from left to right (Rahn and Perren 1975).

c Osteon: Schematic diagram. The cutter head at the right tip with osteoclasts and the conical surface with osteoblasts towards the left is visualized (Perren et al. 1981).

d Gap healing: Under stable conditions (due to nearby contact) a gap fills directly with mature bone of similar structure but of different orientation than the original lamellar bone. This bone is later remodeled to a structure and orientation similar to lamellar bone, i.e., gap healing. The next step in this process consists of internal remodeling through the gap and/or from the gap into the cortex (plugging) (Perren and Cordey 1980).

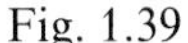

Fig. 1.39

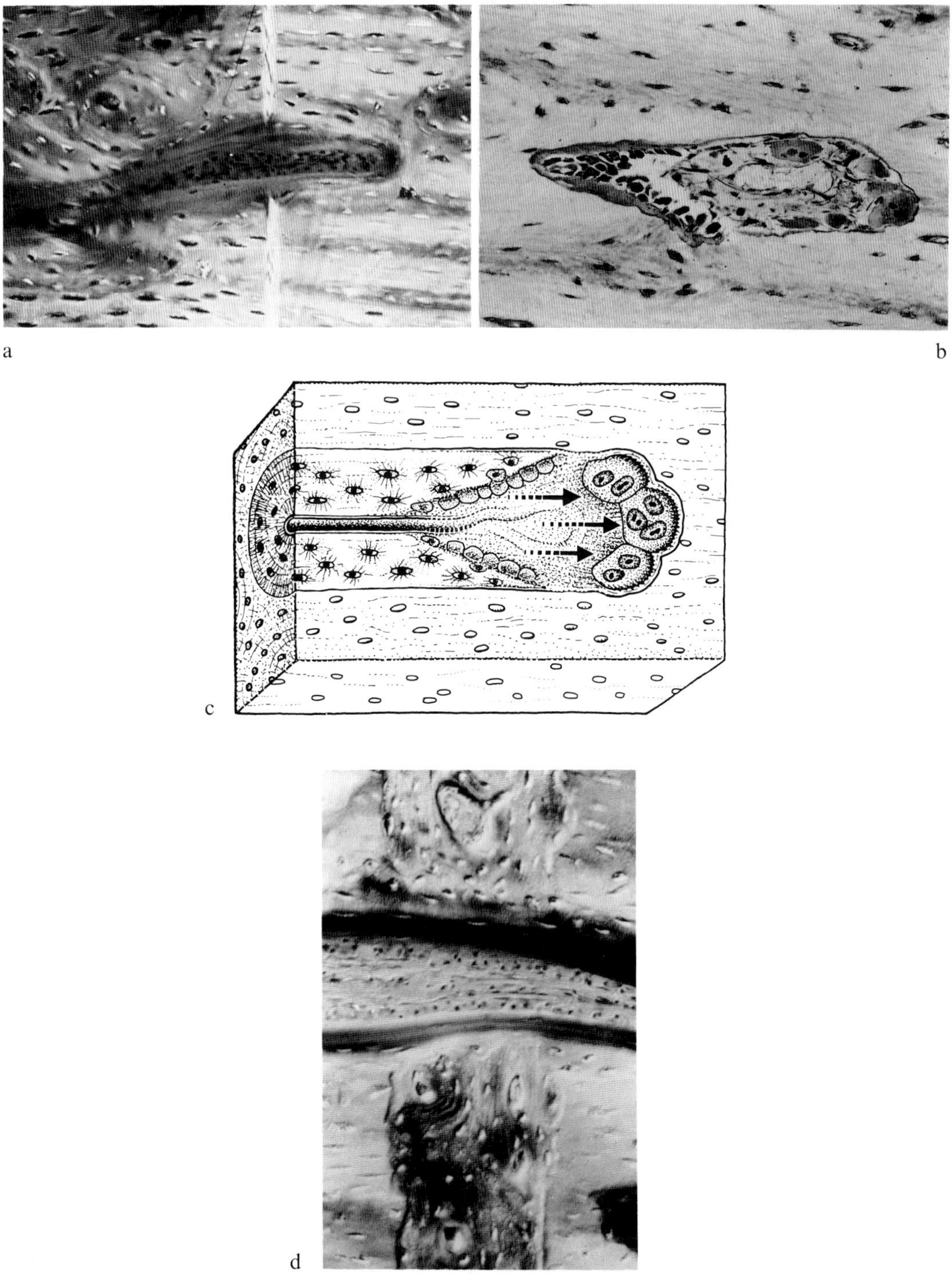

a

b

c

d

1.3.3.6 Relevance of Different Types of Healing

The different types of bone healing are of considerable scientific interest. The physician in charge of the fracture treatment can argue that the only goal for treatment is the solid union of a correctly reduced bone with maintained joint function (thus avoiding soft tissue complications). The important difference between direct and indirect healing is that direct healing does not proceed with fragment end shortening. Such shortening can easily be taken up by a gliding splint such as the intramedullary nail. Fixation by intramedullary nailing does not require absolute stability. Compression fixation of single fractures by lag screws in combination with a neutralization plate does not tolerate even minimal instability. The type of plate used in the bridge or wave mode ("biological fixation"; see p. 2) with preservation of the fragment blood supply neither provides nor requires absolute interfragmental stability and greatly extends the indication for plate fixation.

1.3.3.7 Controlling Mechanisms of Bone Healing

Fracture healing can proceed in many different ways. It is now well documented that instability results in callus formation, fragment end resorption, and indirect bone formation via soft repair tissues. Under conditions of maintained stable contact, bone heals internally with minimal or no callus, without fragment end resorption and with direct bone formation. The fracture circumstances dictate which type of healing offers the most advantages.

1.3.4 Scientific Background of Development

The specific characteristic of the AO development of principles, techniques, implants and instruments is close collaboration of research on the one hand and practical surgical work on the other hand. The Laboratory for Experimental Surgery in Davos, the central research facility of the AO, has recently contributed to the following developments. Similar developments from other AO research and development groups are equally important.

Fig. 1.40 Klaue's experiment demonstrating the loss and recovery of lag screw compression.

a When a conventional fully threaded lag screw (i.e., a screw within a gliding hole) is applied in an inclined position, wedging of the threads within the gliding hole occurs and a considerable part (more than 50%) of the potential compression is lost.

b Using a shaft screw with a shaft diameter corresponding to the outer diameter of the screw thread, wedging is avoided and optimal compression achieved.

c The measured values of interfragmental compression exerted by the two different types of screws. The *black bars* correspond to a, the *hatched bars* to b. The new shaft screw is 60% more efficient than the fully threaded inclined lag screw.

Fig. 1.40

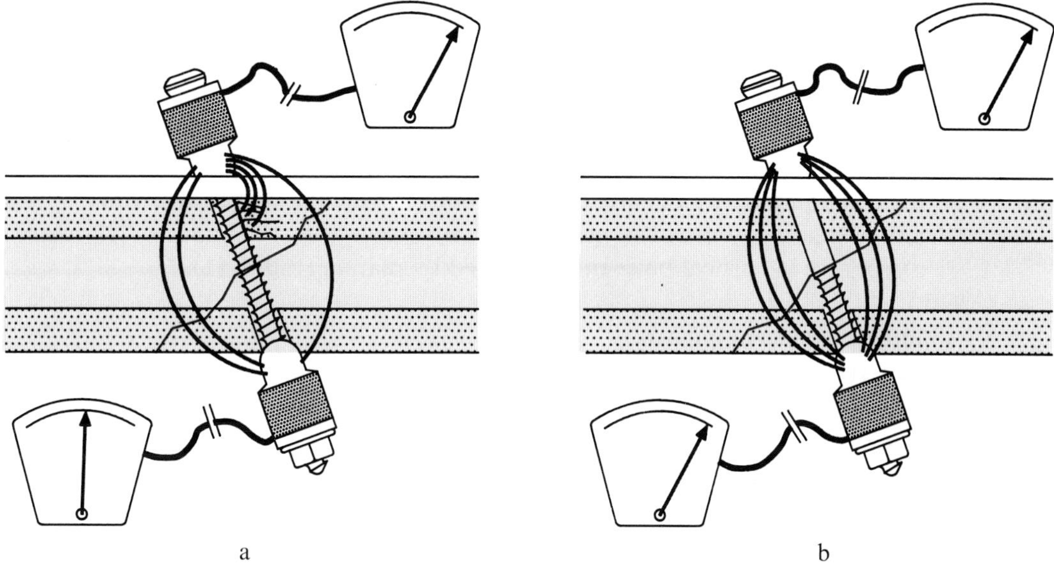
a
b

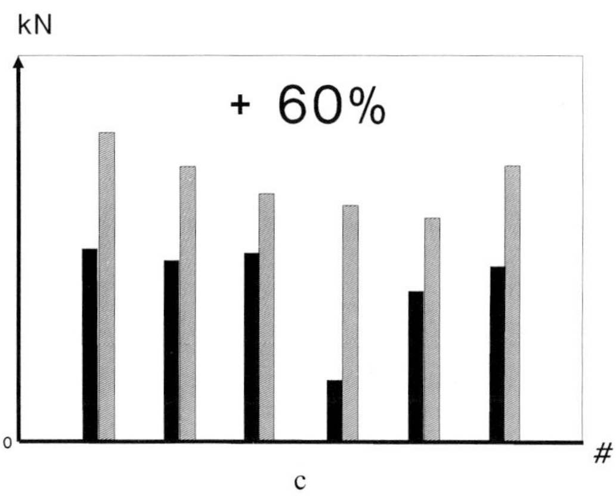

c

1.3.4.1 The Concept of Biological Plating: The LC-DCP

The scientific observations of biomechanics and biology of bone lead to the new concept of biological plating (see also p. 108): *The newly designed LC-DCP*[15] *stands for a new approach to plate fixation: reduced trauma to bone, preservation of blood supply, avoidance of producing stress risers at implant removal, and excellent tissue tolerance were the goals to be realized.* The LC-DCP is technically a further development of the DCP (Perren et al. 1969c). It is based mainly on the experimental work of Klaue (1982) and Klaue and Perren (1982), who developed its predecessor, the DCU (dynamic compression unit). In the DCU the lag screws applied through the plate are about twice as efficient as the conventional inclined lag screws. The symmetrical self-compressing plate hole and the deletion of the elongated distance between the innermost screw holes make the DCU more versatile for use in any fracture type, disregarding the hitherto "standard" transverse osteotomy in cortical bone rarely treated by plating (Fig. 1.41).

The new concept aims at:

1. *Minimal surgical damage* to blood supply.
2. *Improved healing* in the critical zone covered by the plate.
3. Minimal damage to the bone lining the plate *to reduce the risk of refracture* following plate removal.
4. *Optimal tissue tolerance* of the implant by selection of pure titanium as an implant material.

As outlined in Fig. 1.40, when using a shaft screw (originally designed as an inclined plate screw for use with the DCU or LC-DCP) to replace the fully threaded inclined lag screw, about 50% of compression – lost due to wedging of the fully threaded screw – is salvaged.

This type of shaft screw, originally designed for the inclined plate screw in the DCU or LC-DCP, can be used as a free lag screw. It provides more efficient compression than a normal lag screw. Here once again secondary wedging within the gliding hole is prevented.

Grooves on the undersurface of the LC-DCP serve three purposes:

(1) They improve blood circulation by minimizing the damage due to contact between plate and bone. (2) They allow for a small bone bridge beneath the plate at a place which is otherwise weak due to a stress concentration effect of the nonhealed fracture gap at the periosteal surface. (3) They result in more even distribution of the stiffness of the plate than in conventional plates, where the cross section at the screw holes is softer and weaker, while the full rectangular cross section between the screw holes is

---

Fig. 1.41 Histological appearance of bone healing with the DCU.

Sheep tibia 56 days after surgery (Klaue et al. 1982). Intensive remodeling of the oblique osteotomy is seen mainly as a band lining the osteotomy (Area "A"). Little remodeling is seen immediately deep to the plate with smooth undersurface (Area "B"). Where the shaft of the screw is in direct contact (Area "C"), intensive remodeling is observed. Where the shaft of the screw does not touch the clearance hole (Area "D"), minimal remodeling is seen. In the contact area around the thread of the lag screw (Area "E"), intensive remodeling is visible. Though the overall pattern of remodeling is "patchy", it best correlates with local conditions of blood supply. It is noteworthy that the band of remodeling providing healing is obviously related to temporary loss and recovery of blood supply rather than to changes of mechanical load or to an unknown signal radiating from the fracture site. Direct or primary healing therefore seems to be rather a by-product than a direct biological response to the fracture.

Fig. 1.41

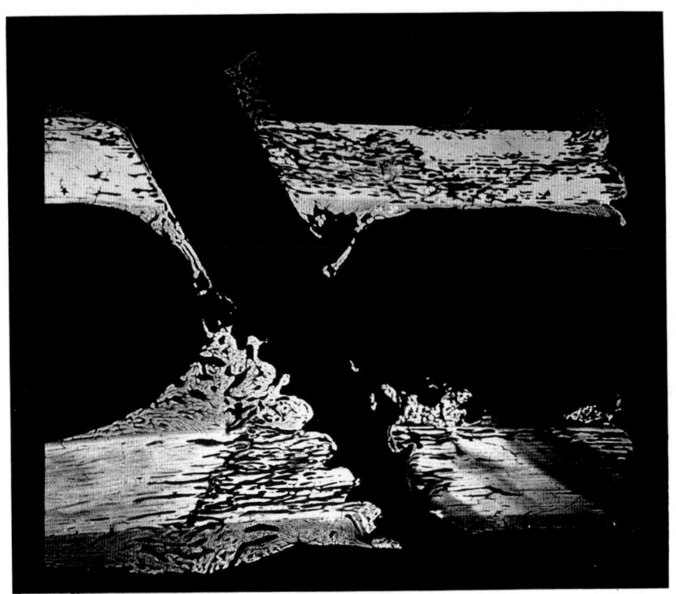

markedly stiffer, i.e., more resistant to bending and torque. The difference in stiffness results in a relatively increased load within the weak spot at the screw holes.

The healing pattern of bone plated with the LC-DCP displays a more abundant bone formation with a circumferential shell of mature callus bone (Fig. 1.43), especially around the fracture site. The fracture gap exhibits a band of remodeling and not fracture surface resorption (which could lead to breakdown of stability). The contact of the plate with the bone is limited and the plate-induced remodeling is small. The bone porosis induced by the LC-DCP ranges between the extremes shown in Fig. 1.37a (conventional plate, smooth undersurface) and Fig. 1.37c (plate does not touch bone at all).

Apparently, a larger screw hole remains after removal of the shaft screw. However, one should consider that the outer diameter of the hole with a fully threaded screw is the same as that with a shaft screw. The fully threaded screw, though, allows for filling in of the threads. The mechanical difference with respect to the strength of the bone is negligible.

The X-ray of a diaphysis plated with a conventional plate with smooth undersurface (Fig. 1.42e) illustrates the problem: at the periosteal surface, facing the undersurface of the plate, the fracture gap shows a small defect. Since, whenever possible, the plate is placed at the tension side of the bone for best resistance to fatigue failure and for best stabilization according to the tension band principle, this defect is at the worst place possible, when considering plate removal. The photoelastic model of a beam under bending load with the defect at the tension side is shown in Fig. 1.42g: the harmful stress concentration is disclosed.

Fig. 1.42 The developments in AO internal fixation plates. In a–d upper (*left*) and lower (*right*) surfaces are shown.

a The round hole plate (Müller et al. 1963). The conically undercut screw head allows for only a perpendicular position of the screw. The distance between the inner screw holes is larger. The plate undersurface is smooth.

b The dynamic compression plate DCP (Perren et al. 1969c). The spherical contact geometry allows for 20° of tilting of the screw along the long axis of the bone.

c The dynamic compression unit DCU (Klaue and Perren 1982). The completely symmetric screw holes are distributed at even distances throughout the plate. Symmetric screw holes with oblique undercut for improved range of inclination.

d The limited-contact dynamic compression plate LC-DCP (Perren et al. 1989) viewed from above: symmetric arrangement of the screw holes without a solid elongation between the innermost screw holes. The screw holes themselves are symmetrical and are provided with two sloped cylinders. Lateral undercuts allow for bone formation at the plate (tension) side of the periosteal surface. Less damage to blood supply results, and the trapezoid cross section allows for easier and less traumatic removal of the plate.

e A clinical case in which a plate with smooth undersurface had been used: defect in fracture healing immediately beneath the plate. This defect acts as a stress riser and increases the mechanical stress locally. (Courtesy of S. Kessler).

f Following plate removal, a refracture originated at the stress concentration. Removal had been too early for this type of plate.

g The photoelastic model shows a stress concentration under mechanical loading near a small defect at the surface of a cantilever beam loaded in bending.

Fig. 1.42

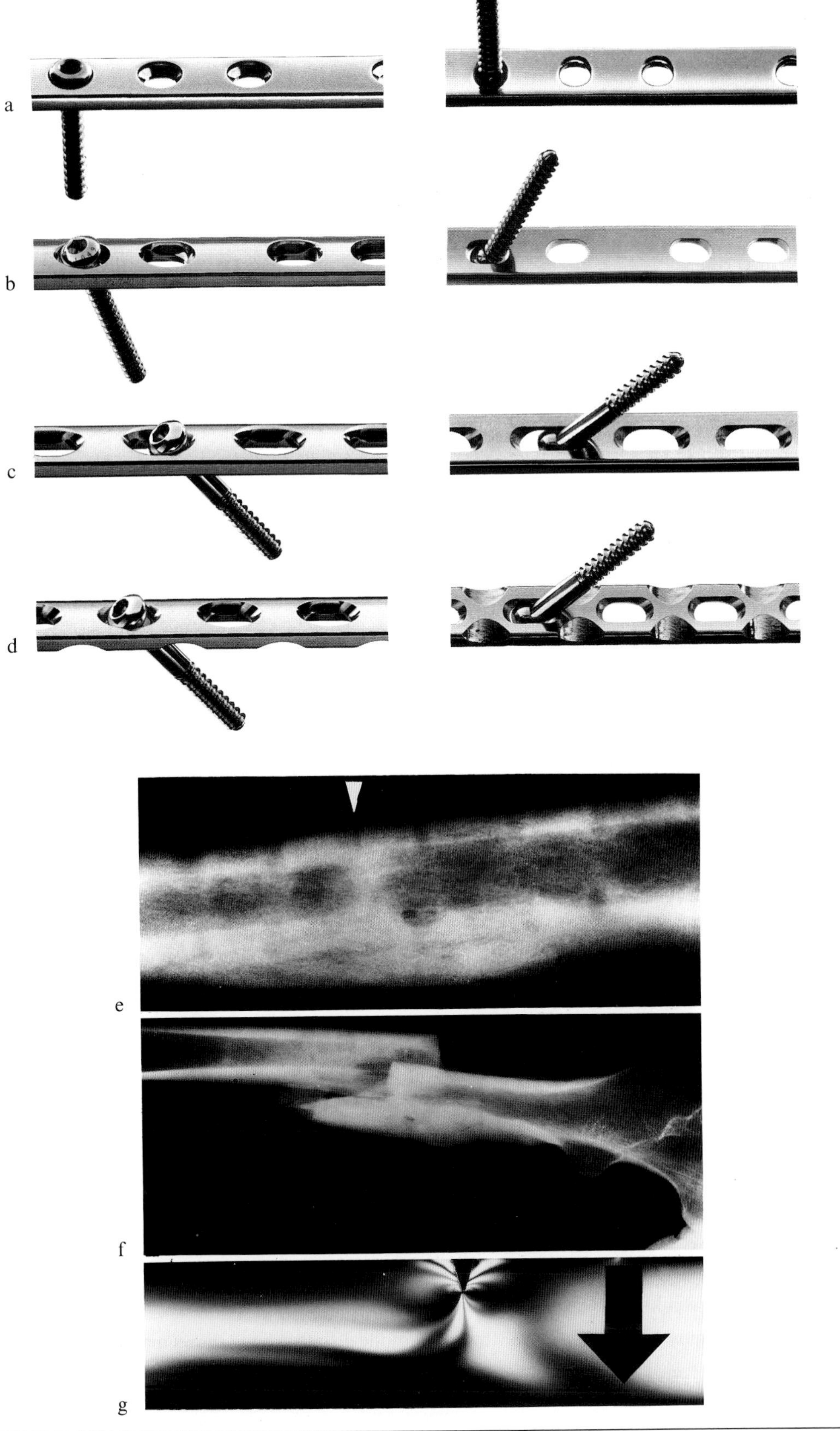

Fig. 1.43 Bone healing and minimal early temporary porosis with the LC-DCP.

a Fracture of sheep tibia plated with LC-DCP. An oblique shaft screw and a nearby single cortex plate screw were used.

b Three months after operation: clinical X-ray before sacrifice.

c Three months after operation: the X-ray of the dissected bone shows marked bone density in the fracture area.

d The microradiograph of the undecalcified cross section shows minimal early temporary porosis beneath the plate and in the next quadrant. A shell of mature callus is seen lining the periosteal surface.

Fig. 1.43

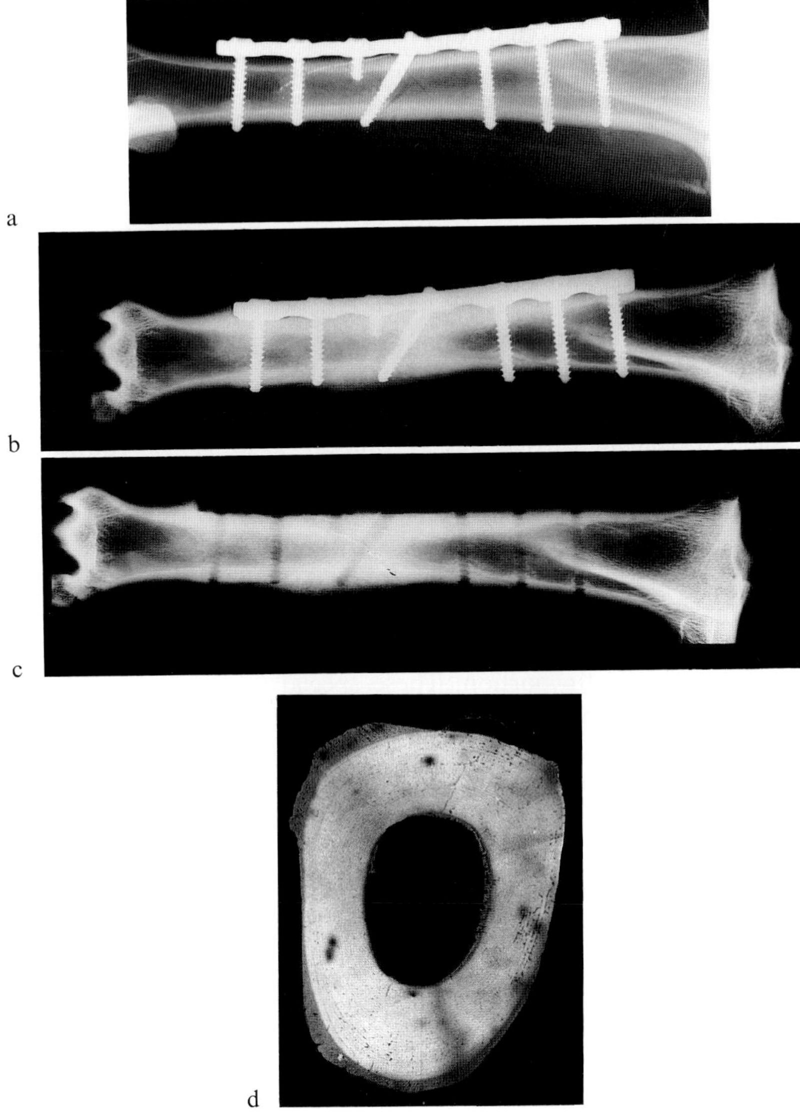

1.3.4.2 Improved Effectiveness of External Fixator Pins

In the past decade it has become clear that pin loosening and pin tract infections can be significantly reduced (Behrens 1982, 1989) by (1) using larger pins and (2) generating radial preload with the inserted pins.

Based on early clinical experience (Behrens 1982) the AO introduced, in 1984, short-threaded Schanz screws with a core diameter of 3.5 mm and a shaft diameter of 4.5 mm. These screws provided excellent purchase in cortical bone while making the smooth shaft of 4.5 mm the effective pin diameter in the near cortex. These Schanz screws were considerably stiffer than the 5-mm screws previously used, where the threaded portion (core diameter of 4.0 mm) engaged in both cortices.

Clinical experience in the early 1980s indicated that using pins with short threads inserted in pin holes smaller than the shaft diameter lowered the empirical rate of pin tract infections and loosening (Behrens 1982). With these systems, misfits between drill hole and pin shaft (radial preload) of somewhere between 0.5 mm and 1.0 mm were created (Behrens 1986, 1989). On closer examination of this issue, Gasser (1989) predicted on theoretical grounds that mismatches between core and shaft diameter of 0.1–0.2 mm would be highly effective, yet small enough to prevent mechanical disruption of the surrounding cortex. Hyldahl et al. (1989) further established the effectiveness of radial preload using a pneumatically operated pin motion system in the sheep tibia (see p. 50), while similar experiments carried out by Biliouris et al. (1989) confirmed Gasser's theoretical prediction (Fig. 1.44).

Based on these insights, a new AO Schanz-type screw for unilateral external fixation has been developed (Fig. 1.45). It has a 3.4-mm core diameter and a 4.5-mm outer diameter of the thread near the trocar tip. A very shallow thread with 4.7-mm core diameter and 5.0-mm outer diameter connects to the 5-mm drive shaft. The portion of the screw with the shallow thread produces forward propulsion of the pin until the far cortex is engaged by the tip portion. These special design features result in a 0.2-mm misfit for all parts of the new Schanz screw. It is, therefore, not a conical screw but a conically preloaded cylindrical screw, which avoids the disadvantage of the conical threads, namely that they require a predetermined position along the long axis of the screw, i.e., a predetermined position in relation to the depth within the bone.

In the meantime, a uniforme design of the Schanz screw has been adopted. It axerts radial preload on both cortices and requires only drilling of both cortices to 4.5 mm. This simplifies Schanz screw application significantly (see Chap. 5).

Fig. 1.44 The effect of different degrees of pin oversize upon pin loosening in experimental external fixation (Biliouris et al. 1989).

a An exact fit between pin and bone results in pin loosening without prior mechanical damage to the interfacing bone.

b Oversize of 0.1 mm results in the best bone structure and avoidance of pin loosening due to adequate fit.

c Oversize of 0.3 mm results in mechanical damage, instability, and consequent micromotion-induced bone resorption.

d Oversize of 0.5 mm results in massive mechanical destruction of bone by overload.

Fig. 1.44

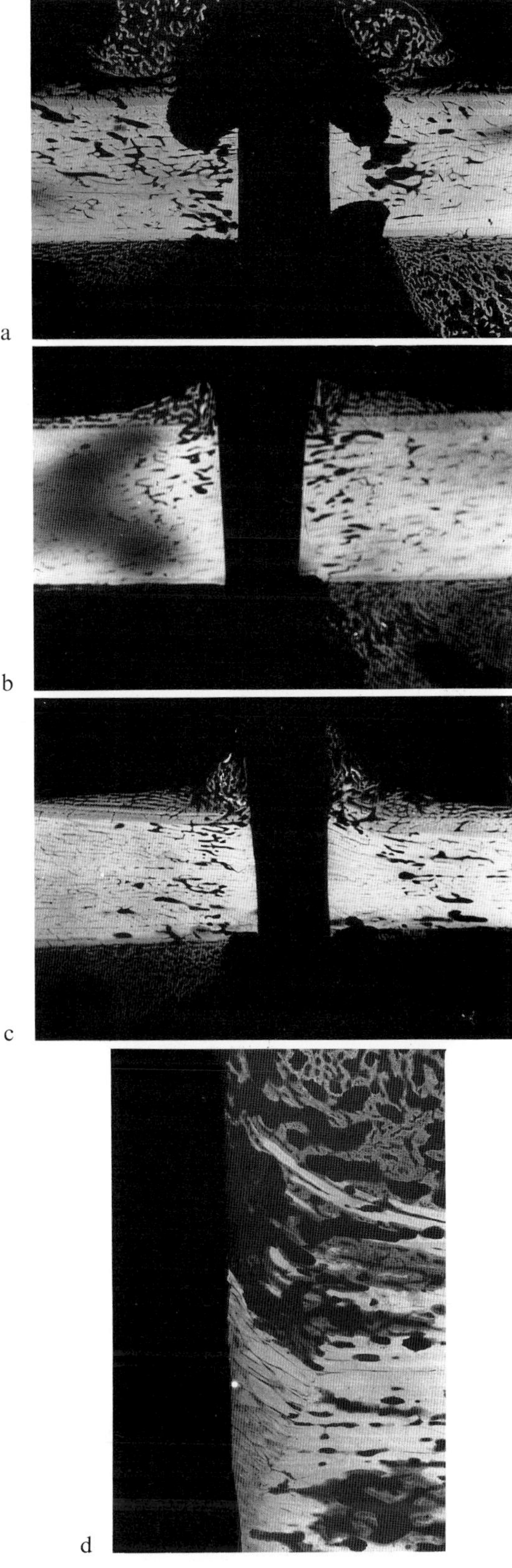

1.3.4.3 The Development of "Tube-to-Tube" Clamps as an Example of the Development Within the AO Group's Technical Commissions

A recent contribution to external fixation consists in the "tube-to-tube" fixation as realized by Fernández Dell 'Oca (1989). Tube-to-tube fixation allows for very versatile assembly of the tubes which connect the pins. According to the philosophy of the AO group, the fragments of the fracture are fixed subsequent to appropriate reduction. Therefore, extensive secondary corrections are actually a less important indication for tube-to-tube fixation. More important is the possibility to apply pins in distinctly different planes. A good example for such application is the external fixation of the humerus, where damage to the radial nerve can best be avoided by applying the pins in two planes, at right angles to each other. Tube-to-tube fixation is a typical example of AO ingenuity: versatility is achieved without complicated additions to the system of instrumentation and implants. In spite of the extended possibilities offered, the system remains simple and can be taught and learned with little effort. Quality and simplicity are equally important guidelines for the development of implants and instruments. The technical commissions of the AO group each consist of medical specialists, researchers, and technical staff, whose purpose it is to develop principles, techniques, and necessary instrumentation as well as implants and to monitor their clinical performance.

Fig. 1.45 The new AO Schanz-type screws for unilateral external fixation.

a Combined deep- and shallow-thread Schanz type screw. The thread near the tip has a 4.5-mm outer and 3.2-mm core diameter, the tip is self-cutting. The shaft is 4.6 mm in diameter and connects with a conical part. It is furthermore provided with a shallow thread to engage and drive the screw forwards when the thread near the tip has not yet engaged in the far cortex. This Schanz screw is designed for use in cortical bone providing automatic radial preload. It is used wherever the axial holding strength requires priority.

b Shallow-thread Schanz-type screw. This screw is provided with only a shallow thread and is especially designed for use in cancellous bone where large transverse surfaces are present (good strength in relation to a force acting perpendicularly to the long axis). This screw is of advantage wherever the resistance to transverse forces has priority over the axial holding strength (e.g., in short metaphyseal fragments).

Fig. 1.45

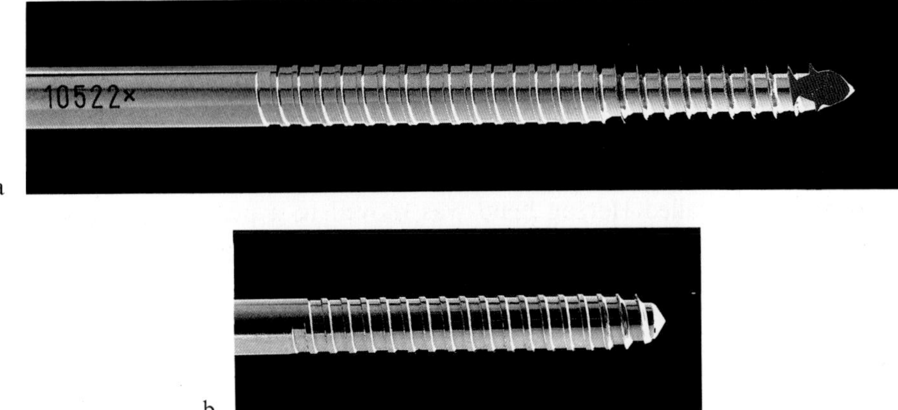

1.3.4.4 The New Design of the Nails

The use of interlocking intramedullary nails, as proposed by Küntscher, Klemm and Schellmann (1972), Kempf et al. (1978), and others, requires a stronger implant, a nail stiffer than the one used for conventional nailing. In the classical indication for interlocked nailing, the shape of the nail plays a minor role, If there is little fragmentation, the bone does not tolerate a misfit and fails upon insertion unless a smaller diameter is selected.

The shape of the medullary cavity of the femur was studied by Winquist et al. (1984) and Zuber et al. (1988). Based on these measurements, the AO universal nail for the femur has a bending radius of 1500 mm (Fig. 1.46a, b). Its cross section is completely slotted to avoid stress concentrations usually encountered at the end of a partial slot (Beaupre et al. 1984). The point of insertion has been reconsidered as well, based on image reconstruction (Zuber et al. 1988). In spite of the new slot geometry, the conical drive connection could be maintained because of a "key lock" construction by Mathys and Cotting (1986).

An anatomical study by Heini (1988) provided the need of a new shape of the tibia nail. The so-called Herzog bend was moved to a point one-third of the way down the total length of the nail from the proximal end (Fig. 1.46c, d). A sledge construction for the tip of the nail was added based upon computer studies of the fit between the medullary cavity and the nail.

Fig. 1.46 The new shape of the intramedullary nails based upon the study of the shape of the medullary cavity.

a The data obtained by Zuber et al. (1988) for the shape of the femur nail are based upon measurements of the inner shape of the femur.

b The insertion point of the femur nail would ideally be located at *a*, but for safety reasons the insertion point (*p*) is recommended. The former more lateral point of insertion (*t*) leads to a bending load, resulting in twisting of the slotted nail.

c The data obtained by Zuber: the average radius of the bend of the medullary cavity is between 800 and 1500 mm. For the femur nail the upper limit of this range was selected.

d The data obtained by Heini for the shape of the tibia nail: the misfit of the old nail with the Herzog bend and the better alignment of the new shape are demonstrated. The fit was obtained using CAD (computer-aided design techniques).

e The corresponding shapes of the tibia nail: the tibia, the old, and the new nail (*top*) are displayed.

Fig. 1.46

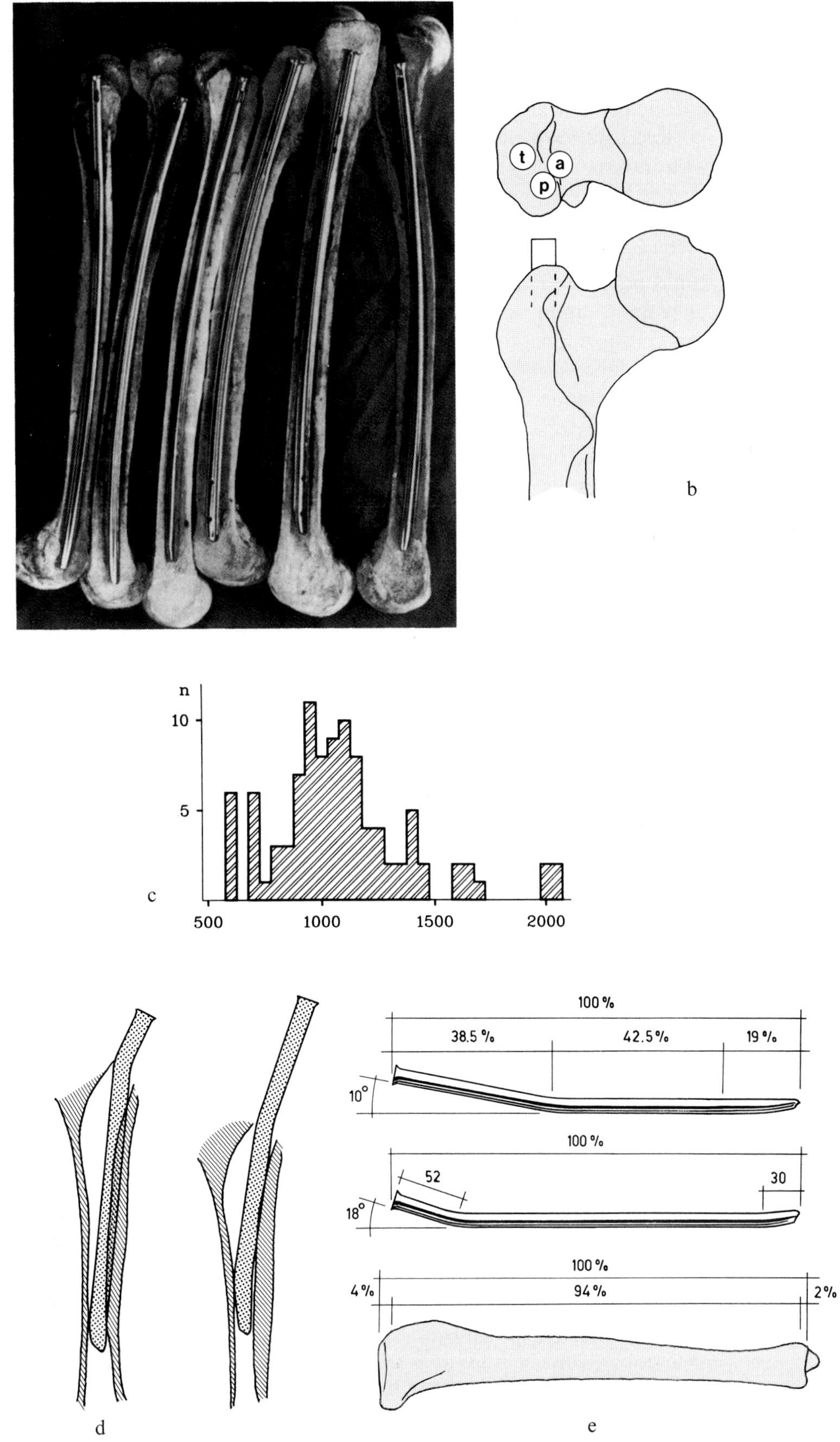
a
t
a
p
b
n
10
5
c
500
1000
1500
2000
100 %
38.5 %
42.5 %
19 %
10°
100 %
52
30
18°
100 %
4 %
94 %
2 %
d
e

1.3.4.5 Unreamed Intramedullary Nailing

Conventional (with reaming, without interlocking) intramedullary nailing in severely open fractures was considered for many years to be dangerous. The risk of intramedullary infection was considered to be to high in relation to advantages gained by the nailing.

Recently, however, Wiss et al. (1986) and Helfet (1989) have reported good results with intramedullary nailing of severe open shaft fractures. The procedure used consisted in inserting a comparably small diameter nail into a medullary cavity which had not been previously reamed.

The question arose of whether reaming has an effect upon bone circulation which could be deleterious in severe open fractures. Klein et al. (1989) studied the acute effect of reaming upon bone circulation (Fig. 1.46). Comparing unreamed nailed and reamed nailed beagle tibia, they used procion red (Rahn 1986) as an intravital dye. The hypothesis was that insertion of the nail temporarily results in complete damage to the medullary blood circulation. It was demonstrated that intact dog tibia were largely able to compensate for the lack of medullary circulation through periosteal circulation. The reamed bones showed large deficits of blood circulation 7 h after reaming and nailing.

These results prove that the cortical circulation is preserved by unreamed nailing to a good degree. This explains why an unreamed nail might successfully be used for the treatment of severe open fractures. Unreamed nailing without interlocking — as long found with small Küntscher nails — lacks the necessary torsional stability. Closely fitting nails, as required in noninterlocked nailing, may jam upon insertion.

In conventional nailing of fractures, the reduction of blood circulation due to reaming plays a less important role than the necessarily reduced strength and stiffness of a smaller nail. The risk of explosion fractures upon insertion, without reaming, of a solid nail must also be carefully considered.

Fig. 1.47 The new AO unreamed medullary nail: the study of blood circulation by Klein (1990).

a The dog experiment with the two nails in situ, a larger nail after reaming and a smaller one inserted without prior reaming.

b Two cross sections of the bone showing the blood circulation with (*left*) and without (*right*) reaming. The circulation is markedly better without reaming. (Courtesy of B.A. Rahn).

c The same cross sections but with expansion of the blood vessels to show which area is perfused and nourished by diffusion, based upon the hypothesis that to about a 100 μm radius around a blood vessel, living cells can survive. (Courtesy of B.A. Rahn).

d The loss of blood circulation within the cross sections of the cortical bone nailed with (*left column*) and without (*right column*) reaming for each animal (intravital marker: procion red).

Fig. 1.47

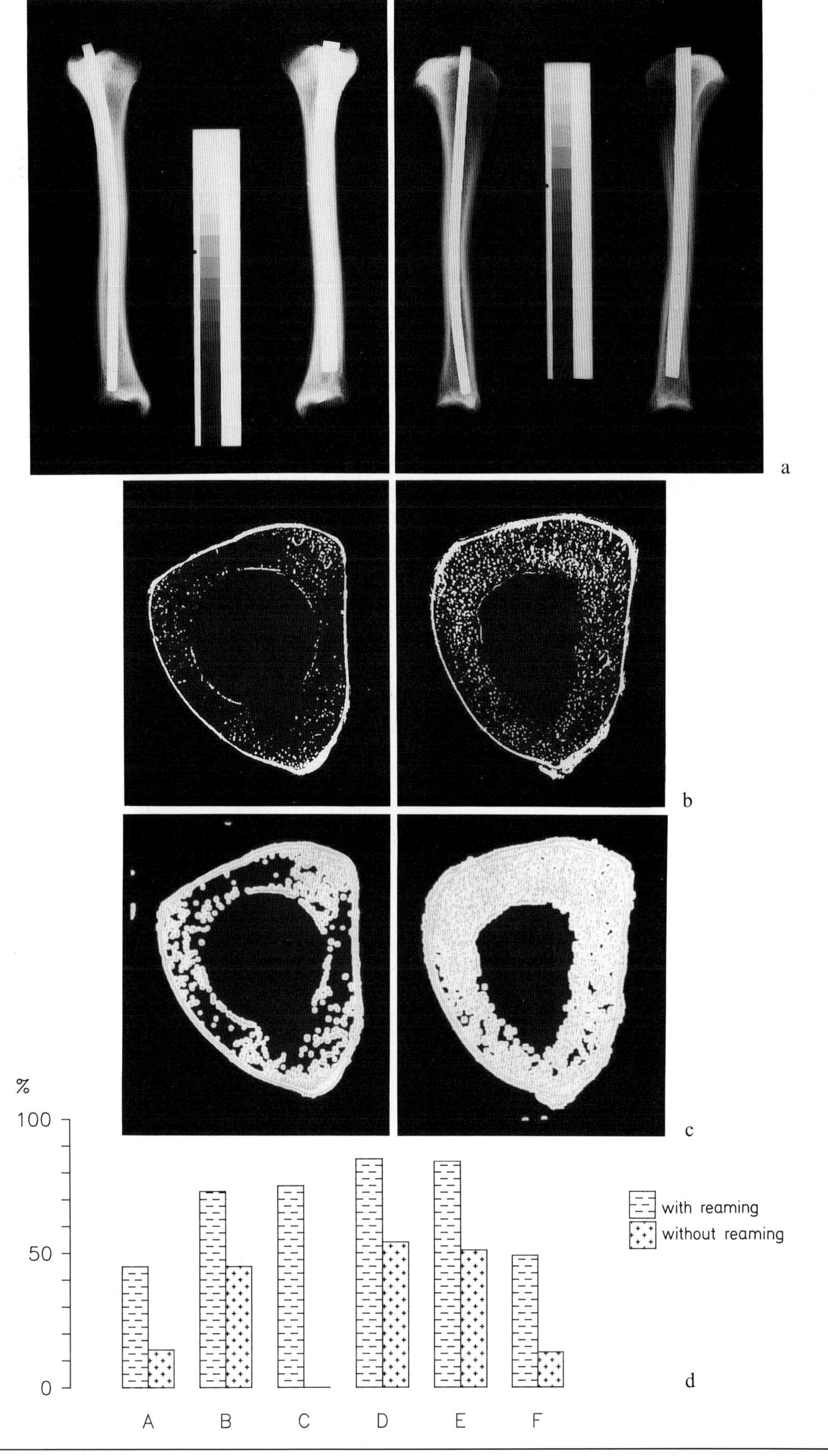

1.3.4.6 Instrumented Nail for Telemetry

The problem of designing implants for use in the human consists in the lack of precise data on loading of the bone and the implants. While data is available for experimental animals, where bending and torque was measured in vivo (Cordey et al. 1980), too little is known concerning the loading of the human skeleton under conditions comparable to the situation of fracture treatment in long bones.

The project (Schneider et al. 1988), telemetry (Genge et al. 1988), and clinical application (Michel 1990) of an intramedullary telemetry nail for use in fixation of human femur fractures was undertaken. A hollow nail which was hermetically sealed by welding contained the power module, the analog to digital conversion, the scanner/multiplexer and the transmitter. The power for the transmitter was fed inductively between a coil placed around the thigh and one within the nail. The eight channels of the telemetry were transmitted digitally. The data, sampled at intervals, were measured with precision and repeatability.

The interlocking nail with a 16-mm diameter allows fixation of multifragmentary and complex fractures (Fig. 1.48a, b), which (soon after fixation) transmit the entire load placed upon the femur to the nail. The measurement therefore reflects the pattern of loading during rehabilitation and after healing has taken place. The load placed upon the nail after healing has occurred is important in regard to possible implant fatigue.

The measurements made (Fig. 1.48c) show unloading of the nail starting as early as in the 4th week and progressing with a short inversion between the 5th and 6th weeks.

Fig. 1.48 Telemetry nail used in the human femur. The nail is used to determine the load in vivo during rehabilitation and after healing has taken place.

a X-rays taken at surgery show the fracture and the nail in situ. The interlocked nail spans a multifragmentary, complex femur midshaft fracture.

b X-rays taken 6 weeks after surgery.

c Results of the measurements between 22 and 107 days after surgery in a human patient. The three components of the moment (Nm) and the three components of the force (N) are plotted for weekly intervals under weight-bearing of 250 N. As expected, the healing process coincides with unloading, which shows discontinuities (e.g., around the 5th and 8th weeks). At the end of the 3-month period there is still a significant transmission of axial forces. This fact will have to be considered when the decision is made to remove the interlocking bolts.

Fig. 1.48

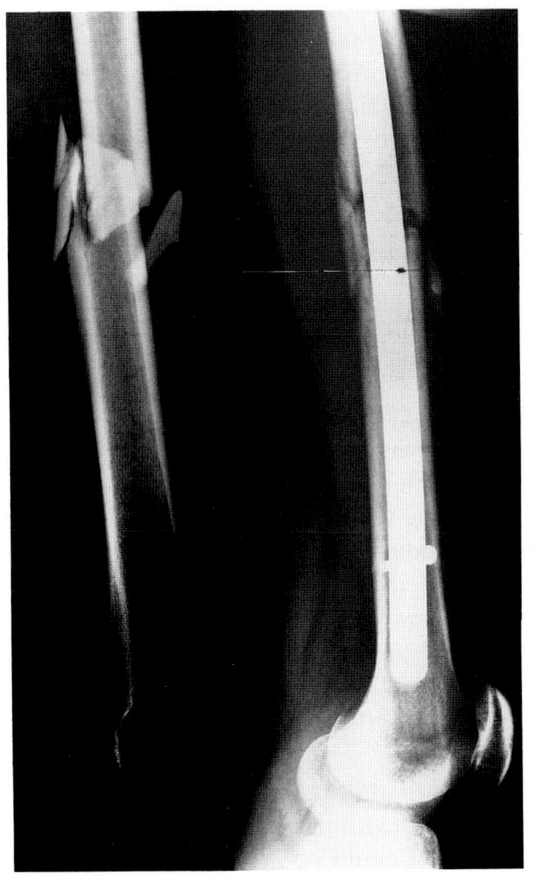
a
b

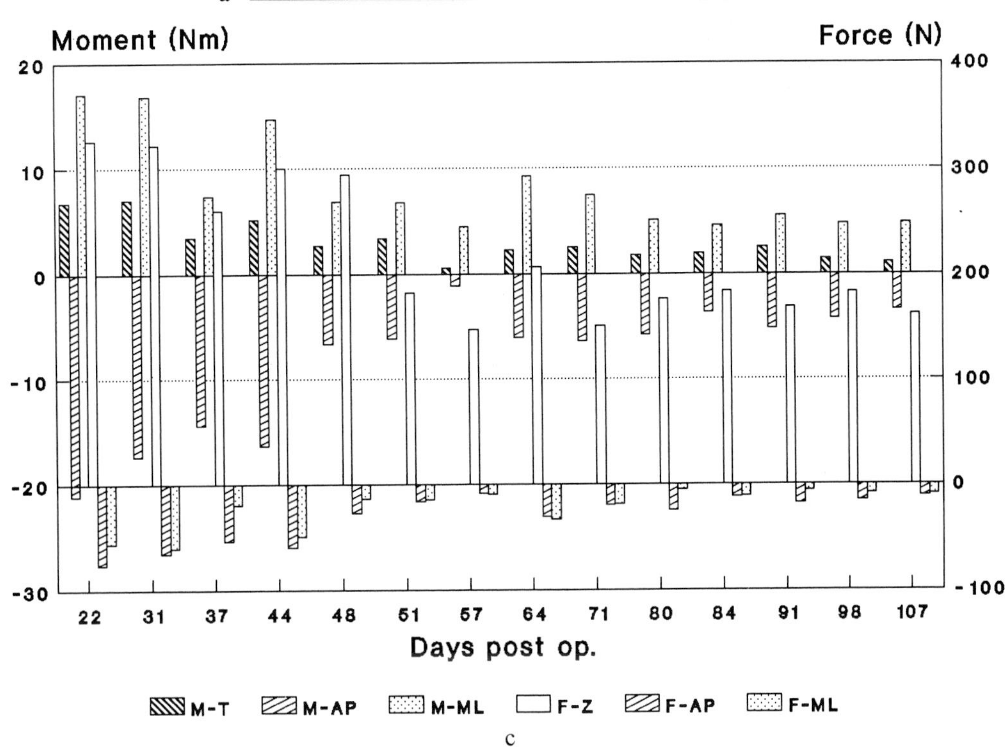
Moment (Nm)
Force (N)
20
10
0
-10
-20
-30
400
300
200
100
0
-100
22 31 37 44 48 51 57 64 71 80 84 91 98 107
Days post op.
M-T M-AP M-ML F-Z F-AP F-ML

c

1.3.4.7 Distraction Osteogenesis

Bone defects resulting from, for example, infected non-unions, require prolonged treatment with bone grafting in most cases. The most efficient way to produce bone would be autologous grafting with optimal vascular support and soft tissue connection. Bone segment transportation according to Ilizarov (1989) ideally fulfills these requirements: In one or both fragments adjacent to a defect, an osteotomy is performed. The resulting bone segment is then transported (1 mm/day) along the long axis of the bone to close the defect. The newly formed gap behind the segment fills with bone. Once the transported segment has closed the defect, it unites readily with the opposite fragment. This type of autologous local bone grafting has gained wide acceptance for the treatment of desperate cases. In a similar way malformations and malalignment may be treated by bone lengthening and correction.

Ilizarov has realized, in a clinically reliable and reproducible way, what before him Kirschner (1916), Bier (1918), Putti (1918), Anderson (1936) demonstrated but for which they could find no wide application. While Ilizarov's ingenious method is performed with an apparatus that allows for easy three-dimensional corrections, the requirement of multiple transfixing wires, the comparably large rings and the long duration of fixation has led others to study the feasibility of bone transportation with simpler devices which are more acceptable to today's demanding patient. Rüter and Brutscher (1988) have established the clinical usefulness of a device which allows for transportation without transfixing wires. Their procedure completely avoids cutting of the wires through soft tissues. Regazzoni (1989) has recently demonstrated the use of the AO unilateral external fixator supplemented with a simple nut for transportation along the conventional AO spindle.

Rüter et al. (1989) studied the use of wires applied along the bone in animal experiments utilizing full osteotomies and corticotomies. Figure 1.49 shows the result in the sheep. Transportation could be achieved reliably. Once the transported fragment closed the defect, solid union occurred without further internal fixation. Long-lasting fixation using transcutanously connected external devices was felt to be in need of improvement. Brunner et al. (1989, 1990) have devised a method of transportation using an intramedullary nail, whereby the transport is achieved using the method of noncutting wires explained in Fig. 1.49b. The small and simple external frame helps to achieve the distraction of the fragments; the intramedullary rod provides splinting. After transportation has come to an end, the external part is removed and the intramedullary rod left in place. Tepic (1989) has developed a method for continuous transportation of the fragment. It consists of a bar which includes a battery-operated spindle device. Korcinek (1989) demonstrated the formation of a more homogeneous bone in dogs and in man with continuous distraction according to Tepic.

Fig. 1.49 Distraction osteogenesis according to Ilizarov.

a The new method of Rüter and Brutscher (1988) using noncutting wires, with X-ray and CT immediately after surgery and 3 months later. Transportation is achieved using elements of the conventional AO external fixator with carbon fiber bars supplemented with two ratchets. *Center*, before transportation; *right*, after complete transportation.

b The recent method of Brunner and coworkers combining the above-mentioned method with an intramedullary nail. The apparatus (*left*) consists of a small bilateral AO external fixator frame supplemented with two small Wagner external fixators to allow transport of the segment using a pair of tension wires. *Center*, the situation before transportation of a segment to close a 45-mm-long defect. *Right*, after 32 weeks the gap has filled with homogeneous, tubular bone. The defect is solidly healed.

c–e See p. 92.

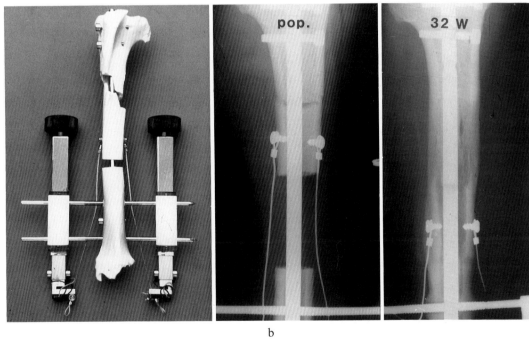

Fig. 1.49

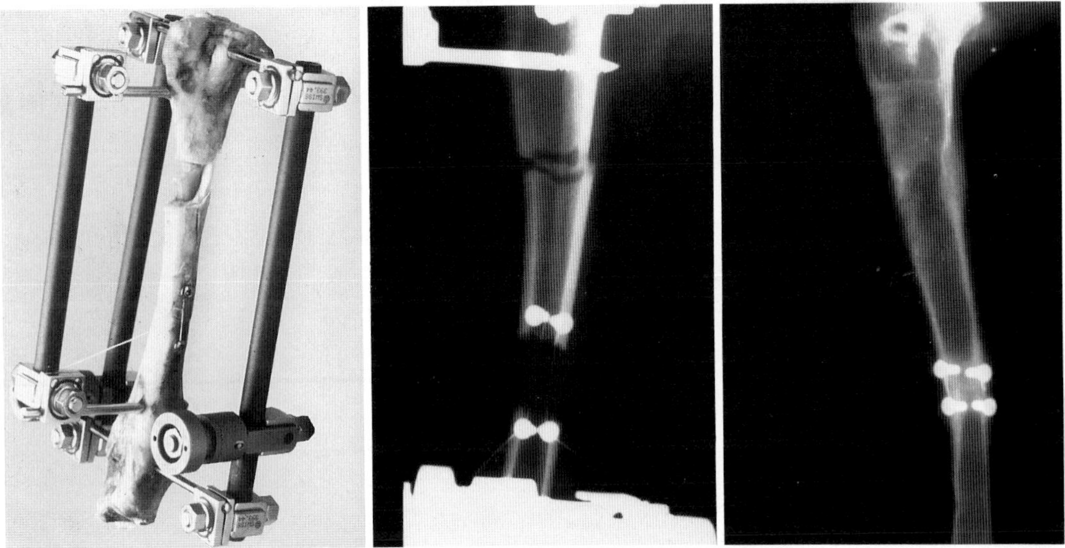

a

b

Fig. 1.49 Distraction osteogenesis according to Ilizarov (continued).

c Rüter and Brutscher radiologically quantified the difference between corticotomy (*filled symbols*) and osteotomy (*open symbols*). A relatively small difference was found.

d The cross sections obtained by quantitative computed tomography of the transported segment shown in b and c. The bone within the gap shows a normal shape with temporarily lesser density (Brunner et al. 1989).

e The motor-driven rod of Tepic for continuous distraction. The study by Korcinek (1989) seems to demonstrate the superiority of continuous distraction. At 6 weeks after surgery the gap is filled with more homogeneous bone.

Fig. 1.49

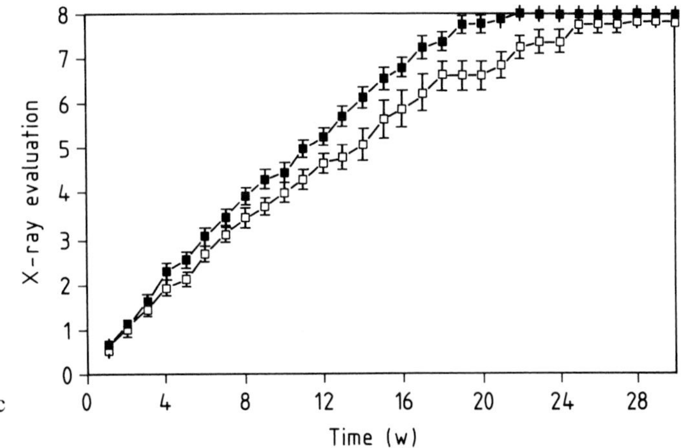
X-ray evaluation
Time (w)
0
1
2
3
4
5
6
7
8
0
4
8
12
16
20
24
28

c

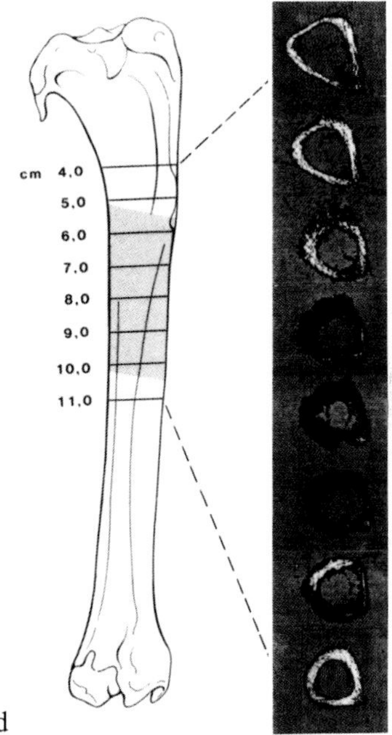
cm 4,0
5,0
6,0
7,0
8,0
9,0
10,0
11,0

d

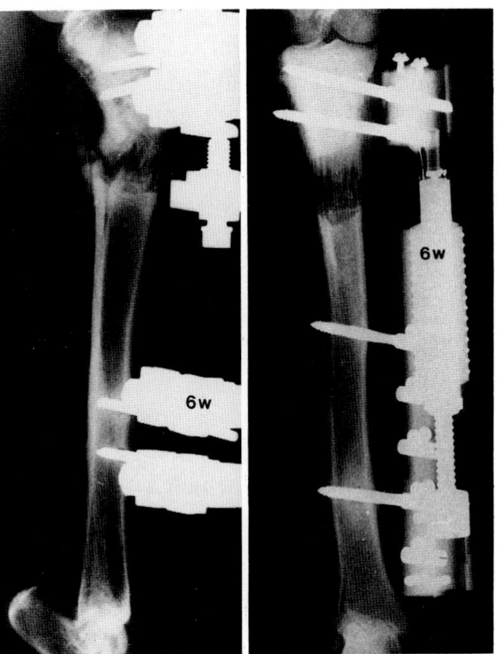
6w
6w

e

1.3.5 Implant Materials

The materials for internal fixation implants must, first of all, perform their task of providing temporary fixation of the fracture to allow for functional treatment. Here good fatigue resistance is required. They must be ductile so as to maintain strength after having been adapted to the bone surface. The stress relaxation by the implants should be minimal, to maintain compression. The material should not degrade in an uncontrolled way. Last, but not least, the implant material must be available continuously, at defined quality, and at an acceptable price, while allowing appropriate qualities for machining and contouring at surgery.

1.3.5.1 Metals

Metals are used as implant materials because they are strong, ductile, i.e., may be shaped to fit the bone surface, and their biocompatibility is generally acceptable. Today's internal fixation implants are made mainly of stainless steel or of pure or alloyed titanium.

Steel

Steel consists mainly of iron, chromium, and nickel. It corresponds to international standards (ISO TC150 5832/1) which define two grades of carbon content and four grades of cold work, from annealed to extra hard. Steel is today's all-round material with a good combination of strength, ductility, and price. Its corrosion resistance and compatibility are fair.

Pure Titanium

Commercially pure titanium (c.p. Ti) consists of titanium and oxygen. Titanium is extremely insoluble and subsequently is inert and compatible. According to Steinemann (1988) the body is saturated with titanium and, therefore, no additional soluble titanium can become active. Cases of sensitization as reported for nickel have not been observed, to our knowledge, when only c.p. titanium was used as implant material. It is available today in grades which combine good strength and ductility (ISO TC150 5832/2). Its price, however, is higher than that of steel.

Titanium-6-Aluminum-4-Vanadium Alloy

Ti6A14V, an alloy of titanium, aluminum and vanadium, offers excellent strength and fair ductility (ISO TC150 5832/3). The material is used extensively in industrial applications where light constructions must be strong (e.g., in airplanes). The corrosion characteristics of Ti6A14V are excellent. For any alloy, the risk of sensitization to one of the components increases with their number. As an element vanadium is known to be about 10 times more toxic than nickel. Other titanium alloys aim at strength (e.g., TiAlFe or TiAlNb) or at a combination of strength and ductility (Ti-beta alloys).

Other Alloys

Chrome-cobalt alloys no longer find wide application in internal fixation. Tantalum and niobium have been proposed as implant material but have, to date, not found widespread application due to their lack of important advantages.

Corrosion

Metals undergo corrosion in body fluids. Implant metals are invariably of the kind which are protected from corroding by a passive layer consisting of nonsoluble corrosion products. Corrosion is increased when a metal component frets against another metal component of the implant. Steinemann (1977) has demonstrated this effect to increase corrosion by a factor of 100. This observation underlines the importance of stable fixation (see p. 14).

1.3.5.2 Other Implant Materials

Polymeric Materials

Polymeric materials have been proposed to replace metals in internal fixation implants. If avoidance of corrosion is the goal, one must also bear in mind that the problem of uncontrolled leakage of components (e.g., plasticizers) from polymeric materials has not been solved yet. The strength of polymeric materials (e.g., carbon fiber reinforced ones) may be high, but it is unlikely that, at the same time, ductility is maintained and stress relaxation avoided.

Biodegradable Polymeric Materials

Metals are often surgically removed from the body once the bone is able to carry the load. To avoid the second operation, Rokkanen et al. (1985) have proposed using biodegradable polymeric materials, so that the implant dissolves after a certain time in the body. No such material has yet become available for use with conventional techniques of internal fixation which combines adequate strength, ductility, maintenance of compression and degradability without marked tissue reaction. Tissue tolerance, especially the local effects on infection resistance, is still an unsolved problem. With some materials an incidence of about 10% of formation of "sterile cysts" is reported. Some of them showed secondary infection. Hoffmann et al. (1989) considered the observed rate of complications as being unacceptable.

Ceramic Materials

Different materials, such as hydroxyapatite and tricalcium phosphate, are available with a variety of mechanical properties. They are used for replacement and for improved bone ongrowth to the implant. Brittleness and limited strength restrict their use as material for internal fixation.

Aluminum oxide ceramics, as well as ceramics based on other metals, offer high strength and smooth surfaces, which are important in prosthetic replacement but less so in internal fixation. With respect to tissue tolerance these materials are very inert, a quality shared by the passive layer of commercially pure titanium.

1.4 AO Teaching

1.4.1 AO Courses

Internal fixation requires intelligence *and* skill, i.e., basic biological and mechanical understanding, careful preoperative planning, and a high standard of surgical perfection. To function adequately the trauma surgeon must understand the scientific basis, the principles, the instrumentation, and the implants. Furthermore, optimal internal fixation requires preoperative planning and manual skills, in order to achieve the best results with the least tissue damage. The goal of AO courses from the very beginning was to teach the scientific basis of fracture treatment and healing as well as the development of manual skills. Initially, the instruments were available only to surgeons who had taken at least a basic course. This policy could not be maintained for very long. Over 30 years, 450 courses have been given for 60000 surgeons and 490 courses for 42000 nurses (Fig. 1.50). AO courses are available at a basic or advanced level. They can also be directed at problem solving with advanced groups. Other courses address specific fields, such as hand, spine, or pelvic surgery. AO courses are also available for veterinary surgeons, who have found them successful and stimulating.

The 80 courses given in Davos, attended by 20000 participants, have led to the development of various teaching aids and particularly, to the possibility of hands-on teaching to large classes. Today the courses, given in a large number of countries, have contributed greatly to the refinement in teaching basic principles as well as basic skills.

1.4.2 AO Workshops

In 70 clinics, workshops for the development of manual skills have been installed to allow the surgeon to instruct his team of doctors and nurses on a continuous basis (Fig. 1.51).

1.4.3 AO Fellowships

Nothing can replace hands-on experience and on-site evaluation. Through AO International, 150 fellowships are granted annually, each lasting for 2–3 months. They are available at clinics run by experienced "AO surgeons." To date 1700 fellows have taken the opportunity to observe surgery, discuss indications and operative techniques, and study the results.

Fig. 1.50 Programs of various AO courses.

Fig. 1.51 Installation of an AO workshop.

Fig. 1.50

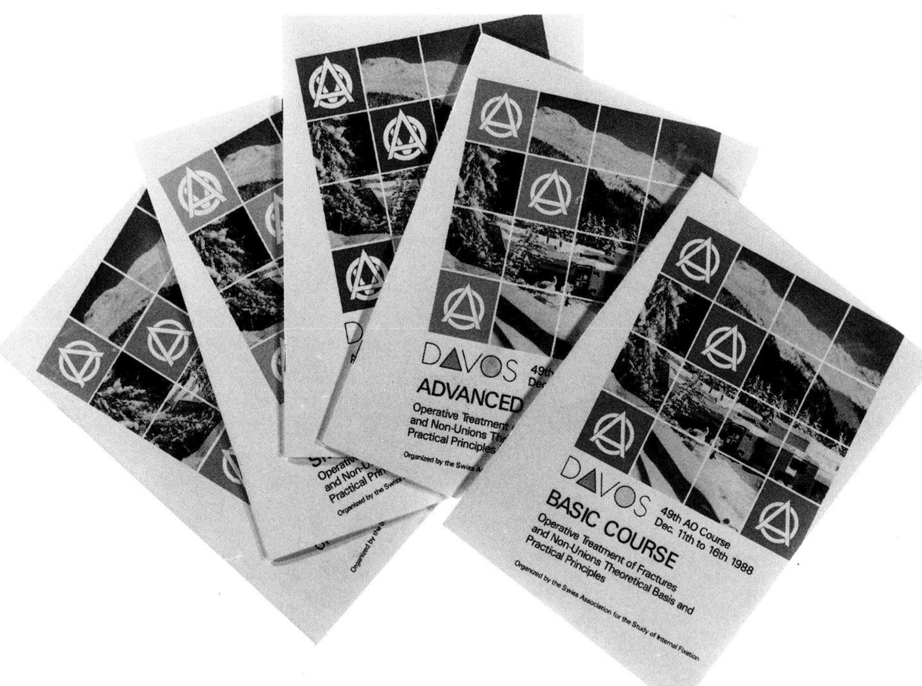

Fig. 1.51

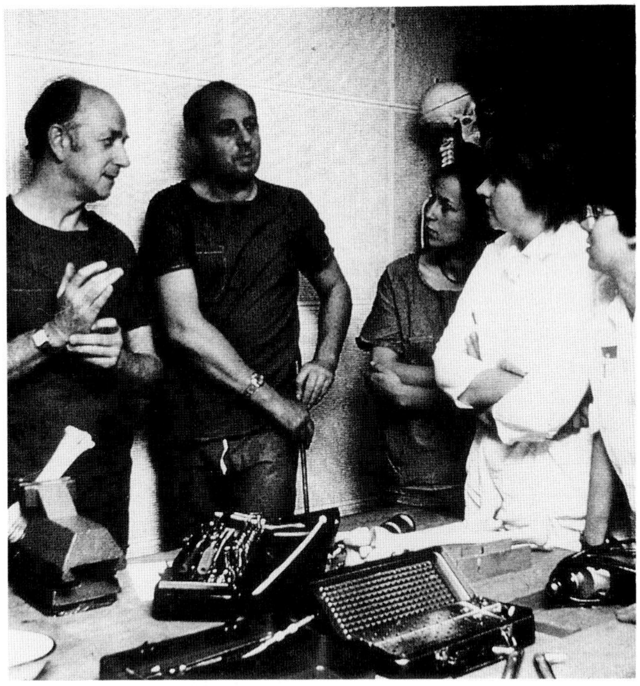

1.4.4 AO Research Grants

The purpose of AO research grants is to support basic and applied research in different laboratories and clinics. This often facilitates later applications for research grants from national institutions.

1.4.5 AO Video Tapes

The braining of a large number of trauma and orthopedic surgeons has created the need for optimal audiovisual instruction material. The Davos video team, working at the Laboratory for Experimental Surgery (Fig. 1.52), has produced 275 master videotapes for instructional purposes in the last 5 years, with a total of 7500 copies. These tapes are updated each year and supplemented with short technical "flashes."

Fig. 1.52 The video facilities of the laboratory at Davos.

a The studio.

b The editing desk.

c The collection of original tapes.

Fig. 1.52

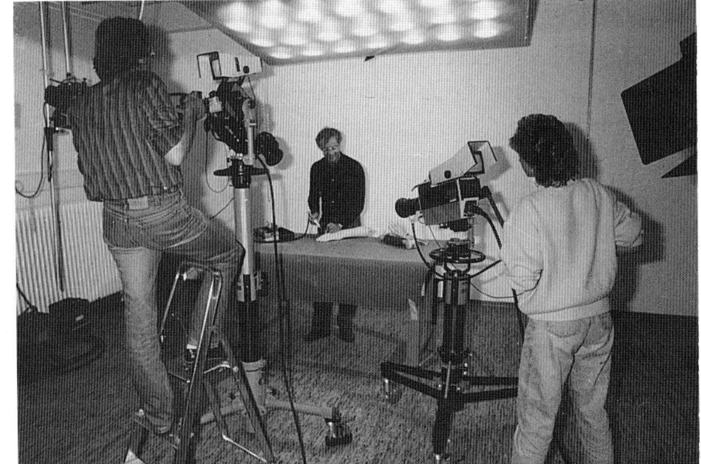

a

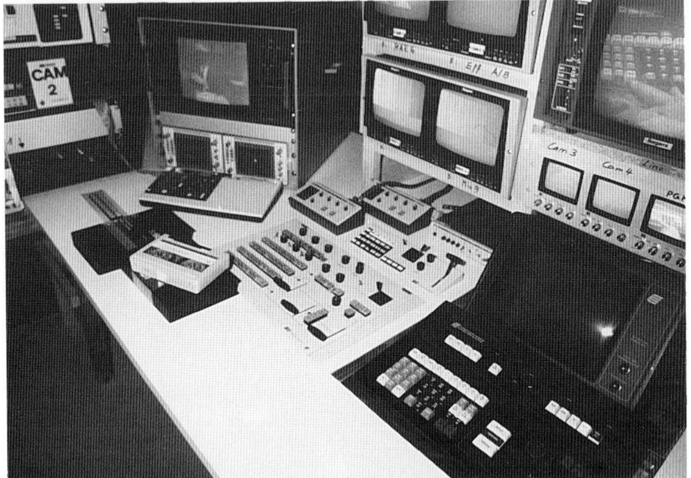

b

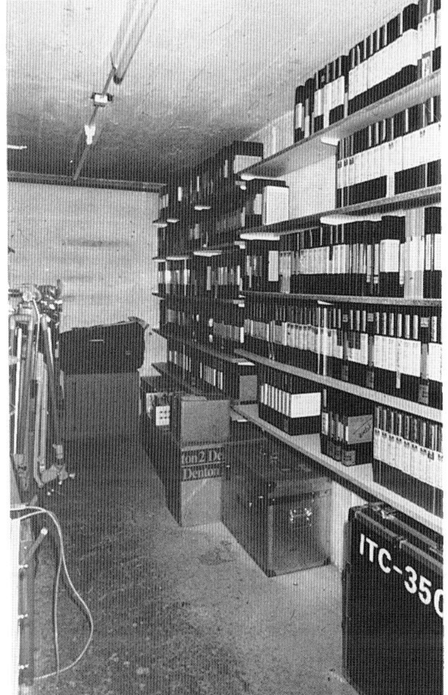

c

1.4.6 AO Artificial Bones and Limbs

Though the first courses were given using human cadaver bones, it soon became necessary to develop an artificial bone with appropriate mechanical properties, which would allow the production of realistic fractures and would give the characteristic sensation during drilling, tapping and tightening of the implants. These artificial bones were developed as a result of a collaboration between the Laboratory for Experimental Surgery in Davos and the Contraves Company of Zürich. They are now produced in Filisur, near Davos, by Synbone. More than 300000 bones of 72 different varieties have been used at the AO courses. The artificial bones are also available as teaching and exercise tools for use in clinics, especially for preoperative planning and surgical simulation. The bones are provided to the surgeons by the laboratory at net cost (Fig. 1.53).

Special anatomical models have been developed which facilitate teaching and learning of the different approaches in the leg and arm (Fig. 1.54).

Fig. 1.53 The artificial bones developed especially for the AO courses.

a The range of bones. A total of 72 bones and/or fractures are available.

b A model of a wedge fracture. The fracture pattern is very realistic.

c A model of tension band wiring of the olecranon, an exercise performed at the AO courses.

Fig. 1.54 The artificial limbs developed by Baldomero and Rüedi for simulation of surgical approaches. The bones, muscles, and major nerves and blood vessels are modeled.

a Artificial thigh.

b Artificial arm.

Fig. 1.53

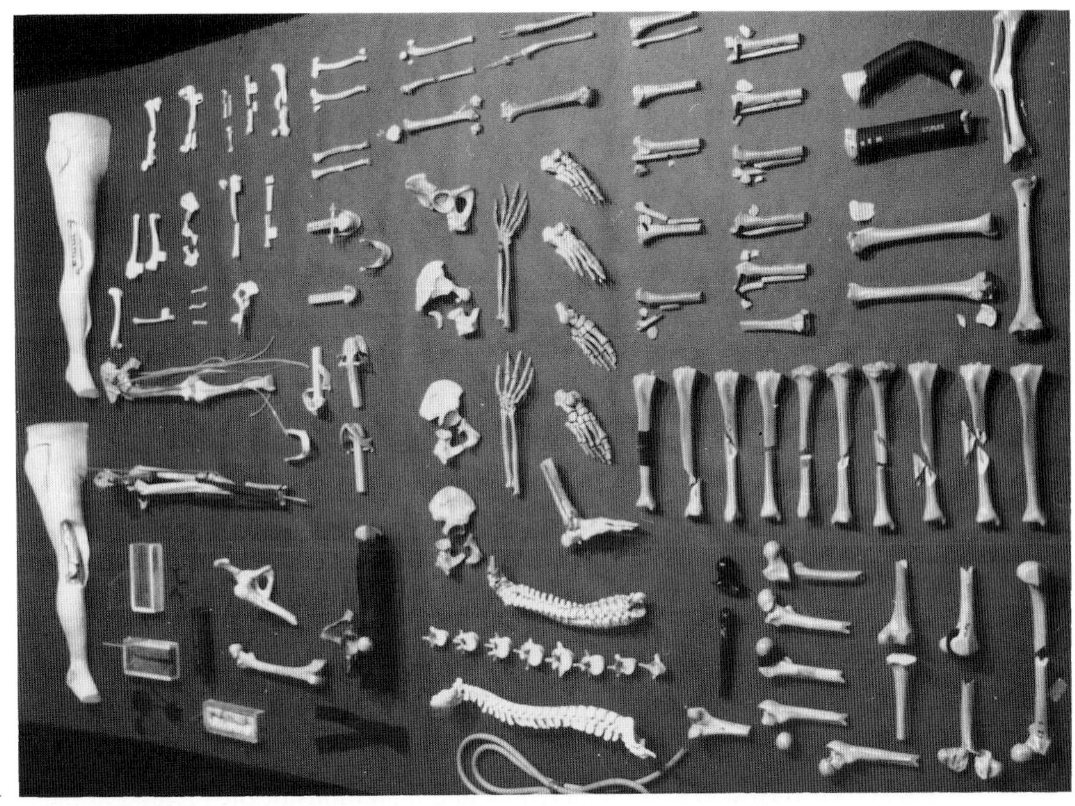

a

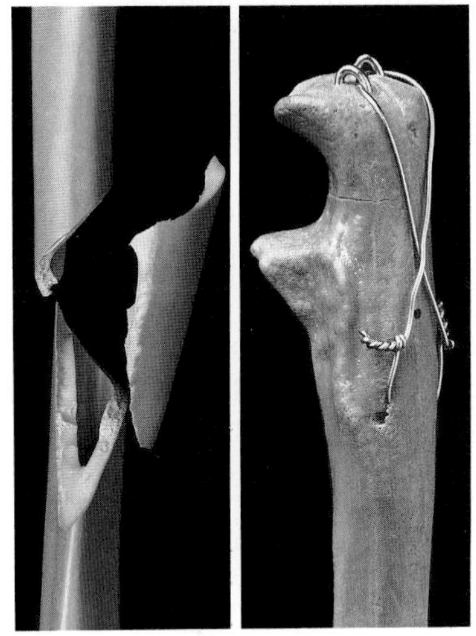

b c

Fig. 1.54

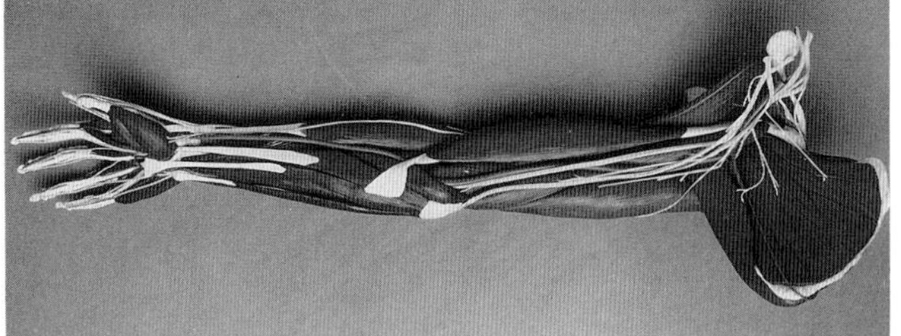

a

b

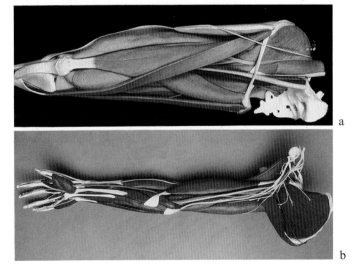

1.5 Documentation

The backbone of the AO method is the documentation of over 150000 operative cases; 500000 code sheets have been completed and entered into computer files for analysis. Over 1200000 radiographs, including those taken before and after operation and at 4 and 12 months after surgery, have been microfilmed, printed, and fixed on to punch cards. It is through this detailed, painstaking documentation that members of the AO have been able to assess the potential, as well as the results, of the methods and to eliminate certain mistakes. This kind of follow-up required a great deal of patience and excellent organization. The arduous task turned out, in the long run, however, to be most worthwhile. The study of failures was particularly valuable. We established the rule that a single failure following from the correct application of the method, and not from its misuse, required re-evaluation and perhaps redesign of the technique. Over the years, many of the procedures have been gradually changed and improved, expanded in scope, and newly standardized.

The systematic analysis of failures has shown that the majority of these were due to a disregard of biomechanical principles: most failures are preventable. Whenever a surgical procedure has been developed to the point that success or failure can be predicted, and success reliably achieved if sufficient care is taken, then the procedure can be considered dependable. This does not mean, however, that these procedures are easy and that everyone is capable of carrying them out. On the contrary, years of practice and experience are required in order to master all the intricacies of the AO method.

Everyone who uses the AO method should perform a follow-up evaluation at 4 and 12 months of all patients so treated. This is the only way that surgeons can critically assess their own skill and the potential and limitations of the method in their own hands. They will also come to recognize complications and will learn to treat them promptly.

The documentation of the 1990s is to be carried out at AO clinics using a decentralized documentation system. An optical reader helps to transfer the data from the code sheets to a database on a personal computer.

The new equipment allows immediate access to one's patient database. The desired information can be retrieved for history, reports, letters, statistics, etc. Together with the completed follow-up, the data will be transferred to the AO Documentation Center. Data are transferred in both directions using code sheets, floppy disks, or electronic links with modems and international computer networks.

The radiographic data are recorded by photographic and/or video techniques. Image enhancement is used to improve and standardize image quality. Image analysis may be applied as a diagnostic tool, once the adequate software is available.

With this system it is possible to improve efficiency in the clinic and to reduce paperwork. At the same time a method for quality control is directly located in the clinic.

Fig. 1.55 AO documentation.

a A punch card showing the most important information on one side with the microfilms of the radiographs pasted on the back. The data are recorded on film using video image enhancement techniques.

b The three AO code sheets: for the initial hospitalization, for the 4-month follow-up, and for the final review.

Fig. 1.55

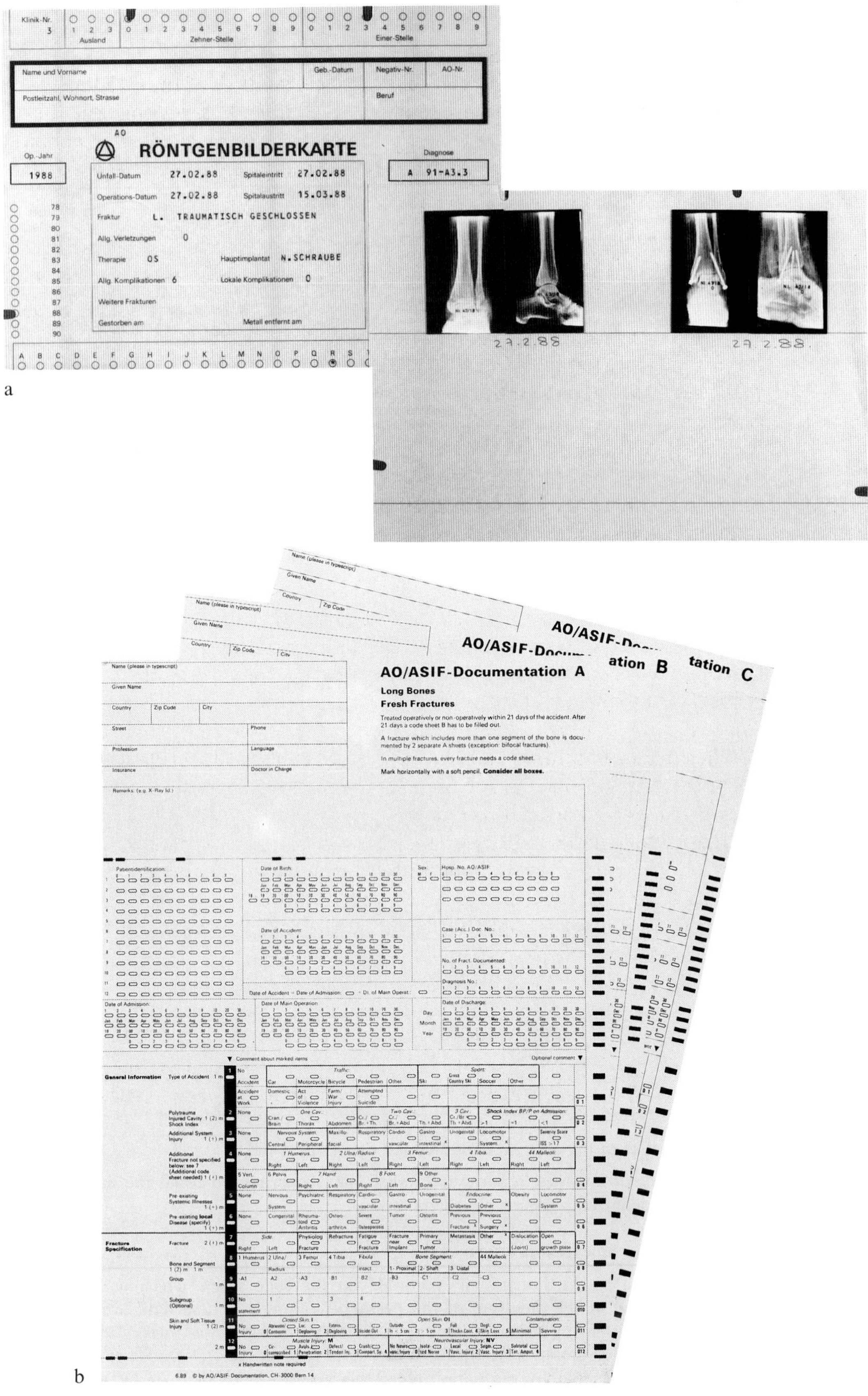

Röntgenbilderkarte (a)

Klinik-Nr. 3	Ausland 1 2 3	Zehner-Stelle 0 1 2 3 4 5 6 7 8 9	Einer-Stelle 0 1 2 3 4 5 6 7 8 9

Name und Vorname	Geb.-Datum	Negativ-Nr.	AO-Nr.
Postleitzahl, Wohnort, Strasse		Beruf	

AO

RÖNTGENBILDERKARTE

Op.-Jahr: 1988

Diagnose: A 91-A3.3

Unfall-Datum	27.02.88	Spitaleintritt	27.02.88
Operations-Datum	27.02.88	Spitalaustritt	15.03.88
Fraktur	L. TRAUMATISCH GESCHLOSSEN		
Allg. Verletzungen	0		
Therapie	OS	Hauptimplantat	N. SCHRAUBE
Allg. Komplikationen	6	Lokale Komplikationen	0
Weitere Frakturen			
Gestorben am		Metall entfernt am	

78 79 80 81 82 83 84 85 86 87 88 89 90

A B C D E F G H I J K L M N O P Q R S

27.2.88 27.2.88

a

AO/ASIF-Documentation A (b)

Name (please in typescript) · Given Name · Country · Zip Code · City · Street · Phone · Profession · Language · Insurance · Doctor in Charge

Remarks: (e.g. X-Ray Id.)

AO/ASIF-Documentation A

Long Bones

Fresh Fractures

Treated operatively or non-operatively within 21 days of the accident. After 21 days a code sheet B has to be filled out.

A fracture which includes more than one segment of the bone is documented by 2 separate A sheets (exception: bifocal fractures).

In multiple fractures, every fracture needs a code sheet.

Mark horizontally with a soft pencil. **Consider all boxes.**

AO/ASIF-Documentation B

AO/ASIF-Documentation C

Patientidentification · Date of Birth · Sex · Hosp. No. AO/ASIF · Date of Accident · Case (Acc.) Doc. No. · No. of Fract. Documented · Diagnosis No. · Date of Admission · Date of Main Operation · Date of Discharge

General Information: Type of Accident · Polytrauma Injured Cavity · Shock Index · Additional System Injury · Additional Fracture not specified below · Pre-existing Systemic Illnesses · Pre-existing local Disease (specify)

Fracture Specification: Fracture · Bone and Segment · Group · Subgroup (Optional) · Skin and Soft Tissue Injury

x Handwritten note required

6.89 © by AO/ASIF-Documentation, CH-3000 Bern 14

b

Fig. 1.56 Examples of data of the code sheet printed for use of the clinic.

Different types of histories, reports and letters may be produced using the data from the code sheets stored on the decentralized personal computer.

Fig. 1.57 Decentralized documentation system of the 1990s.

The data on the patient are initially recorded on the code sheets which will be read by the optical reader and stored in the database of the personal computer. These data are then made available to the centralized system by means of floppy disks or via modem and international networks. One copy of the punch card is stored in the clinic and one is sent to the AO Documentation Center. The clinic can use centralized data by means of interactive access via modem or by receiving data on floppy disks.

Fig. 1.56

AO/ASIF Test Clinic
Main Street 1990
2000 Big Town

Dr.
J. Newtester
Alley 77
2000 Big Town

CASE REPORT for Phamily Physician of
Demonstration John, born 10/31/1948, Photographer, CH-3000 Bern, Belpstr. 24

General Information:

Date of admission at our hospital was 04/12/1989
Date of discharge 04/24/1989

He had a domestic accident on 04/12/1989 with no polytrauma. Shock index on admission was)1. There was no additional system injury, no additional fracture, no pre-existing systemic illnesses, no pre-existing local disease.

Fracture Specification:

Left side physiological fracture (42-A3) of tibia diaphysis, simple fracture, transverse, fibula intact.

Skin and soft tissue injury (I1,M0,NVO):
No skin breakages, but contusion (I1), no muscle injury (M0), no neurovascular injury (NVO)

Treatment:

Date of main operation was 04/12/1989. Open reduction on fracture table. The procedure was an internal fixation alone with an unlocked universal nail as main implant. Implant material: steel. Function of implant is internal splintage. There were no intraoperative findings, no peroperative findings. Duration of procedure was below 60 minutes. Anesthesia: general, no volume substitution was necessary. Assessment reduction: anatomical. Assessment reduction: stable.

Aftertreatment:

Standard wound care proceedings. Thromboembolic prophylaxis with dextran.

Discharge from hospital:

As walking aids are two crutches used. Patient for further treatment transferred to family physician. No special documentation prepared. AO/ASIF-Follow-up is planned for: 04/1990.

The patient has to go twice a week to special physiotherapy. For special or additional information please contact me or my assistant, Dr. Test.

Big Town, 04/24/1989

Dr. G. Tester

Fig. 1.57

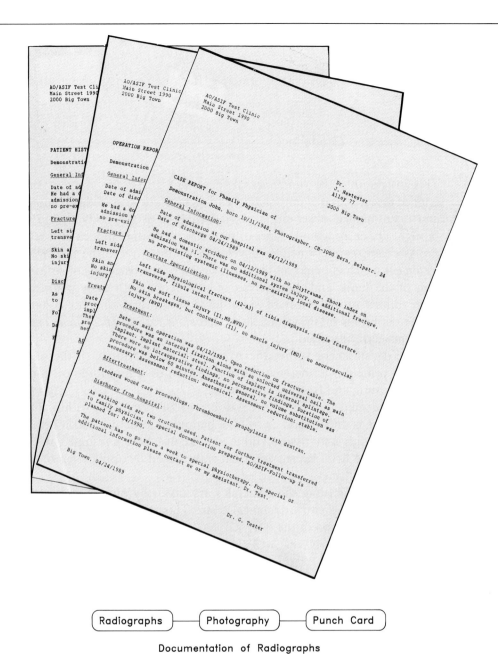

Radiographs — Photography — Punch Card

Documentation of Radiographs

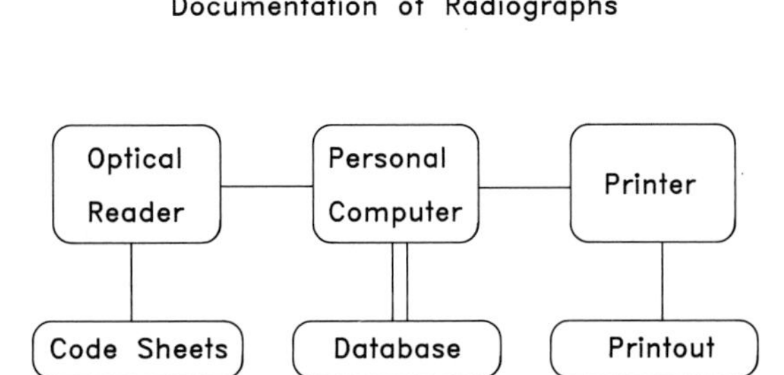

Decentralized Documentation System

1.6 Development

Development includes that of principles, techniques, instruments, and implants.

1.6.1 Principles and Guidelines

This insight into the fundamental facts that guide development stems from basic and applied research and from practical experience. The knowledge is compiled through careful and open-minded observation of the reaction of the body tissues to different changes brought about by various types of trauma and distinct modes of treatment.

As examples of principles developed we may quote the principle of *early functional treatment* which is based on the observation of the reactions of soft tissues to immobilization of the limbs and the analysis of the reactions to early pain-free mobilization. The observations of the effect of suboptimal restoration of joint congruence have resulted in the definition of the principle of *complete restitution of joint anatomy* as a basis for best long-term function.

The development within the AO group gives priority to the scientific establishment of basic principles rather than to production of a multitude of implants, one for every bone, location, and fracture conceivable.

A basic guideline for the development of principles within the AO group is that injured bone is understood as being a biological structure which depends on its biological interaction with soft tissues. Bone should not be confounded with a piece of broken furniture to be first cleaned and then embellished by application of individual but largely "unnecessary fittings" (Weber, pers. comm.).

Decisions regarding the principles are taken by physicians and scientists assisted by a competent and creative technical team. This interdisciplinary group forms the general technical commission of the AO.

1.6.2 Techniques

The manner of accomplishing internal fixation according to the principles must satisfy the criteria of *simplicity and safety*. The different techniques such as plating, nailing, external fixation, wiring, etc. rely on the understanding of the bone reaction to the prevailing mechanical and biological ("biomechanical") conditions. On the one hand, in conventional plating (with the exception of, for example, biological plating) unloading of the plate, degree of corrosion, mechanical fatigue of the implant, type as well as rate of bone healing, and susceptibility to infection depend much on the degree of stability of fixation achieved. On the other hand, the stability achieved with noninterlocked nailing, and to a certain extent that achieved with interlocked nailing, is less critical.

With respect to the selection of the optimal technique, the type of fracture and the conditions of the soft tissues obviously play an important role. Other factors, such as the skill of the surgeon, the surgical environment (help provided, conditions of asepsis), the instruments and implants available, and cooperation by the patient are important and variable elements to be taken into consideration.

1.6.3 Instrumentation and Implants

The tools and the implants must be simple and of high quality. The surgeon must have an armamentarium at hand which puts him in a position to deal with the widest variety of fractures. The instrumentation must be understood and therefore be taught and learned. The interaction and the function of the set of instruments and implants must satisfy the criteria of *simplicity and completeness*. Good results depend on the selection of the material, the appropriate grade (degree of cold work, purity, etc.) and the excellence of its construction. Instruments and implants must be used for the applications for which they have been developed. Only the creative expert may take advantage of other possible uses. The dimensions of the instruments must be carefully adapted to those of the implants. This is the reason why mixing instruments and implants from different producers may lead to unexpected problems, when, for example, the nominal dimensions fit, but the tolerances are different.

We do not recommend repeated use of the implants. They are not designed for reuse, and one cannot estimate the degree of fatigue the implant has undergone during an earlier period of use.

1.6.4 The Technical Commissions of the AO

Developments under the aegis of the AO are controlled by the technical commissions. The "large" technical commission sets the long-term goals and guidelines and coordinates of smaller technical commissions. The latter deal with problems in special areas such as small fragment surgery, maxillofacial surgery, spine surgery, joint surgery, pelvic surgery, and veterinary surgery. An additional group deals with the development of new materials.

At the AO research center in Davos a group develops prototypes based on the insights provided by the scientists. Each manufacturer of AO products has a group for product development. To coordinate the efforts of all these groups is a further task of the technical commission.

A development is activated by a single person, be it scientist or physician, who works with a member of the prototype or product development group. Once such a team has developed something they consider to be worth testing, the technical commission organizes the tests in the laboratories and hospitals. Care is taken that the clinics selected for performance of the tests provide a complete test of the different intended types of use under realistic conditions. The results are reported to and judged by the technical commission. The AO works as a group; therefore, the inventor's name will not appear on the final product and private reimbursement, apart from compensation for the costs of the development, is excluded. However, the AO will readily support ongoing research, teaching, and fellowships at the inventor's facility. In this way a safeguard is provided against private interests which could impede critical and realistic evaluation of the potential and the possible shortcomings of a technique, instrument, or implant. In a similar way, special scientific achievements are awarded the AO Prize, and inventions are awarded the AO Inventors Prize or the AO Recognition Prize.

1.7 Glossary

Absolute stability: The compressed surfaces of the fracture do not displace under applied functional load. The definition of absolute stability applies only to a given time and a given site: some areas of a fracture may displace in relation to each other, other areas of the fracture may not, and different areas may exhibit different displacement at different times. Practically the only method of achieving absolute stability consists in the application of interfragmental compression. The compression stabilizes by preloading and by producing friction (Perren 1972).

Biological internal fixation, biological plating (Mast et al. 1989): In internal fixation a delicate balance exists between the degree of stabilization and that of surgical trauma. The benefits of each must be pondered. Biological fixation favors the preservation of the blood supply and thus optimizes the healing potential of bone and soft tissues. It provides sufficient stability for multifragmentary fractures to heal in correct alignment. For protection of the implants from overload it relies on early biological reaction (callus formation).

If simple fractures are plated, stable fixation to prevent induction of bone surface resorption is required. In single fractures with closely adapted fracture surfaces, minimal motion generates high strain. High strain induces bone surface resorption in contact areas. When locking splints (see p. 24) or nongliding splints (see p. 28) are used for fracture fixation reliable results are produced by stability which prevents loosening. Surgical exposure required for stabilization of a simple fracture is limited and therefore less detrimental to the blood supply and healing of the fracture.

Multifragmentary fractures and complex fractures are less demanding in respect to stability. Here instability produces small amounts of strain due to (1) larger fracture gaps and (2) distribution of strain over several, serially located fracture gaps. Surgical exposure required for stable fixation of multifragmentary fractures would be extensive with consequent important disturbance of blood supply. Therefore in plating of simple fracture, stability is an important goal to achieve, while in multifragmentary fractures biology takes precedence.

Blood supply to cortical bone (restoration of): Cortical bone which has been completely deprived of blood supply for an extended period of time becomes necrotic. It may be revascularized by regrowth of blood vessels without marked widening of the haversian canals (Pfister et al. 1979), or by newly formed haversian canals. The restoration by neoformation of haversian canals is a process with a marked lag period and relatively low speed (0.1 mm/day, Schenk 1987). Bone may be revascularized by resorption and replacement with newly formed, vascular bone (creeping substitution).

Buttress: When the trauma results in impaction of the bone (e.g., at the distal metaphysis of the tibia) a defect remains after fracture reduction. An implant (plate, external fixator, or interlocking nail) then temporarily carries functional load while it maintains the shape of the bone.

Callus: A reparative tissue made of connective, cartilaginous, or bony tissue (or any combination thereof). Callus formation may be induced by any irritation – chemical (Küntscher 1970), infection and/or instability (Hutzschenreuter et al. 1969) or others. In internal fixation the appearance of callus is therefore little appreciated, as a sign of an unwanted condition. Callus, though, is always welcome as a repair tissue.

Complete articular fracture: The articular surface is completely dissociated from the diaphysis.

Complex fracture: Fracture in which after reduction there is no contact between the main fragments.

Compression: The act of pressing together. It results in deformation (shortening like a spring) and in improvement or creation of stability. Compression is used (1) to provide stability of fixation where motion-induced resorption must be prevented, and (2) to protect the implants and to improve their efficiency by unloading them. Unloading is achieved through restoration of the load-bearing capacity of the bone. Any fixation taking advantage of the load-bearing capacity of fragments of a fracture bone can withstand appreciable amounts of load without mechanical failure or temporary micromotion within the fracture. This is the main reason for using careful reduction and application of compression. Compression furthermore helps to restore dynamic loading of the bone fragments, a process for which stable contact of the fracture fragments is a prerequisite.

If the implant (screw, plate) bridging the fracture is applied under tension the fracture focus undergoes an equal amount of compression. The compression is used to help stabilize the fracture. We have not observed any "magic biological effect" of compression.

Contact healing: A healing which occurs between two fragment ends of a fractured bone, at circumscribed places which are maintained in motionless contact. The fracture is then repaired by direct internal remodeling. Contact healing may be observed additionally where the gap is only a few micrometers wide.

Debricolage: A French term signifying the process of mechanical failure of an internal fixation prior to the onset of solid bone bridging.

Direct healing: A type of fracture healing observed with stable internal fixation. It is characterized by:
1. Absence of callus formation specific to the fracture site.
2. Absence of bone surface resorption at the fracture site.
3. Direct bone formation, i.e., without intermediary repair tissue.

Direct fracture healing was formerly called "primary" healing in some countries. Today we avoid the term primary so as not to grade the quality of fracture healing. Two types of direct healing are distinguished: contact healing (q.v.) and gap healing (q.v.).

Extra-articular fractures: The fracture does not involve the articular surface, but it may be intracapsular.

Far (trans-) cortex: The cortex away from the plate. The consequences of a defect within the far cortex are much more important than those of a defect in the near cortex. The difference is due to the larger lever arm of the far cortex.

Fracture: A sudden rupture of a structure which occurs whenever the internal stress produced by load exceeds the limits of strength. Depending on the type of load – compressive, flexural, torsional, shear, or any combination thereof – a typical fracture pattern is observed (impaction, transverse fracture, spiral fracture, avulsion, etc.). The complexity of the fracture depends mainly upon the amount of energy stored prior to fracture.

Fracture disease: A condition characterized by pain, swelling, and other signs of dystrophy such as patchy bone loss and stiffness of joints (Lucas-Championnière 1907). Fracture disease (synonym: Sudeck's atrophy) can best be avoided by stable fixation to reduce irritation and by early active movement and, when possible, immediate or at least partial weight-bearing by the injured limb (Allgöwer 1978).

Gap healing: The healing process taking place between two fragment ends kept in stable relative position with a small gap between the fragment ends. Gap healing progresses in two phases: (1) the filling of the gap with lamellar bone of different orientation than the bone of the fragments, (2) the subsequent remodeling of the newly filled bone from within the gap into the fragments (plugging) or crossing from one fragment through the newly filled bone into the other fragment (remodeling).

Gliding hole: When a fully threaded screw is used as a lag screw, the cortex under the screw head should not engage. This can be accomplished by overdrilling the near cortex screw hole to at least the size of the outer diameter of the screw thread.

Gliding splint: A splint (e.g., conventional nail) which allows for axial shortening. Such a splint provides the possibility for coaptation under conditions of fragment end shortening due to bone surface resorption.

Goal of fracture treatment: According to Müller et al. (1963), the goal of fracture treatment is to restore optimal function of the limb in respect to mobility and load-bearing capacity. The goal is furthermore to avoid early disturbances such as Sudeck's atrophy (fracture disease) and late sequels such as post-traumatic arthrosis.

Healing: Restoration of the original integrity. Theoretically the healing process after a bone fracture would last many years, until internal fracture remodeling subsides. For practical purposes healing is considered completed when the bone has regained its normal stiffness and strength.

Impacted fracture: A fracture in which the cortex or articular surface is driven into the cancellous bone.

Indirect healing: Bone healing as observed in nontreated or nonstably treated fractures. Callus formation is predominant, the fracture fragment ends are resorbed, and bone formation results from a process of transformation of fibrous and/or cartilaginous tissue to bone.

Interfragmental compression (effect of): Static compression applied to a fracture area stabilizes the fragments and thus reduces irritation. Bone surface resorption is then absent. No proof has been found that compression per se has an effect upon internal remodeling of the cortical bone (Matter et al. 1974).

Interlocking nail: A nail provides some degree of stability mainly by its (flexural) stiffness. A conventional nail allows the fragments to slide along the nail; the fracture must therefore be provided with a solid support against shortening. For the treatment of complex fractures the nail can be interlocked to prevent shortening and rotation.

Lag screw: The lag screw produces interfragmental compression by compressing the bone under the screw head against the fragment in which the screw threads are anchored. Interfragmental compression will be reduced by engagement (wedging) of the screw threads with the walls of the gliding hole. Anchorage in the near fragment can be avoided by the use of a shaft screw. This method is required to maintain efficient compression when the lag screw is applied through the plate in an inclined position.

Locking splint: An implant (e.g., plate) acting as splint which, when somewhat loosened by interface resorption, does not allow coaptation. Therefore, when using a locking splint for fixation of a simple and adapted fracture, interfragmental displacement should be avoided to prevent bone surface resorption with consequent biological loosening of the fixation. Such loosening without possible coaptation may result in a mechanically induced non-union. This is a problem after plating, while after locked nailing the mere removal of the locking pins allows for maintenance of the splinting while gliding along the long axis of the nail is permitted.

Multifragmentary fracture: A term reserved usually for extra-articular and articular fractures which have one or more completely dissociated intermediate fragments.

Near (cis-) cortex: The cortex near the plate. In respect to bending the near cortex contributes little to stability of fixation. When – e.g., in wave plate application – the distance between the plate and the near cortex is increased, the bone and the repair tissues gain better leverage.

Neutralization: An implant (plate, external fixator, or nail) which acts based upon its stiffness is said to "neutralize" the effect of the functional load. The implant carries a major part of the functional load and thus protect, e.g., a screw fixation. It does not actually "neutralize" but does minimize the effect of the forces (see Protection).

Partial articular fracture: The fracture involves only part of the joint while the remainder remains attached to the diaphysis.

Pin loosening: The pins of external fixator frames serve to stabilize the fragments of a fracture. Stability depends, among other things, upon the contact between pin and bone. If bone surface resorption at the pin-bone interface occurs, stability is reduced. Pin loosening is less important in respect of loss of stability but is important in respect of its deleterious effect upon pin tract infection.

Prebending of plate: Exactly contoured plates produce asymmetric compression, i.e., the near cortex is more compressed than the far cortex. The latter may not be compressed at all. In respect of stabilization against torque and bending the compression of the far cortex is more important than that of the near cortex. To provide compression of the far cortex the plate is applied after exact contouring but with an additional bend of the plate segment bridging the fracture. The bend is such that the midsection of the plate is elevated from the bone surface prior to fixation to the bone. Prebending is an important tool to increase stability in small and/or porotic bones.

Precise reduction: The exact adaptation of fracture fragments (hairline adjustment). It should result in complete restoration of anatomy and optimal late function. It should be noted that overall stability does not depend on precise reduction, but precise reduction more reliably results in stability and increased strength of fixation.

Preload: The application of interfragmental compression keeps the fragments together until a tensile force exceeding the compression (preload) is applied.

Protection: While the term "neutralization" has often been used in plate and screw fixation, the term "protection" should replace it. In reality nothing is neutralized. In plate fixation the plate reduces the load placed upon the screw fixation. It therefore protects the screw fixation from overload.

Pure depression: An articular fracture in which there is only depression of the articular surface without a split.

Pure split: An articular fracture in which there is an articular split without any additional cartilaginous lesion.

Refracture: A fracture occurring after the bone has solidly bridged, at a load level otherwise tolerated by normal bone. The resulting fracture line may coincide with the original fracture line or it may be located remote from the original fracture, but within the area of bone undergoing changes due to fracture and treatment.

Relative stability: An internal fixation construct that allows small amounts of motion in proportion to the load applied. This is the case with a fixation which depends only on the stiffness of the implant (such as a nail bridging a fracture without exerting compression). It will always show deformation or displacement which is inversely proportional to the stiffness of the implant. Such motion is always present but harmless in nail fixation. According to the philosophy of the AO/ASIF group, plate fixation is more reliable if motion is prevented. (Callus as a sign of unwanted instability is then absent.)

Rigid fixation: A fixation of a fracture which allows little deformation under load.

Rigid implants: In general implants are considered to be rigid when they are made of metals. The implant geometry is more important than the stiffness of the material. Most implants made of metal are much more flexible than the corresponding bone.

Rigidity: This term is often used synonymously with stiffness. According to Timoshenko (1941) it should be used when related to shear (e.g., in the interface of plate and bone).

Simple (single) fracture: A disruption of bone (diaphyseal, extraarticular, articular) with two main fragments.

Splinting: Reducing the mobility of a fracture by coupling a stiff body to the bone fragments. The splint may be external (plaster, external fixators) or internal (internal fixation plate, intramedullary nail).

Split depression: A combination of split and depression in an articular fracture.

Spontaneous healing: The healing pattern of a fracture without treatment. Solid healing is observed in most cases but malalignment frequently results.

Stable fixation: A fixation which keeps the fragments of a fracture in motionless adaptation at least for joint movement. While a mobile fracture produces pain with any attempts to move the limb, stable fixation allows early painless mobilization. Thus stable fixation minimizes irritation, which may eventually lead to fracture disease.

Stability of fixation: This is characterized by lack of motion at the fracture site (i.e., little or no displacement between the fragments of the fracture). In technical terms, stability describes the tendency to revert to a condition of low energy.

Stiffness: The resistance of a structure to deformation. The higher the stiffness of an implant the smaller its deformation, the smaller the displacement of the fracture fragments, the smaller the straining of the repair tissue. Reduced but not abolished strain promotes healing.

Stiffness and material properties: The stiffness of a structure depends on its Young's modulus of elasticity. An increasing Young's modulus affects the deformation of the material by its first power.

Stiffness and geometrical properties: The thickness affects the deformability by its third power. Changes in geometry are therefore much more critical than the changes of material properties, a fact which is often overlooked by nonengineers. Thus, if flexible fixation is a goal, it can be achieved better by a small change of the dimensions than by using a "less rigid" material.

Strain: Relative deformation of, e.g., a repair tissue. Motion at the fracture site in itself is not the important feature, but the resulting relative deformation, which is called strain ($\delta L/L$). As strain is a relative unit (displacement of fragments divided by width of fracture gap), very high levels of strain may be present within small fracture gaps under conditions where the displacement may even not be visible. This possibility must always be considered.

Strain induction: Tissue deformation may – among other things – result in induction of callus. This is an example of a mechanically induced biological reaction. For those reactions triggered by strain, such as callus formation and bone surface resorption, a lower limit of strain, the minimum strain, is to be considered.

Strain tolerance: This determines the tolerance of the repair tissues to mechanical conditions. No tissue can be formed under conditions of strain which exceed the elongation at rupture of the tissue. Above the critical level, the straining of tissues will destroy the tissue once formed or will prevent its formation.

Strength: The ability to withstand load without structural failure. The strength of a material can be reported as ultimate tensile strength, as bending strength or as torsional strength. The local criterion for failure of bone or implants is expressed in units of force per unit of area: stress, or (equivalent) deformation per unit length; strain, or elongation at rupture.

Stress protection: This term, initially used to describe bone reaction to reduced functional load (Allgöwer et al. 1969) is used today mainly to express the negative aspects of stress relief of bone. The basic assumption is that bone deprived of necessary functional stimulation by changing mechanical load becomes less dense or strong (Wolff's law, Wolff 1893, 1986). Stress protection is often used synonymously with stress shielding, i.e., in a purely mechanical sense. It is often used to characterize bone loss – implying a negative reaction to stress shielding. With regard to internal fixation of cortical bone, stress protection seems to play a fairly unimportant role compared with vascular considerations.

The *early bone loss* which was hitherto attributed to stress protection can be explained on the basis of temporary lack of blood supply. The necrotic area then is remodeled by osteons which originate from the area with good blood supply. Remodeling goes along with temporary osteoporosis. Measurements of *late bone loss* under clinical conditions of internal fixation in the human using quantitative computed tomography show very little bone loss at the time of implant removal (Cordey et al. 1985).

In summary, bone may react to unloading but this plays a minor role in internal fixation of cortical bone fractures.

Stress shielding: When internal fixation relies upon screws and plates, according to the AO/ASIF group the stability of fixation is achieved by interfragmental compression exerted mainly by the lag screws. Such stabilization by lag screw is very stable but provides safety under functional load only in some special situations (long spiral fractures, metaphyseal fractures, etc.). A plate providing protection (or neutralization) is therefore often added. The function of such a plate is to reduce the amount of peak load applied to the screw fixation. Protection is provided based upon the stiffness of the plate. The plate shields the fractured and temporarily fixed bone.

Tension band: An implant (wire or plate) functioning according to the tension band principle: when the bone undergoes flexural load and with the implant attached to the convex surface, it carries tensile force; the bone, especially the far cortex, is then dynamically compressed. The plate is able to resist very large amounts of tensile force, while the bone best resists compressive load.

Vascularity: A tissue is vascularized if it contains blood vessels connected to the main circulatory system. Blood vessels may be shut off temporarily from the circulatory system. We consider a tissue to be nonvascular if there are no vessels, as in cartilage, or if the vessels present are not functioning, e.g., obliterated by thrombosis.

Wedge fracture: Fracture with a third fragment in which after reduction there is some direct contact between the main fragments.

References

Aeberhard HJ (1973) Der Einfluß der Platten-Überbiegung auf die Torsionsstabilität der Osteosynthese. Inaugural dissertation, University of Bern

Allgöwer M (1978) Cinderella of surgery – fractures? Surg Clin North Am 58:1071–1093

Allgöwer M, Ehrsam R, Ganz R, Matter P, Perren SM (1969) Clinical experience with a new compression plate "DCP". Acta Orthop Scand [Suppl] 125:45–63

Anderson R (1936) Femoral bone lengthening. Am J Surg 31:479

Ashhurst DE (1986) The influence of mechanical conditions on the healing of experimental fractures in the rabbit. A microscopical study. Phil Trans R Soc Lond 313:271–302

Bagby GW, James JM (1957) An impacting bone plate. Staff meeting, Mayo Clinic 32:55–57

Barraud GE (1982) De la stabilité des osteotomies spiroides in vitro fixées par différents vissages avec ou sans plaque de protection. Inaugural dissertation, University of Bern

Beaupre GS, Schneider E, Perren SM (1984) Stress analysis of a partially slotted intramedullary nail. J Orthop Res 2:369–376

Behrens F (1982) Personal communication

Behrens F (1989) General theory and principle of external fixation. Clin Orthop 241:15–23

Behrens F, Searls K (1986) External fixation of the tibia. Basis concepts and prospective evaluation. J Bone Joint Surg [Br] 68:246–254

Bier A (1918) Beobachtungen über die Regeneration beim Menschen. Dtsch Med Wochenschr 44:281–284

Biliouris T, Schneider E, Rahn BA, Gasser B, Perren SM (1989) The effect of radial preload on the implant-bone interface: a cadaveric study. J Orthop Trauma 3:323–332

Blümlein H, Cordey J, Schneider UA, Rahn BA, Perren SM (1977) Langzeitmessung der Axialkraft von Knochenschrauben in vivo. Med Orthop Tech 97:17–19

Böhler L (1938) Technik der Knochenbruchbehandlung. Maudrich, Wien

Border J, Allgöwer M, Hansen T, Rüedi T (1990) Blunt multiple trauma: comprehensive pathophysiology and care. Dekker, New York

Brennwald J (1976) Personal communication (see also Stadler et al. 1982)

Brennwald J, Matter P, von Arx C, Cordey J, Perren SM (1975) Peroperative Messung des Drehmomentes an Knochenschrauben. Unfallmed Berufskr 3:123–126

Brunner CF, Weber BG (1981) Besondere Osteosynthesetechniken. Springer, Berlin Heidelberg New York

Brunner U, Schweiberer L, Cordey J, Rahn B, Perren SM (1990) Treatment of large bone defects using segment bone transportation with nail fixation: experimental study. Transactions of 36th Annual Meeting of ORS, New Orleans

Brunner U, Kessler S, Cordey J, Rahn B, Schweiberer L, Perren SM (1990) Defektbehandlung langer Röhrenknochen durch Distraktionsosteogenese (Ilizarov) und Marknagelung. Theoretische Grundlagen, tierexperimentelle Ergebnisse, klinische Relevanz. Unfallchirurg 93:244–250

Brutscher R, Rueter A, Perren SM (1989) Der Stellenwert der Corticotomie und Osteotomie nach Segmentverschiebung bei der Behandlung von Knochendefekten. 53. Jahrestagung, Deutsche Gesellschaft für Unfallheilkunde, Berlin

Claes L, Burri C, Kinzl L, Fitzer E, Hüttner W (1980) Less rigid fixation with carbon fibre reinforced materials: mechanical characteristics and behavior in vivo. In: Uhthoff HK, Stahl E (eds) Current concepts of internal fixation of fractures. Springer, Berlin Heidelberg New York, pp 156–159

Claes L, Palme U, Palme E, Kirschbaum U (1982) Biomechanical and mathematical investigations concerning stress protection of bone beneath internal fixation plates. In: Huiskes R, van Campen DH, de Vijn JR (eds) Biomechanics: principles and applications. Martinus Nijhoff, The Hague, pp 325–330

Claudi B, Schläpfer F, Cordey J, Perren SM, Allgöwer M (1979) Die schräge Plattenzugschraube – In-vitro-Messungen der Stabilität an queren Osteotomien des Tibiaschaftes. Helv Chir Acta 46:177–182

Cochran GVB (1969) Effects of internal fixation plates on mechanical deformation of bone. Surg Forum Orthop Surg 20:469–471

Cordey J (1987) Analyse mécanique de l'ostéosynthèse par plaque. PhD thesis, Faculté des Sciences de l'Université de Lausanne

Cordey J, Schnetzer M, Brennwald J, Regazzoni P, Perren SM (1980) Direct in vivo measurements of torque and bending in sheep tibiae. In: Uhthoff HK, Stahl E (eds) Current concepts of internal fixation of fractures. Springer, Berlin Heidelberg New York, 78–87

Cordey J, Schwyzer HK, Brun S, Matter P (1985) Bone loss following plate fixation of fractures? Helv Chir Acta 52:181–184

Cordey J, Perren SM, Steinemann S (1987) Parametric analysis of the stress protection in bone after plating. In: Bergmann G, Kölbel R, Rohlmann A (eds) Biomechanics: basic and applied research. Martinus Nijhoff, Dordrecht, pp 387–392

Coutts RE, Akeson WH, Woo S, Matthews JV, Gonsalves M, Amiel D (1976) Comparison of stainless steel and composite plates in the healing of diaphyseal osteotomies of the dog radius: report on a short term study. Orthop Clin North Am 7:223–229

Craig J: Unpublished work from the Laboratory for Experimental Surgery, Davos, Switzerland

Danckwardt-Lilliestrom G, Grevsten S, Olerud S (1972) Investigation of effect of various agents on periosteal bone formation. Ups J Med Sci 77:125–128

Danis R (1947) The operative treatment of bone fractures. J Int Chir 7:318–320

Danis R (1979) Théorie et pratique de l'ostéosynthèse. Masson, Paris

Diehl K (1975) Stabilität und Beanspruchung von Osteosynthesen des Ober- und Unterschenkels bei der Frühmobilisation. Unfallheilkunde 79:81–89

Eisner HP, Barraud GE, Johner RT, Cordey J (1985) Optimal insertion of lag screws for internal fixation of spiral fracture of the tibia. Biomechanics 1:543

Fernández Dell'Oca AA (1989) Modular external fixation in emergency with the AO tubular system. Intergraf, Montevideo

Ganz R, Brennwald J (1987) L'ostéosynthèse à compression du tibia du lapin. Etude de la revascularisation du canal medullaire et de la corticale sous fixation stable. In: Boitzy A (ed) Ostéogenèse et compression. Huber, Bern, pp 166–173

Ganz R, Perren SM, Rüter A (1975) Mechanical induction of bone resorption. Fortschr Kiefer Gesichtschir 19:45–48

Gasser B (1989) Personal communication. ME Müller Institut für Biomechanik, Bern, Switzerland

Gautier E (1988) Belastungsveränderung des Knochens durch Plattenosteosynthese. Dissertation, University of Bern

Gautier E, Cordey J, Lüthi U, Mathys R, Rahn BA, Perren SM (1983) Knochenumbau nach Verplattung: biologische oder mechanische Ursache? Helv Chir Acta 50:53–58

Gautier E, Cordey J, Mathys R, Rahn BA, Perren SM (1984) Porosity and remodelling of plated bone after internal fixation: result of stress shielding or vascular damage? Elsevier Science, Amsterdam
Gautier E, Rahn BA, Perren SM (1986) Effect of steel versus composite plastic plates on internal and external remodeling of intact long bones. Orthop Trans 10:391
Genge M, Schneider E, Michel MC, Genge H, Perren SM (1988) Hochauflösende implantierbare Telemetrie-Anlage für statische Belastungsmessungen. European Telemetry Conference. Döring-Druck, Braunschweig, pp 288–296
Goodship AE, Kenwright J (1985) The influence of induced micromovement upon the healing of experimental fractures. J Bone Joint Surg [Br] 67:650–655
Gotzen L, Huetter J, Haas N (1980) The prebending of AO plates in compression osteosynthesis. In: Uhthoff HK, Stahl E (eds) Current concepts of internal fixation of fractures. Springer, Berlin Heidelberg New York, pp 201–210
Gotzen L, Haas N, Strohfeld G (1981) Zur Biomechanik der Plattenosteosynthese. Unfallheilkunde 84:439–443
Gunst MA, Suter C, Rahn BA (1979) Die Knochendurchblutung nach Plattenosteosynthese. Helv Chir Acta 46:171–175
Haas N, Gotzen L, Riefenstahl L (1985) Biomechanische Untersuchungen zur Plattenfixation an die Hauptfragmente. Orthopedics 123:591
Hayes WC (1980) Basic biomechanics of compression plate fixation. In: Uhthoff HK, Stahl E (eds) Current concepts of internal fixation of fractures. Springer, Berlin Heidelberg New York, pp 49–62
Hayes WC, Perren SM (1971) Flexural rigidity of compression plate fixation of fractures. Proceedings, Second Nordic Conference on Medical and Biological Engineering, pp 242–244
Heini PF (1988) Untersuchungen der Tibia-Innenform im Zusammenhang mit der Marknagelung. Inaugural dissertation, University of Bern
Heitemeyer U, Hierholzer G (1985) Die überbrückende Osteosynthese bei geschlossenen Stückfrakturen des Femurschaftes. Akt Traumatol 15:205–209
Helfet DL, DiPasquale TG, Howey TD, Sanders R, Zinar D, Popman D, Brooker A (1990) The treatment of open and/or unstable tibial fractures with an unreamed double-locked tibial nail. AAOS, New Orleans
Hente R (1989) Personal communication
Hertel R (1984) Beanspruchung von Osteosyntheseplatten mit schraubenfreiem Plattenloch. Inaugural dissertation, University of Bern
Hoffmann R, Krettek C, Haas N, Tscherne H (1989) Die distale Radiusfraktur. Frakturstabilisierung mit biodegradablen Osteosynthese-Stiften (Biofix). Experimentelle Untersuchungen und erste klinische Erfahrungen. Unfallchirurg 92:430–434
Huiskes R, Chao EYS, Crippen TE (1985) Parametric analyses of pin-bone stresses in external fracture fixation devices. J Orthop Res 3:341–349
Hutzschenreuter P, Perren SM, Steinemann S, Geret V, Klebl M (1969) Some effects of rigidity of internal fixation on the healing pattern of osteotomies. Injury 1:77–81
Hyldahl C, Pearson S, Tepic S, Perren SM (1988) Induction and prevention of pin loosening in external fixators in the sheep tibia. Orthop Trans 12:378
Ilizarov GA (1989) The tension-stress effect on the genesis and growth of tissues. Clin Orthop 238:249–281
Jörger KA (1987) Akute intrakortikale Durchblutungsstörung unter Osteosyntheseplatten mit unterschiedlichen Auflageflächen. Inaugural dissertation, University of Bern
Johner RT, Joerger K, Cordey J, Perren SM (1989) Rigidity of pure lag-screw fixation as a function of screw inclination in an in vitro spiral osteotomy. Clin Orthop 178:74–79
Kempf I, Grosse A, Lafforgue D (1978) L'apport du verouillage dans l'enclouage centro-medullaire des os longs. Rev Chir Orthop 64:635–651
Kessler SB, Perren SM, Hallfeldt KKJ, Madelkow H (1988) Refrakturen nach operativer Frakturenbehandlung. Biologische Aspekte. Hefte Unfallheilkd 194:13–27
Kirschner M (1916) Die künstliche Verlängerung von Beinen, die nach Frakturen, namentlich nach Schußfrakturen, mit starker Verkürzung geheilt sind. Beitr Klin Chir 100:329–370
Klaue K (1982) The Dynamic Compression Unit (DCU) for stable internal fixation of bone fractures. Dissertation, University of Basel
Klaue K, Perren SM (1982) Fixation interne des fractures par l'ensemble plaque-vis à compression conjuguée (DCU). Helv Chir Acta 49:77–80
Klaue K, Frigg R, Perren SM (1985) Die Entlastung der Osteosyntheseplatte durch interfragmentäre Plattenzugschraube. Helv Chir Acta 52:19–23
Klein MPM (1990) Aufbohren oder nicht Aufbohren? Zirkulationsstörung durch Marknagelung an der Hundetibia. Dissertation, University of Basel

Klein M, Rahn BA, Frigg R, Kessler S, Perren SM (1989) Die Blutzirkulation nach Marknagelung ohne Aufbohren. Proceedings, Berhard Küntscher Kreis, Vienna

Knets IV, Pfafrod GO, Saulgozis JZ (1980) Deformation of hard biological tissue (in Russian). Zinatne, Riga

Korcinek K (1989) Personal communication

Krompecher S, Kerner E (1979) Callus formation. Symposium on the biology of fracture healing. Academiai Kiado, Budapest

Küntscher G (1970) Das Kallus-Problem. Enke, Stuttgart

Küntscher GA, Klemm KA, Schellmann WDA (1972) Locking of the intramedullary nail with threaded bolts. SICOT 12:33

Lane WA (1913) The operative treatment of fractures. Medical Publishing, London

Lanyon LE, Rubin CT (1985) Functional adaptation in skeletal structures. Belknap Press, Harvard University Press, Cambridge, Mass, pp 1–25

Latta LL, Sarmiento A, Tarr RR (1980) The rationale of functional bracing of fractures. Clin Orthop 146:28–36

Leu D, Bilat C, Rüedi T (1989) Refrakturen nach Metallentfernung. Eine Nachkontrolle von operierten Tibiafrakturen. Unfallchirurg 92:399–400

Lucas-Championnière J (1907) Les dangers de l'immobilisation des membres – fragilité des os – altération de la nutrition du membre – conclusions pratiques. Rev Méd Chir Pratique 78:81–87

Lüthi UK, Rahn BA, Perren SM (1982) Implants and intracortical vascular disturbances. 28th Annual ORS Meeting, p 337

Mast J, Jakob R, Ganz R (1989) Planning and reduction techniques in fracture surgery. Springer, Berlin Heidelberg New York

Mathys R, Cotting A (1986) USA patent, 4, 628, 920

Matter P, Brennwald J, Perren SM (1974) Biologische Reaktion des Knochens auf Osteosyntheseplatten. Helv Chir Acta [Suppl] 12:1

Michel M (1990) Die klinische Anwendung der Marknagel-Telemetrie. Dissertation, University of Bern

Moor R, Tepic S, Perren SM (1989) Hochgeschwindigkeits-Film-Analyse des Knochenbruchs. Z Unfallchir 82:128–132

Moyen BJ, Lahey PJ, Weinberg EH, Harris WH (1978) Effects on intact femora of dog of the application and removal of metal plates. J Bone Joint Surg [Am] 60:940–947

Müller KH, Witzel U (1984) Die Brückenplatte zur Osteosynthese bei ossären Schaftdefekten des Femur nach Fehlschlägen von Plattenosteosynthesen. Unfallheilkunde 87:1–10

Müller ME, Allgöwer M, Willenegger H (1963) Technik der operativen Frakturenbehandlung. Springer, Berlin

Müller ME, Schneider R, Allgöwer M (1984) 25 Jahre Schweizerische Arbeitsgemeinschaft für Osteosynthesefragen (AO). Swiss Med 6:51–54

Pauwels F (1958) Über die therapeutische Anwendung neuer Erkenntnisse auf dem Gebiet der funktionellen Anatomie bei Erkrankungen des Stütz- und Bewegungsapparates. Aschoff Vorlesung, Freiburg i. Breisgau

Pauwels F (1965) Gesammelte Abhandlungen zur funktionellen Anatomie des Bewegungsapparates. Springer, Berlin Heidelberg New York

Pauwels F (1980) Biomechanics of the locomotor apparatus. Springer, Berlin Heidelberg New York

Perren SM (1971) Biomécanique de la compression interfragmentaire. In: Boitzy A (ed) Ostéogenès et compression. Huber, Bern, pp 136–145

Perren SM, Boitzy A (1978) La différenciation cellulaire et la biomécanique de l'os. Anat Clin 1:13–28

Perren SM, Cordey J (1977) Die Gewebsdifferenzierung in der Frakturheilung. Monatsschr Unfallheilkd 80:161–164

Perren SM, Cordey J (1980) The concept of interfragmentary strain. In: Uhthoff HK, Stahl E (eds) Current concepts of internal fixation of fractures. Springer, Berlin Heidelberg New York, pp 63–77

Perren SM, Huggler A, Russenberger M, Straumann F, Müller SM, Allgöwer M (1969a) Cortical bone healing. A method of measuring the change in compression applied to living cortical bone. Acta Orthop Scand [Suppl] 125:5–16

Perren SM, Huggler A, Russenberger M, Allgöwer M, Mathys R, Schenk R, Willenegger H, Müller ME (1969b) Cortical bone healing. The reaction of cortical bone to compression. Acta Orthop Scand [Suppl] 125:17–28

Perren SM, Russenberger M, Steinemann S, Müller ME, Allgöwer M (1969c) A dynamic compression plate. Acta Orthop Scand [Suppl] 125:31–41

Perren SM, Hayes WC, Eliasson E (1974) Biomechanik der Plattenosteosynthese. Med Orthop Tech 94:56–61

Perren SM, Ganz R, Rüter A (1975) Oberflächliche Knochenresorption um Implantate. Med Orthop Tech 95:6–10

Perren SM, Rahn BA, Lüthi U, Gunst MA, Pfister U (1981) Aseptische Knochennektrose: sequestrierender Umbau? Orthopäde 10:3–5

Perren SM, Klaue K, Frigg R, Predieri M, Tepic S (in prep) The concept of biological plating: the limited-contact dynamic compression plate, LC-DCP. Orthop Trauma

Pfister U (1983) Biomechanische und histologische Untersuchungen nach Marknagelung der Tibia. Fortschr Med 101 (37):1652–1659

Putti V (1918) La trazione per doppia infissione d l'allungamento operative dell'arto inferiore. Chir Org Mov, vol II:421

Rahn BA (1987) Direct and indirect bone healing after operative fracture treatment. Otolaryngol Clin North Am 20:425–440

Rahn BA, Perren SM (1975) Die mehrfarbige Fluoreszenzmarkierung des Knochenanbaus. Chem Rundschau 29:12–15

Rahn BA, Gallinaro P, Schenk R, Baltensperger A, Perren SM (1971) Compression interfragmentaire et surcharge locale de l'os. In: Boitzy A (ed) Ostéogenèse et compression. Huber, Bern, pp 146–153

Rahn BA, Bacellar FC, Trapp L, Perren SM (1980) Methode zur Fluoreszenz – Morphometrie des Knochenanbaus. Aktuel Traumatol 10:109–115

Regazzoni P (1982) Osteosynthesen an Röhrenknochen: technische und biologische Untersuchungen zur Stabilität und Heilung. Habilitationsschrift, University of Zürich

Regazzoni P (1989) Das Ilizarov-Konzept mit einem modularen Rohrfixateur. Operat Orthop Traumatol 1:90–93

Rhinelander FW (1978) Physiology of bone from the vascular viewpoint. Society for Biomaterials, San Antonio, Texas 2:24–26

Rhinelander FW, Wilson JW (1982) Blood supply in developing mature and healing bone. In: Summer-Smith G (ed) Bone in clinical orthopaedics. Saunders, Philadelphia

Rokkanen P, Böstman O, Vainionpää S, Vihtonen K, Törmälä P, Laiho J, Kilpikari J, Tamminmäki M (1985) Biodegradable implants in fracture fixation: early results of treatment of fractures of the ankle. Lancet 1:1422–1424

Rüter A, Brutscher R (1988) Die Behandlung ausgedehnter Knochendefekte am Unterschenkel durch die Verschiebeosteotomie nach Ilizarov. Chirurg 59:357–359

Sarmiento A (1980) Nichtoperative funktionelle Frakturbehandlung. Springer, Berlin Heidelberg New York

Schatzker J, Tile M (1987) The rationale of operative fracture care. Springer, Berlin Heidelberg New York

Schenk RK, Willenegger H (1963) Zum histologischen Bild der sogenannten Primärheilung der Knochenkompakta nach experimentellen Osteotomien am Hund. Experientia 19:593

Schenk R (1987) Cytodynamics and histodynamics of primary bone repair. In: Lane JM (ed) Fracture healing. Churchill Livingstone, New York

Schneider E, Genge M, Wyder D, Mathys R Jr, Perren SM (1988) Telemetrized interlocking nail for in vivo load determination in the human femur. European Telemetry Conference. Döring-Druck, Braunschweig, pp 272–279

Stadler J, Brennwald J, Frigg R, Perren SM (1982) Induction of bone surface resorption by motion. An in vivo study using passive and active implants. Second International Symposium on Internal Fixation of Fractures, Lyon, pp 62–64

Steinemann SG (1977) Corrosion of implants – in vivo and in vitro tests. Société Européenne pour les biomatériaux

Steinemann SG, Mäusli PA (1988) Titanium alloys for surgical implants – biocompatibility from physicochemical principles. Sixth World Conference on Titanium, Cannes

Tayton K, Johnson-Nurse C, McKibbin B, Bradley J, Hastings G (1982) The use of semi-rigid carbon fibre reinforced plastic plates for fixation of human fractures. J Bone Joint Surg [Br] 64:105

Tepic S (1989) Personal communication

Timoshenko S (1941) Strength of materials. van Nostrand, Princeton

Timoshenko S (1968) Résistance des matériaux. Dunod, Paris

Tonino AJ, Davidson CL, Klopper PJ, Linclau LA (1976) Protection from stress in bone and its effects. Experiments with stainless steel and plastic plates in dogs. J Bone Joint Surg [Br] 58:107–113

Uhthoff HK, Dubuc FL (1971) Bone structure changes in the dog under rigid internal fixation. Clin Orthop 81:165–170

Vattolo M (1986) Der Einfluß von Rillen in Osteosyntheseplatten auf den Umbau der Kortikalis. Dissertation, University of Bern

von Arx C (1975) Schubübertragung durch Reibung bei Plattenosteosynthesen. AO-Bulletin, pp 1–34

von Recum AF (ed) (1986) Handbook of biomaterials evaluation (section on intra vitam staining techniques). Macmillan, New York
Weber BG Personal communication
Weber BG, Brunner C (1981) The treatment of nonunions without electrical stimulation. Clin Orthop 161:24–32
Weber BG, Cech O (1973) Pseudarthrosen. Pathophysiologie – Biomechanik – Therapie – Ergebnisse. Huber, Bern
Winquist RA, Hansen ST, Clawson DK (1984) Closed intramedullary nailing of femoral fractures. A report of five hundred and twenty cases. J Bone Joint Surg [Am] 66:529–539
Wiss DA, Segal D, Gumbs VL, Salter D (1986) Flexible medullary nailing of tibial shaft fractures. J Trauma 26:1106–1112
Wolff J (1892) Das Gesetz der Transformation der Knochen. Hirschwald, Berlin
Wolff J (1986) The law of bone remodelling. Springer, Berlin Heidelberg New York
Woo SLY, Akeson WH, Coutts RD, Rutherford L, Jemmott GF, Amiel D (1976) A comparison of cortical bone atrophy secondary to fixation with plates with large differences in bending stiffness. J Bone Joint Surg [Am] 58:190–195
Yamada H, Evans FG (1970) Strength of biological materials. Williams and Wilkins, Baltimore
Zuber K, Schneider E, Eulenberger J, Perren SM (1988) Form und Dimension der Markhöhle menschlicher Femora in Hinblick auf die Marknagelung. Unfallchirurg 91:314–319

Appendix A
The Comprehensive Classification of Fractures of Long Bones

"A classification is useful only if it considers the severity of the bone lesion and serves as a basis for treatment and for evaluation of the results."

MAURICE E. MÜLLER

The Principle of the Classification

The fundamental principle of this classification is the division of all fractures of a bone segment into three types and their further subdivision into three groups and their subgroups, and the arrangement of these in an ascending order of severity according to the morphologic complexities of the fracture, the difficulties inherent in their treatment, and their prognosis.

Which type? ... Which group? ... Which subgroup? ... These three questions, and the three possible answers to each, are the key to the classification.

The *3 types* are labelled A, B and C. Each type is divided into *3 groups:* A1, A2, A3; B1, B2, B3; C1, C2, C3. Thus there are 9 groups. As each group is further subdivided into *3 subgroups*, denoted by a number .1, .2, .3, there are 27 subgroups for each segment. The subgroups represent the 3 characteristic variations within the group.

The colours green, orange, and red, as well as the *darkening arrows,* indicate the *increasing severity:* A1 indicates the simplest fracture with the best prognosis and C3 the most difficult fracture with the worst prognosis. Thus when one has classified a fracture one has established its severity and obtained a guide to its best possible treatment.

For further details regarding the subgroups and qualifications of the classification please refer to: *The Comprehensive Classification of Fractures of Long Bones*. M.E. Müller, S. Nazarian, P. Koch, J. Schatzker. Springer-Verlag, Berlin-Heidelberg-New York, 1990

Fig. 1 The principle of the classification represented schematically.

Fig. 1

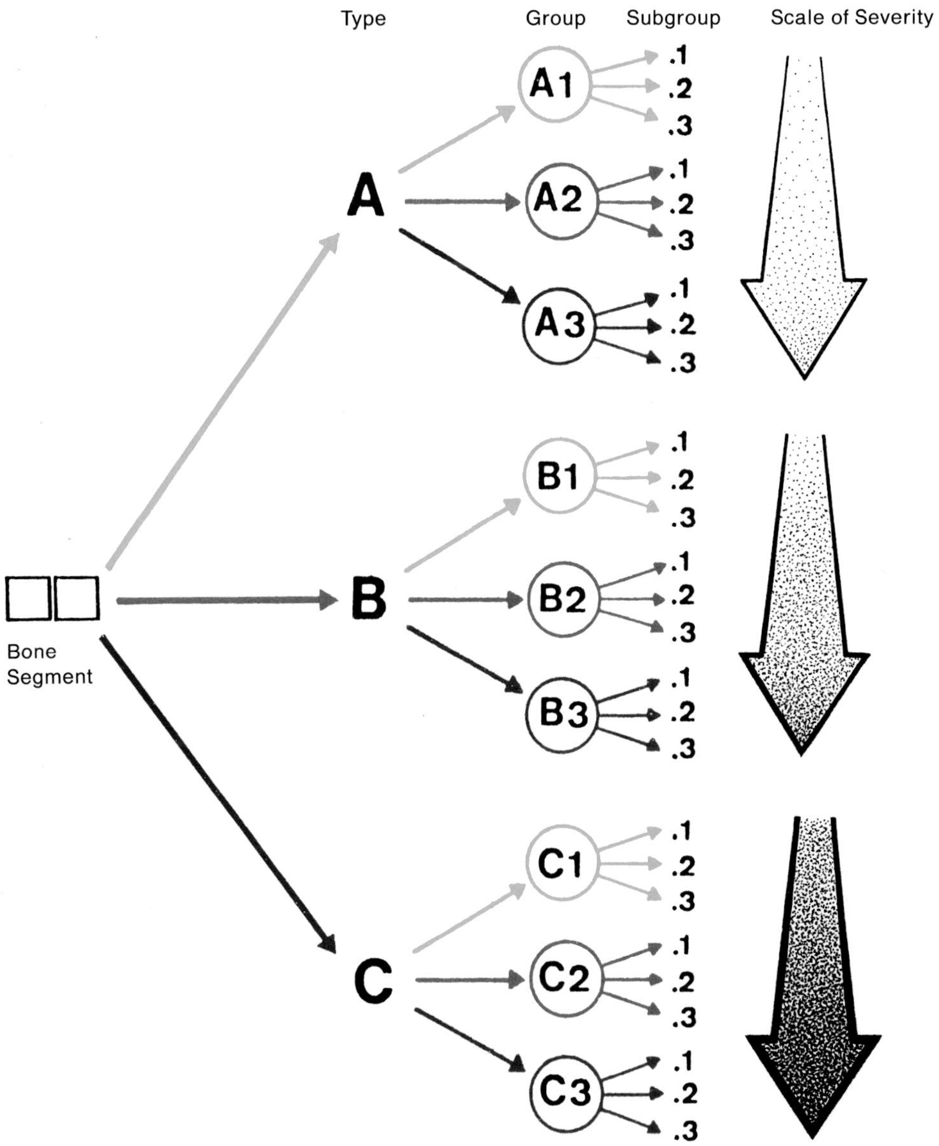

Type Group Subgroup Scale of Severity

A
A1 .1 .2 .3
A2 .1 .2 .3
A3 .1 .2 .3

B
B1 .1 .2 .3
B2 .1 .2 .3
B3 .1 .2 .3

C
C1 .1 .2 .3
C2 .1 .2 .3
C3 .1 .2 .3

Bone Segment

The Anatomic Location

This is designated by two numbers, one for the bone and one for its segment.

The Long Bones

Ulna and radius, and tibia and fibula are each considered as one bone. Therefore we have four long bones.

1 = humerus, 2 = radius/ulna, 3 = femur, 4 = tibia/fibula

The Bone Segments

Each long bone has three segments: the proximal, the diaphyseal, and the distal segment (Fig. 2). The malleolar segment is an exception and is classified as the fourth segment of the tibia/fibula (44-).

The segments are designated by numbers: 1 = the proximal, 2 = the middle, and 3 = the distal segment.

The proximal and distal segments of long bones are each defined by a square whose sides are the same length as the widest part of the epiphysis (exceptions: 31- and 44-).

Before a fracture can be assigned to a segment, one must first determine its center. In a simple fracture the center is at the level of the broadest part of the wedge. In a complex fracture the center can only be determined after reduction.

Any fracture associated with a displaced articular component is classified as an articular fracture. If the fracture is associated only with an undisplaced fissure which reaches the joint, it is classified as metaphyseal or diaphyseal depending on the location of its center.

Remark:
A long bone is usually divided into two epiphyseal, two metaphyseal, and one diaphyseal segment. In this classification the metaphysis and the epiphysis are considered as one segment because the morphology of the fracture in the metaphysis influences the treatment and the prognosis of the articular fracture. To determine the limit between the diaphyseal and the proximal and distal segment, the above-mentioned system of squares is applied.

Fig. 2 The numbering of all bones or bone groups. The four long bones are specified with a circle.

Fig. 3 The segments of the four long bones. The proximal and distal segments are defined by a square (exception: proximal femur).

Fig. 2

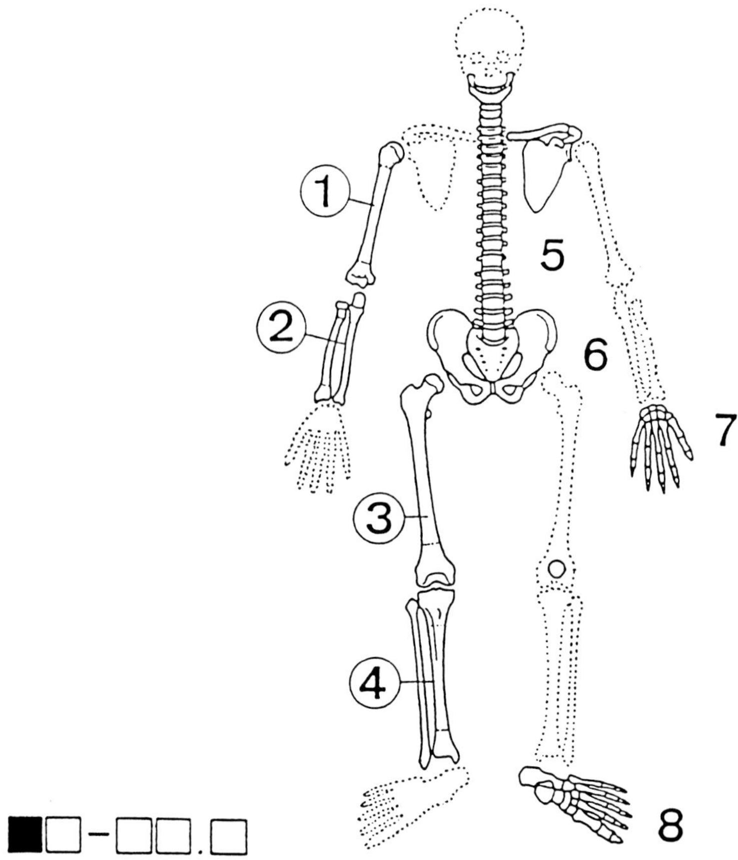
1
2
3
4
5
6
7
8

Fig. 3

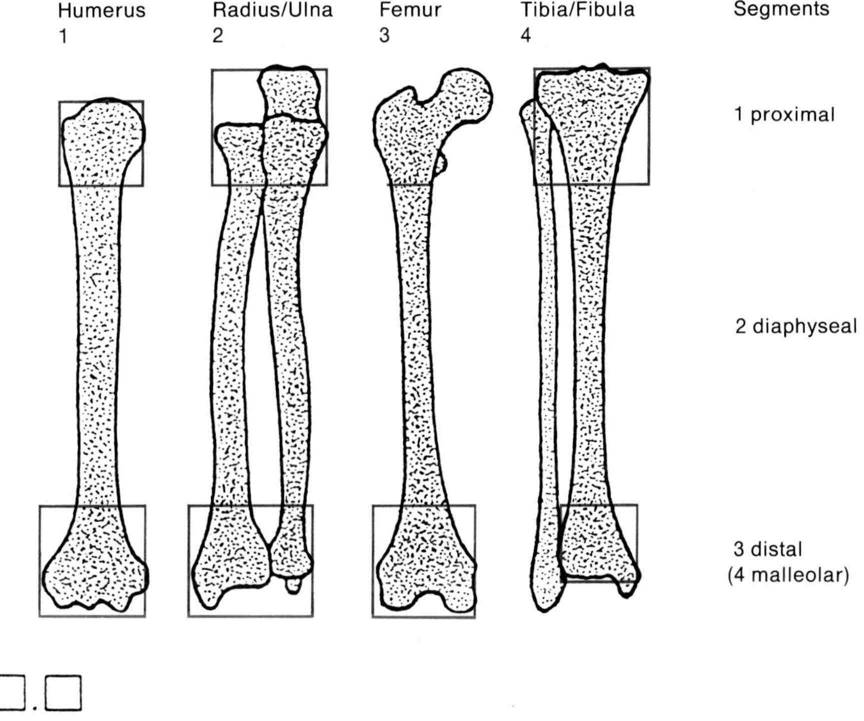
Humerus
1
Radius/Ulna
2
Femur
3
Tibia/Fibula
4
Segments
1 proximal
2 diaphyseal
3 distal
(4 malleolar)

The Fracture Types

Diaphyseal Segment

All fractures of the diaphyseal segment (see Glossary) are either "simple" (type A) or "multifragmentary". Multifragmentary fractures are either "wedge" fractures (type B) or "complex" fractures (type C).

Proximal and Distal Segments

In the proximal and distal segments the fractures are either "extra-articular" (type A) or "articular". The articular fractures are either "partial articular" (type B) or "complete articular" (type C).

The 3 *exceptions* are: the *proximal humerus* (A = extra-articular unifocal, B = extra-articular bifocal, and C = articular), the *proximal femur* (A = trochanteric area, B = neck, C = head), and the *malleolar segment* (A = infrasyndesmotic, B = transsyndesmotic, and C = suprasyndesmotic).

The Coding of the Diagnosis

The diagnosis of a fracture is obtained by combining its anatomic location with its morphological characteristic.

The answers to the questions "Where?" ... and "What?" ... are the key to the diagnosis.

An alpha-numeric coding system was chosen to express the diagnosis in order to facilitate computer storage and retrieval. Two numbers are used to express the location of the fracture. These are followed by a letter and two numbers which express the morphological characteristics of the fracture (Fig. 5).

Example of the coding of a fracture of a diaphyseal segment: 32-B2.1

3	2-	B	2	.1
Femur	diaphysis	wedge fracture	bending wedge	subtro-chanteric

Example of the coding of a fracture of a distal segment: 33-C3.2

3	3-	C	3	.2
Femur	distal	complete articular fracture	multi-fragmentary	metaphyseal multi-fragmentary

---

Fig. 4 The fracture types of the diaphyseal (A = simple, B = wedge, C = complex) and of most of the proximal and distal segments (A = extra-articular, B = partial articular, C = complete articular) of long bones.

Fig. 5 Alpha-numeric coding of the diagnosis (= location + morphological characteristic).

Fig. 4

A
B
C
A
B
C

Fig. 5

Diagnosis
where?
what?
Bone
1 2 3 4
Segment
1 2 3 (4)
Type
A B C
Group
1 2 3
Sub-
group
.1 .2 .3

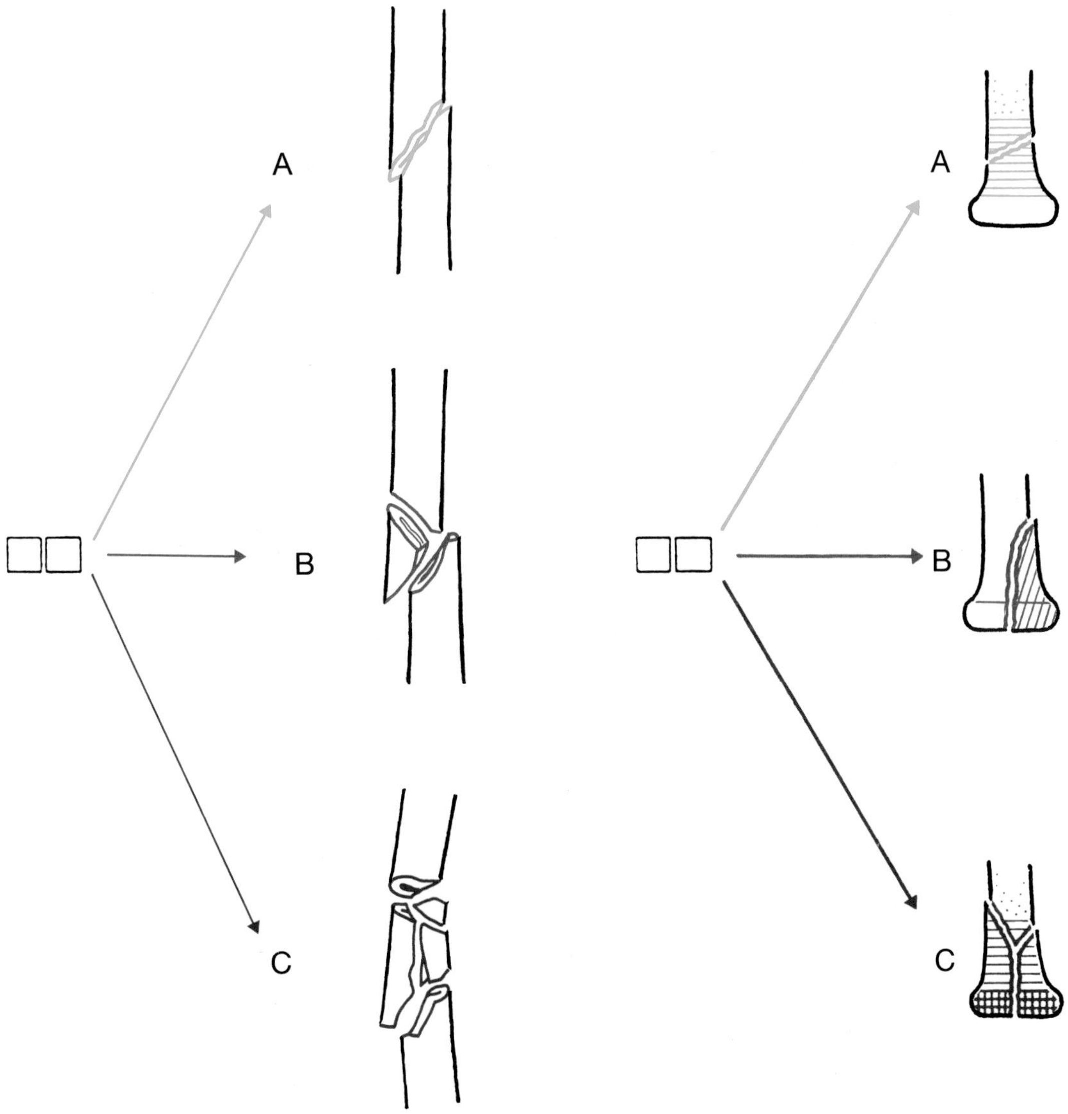

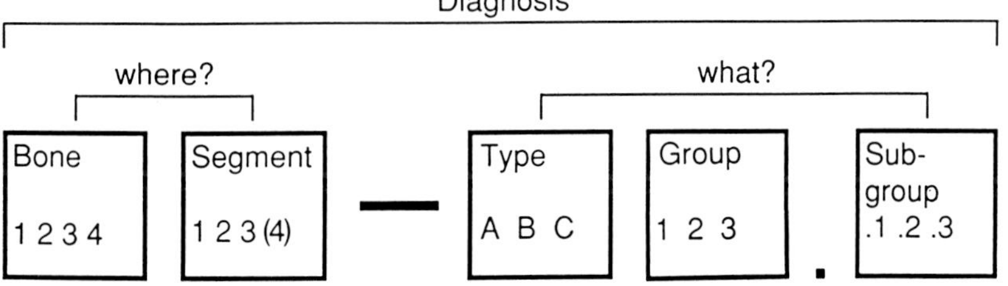

11- Humerus Proximal

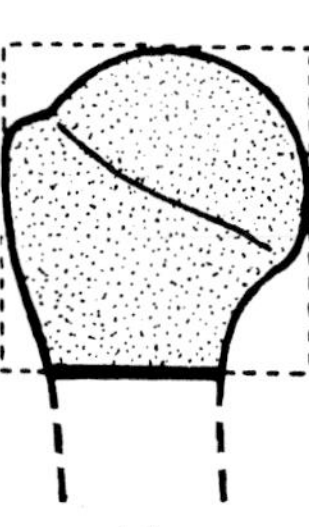

A = Extra-articular unifocal fracture

-A1 Extra-articular unifocal fracture, tuberosity
- .1 greater tuberosity, not displaced
- (.2) greater tuberosity, displaced
- .3 with a glenohumeral dislocation

-A2 Extra-articular unifocal fracture, impacted metaphyseal
- .1 without frontal malalignment
- (.2) with varus malalignment
- .3 with valgus malalignment

-A3 Extra-articular unifocal fracture, non-impacted metaphyseal
- .1 simple, with angulation
- (.2) simple, with translation
- .3 multifragmentary

B = Extra-articular bifocal fracture

-B1 Extra-articular bifocal fracture, with metaphyseal impaction
- (.1) lateral + greater tuberosity
- .2 medial + lesser tuberosity
- .3 posterior + greater tuberosity

-B2 Extra-articular bifocal fracture, without metaphyseal impaction
- .1 without rotatory displacement of the epiphyseal fragment
- (.2) with rotatory displacement of the epiphyseal fragment
- .3 multifragmentary metaphyseal + one of the tuberosities

-B3 Extra-articular bifocal fracture, with glenohumeral dislocation
- .1 "vertical" cervical line + greater tuberosity intact + anterior and medial dislocation
- (.2) "vertical" cervical line + greater tuberosity fractured + anterior and medial dislocation
- .3 lesser tuberosity fractured + posterior dislocation

C = Articular fracture

-C1 Articular fracture, with slight displacement
- (.1) cephalotubercular, with valgus malalignment
- .2 cephalotubercular, with varus malalignment
- .3 anatomical neck

-C2 Articular fracture, impacted with marked displacement
- (.1) cephalotubercular, with valgus malalignment
- .2 cephalotubercular, with varus malalignment
- .3 transcephalic and tubercular, with varus malalignment

-C3 Articular fracture, dislocated
- .1 anatomical neck
- (.2) anatomical neck and tuberosities
- .3 cephalotubercular fragmentation

The subgroup illustrated is indicated by ◯ in the text.

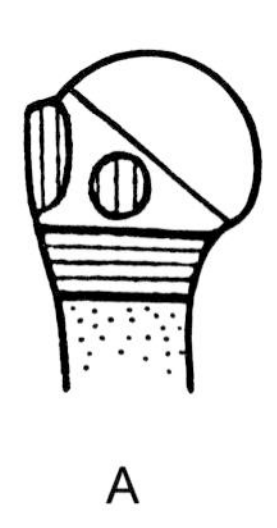
A

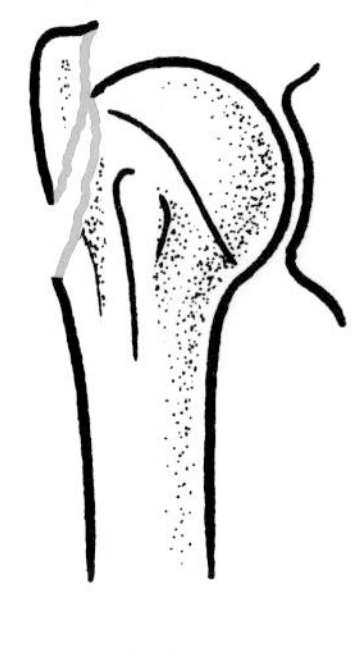
A1

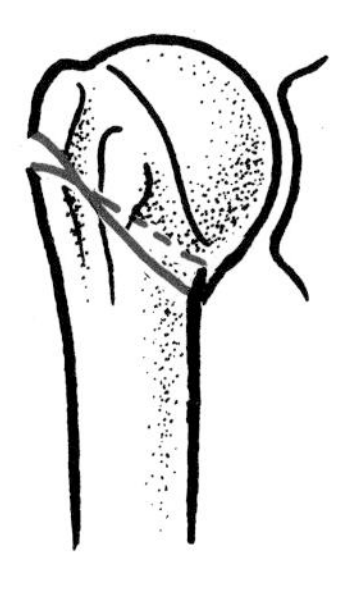
A2

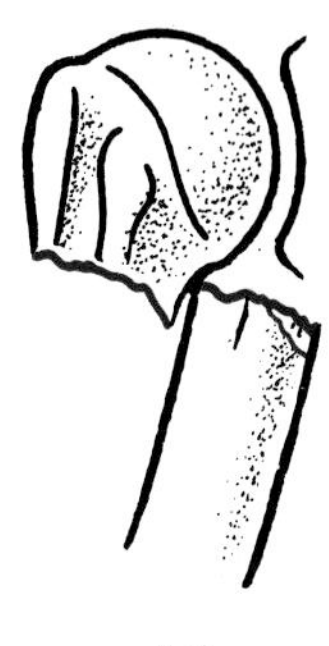
A3

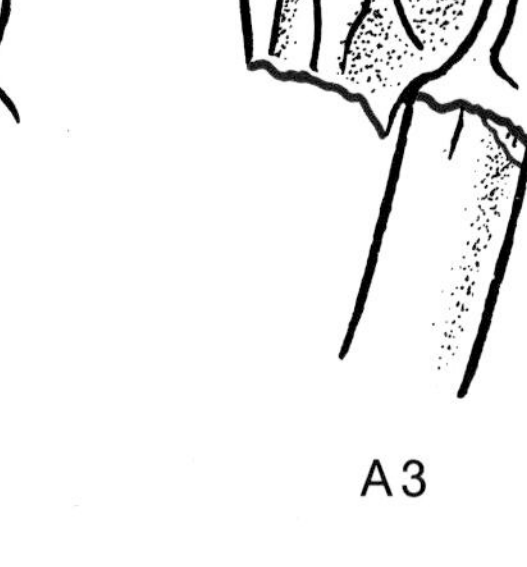

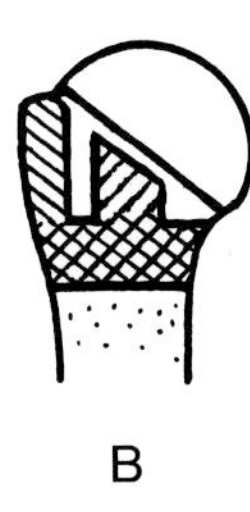
B

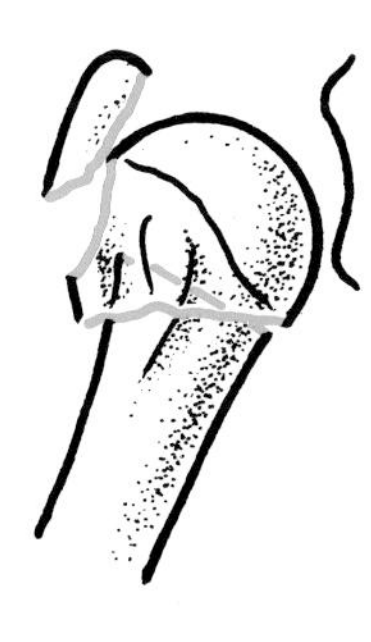
B1

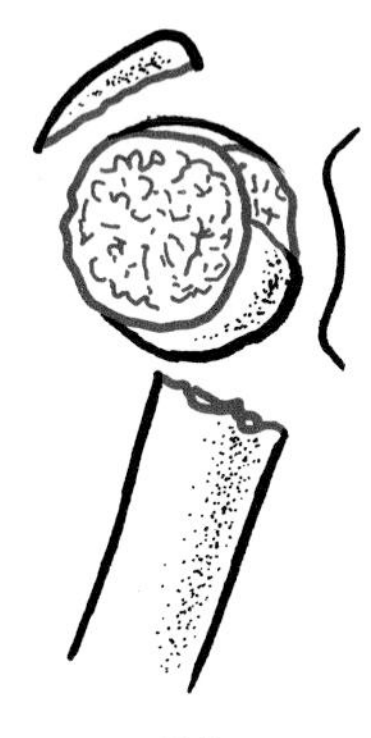
B2

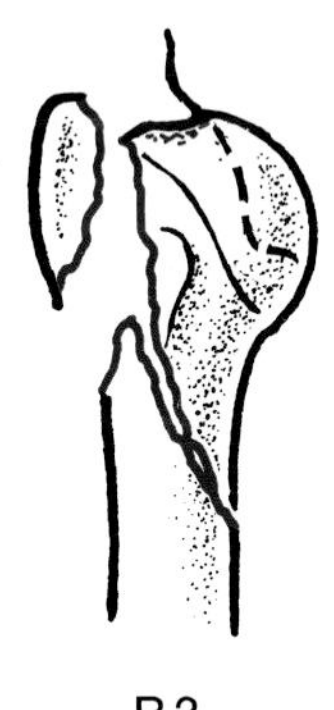
B3

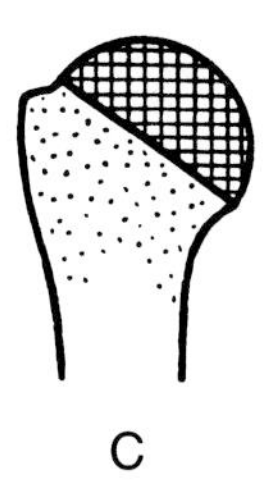
C

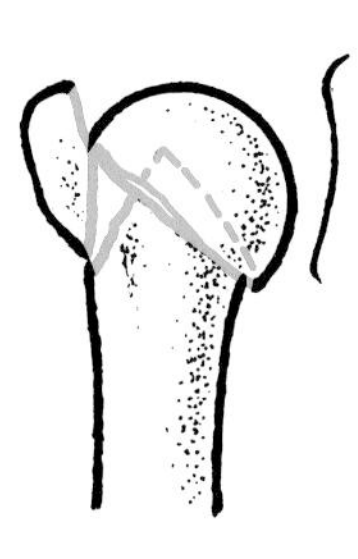
C1

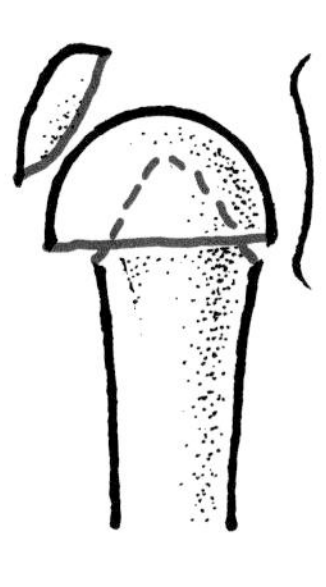
C2

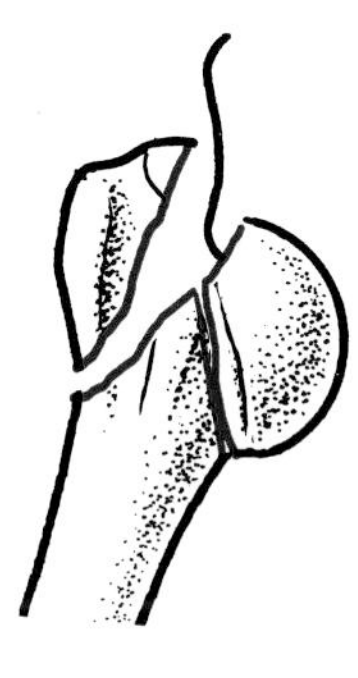
C3

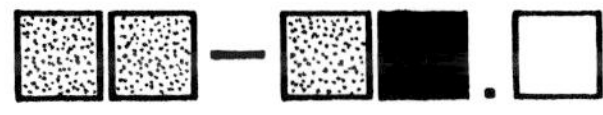

12- Humerus Diaphysis

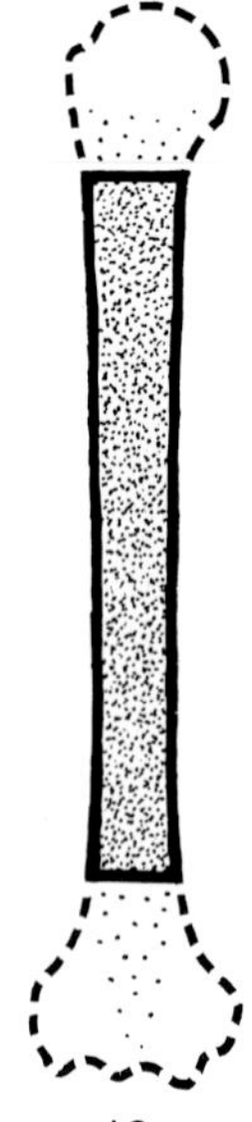

A = Simple fracture

- -A1 Simple fracture, spiral
  - .1 proximal zone
  - (.2) middle zone
  - .3 distal zone
- -A2 Simple fracture, oblique (≥30°)
  - .1 proximal zone
  - (.2) middle zone
  - .3 distal zone
- -A3 Simple fracture, transverse (< 30°)
  - .1 proximal zone
  - (.2) middle zone
  - .3 distal zone

B = Wedge fracture

- -B1 Wedge fracture, spiral wedge
  - .1 proximal zone
  - (.2) middle zone
  - .3 distal zone
- -B2 Wedge fracture, bending wedge
  - .1 proximal zone
  - (.2) middle zone
  - .3 distal zone
- -B3 Wedge fracture, fragmented wedge
  - .1 proximal zone
  - (.2) middle zone
  - .3 distal zone

C = Complex fracture

- -C1 Complex fracture, spiral
  - .1 with two intermediate fragments
  - (.2) with three intermediate fragments
  - .3 with more than three intermediate fragments
- -C2 Complex fracture, segmental
  - (.1) with one intermediate segmental fragment
  - .2 with one intermediate segmental and additional wedge fragment(s)
  - .3 with two intermediate segmental fragments
- -C3 Complex fracture, irregular
  - .1 with two or three intermediate fragments
  - .2 with limited shattering (< 4 cm)
  - (.3) with extensive shattering (≥4 cm)

The subgroup illustrated is indicated by ◯ in the text.

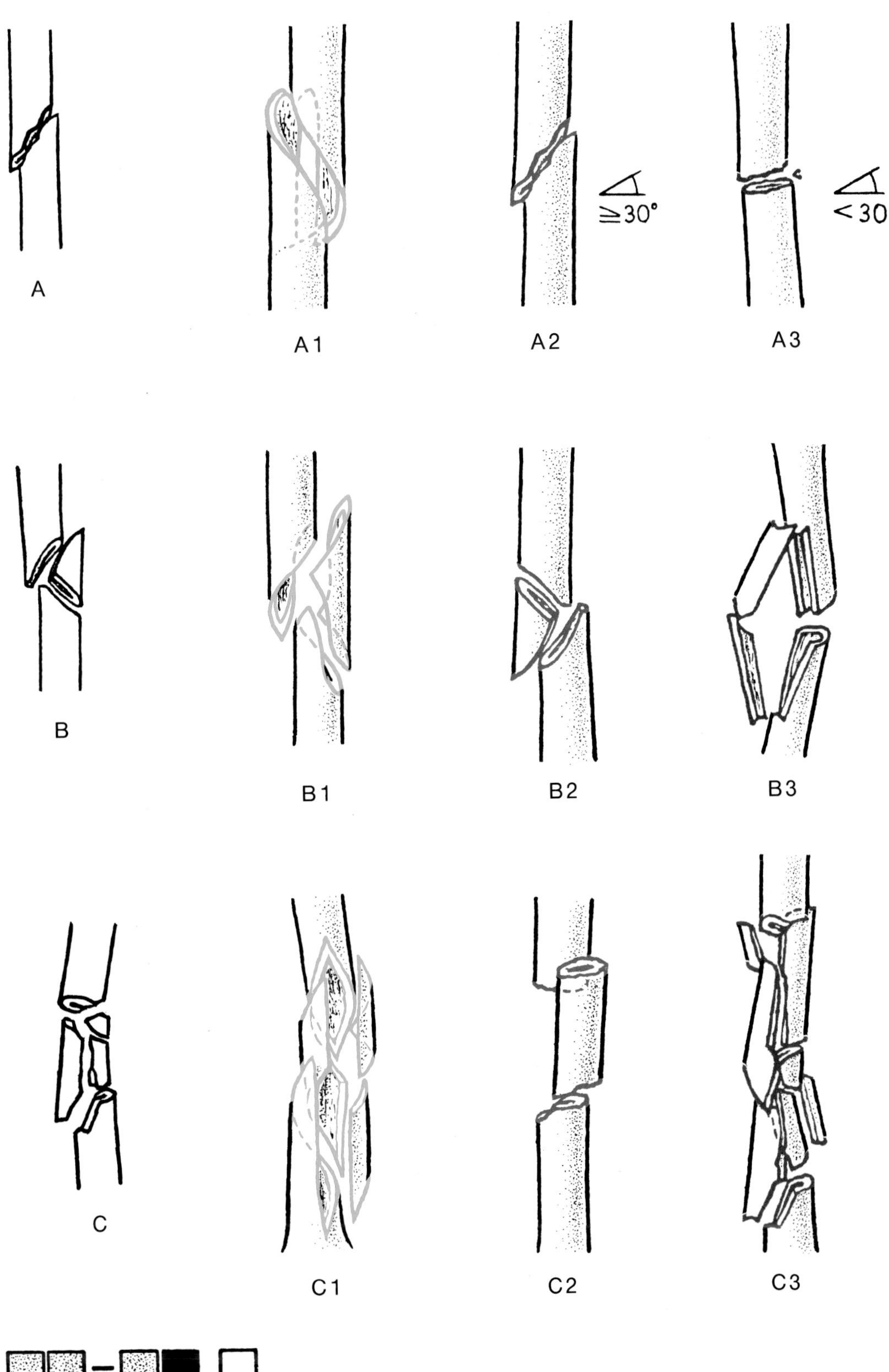
A
A1
A2
≧30°
A3
<30°
B
B1
B2
B3
C
C1
C2
C3

13- Humerus Distal

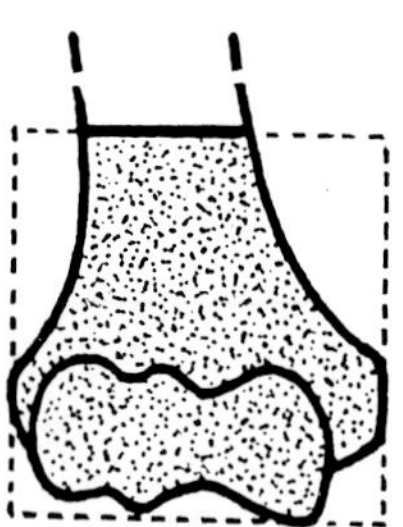

A = Extra-articular fracture

-A1 Extra-articular fracture, apophyseal avulsion
- .1 lateral epicondyle
- (.2) medial epicondyle, non incarcerated
- .3 medial epicondyle, incarcerated

-A2 Extra-articular fracture, metaphyseal simple
- .1 oblique downwards and inwards
- (.2) oblique downwards and outwards
- .3 transverse

-A3 Extra-articular fracture, metaphyseal multifragmentary
- .1 with an intact wedge
- (.2) with a fragmented wedge
- .3 complex

B = Partial articular fracture

-B1 Partial articular fracture, lateral sagittal
- .1 capitellum
- (.2) transtrochlear simple
- .3 transtrochlear multifragmentary

-B2 Partial articular fracture, medial sagittal
- .1 transtrochlear simple, through the medial side (Milch I)
- (.2) transtrochlear simple, through the groove
- .3 transtrochlear multifragmentary

-B3 Partial articular fracture, frontal
- (.1) capitellum
- .2 trochlea
- .3 capitellum and trochlea

C = Complete articular fracture

-C1 Complete articular fracture, articular simple, metaphyseal simple
- .1 with slight displacement
- (.2) with marked displacement
- .3 T-shaped epiphyseal

-C2 Complete articular fracture, articular simple, metaphyseal multifragmentary
- .1 with an intact wedge
- (.2) with a fragmented wedge
- .3 complex

-C3 Complete articular fracture, multifragmentary
- .1 metaphyseal simple
- (.2) metaphyseal wedge
- .3 metaphyseal complex

The subgroup illustrated is indicated by ◯ in the text.

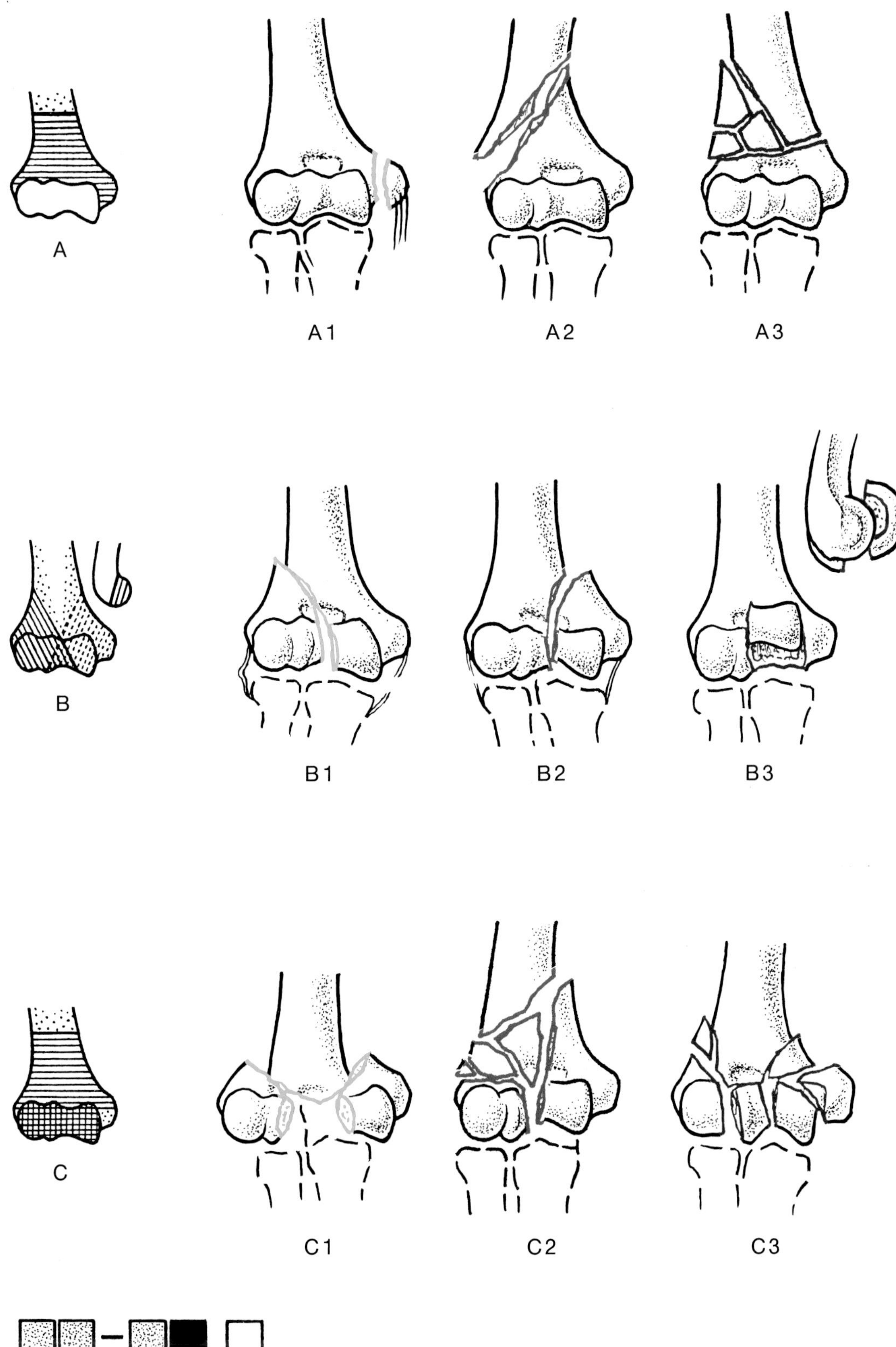
A
A1
A2
A3
B
B1
B2
B3
C
C1
C2
C3

21- Radius/Ulna Proximal

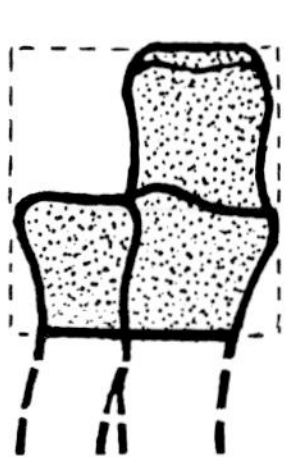

A = Extra-articular fracture

-A1 Extra-articular fracture, of the ulna, radius intact
- .1 avulsion of the triceps insertion from the olecranon
- .2 metaphyseal simple
- (.3) metaphyseal multifragmentary

-A2 Extra-articular fracture, of the radius, ulna intact
- .1 avulsion of the bicipital tuberosity of the radius
- (.2) neck simple
- .3 neck multifragmentary

-A3 Extra-articular fracture, of both bones
- .1 simple of both bones
- (.2) multifragmentary of one bone and simple of the other
- .3 multifragmentary of both bones

B = Articular fracture of one bone

-B1 Articular fracture, of the ulna, radius intact
- (.1) unifocal
- .2 bifocal simple
- .3 bifocal multifragmentary

-B2 Articular fracture, of the radius, ulna intact
- (.1) simple
- .2 multifragmentary without depression
- .3 multifragmentary with depression

-B3 Articular fracture, of the one bone with extra-articular fracture of the other
- .1 ulna, articular simple
- .2 radius, articular simple
- (.3) articular multifragmentary

C = Articular fracture of both bones

-C1 Articular fracture, of both bones, simple
- (.1) olecranon and head of radius
- .2 coronoid process and head of radius

-C2 Articular fracture, of both bones, the one simple and the other multifragmentary
- (.1) olecranon multifragmentary, radial head simple
- .2 olecranon simple, radial head multifragmentary
- .3 coronoid process simple, radial head multifragmentary

-C3 Articular fracture, of both bones, multifragmentary
- .1 three fragments of each bone
- .2 ulna, more than three fragments
- (.3) radius, more than three fragments

The subgroup illustrated is indicated by ◯ in the text.

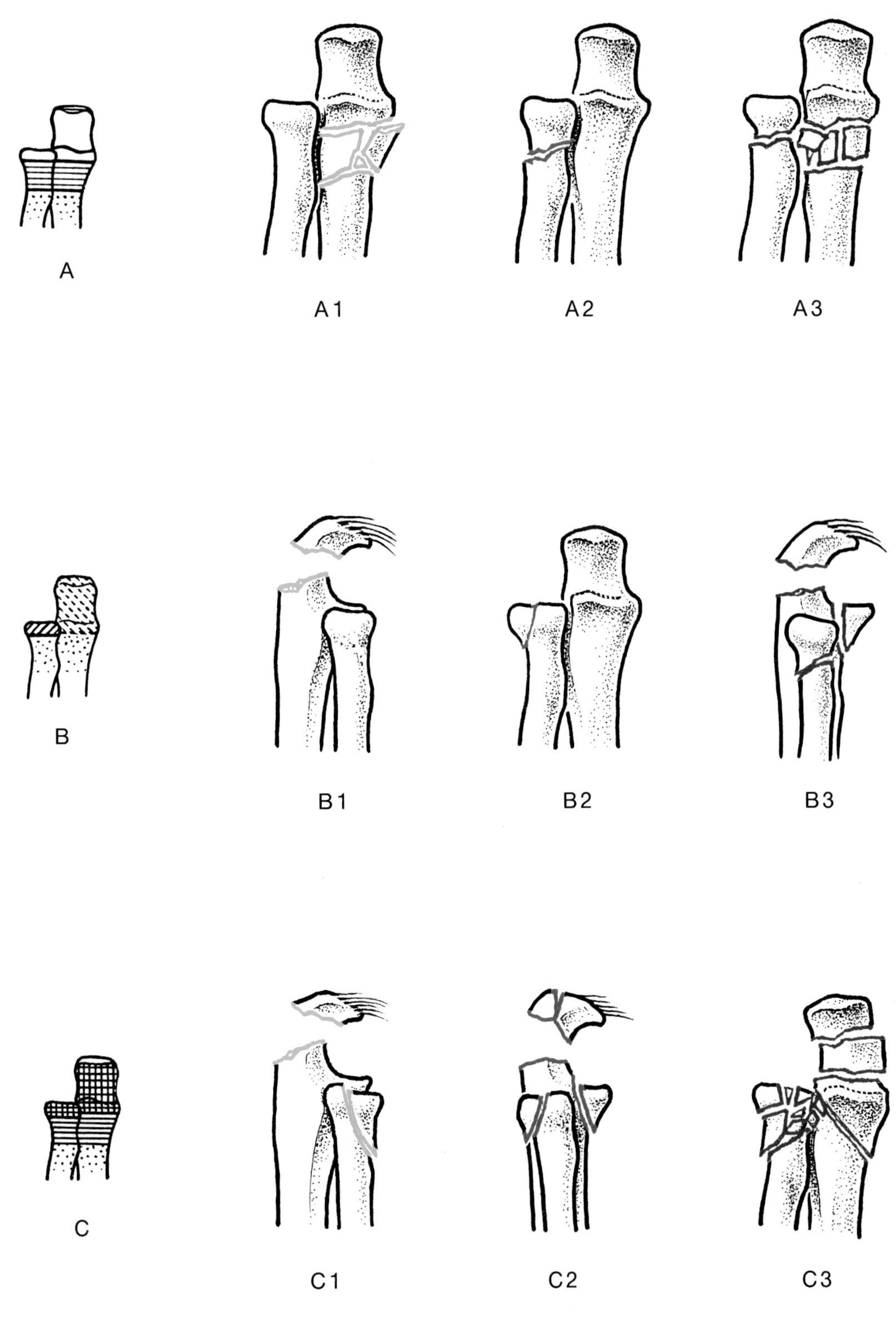
A
A1
A2
A3
B
B1
B2
B3
C
C1
C2
C3

22- Radius/Ulna Diaphysis

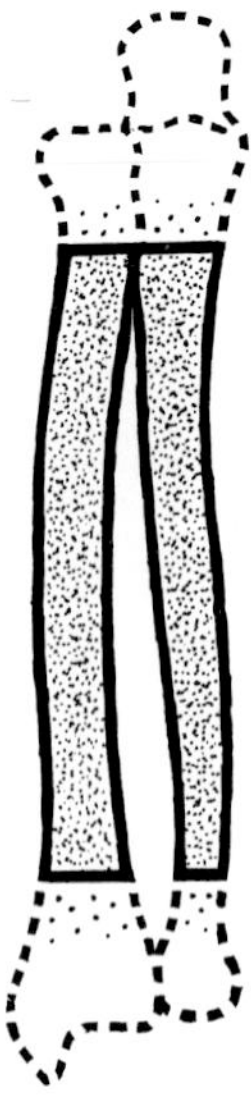

A = Simple fracture

- -A1 Simple fracture, of the ulna, radius intact
  - .1 oblique
  - .2 transverse
  - (.3) with dislocation of the radial head (Monteggia)
- -A2 Simple fracture, of the radius, ulna intact
  - .1 oblique
  - (.2) transverse
  - .3 with dislocation of the distal radio-ulnar joint (Galeazzi)
- -A3 Simple fracture, of both bones
  - .1 radius, proximal bones
  - (.2) radius, middle zone
  - .3 radius, distal zone

B = Wedge fracture

- -B1 Wedge fracture, of the ulna, radius intact
  - (.1) intact wedge
  - .2 fragmented wedge
  - .3 with dislocation of the radial head (Monteggia)
- -B2 Wedge fracture, of the radius, ulna intact
  - (.1) intact wedge
  - .2 fragmented wedge
  - .3 with dislocation of the distal radio-ulnar joint (Galeazzi)
- -B3 Wedge fracture, of the one bone, simple or wedge fracture of the other
  - .1 ulnar wedge and simple fracture of the radius
  - .2 radial wedge and simple fracture of the ulna
  - (.3) ulnar and radial wedges

C = Complex fracture

- -C1 Complex fracture, of the ulna
  - .1 bifocal, radius intact
  - .2 bifocal, radius fractured
  - (.3) irregular
- -C2 Complex fracture, of the radius
  - .1 bifocal, ulna intact
  - (.2) bifocal, ulna fractured
  - .3 irregular
- -C3 Complex fracture, of both bones
  - .1 bifocal
  - .2 bifocal of the one, irregular of the other
  - (.3) irregular

The subgroup illustrated is indicated by ◯ in the text.

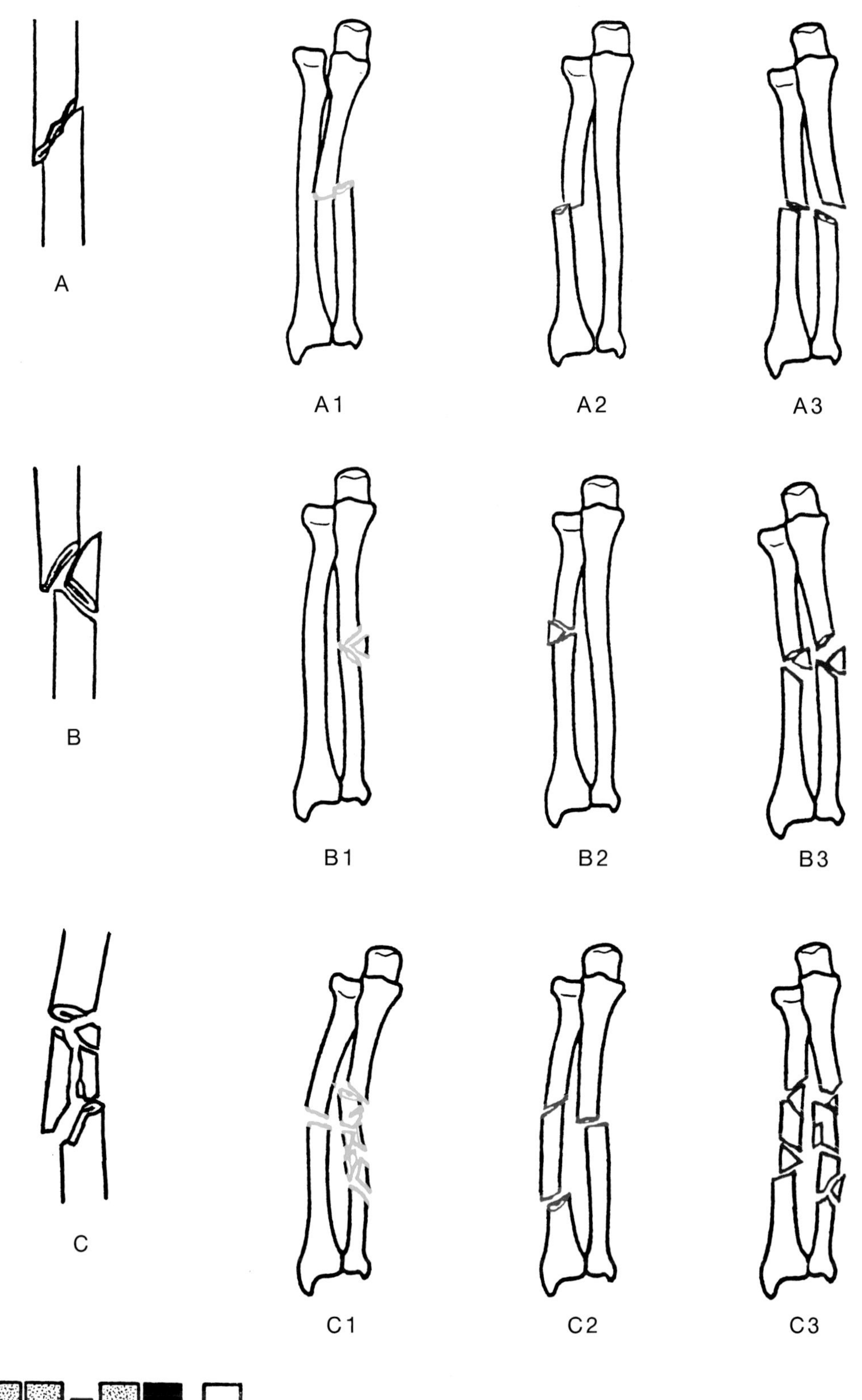
A
A1
A2
A3
B
B1
B2
B3
C
C1
C2
C3

23- Radius/Ulna Distal

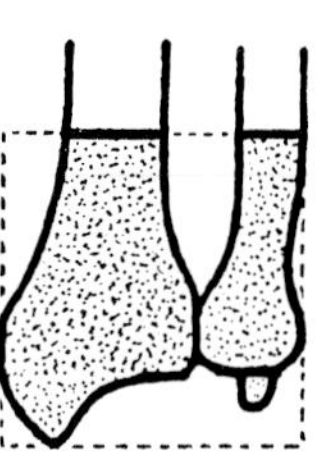

A = Extra-articular fracture

-A1 Extra-articular fracture, of the ulna, radius intact
- .1 styloid process
- (.2) metaphyseal simple
- .3 metaphyseal multifragmentary

-A2 Extra-articular fracture, of the radius, simple and impacted
- .1 without any tilt
- (.2) with dorsal tilt (Pouteau-Colles)
- .3 with volar tilt (Goyrand-Smith)

-A3 Extra-articular fracture, of the radius, multifragmentary
- .1 impacted with axial shortening
- (.2) with a wedge
- .3 complex

B = partial articular fracture

-B1 Partial articular fracture, of the radius, sagittal
- (.1) lateral simple
- .2 lateral multifragmentary
- .3 medial

-B2 Partial articular fracture, of the radius, dorsal rim (Barton)
- (.1) simple
- .2 with lateral sagittal fracture
- .3 with dorsal dislocation of the carpus

-B3 Partial articular fracture, of the radius, volar rim (reverse Barton, Goyrand-Smith II)
- .1 simple, with a small fragment
- (.2) simple, with a large fragment
- .3 multifragmentary

C = Complete articular fracture

-C1 Complete articular fracture, of the radius, articular simple, metaphyseal simple
- .1 postero-medial articular fragment
- (.2) sagittal articular fracture line
- .3 frontal articular fracture line

-C2 Complete articular fracture, of the radius, articular simple, metaphyseal multifragmentary
- (.1) sagittal articular fracture line
- .2 frontal articular fracture line
- .3 extending into the diaphysis

-C3 Complete articular fracture, of the radius, multifragmentary
- .1 metaphyseal simple
- .2 metaphyseal multifragmentary
- (.3) extending into the diaphysis

The subgroup illustrated is indicated by ◯ in the text.

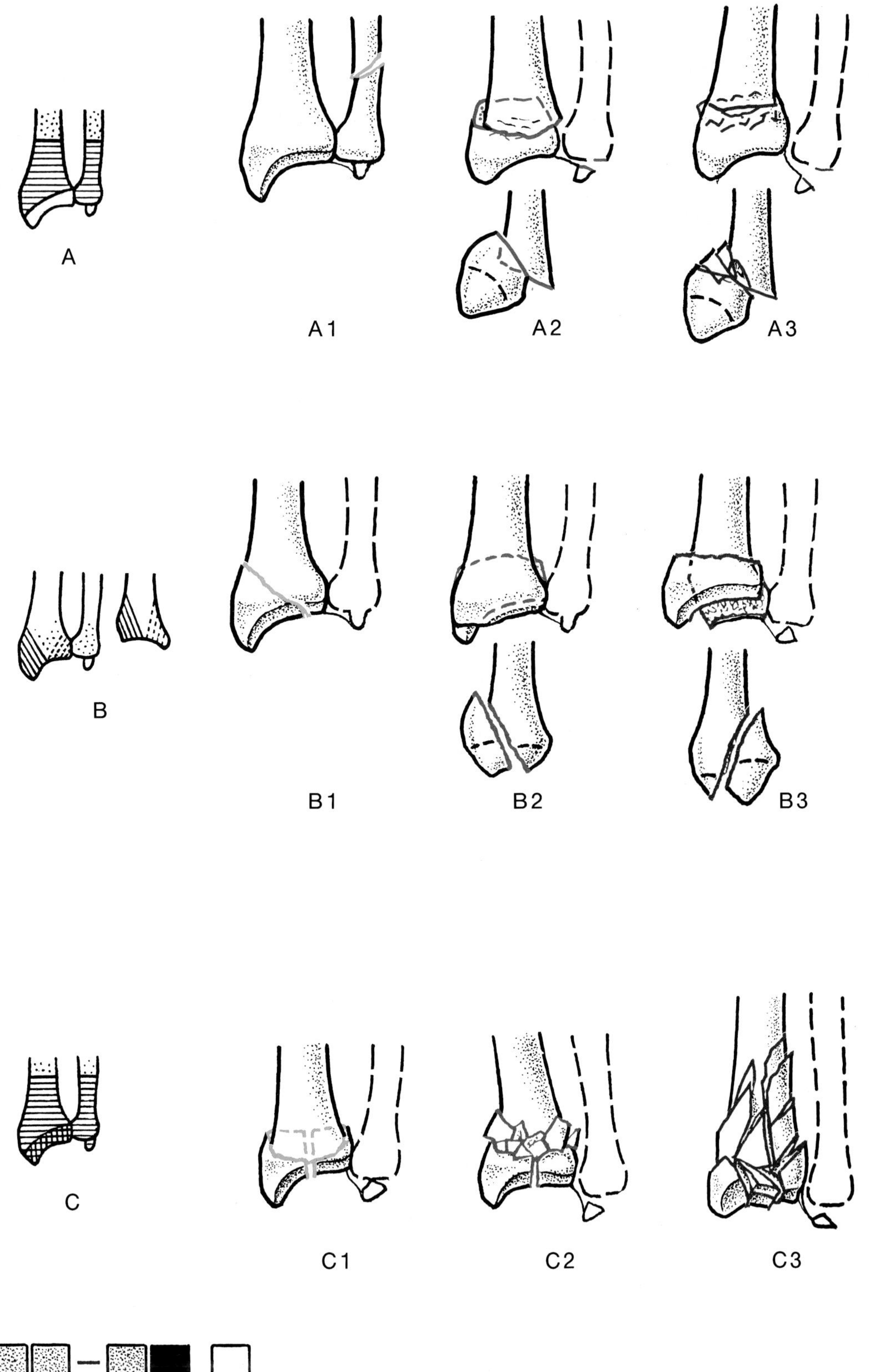
A
A1
A2
A3
B
B1
B2
B3
C
C1
C2
C3

31- Femur Proximal

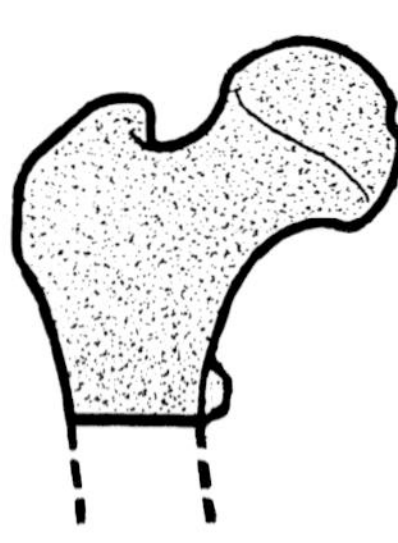

A = Trochanteric area fracture

-A1 Trochanteric area fracture, pertrochanteric simple
- (.1) along the intertrochanteric line
- .2 through the greater trochanter
- .3 below the lesser trochanter

-A2 Trochanteric area fracture, pertrochanteric multifragmentary
- .1 with one intermediate fragment
- (.2) with several intermediate fragments
- .3 extending more than 1 cm below the lesser trochanter

-A3 Trochanteric area fracture, intertrochanteric
- .1 simple, oblique
- (.2) simple, transverse
- .3 multifragmentary

B = Neck fracture

-B1 Neck fracture, subcapital, with slight displacement
- (.1) impacted in valgus $\geq 15°$
- .2 impacted in valgus $< 15°$
- .3 non-impacted

-B2 Neck fracture, transcervical
- .1 basicervical
- .2 midcervical adduction
- (.3) midcervical shear

-B3 Neck fracture, subcapital, non-impacted, displaced
- .1 moderate displacement in varus and external rotation
- .2 moderate displacement with vertical translation and external rotation
- (.3) marked displacement

C = Head fracture

-C1 Head fracture, split
- .1 avulsion of the ligamentum teres
- .2 with rupture of the ligamentum teres
- (.3) large fragment

-C2 Head fracture, with depression
- .1 posterior and superior
- (.2) anterior and superior
- .3 split-depression

-C3 Head fracture, with neck fracture
- .1 split and transcervical neck fracture
- .2 split and subcapital neck fracture
- (.3) depression and neck fracture

The subgroup illustrated is indicated by ◯ in the text.

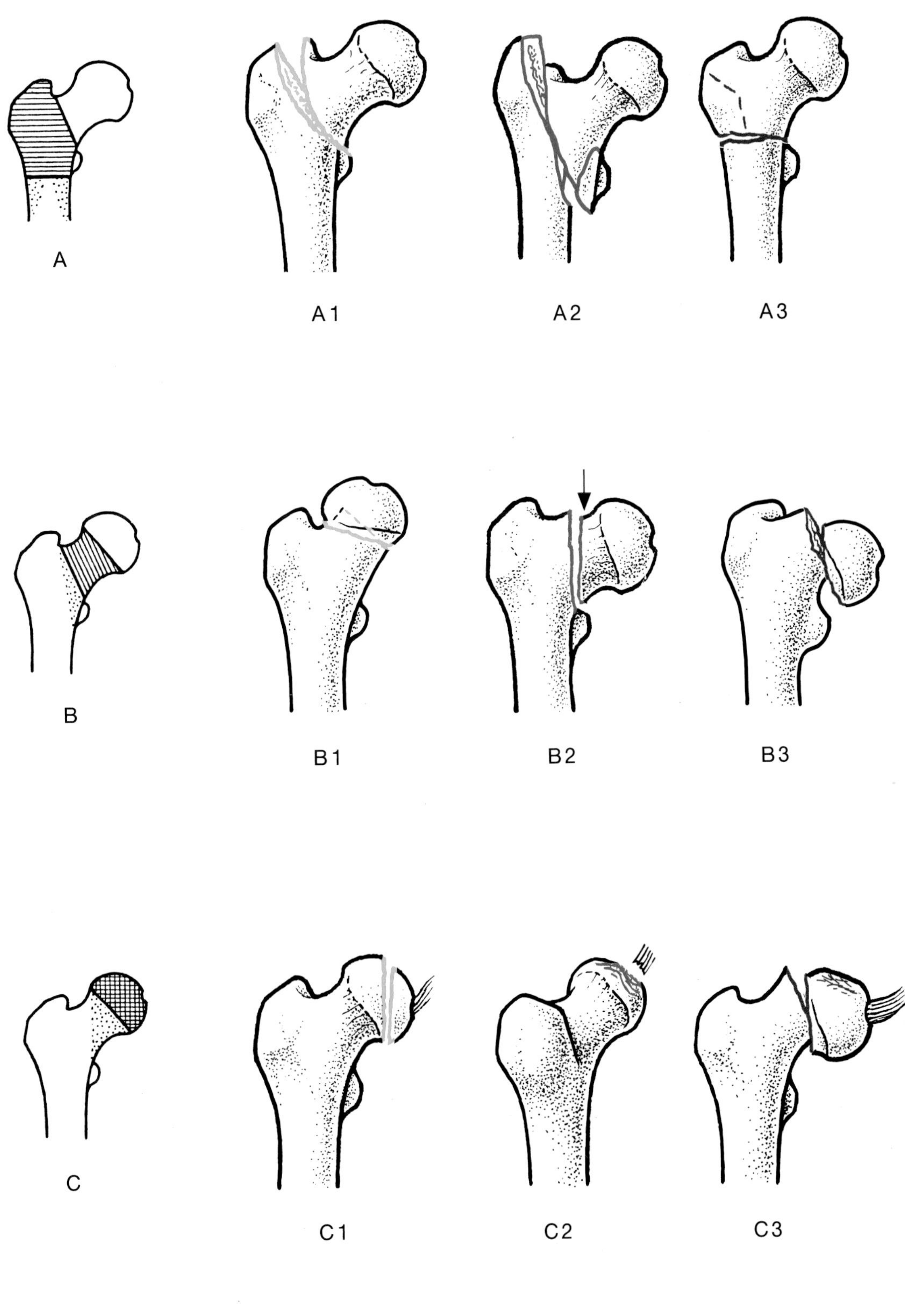
A
A1
A2
A3
B
B1
B2
B3
C
C1
C2
C3

32- Femur Diaphysis

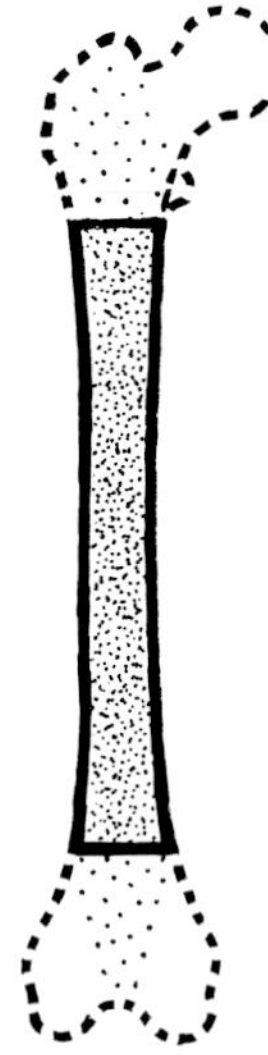

A = Simple fracture

-A1 Simple fracture, spiral
- .1 subtrochanteric zone
- (.2) middle zone
- .3 distal zone

-A2 Simple fracture, oblique ($\geq 30°$)
- .1 subtrochanteric zone
- (.2) middle zone
- .3 distal zone

-A3 Simple fracture, transverse ($< 30°$)
- .1 subtrochanteric zone
- (.2) middle zone
- .3 distal zone

B = Wedge fracture

-B1 Wedge fracture, spiral wedge
- .1 subtrochanteric zone
- (.2) middle zone
- .3 distal zone

-B2 Wedge fracture, bending wedge
- .1 subtrochanteric zone
- (.2) middle zone
- .3 distal zone

-B3 Wedge fracture, fragmented wedge
- .1 subtrochanteric zone
- (.2) middle zone
- .3 distal zone

C = Complex fracture

-C1 Complex fracture, spiral
- .1 with two intermediate fragments
- (.2) with three intermediate fragments
- .3 with more than three intermediate fragments

-C2 Complex fracture, segmental
- (.1) with one intermediate segmental fragment
- .2 with one intermediate segmental and additional wedge fragment(s)
- .3 with two intermediate segmental fragments

-C3 Complex fracture, irregular
- .1 with two or three intermediate fragments
- .2 with limited shattering (< 5 cm)
- (.3) with extensive shattering (≥ 5 cm)

The subgroup illustrated is indicated by ◯ in the text.

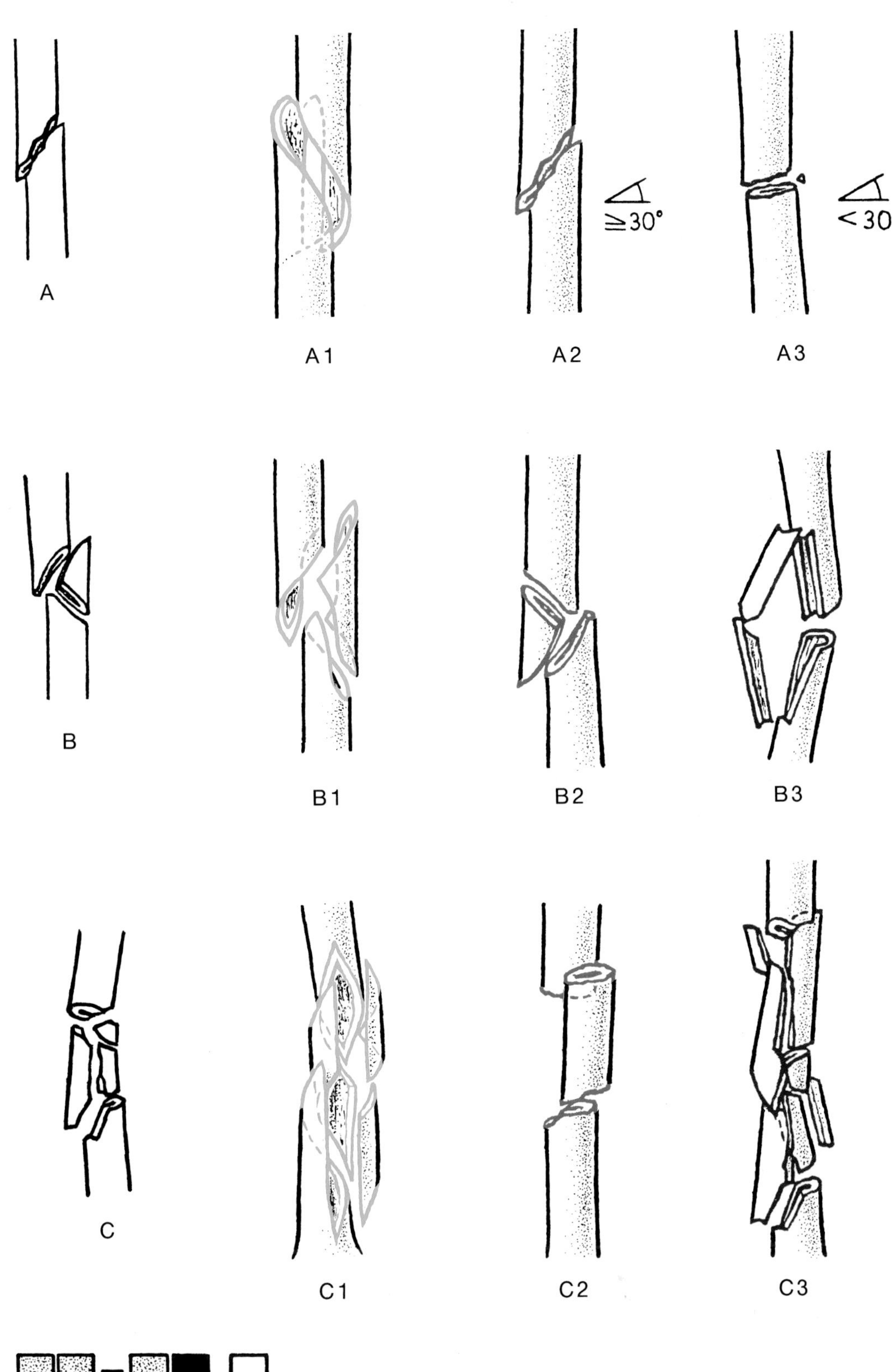

A
A1
A2
≧30°
A3
<30°
B
B1
B2
B3
C
C1
C2
C3

33- Femur Distal

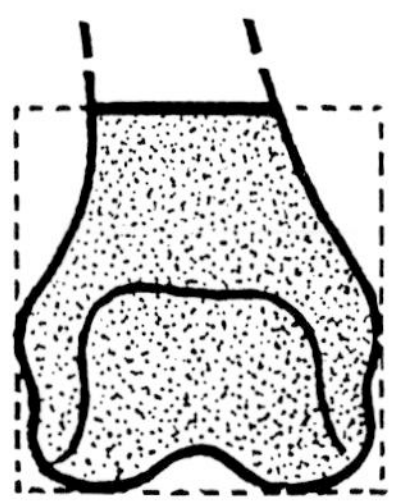

A = Extra-articular fracture

-A1 Extra-articular fracture, simple
- .1 apophyseal
- (.2) metaphyseal oblique or spiral
- .3 metaphyseal transverse

-A2 Extra-articular fracture, metaphyseal wedge
- (.1) intact
- .2 fragmented, lateral
- .3 fragmented, medial

-A3 Extra-articular fracture, metaphyseal complex
- .1 with an intermediate split segment
- (.2) irregular, limited to the metaphysis
- .3 irregular, extending into the diaphysis

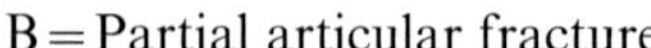

B = Partial articular fracture

-B1 Partial articular fracture, lateral condyle, sagittal
- .1 simple, through the notch
- (.2) simple, through the load-bearing surface
- .3 multifragmentary

-B2 Partial articular fracture, medial condyle, sagittal
- (.1) simple, through the notch
- .2 simple, through the load-bearing surface
- .3 multifragmentary

-B3 Partial articular fracture, frontal
- .1 anterior and lateral flake fracture
- (.2) unicondylar posterior (Hoffa)
- .3 bicondylar posterior

C = Complete articular fracture

-C1 Complete articular fracture, articular simple, metaphyseal simple
- (.1) T- or Y-shaped, with slight displacement
- .2 T- or Y-shaped, with marked displacement
- .3 T-shaped epiphyseal

-C2 Complete articular fracture, articular simple, metaphyseal multifragmentary
- .1 with an intact wedge
- (.2) with a fragmented wedge
- .3 complex

-C3 Complete articular fracture, multifragmentary
- .1 metaphyseal simple
- (.2) metaphyseal multifragmentary
- .3 metaphyseo-diaphyseal multifragmentary

The subgroup illustrated is indicated by ◯ in the text.

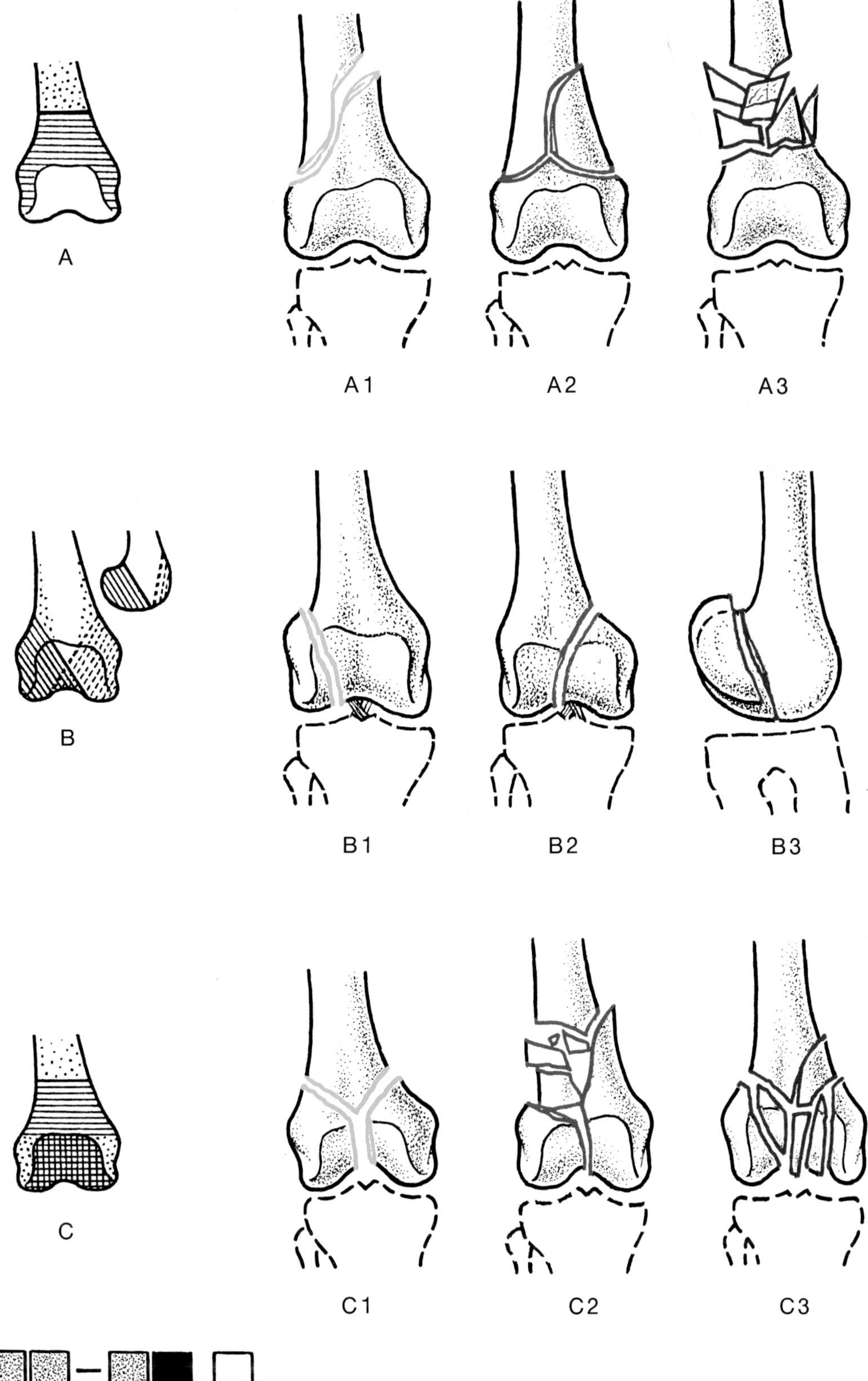
A
A1
A2
A3
B
B1
B2
B3
C
C1
C2
C3

41- Tibia/Fibula Proximal

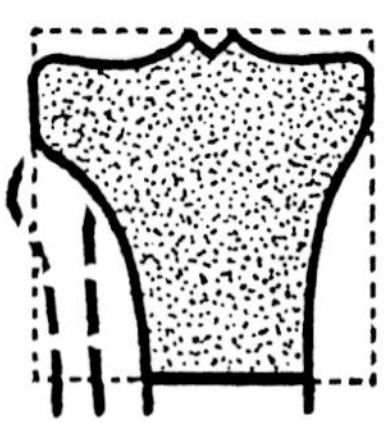

A = Extra-articular fracture

- -A1 Extra-articular fracture, avulsion
  - .1 of the fibular head
  - .2 of the tibial tuberosity
  - (.3) of the cruciate insertion
- -A2 Extra-articular fracture, metaphyseal simple
  - (.1) oblique in the frontal plane
  - .2 oblique in the sagittal plane
  - .3 transverse
- -A3 Extra-articular fracture, metaphyseal multifragmentary
  - .1 intact wedge
  - .2 fragmented wedge
  - (.3) complex

B = Partial articular fracture

- -B1 Partial articular fracture, pure split
  - (.1) of the lateral surface
  - .2 of the medial surface
  - .3 oblique, involving the tibial spines and one of the surfaces
- -B2 Partial articular fracture, pure depression
  - .1 lateral total
  - (.2) lateral limited
  - .3 medial
- -B3 Partial articular fracture, split-depression
  - (.1) lateral
  - .2 medial
  - .3 oblique, involving the tibial spines and one of the surfaces

C = Complete articular fracture

- -C1 Complete articular fracture, articular simple, metaphyseal simple
  - .1 slight displacement
  - (.2) one condyle displaced
  - .3 both condyles displaced
- -C2 Complete articular fracture, articular simple, metaphyseal multifragmentary
  - (.1) intact wedge
  - .2 fragmented wedge
  - .3 complex
- -C3 Complete articular fracture, multifragmentary
  - .1 lateral
  - (.2) medial
  - .3 lateral and medial

The subgroup illustrated is indicated by ◯ in the text.

A

A1

A2

A3

B

B1

B2

B3

C

C1

C2

C3

42- Tibia/Fibula Diaphysis

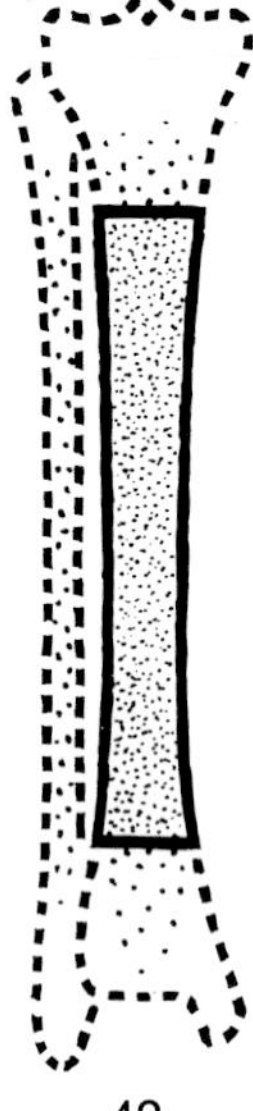

A = Simple fracture

- -A1 Simple fracture, spiral
  - .1 fibula intact
  - .2 fibula fractured at another level
  - .3 fibula fractured at the same level
- -A2 Simple fracture, oblique (≥30°)
  - .1 fibula intact
  - .2 fibula fractured at another level
  - .3 fibula fractured at the same level
- -A3 Simple fracture, transverse (<30°)
  - .1 fibula intact
  - .2 fibula fractured at another level
  - .3 fibula fractured at the same level

B = Wedge fracture

- -B1 Wedge fracture, spiral wedge
  - .1 fibula intact
  - .2 fibula fractured at another level
  - .3 fibula fractured at the same level
- -B2 Wedge fracture, bending wedge
  - .1 fibula intact
  - .2 fibula fractured at another level
  - .3 fibula fractured at the same level
- -B3 Wedge fracture, fragmented wedge
  - .1 fibula intact
  - .2 fibula fractured at another level
  - .3 fibula fractured at the same level

C = Complex fracture

- -C1 Complex fracture, spiral
  - .1 with two intermediate fragments
  - (.2) with three intermediate fragments
  - .3 with more than three intermediate fragments
- -C2 Complex fracture, segmental
  - (.1) with one intermediate segmental fragment
  - .2 with one intermediate segmental and additional wedge fragment(s)
  - .3 with two intermediate segmental fragments
- -C3 Complex fracture, irregular
  - .1 with two or three intermediate fragments
  - .2 with limited shattering (<4 cm)
  - (.3) with extensive shattering (≥4 cm)

The subgroup illustrated is indicated by ◯ in the text.

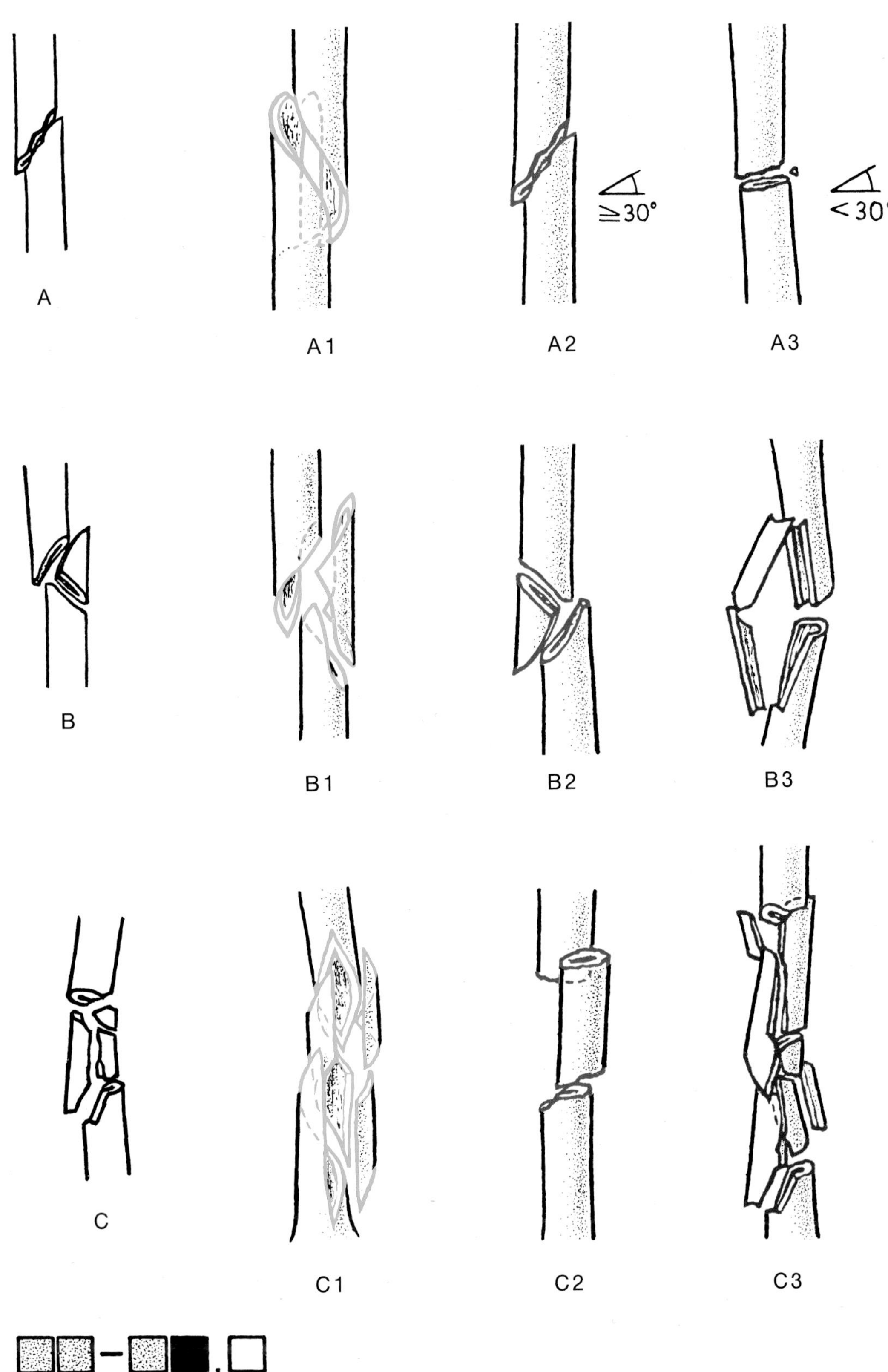
A
A1
A2
≧30°
A3
<30°
B
B1
B2
B3
C
C1
C2
C3

43- Tibia/Fibula Distal

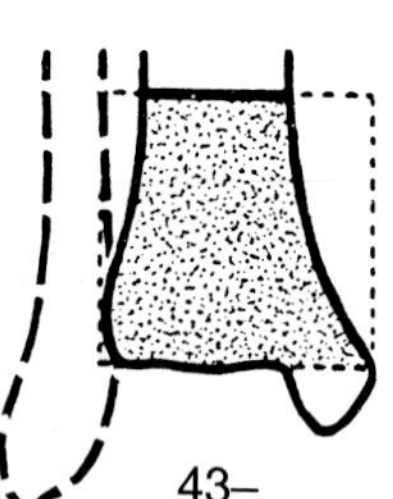

A = Extra-articular fracture

- -A1 Extra-articular fracture, metaphyseal simple
  - .1 spiral
  - .2 oblique
  - (.3) transverse
- -A2 Extra-articular fracture, metaphyseal wedge
  - .1 postero-lateral impaction
  - (.2) antero-medial wedge
  - .3 extending into the diaphysis
- -A3 Extra-articular fracture, metaphyseal complex
  - (.1) three intermediate fragments
  - .2 more than three intermediate fragments
  - .3 extending into the diaphysis

B = Partial articular fracture

- -B1 Partial articular fracture, pure split
  - .1 frontal
  - (.2) sagittal
  - .3 metaphyseal multifragmentary
- -B2 Partial articular fracture, split-depression
  - .1 frontal
  - (.2) sagittal
  - .3 of the central fragment
- -B3 Partial articular fracture, multifragmentary depression
  - (.1) frontal
  - .2 sagittal
  - .3 metaphyseal multifragmentary

C = Complete articular fracture

- -C1 Complete articular fracture, articular simple, metaphyseal simple
  - (.1) without depression
  - .2 with depression
  - .3 extending into the diaphysis
- -C2 Complete articular fracture, articular simple, metaphyseal multifragmentary
  - (.1) with asymmetric impaction
  - .2 without asymmetric impaction
  - .3 extending into the diaphysis
- -C3 Complete articular fracture, multifragmentary
  - .1 epiphyseal
  - (.2) epiphyseo-metaphyseal
  - .3 epiphyseo-metaphyseo-diaphyseal

The subgroup illustrated is indicated by ◯ in the text.

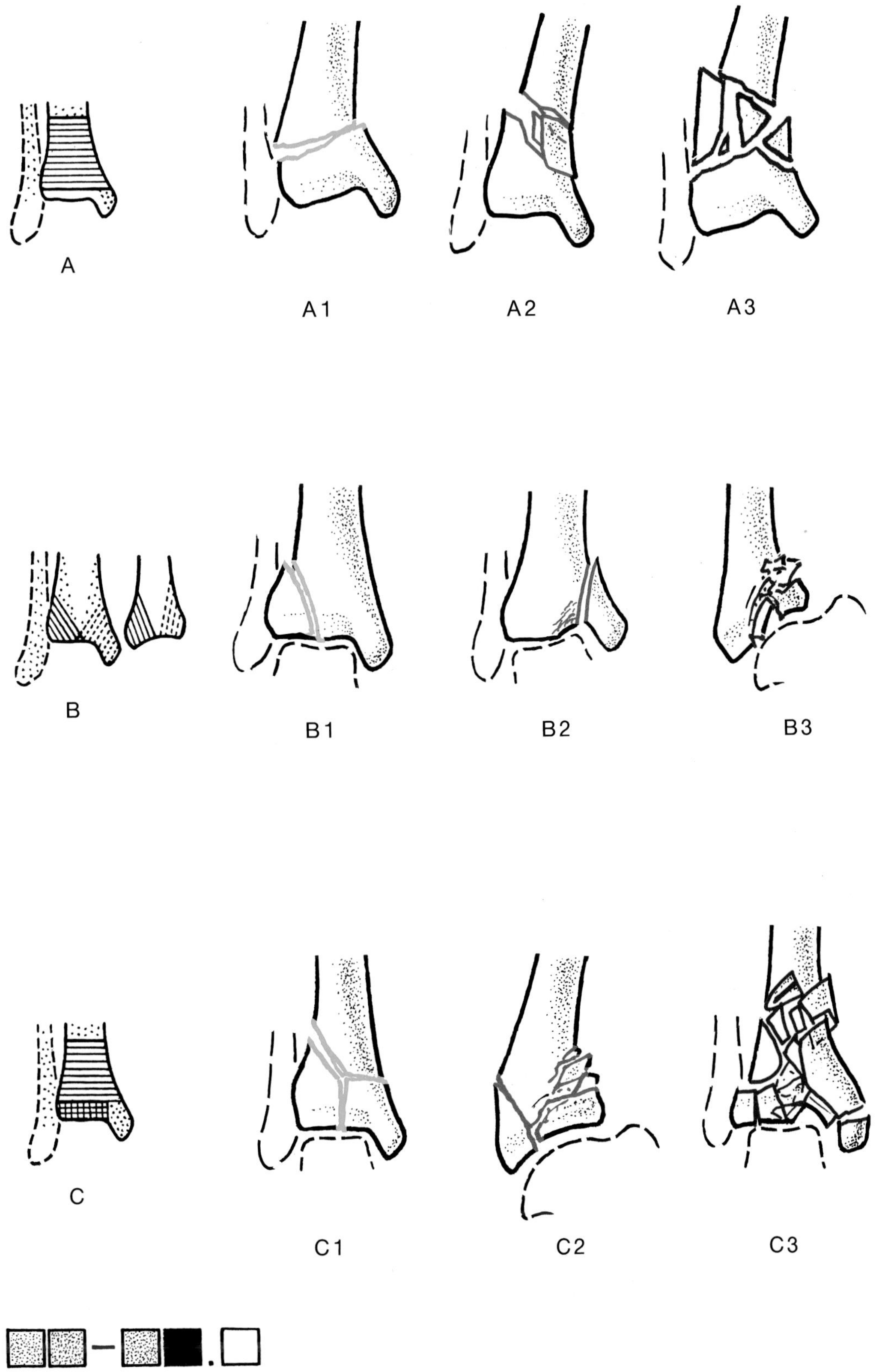

A

A1 A2 A3

B

B1 B2 B3

C

C1 C2 C3

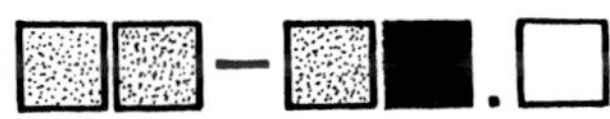

44- Tibia/Fibula, Malleolar Segment

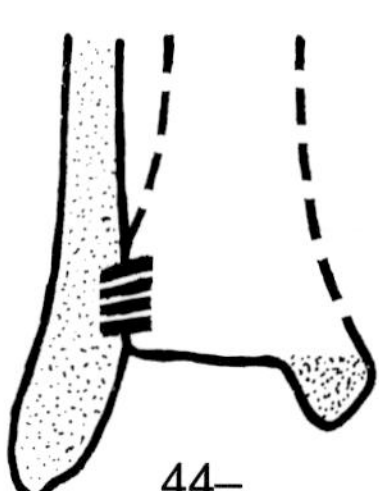

A = Infrasyndesmotic lesion

- -A1 Infrasyndesmotic lesion, isolated
  - .1 rupture of the lateral collateral ligament
  - .2 avulsion of the tip of the lateral malleolus
  - (.3) transverse fracture of the lateral malleolus
- -A2 Infrasyndesmotic lesion, with fracture of the medial malleolus
  - .1 rupture of the lateral collateral ligament
  - .2 avulsion of the tip of the lateral malleolus
  - (.3) transverse fracture of the lateral malleolus
- -A3 Infrasyndesmotic lesion, with postero-medial fracture
  - .1 rupture of the lateral collateral ligament
  - .2 avulsion of the tip of the lateral malleolus
  - (.3) transverse fracture of the lateral malleolus

B = Transsyndesmotic fibular fracture

- -B1 Transsyndesmotic fibular fracture, isolated
  - .1 simple
  - (.2) simple, with rupture of the anterior syndesmosis
  - .3 multifragmentary
- -B2 Transsyndesmotic fibular fracture, with medial lesion
  - .1 simple, with rupture of the medial collateral ligament and rupture of the anterior syndesmosis
  - (.2) simple, with fracture of the medial malleolus and with rupture of the anterior syndesmosis
  - .3 multifragmentary
- -B3 Transsyndesmotic fibular fracture, with medial lesion and a Volkmann (fracture of the postero-lateral rim)
  - .1 fibula simple, with rupture of the medial collateral ligament
  - (.2) fibula simple, with fracture of the medial malleolus
  - .3 fibula multifragmentary, with fracture of the medial malleolus

C = Suprasyndesmotic lesion

- -C1 Suprasyndesmotic lesion, diaphyseal fracture of the fibula, simple
  - (.1) with rupture of the medial collateral ligament
  - .2 with fracture of the medial malleolus
  - .3 with fracture of the medial malleolus and a Volkmann (= Dupuytren)
- -C2 Suprasyndesmotic lesion, diaphyseal fracture of the fibula, multifragmentary
  - .1 with rupture of the medial collateral ligament
  - (.2) with fracture of the medial malleolus
  - .3 with fracture of the medial malleolus and a Volkmann (= Dupuytren)
- -C3 Suprasyndesmotic lesion, proximal fibular lesion
  - .1 without shortening, without Volkmann
  - (.2) with shortening, without Volkmann
  - .3 medial lesion and a Volkmann

The subgroup illustrated is indicated by ◯ in the text.

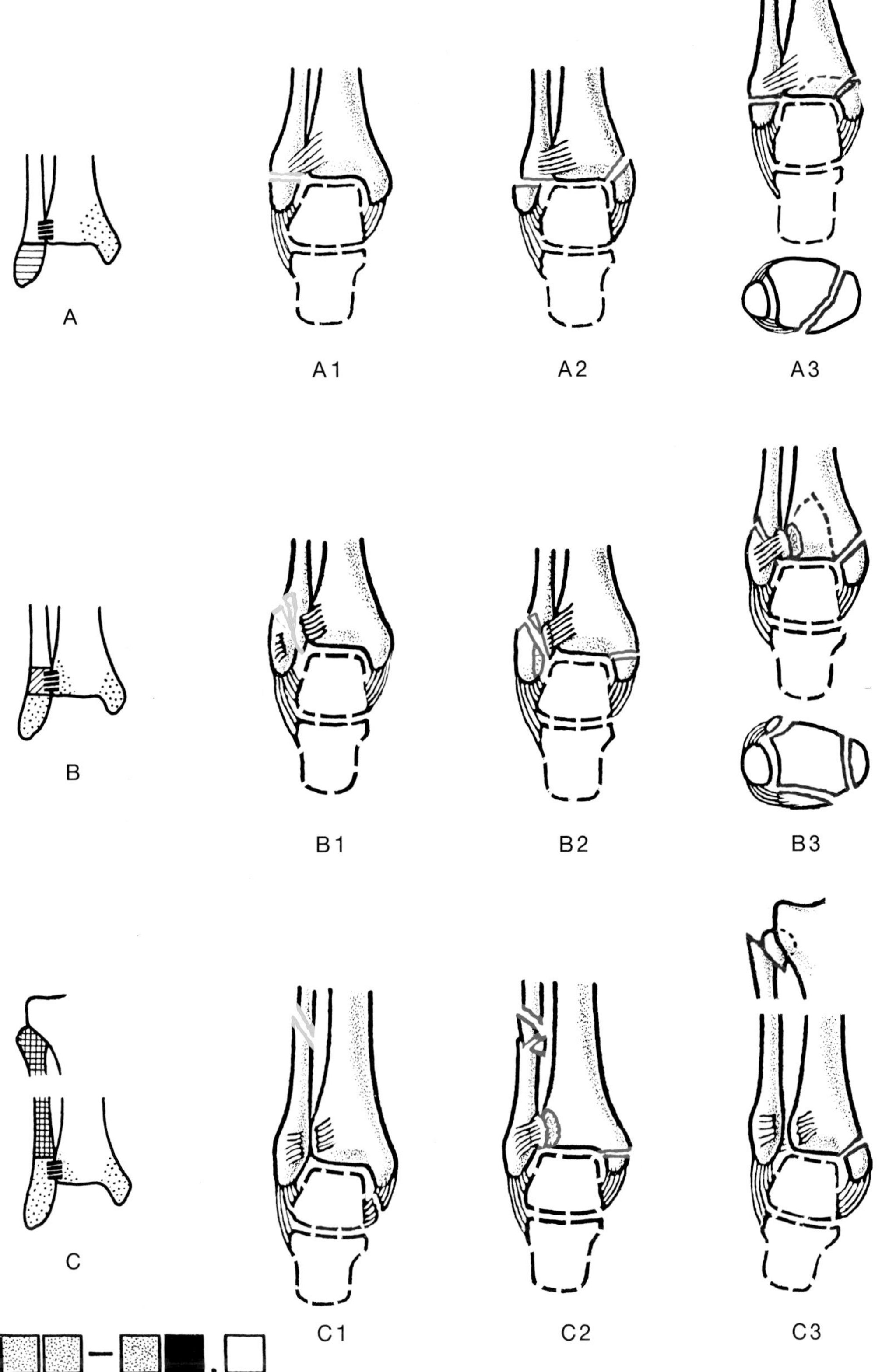
A
A1
A2
A3
B
B1
B2
B3
C
C1
C2
C3

Glossary to Appendix A

All fractures are either *simple* or *multifragmentary*.

simple: A term used to characterize a single circumferential disruption of a diaphysis or metaphysis or a single disruption of an articular surface. Simple fractures of the diaphysis or metaphysis are spiral, oblique or transverse.

multifragmentary: A term used to characterize any fracture with one or more completely separated intermediate fragment(s). In the diaphyseal and metaphyseal segments, it includes the wedge and the complex fractures. The terms *wedge* and *complex* are used only for diaphyseal or metaphyseal fractures.
- *wedge*: A fracture with one or more intermediate fragment(s) in which, after reduction, there is some contact between the main fragments. The spiral or bending wedge may be intact or fragmented.
- *complex*: A fracture with one or more intermediate fragment(s) in which, after reduction, there is no contact between the main proximal and distal fragments. The complex fractures are spiral, segmental or irregular. The term *comminuted* is imprecise and should not be used.

impacted: A stable and usually simple fracture of the metaphysis or epiphysis in which the fragments are driven one into the other.

Specific Terms for the Proximal and Distal Segments

Fractures of the proximal and distal segments are either *extra-articular* or *articular*.

Extra-articular fractures: These do not involve the articular surface, although they may be intra-capsular. They include apophyseal and metaphyseal fractures.

Articular fractures involve the articular surface. They are subdivided into *partial* and *complete*.

Partial articular fractures: The fractures involve only part of the articular surface, while the rest of that surface remains attached to the diaphysis.

Varieties of partial articular fractures:
- *pure split*: A fracture, resulting from a shearing force, in which the direction of the split is usually longitudinal.
- *pure depression*: An articular fracture in which there is pure depression of the articular surface without a split. The depression may be central or peripheral.
- *split-depression*: A combination of a split and a depression, in which the joint fragments are usually separated.
- *multifragmentary depression*: A fracture in which part of the joint is depressed and the fragments are completely separated.

Complete articular fractures: The articular surface is disrupted and completely separated from the diaphysis. The severity of these fractures depends on whether its articular and metaphyseal components are simple or multifragmentary.

Appendix B
Classification of Soft Tissue Injuries

Considering the many different variables that must be included when grading an open or closed fracture, we have combined the widely accepted AO fracture classification for long bones by Maurice E. Müller et al. (1987) with the grading of the skin injury (I for integuments: IC for closed integuments, IO for open integuments), the underlying muscle and tendon injury (MT) and the neurovascular injury (NV).

Scale

1 = Norm (except for open fractures).
2–4 = Increasing severity of lesion.
5 = Something special.

Skin Lesions IC (Closed Fractures)

For the description of the skin lesion the letter "I" was chosen for Integument, which translates well into most Latin and Anglo-Saxon languages. The letters "C" and "O" designate closed and open fractures. Thus, for closed fractures:

IC1 = No skin lesion.
IC2 = No skin laceration, but contusion.
IC3 = Circumscribed degloving.
IC4 = Extensive, closed degloving.
IC5 = Necrosis from contusion.

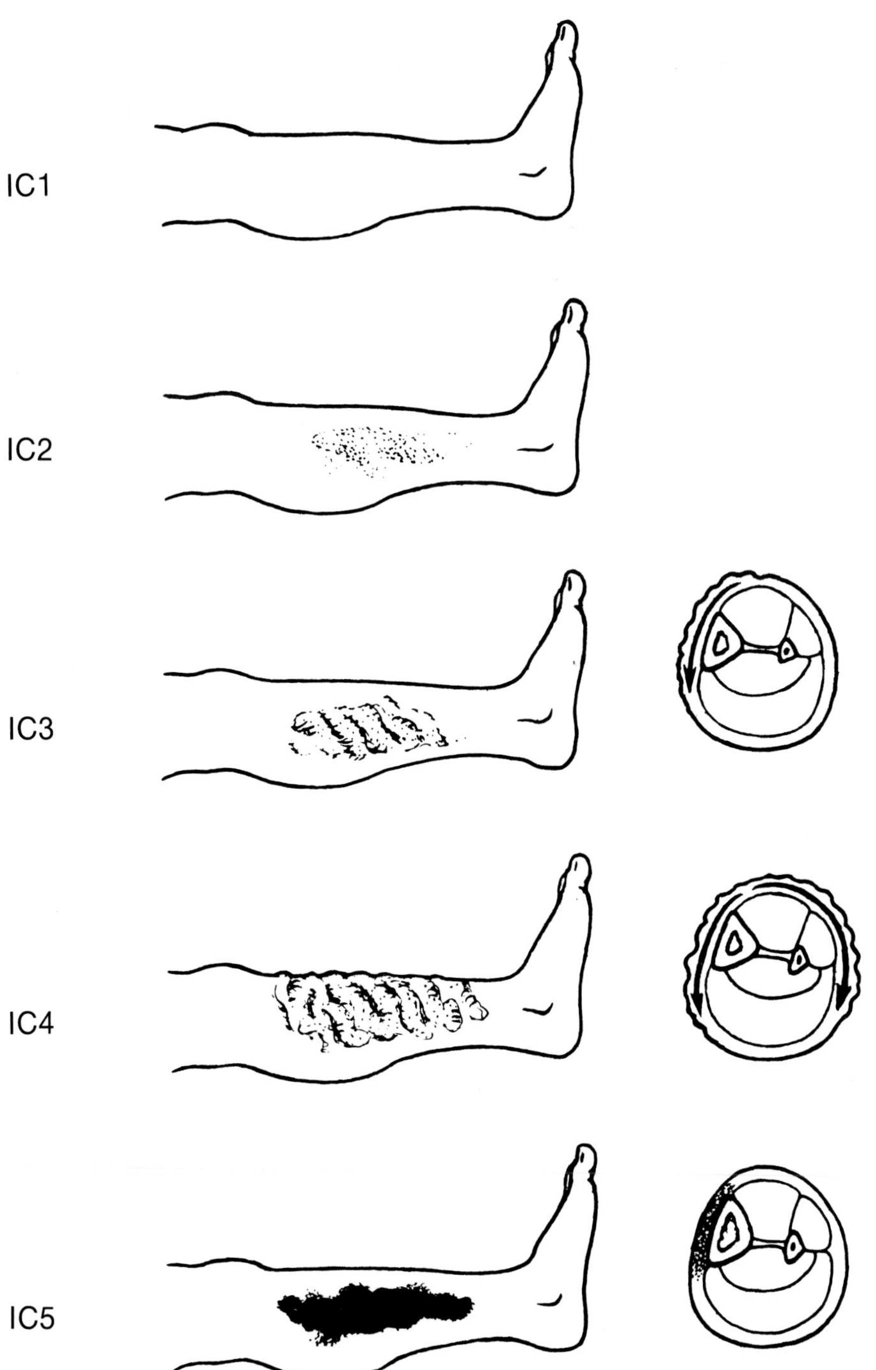
IC1
IC2
IC3
IC4
IC5

Skin Lesions IO (Open Fractures)

IO1 = Skin breakage from inside out.
IO2 = Skin breakage from outside in <5 cm, contused edges.
IO3 = Skin breakage >5 cm, devitalized edges, circumscribed degloving.
IO4 = Full-thickness contusion, abrasion, skin loss.
IO5 = Extensive degloving

This grading of skin wounds fits well with the three-grade system for open fractures but adds a fourth grade for really extensive skin destruction.

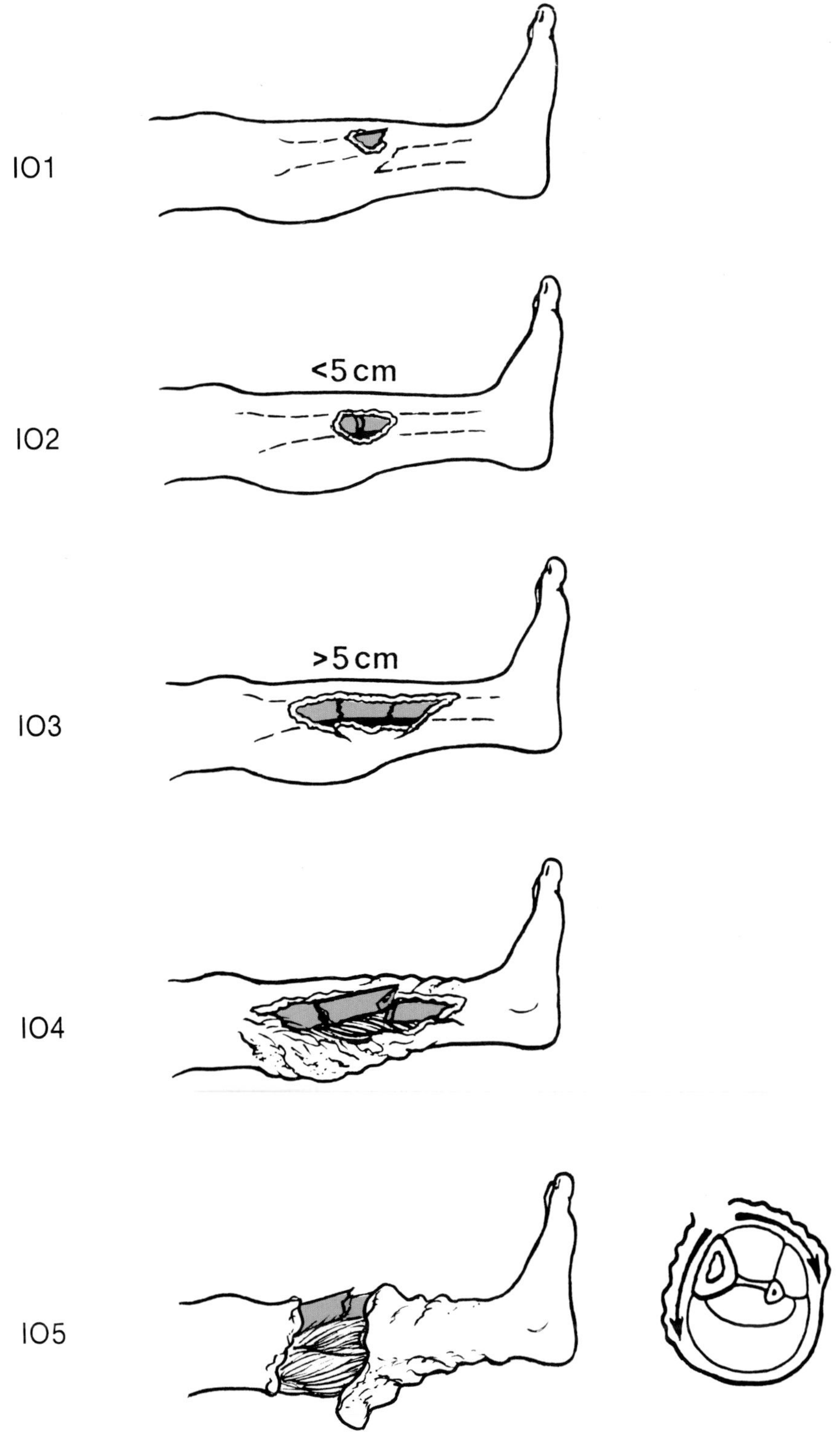
IO1
<5 cm
IO2
>5 cm
IO3
IO4
IO5

Muscle/Tendon Injury (MT)

As there may be considerable injury to the muscle envelope and, rarely, also to the tendons in open as well as in closed fractures, and since this feature is highly prognostic, a grading of the extent of muscle tissue and tendon involvement is considered essential:

MT1 = No muscle injury.
MT2 = Circumscribed muscle injury, one muscle group only.
MT3 = Extensive muscle injury, two or more muscle groups.
MT4 = Avulsion or loss of entire muscle groups, tendon laceration.
MT5 = Compartment syndrome/Crush syndrome.

Neurovascular Injury (NV)

The neurovascular injuries are described with the letter "NV" as follows:

NV1 = No neurovascular injury.
NV2 = Isolated nerve injury.
NV3 = Localized vascular injury.
NV4 = Combined neurovascular injury.
NV5 = Subtotal or total amputation.

Examples

- A simple, closed spiral tibia shaft fracture with no relevant lesions of skin, muscles/tendons, nerves and vessels becomes:
  42-A1/IC1-MT1-NV1.
- A severe open complex irregular tibia shaft fracture with extensive muscular damage and an isolated nerve injury becomes:
  42-C3/IO3-MT2 or 3-NV2 or 3.
- The near-amputation or a complex irregular tibia shaft fracture with extensive skin loss, muscle and tendon damage plus a combined neurovascular injury now becomes:
  42-C3/IO4-MT4-NV5.

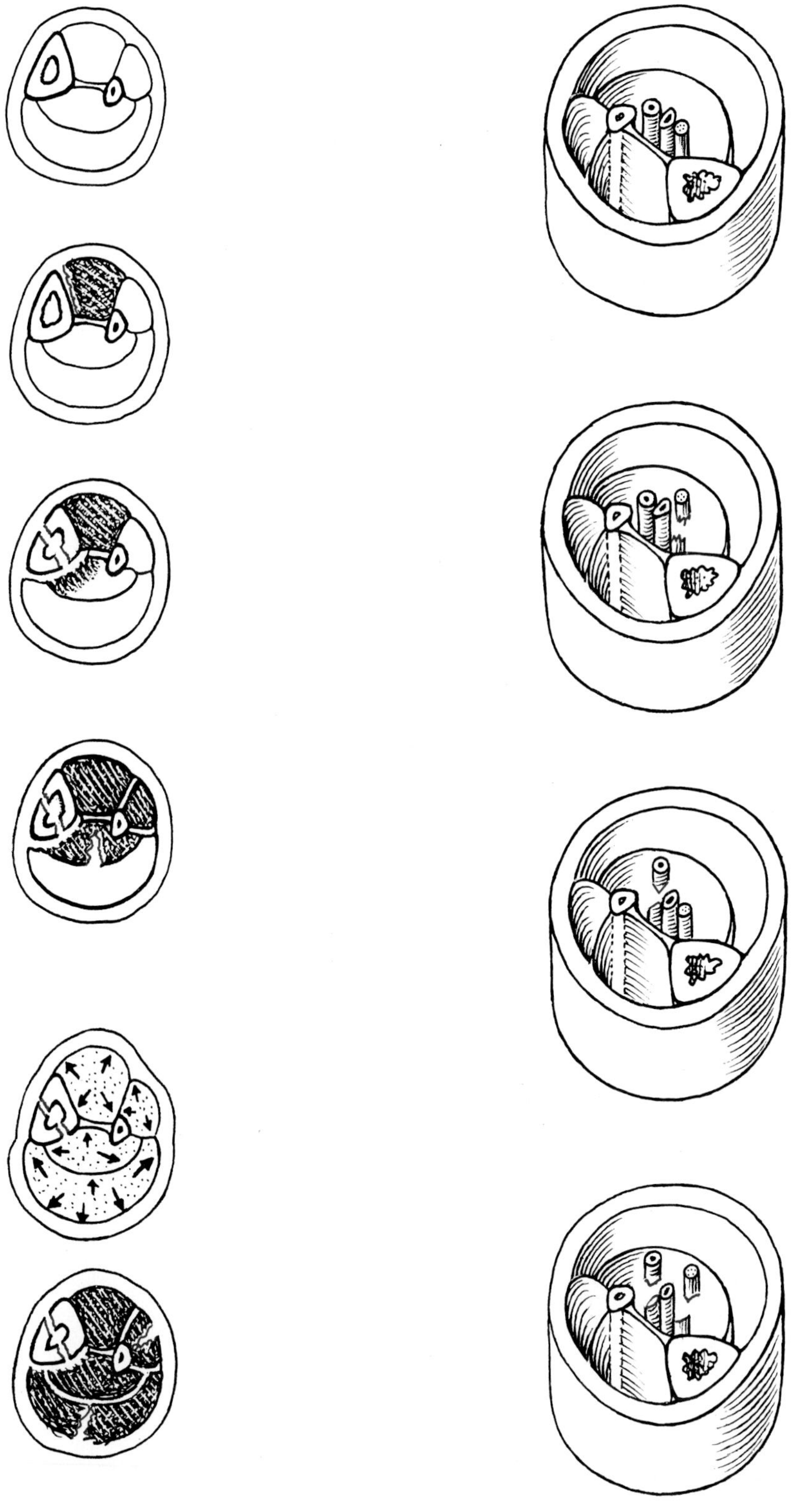

MT1

MT2

MT3

MT4

MT5

NV1

NV2

NV3

NV4

SUBTOTAL } AMPUTATION NV5
TOTAL

Diagnosis of the Injury on Digitized X-Rays

On digitized X-rays the information of the correct diagnosis of the injury (=diagnosis of the bone lesion and of the state of the soft tissue) can be indicated in code form as in the following two examples.

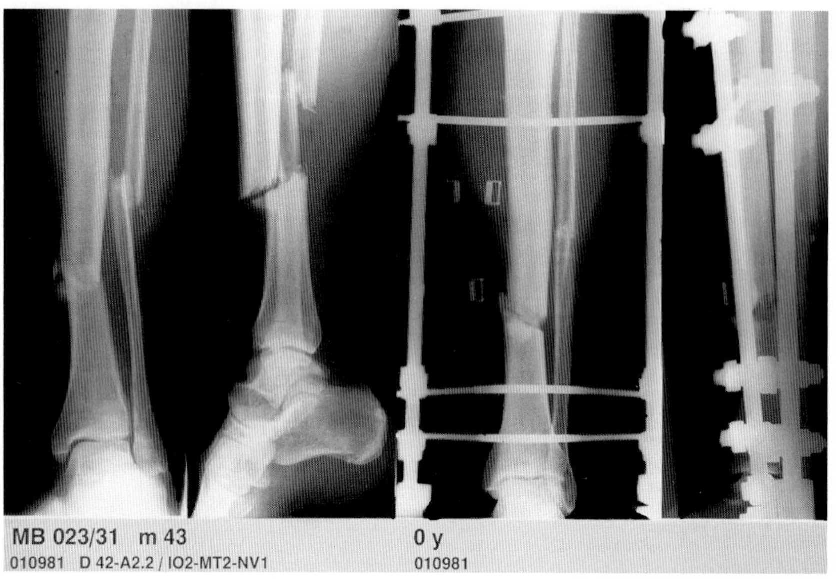

D=Diagnosis of the injury: 42=tibia/fibula diaphysis, A2=simple fracture, oblique ($\geq 30°$), .2=fibula fractured at another level. IO2=Skin breakage from outside in <5 cm, contused edges, MT2=circumscribed muscle injury, one compartment only, NV1=no neurovascular injury.

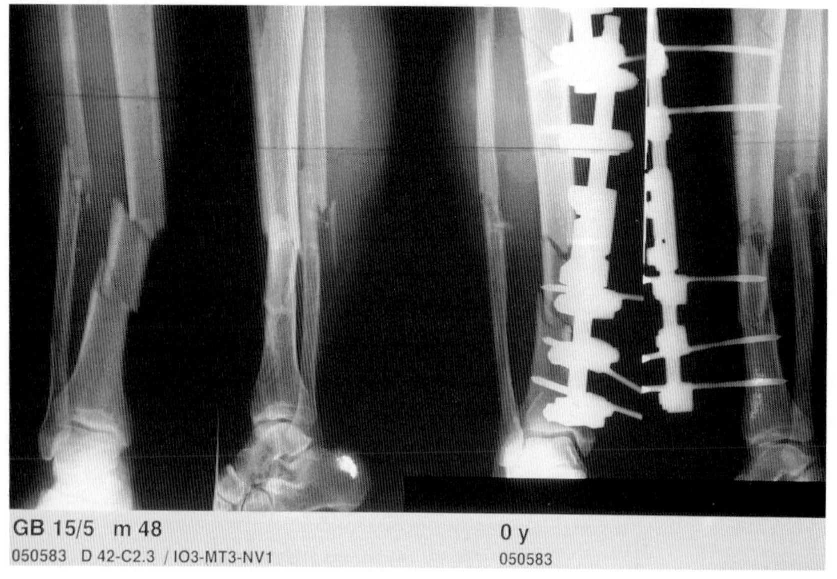

D=Diagnosis of the injury: 42=tibia/fibula diaphysis, C2=complex fracture, segmental, .3=with two intermediate segmental fragments. IO3=Skin breakage >5 cm, increased contusion, devitalized edges, MT3=considerable muscle injury, two compartments, NV1=no neurovascular injury.

2 PREOPERATIVE PLANNING AND PRINCIPLES OF REDUCTION

2.1 Preoperative Planning

The proposed operative procedure should always be planned so that the fracture surgery can be carried out in a smooth and atraumatic manner. The goals of planning are twofold; first, to determine the "desired end result" with a tracing, preoperatively, of the X-rays at the completion of the procedure, and second, to develop the "surgical tactic" which defines the operative steps and their order.

2.1.1 Equipment Needed

It is essential to have the appropriate X-rays, a good viewing box with a strong light source, tracing paper, a goniometer, and colored felt-tip pens.

2.1.2 Technique of Overlay Tracings

This technique demands not only standard X-rays of good quality, but also an adequate evaluation of the patient. Occasionally, further assessment, including oblique or other views, tomography, or computed axial tomography (with or without three-dimensional reconstruction), may be necessary.

2.1.2.1 Planning from the Normal Side

For purposes of comparison, X-rays are required of both the injured and the normal side. The plane of reference is determined by that X-ray projection (usually the AP) which reveals the maximum deformity of fracture displacement.

First, a tracing of the fractured bone is made in the plane of reference. If, for example, this tracing is made in the AP projection and the lateral projection evaluated on the AP tracing, the posterior fracture lines should be differentiated by using dotted lines or a different colored pen. In complex fractures, the fragments may be retraced on a separate piece of tracing paper, increasing the distance between them for easier understanding. Then a tracing of the normal bone is made in the same projection: simple overlay drawing using the normal side as the template is then carried out (Fig. 2.1).

2.1.2.2 Direct Overlay Technique

Tracings of the various fracture fragments on separate sheets of paper allow one to manipulate the tracings directly and individually into reduction.

2.1.2.3 Use of Templates

In both of the techniques described above, one selects the appropriate transparent template preprinted with outlines of standard implants. By overlaying this, one may determine the optimal type and length of the implant and the best positions for the screws.

2.1.2.4 Planning from the Physiological Axes

This technique is mainly applicable to periarticular fractures. It is more difficult, but allows the surgeon to simulate the steps of the reduction and, therefore, more readily to understand the kinetics of the particular case in question. The technique is illustrated in Figs. 2.2–2.4.

2.1.3 Additional Preoperative Planning

When an unfamiliar operation is to be carried out, practising on plastic bones conveys a first-hand "feel" of the surgical procedure and enables one to see how the proposed fixation is accomplished.

2.1.4 Conclusion

Preoperative planning reduces the duration of surgery and the level of frustration. Using the tracings, the operative team can understand the steps of the procedure and ensure that the correct equipment, including the implant, is available.

Fig. 2.1

a A tracing is made of the fracture from the X-ray. In this case, the AP projection was used.

b A tracing is made from a similar projection of the normal or uninjured side.

c If desirable, the fragments appearing on the tracing of the fracture may be separated so that they are more easily appreciated.

d Using a tracing of the normal side, turning it over so that it matches the orientation of the fractured side, simple overlay drawings may be made by manipulating the two sheets of paper such that the normal side tracings overlie recognizable fragments on the fractured side. These fracture lines are then drawn onto the tracing of the normal side.

e This results in an equivalent of an illustration of how the fractured bone will look once it is reduced.

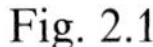

Fig. 2.1

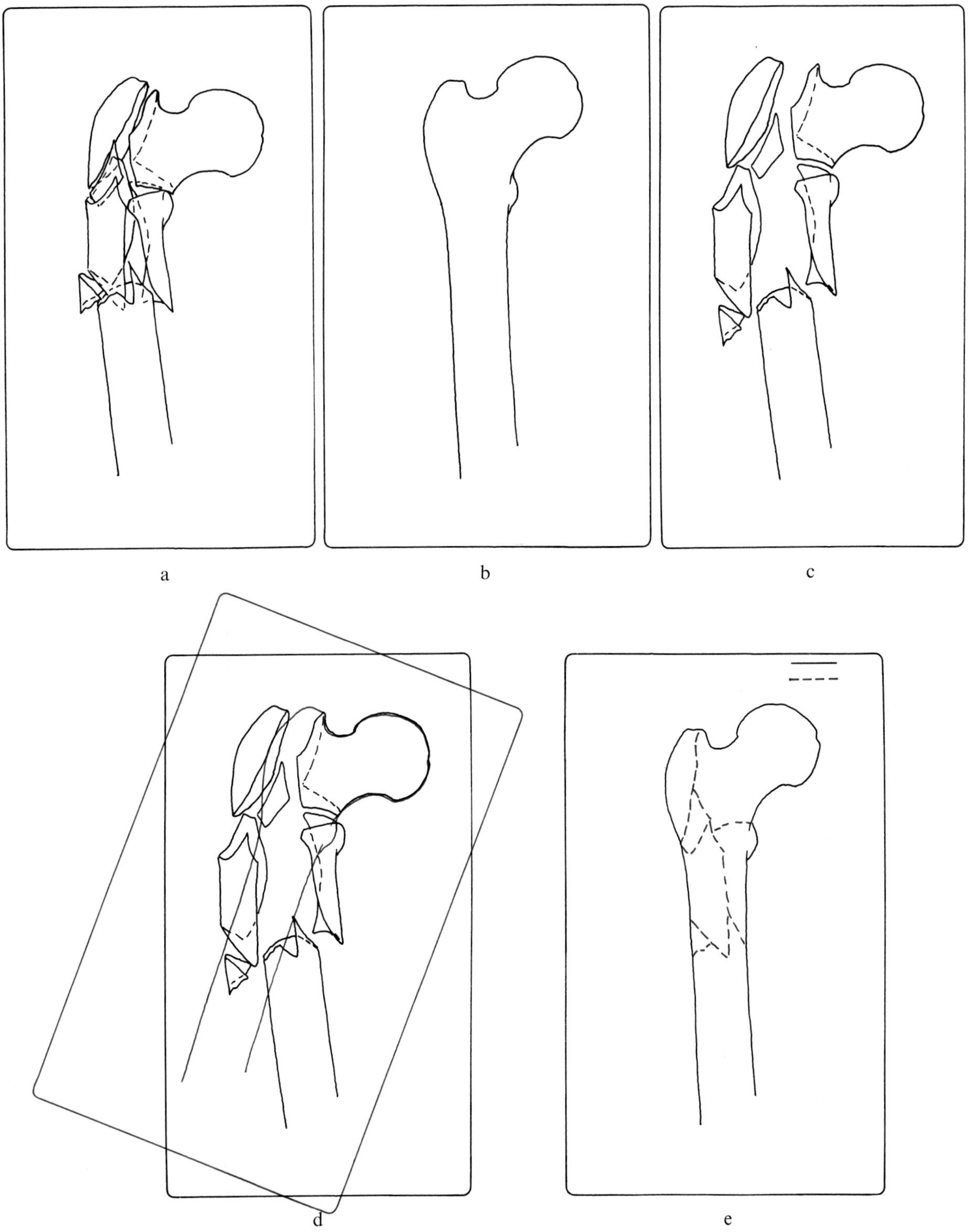

a b c

d e

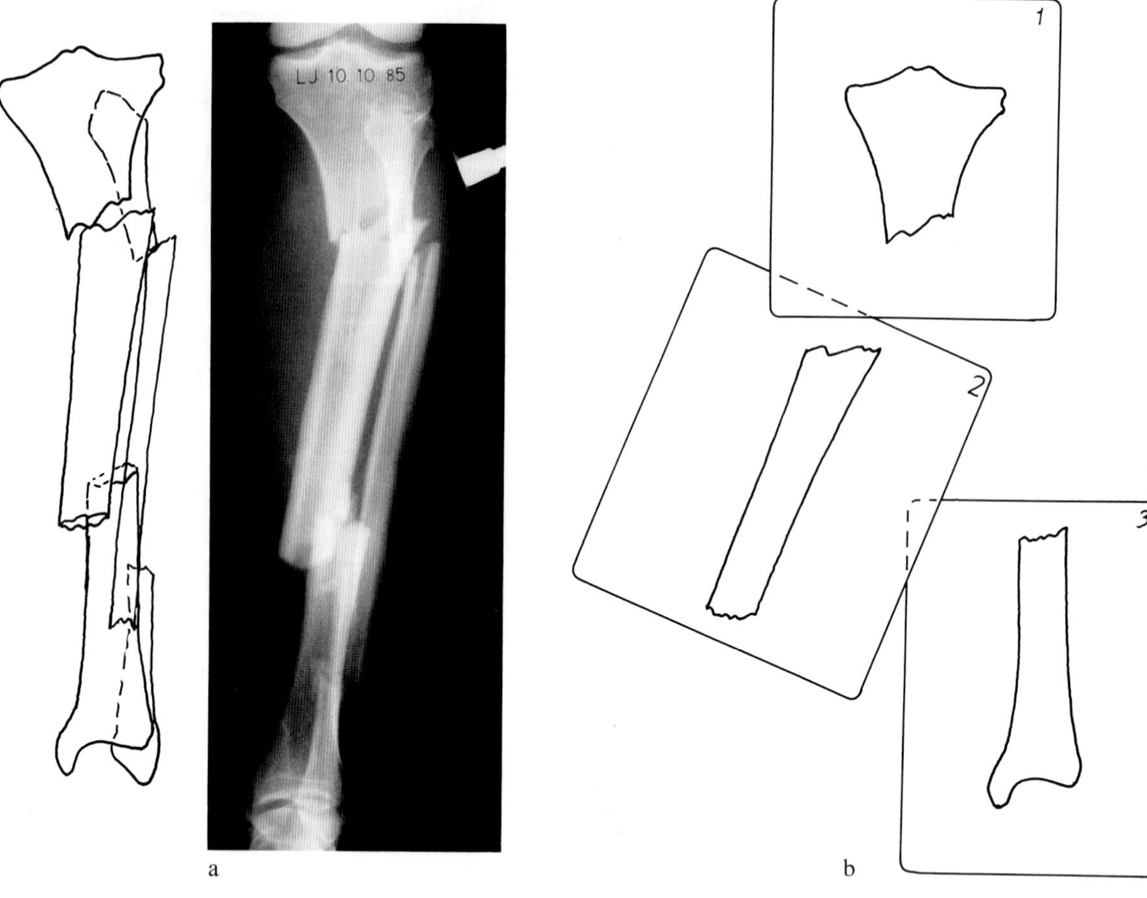

Fig. 2.2

a In a straight bone, the direct overlay technique is a quick method for planning. The fracture, in this case a segmental tibia and fibula fracture, is traced in the AP plane. Since the tibia is a straight bone, and since the fibula fracture is a vassal fracture, the various tibial fragments may be traced on separate pieces of paper and then oriented on a straight line representing the axis.

b The various components of the segmental tibia fracture have been traced on individual pieces of paper.

c A straight line is drawn on an additional piece of paper.

d The fragments are assembled on the axis.

e The final tracing.

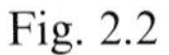

Fig. 2.2

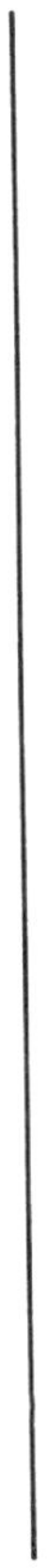

c

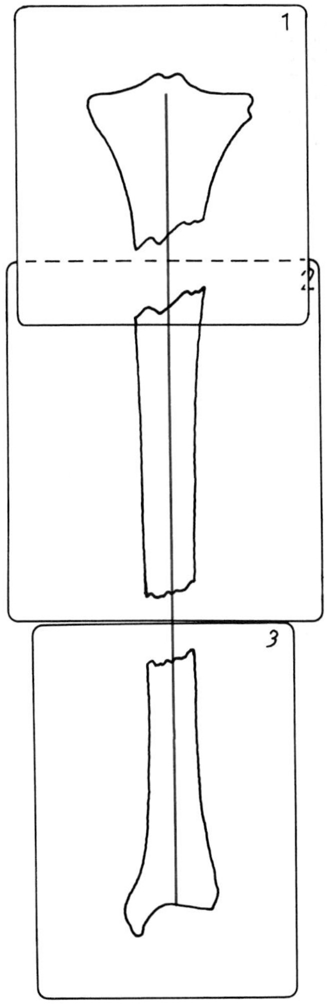

d

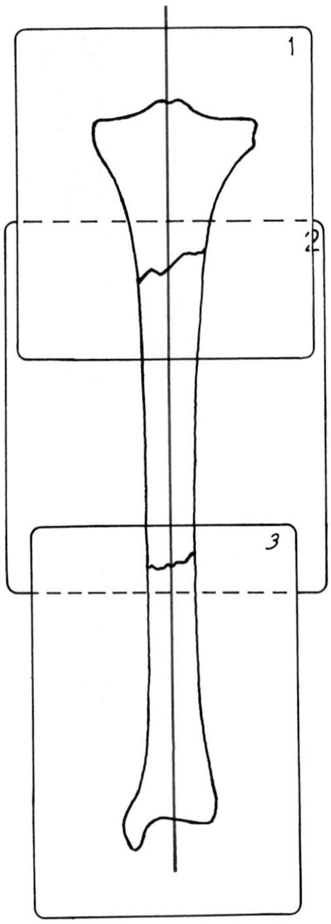

e

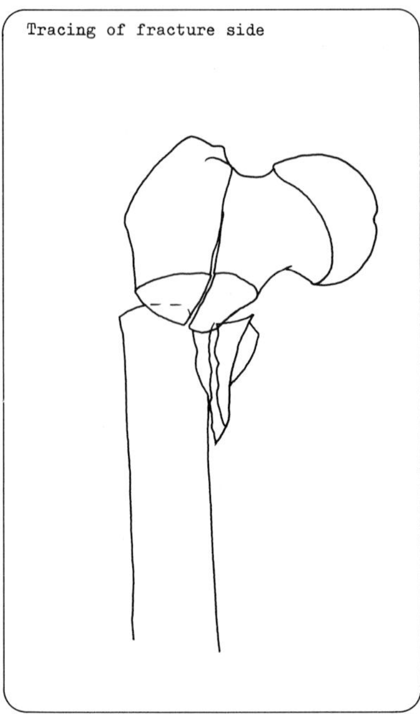

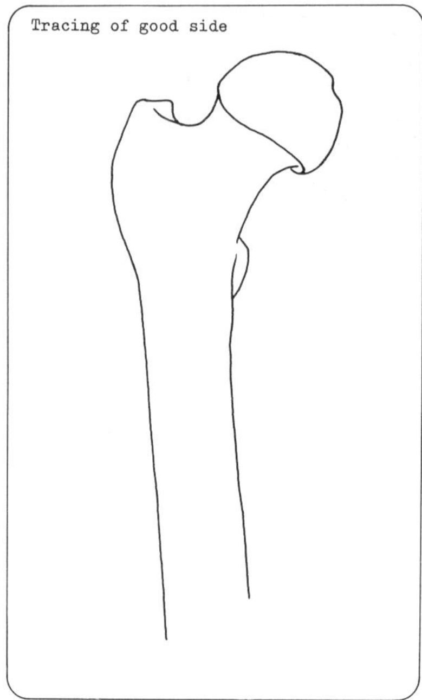

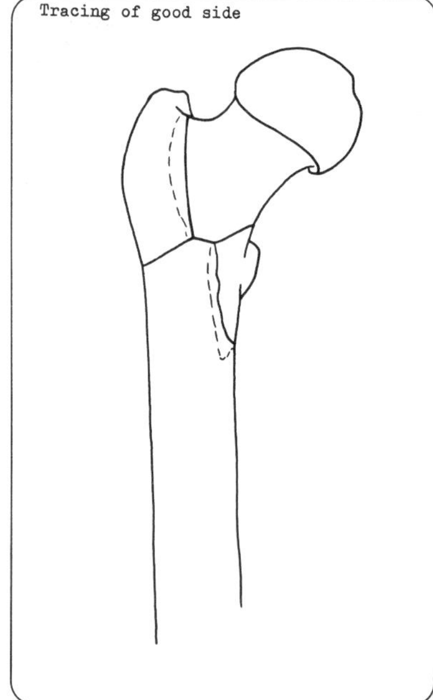

a

Fig. 2.3

a In another example of a complex intertrochanteric fracture, the fracture is traced on a piece of paper. The normal side is traced on a second piece of paper and the drawing turned over to match the fractured side. The fracture lines are transferred to the tracing of the good side as described in Fig. 2.1 d.

b To simulate the actual kinetics of the reduction at surgery, the proximal fragment is traced separately with the template of a 95° angle blade plate overlaid in the proper location.

c The distal fragment is traced separately.

d By overlaying the proximal fragment plus implant and the distal fragment, one may play with the two tracings to see exactly how the reduction may be achieved with the implant. This method of indirect reduction is discussed in this chapter.

e With the fracture reduced and the implant in place, one may ascertain the distance from the tip of the greater trochanter at which the window for the angle blade plate must be made and determine the direction of the seating chisel in the femoral head to ensure that the implant is properly situated. In addition, the proper length of the plate and the location of the lag screws may be planned.

Fig. 2.3

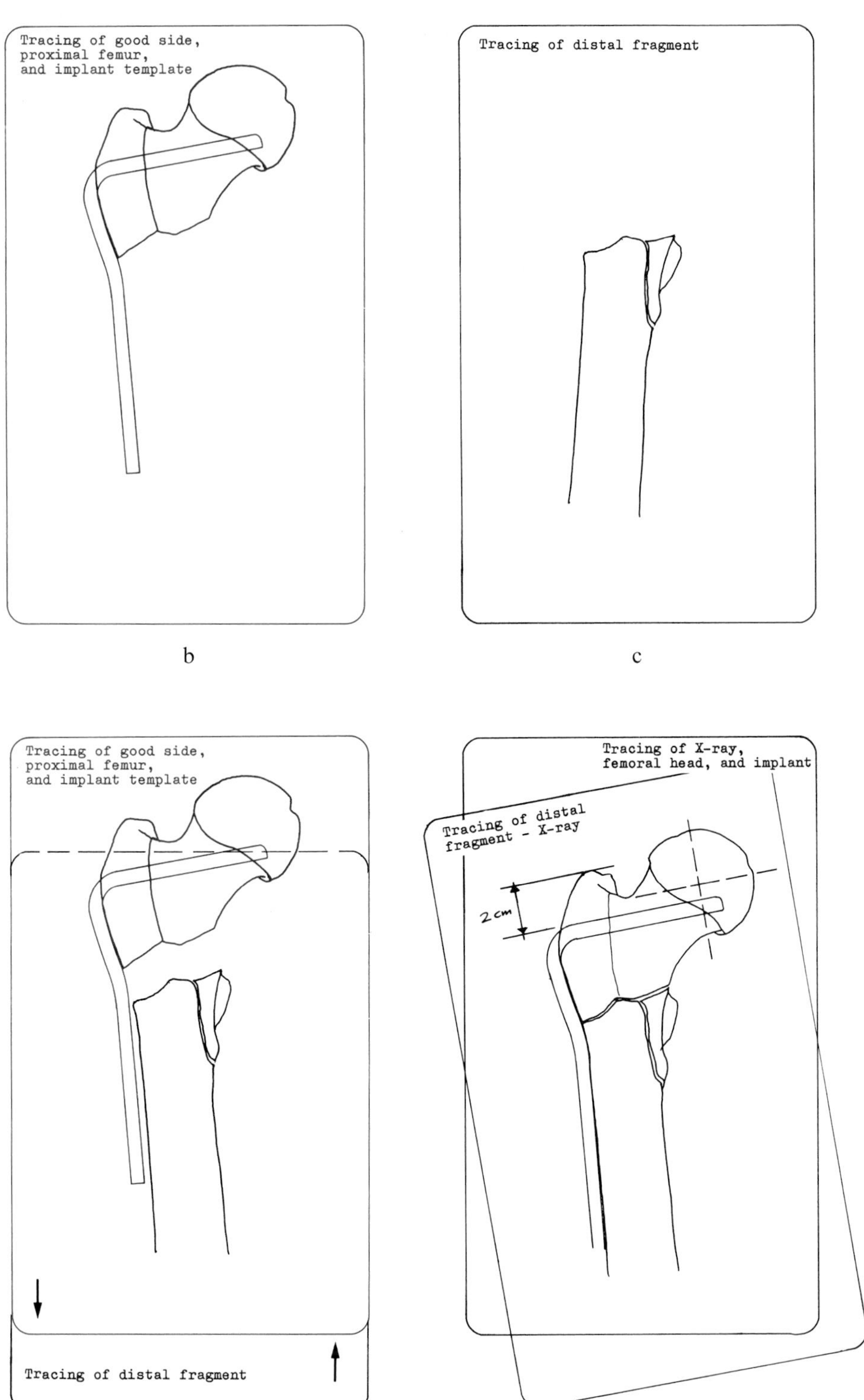
Tracing of good side,
proximal femur,
and implant template
Tracing of distal fragment
b
c
Tracing of good side,
proximal femur,
and implant template
Tracing of distal fragment
Tracing of X-ray,
femoral head, and implant
Tracing of distal
fragment - X-ray
2 cm
d
e

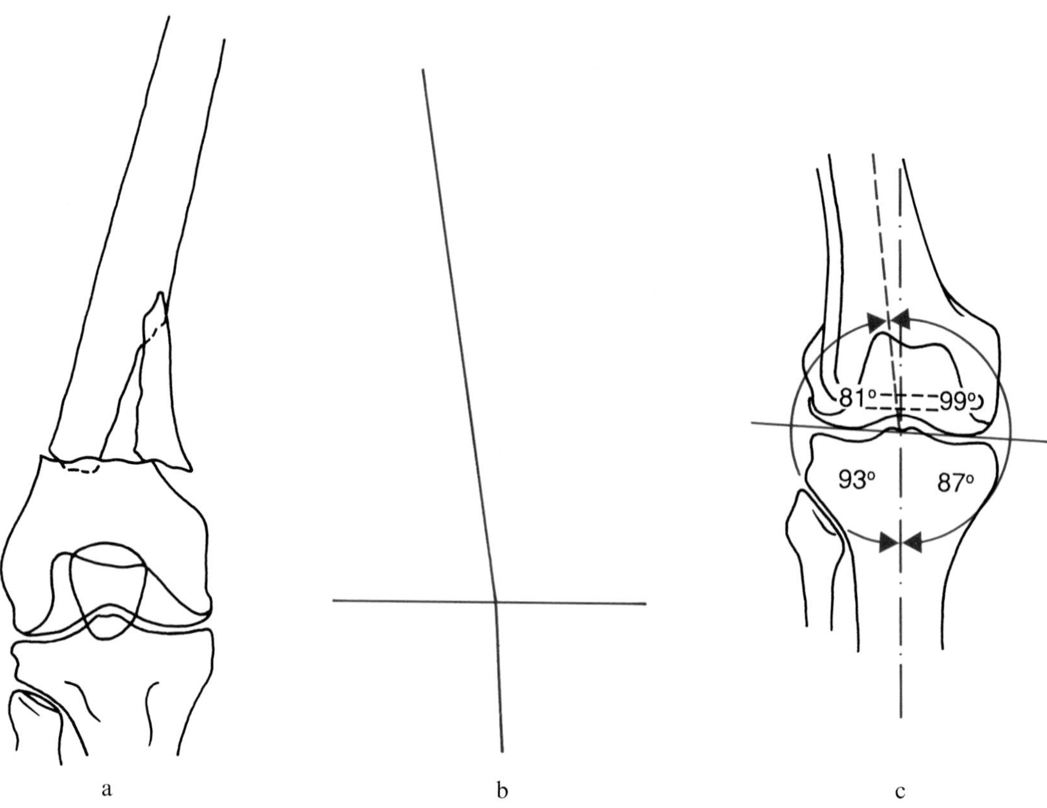

Fig. 2.4

a A tracing of a complex fracture of the distal femur.

b The anatomic axes of the femoral shaft and tibial shaft, crossed by the mechanical axis of the knee joint. The axial relationships will allow us to plan the reduction and fixation of this fracture, which is well treated by a 95° condylar plate.

c The above illustration gives the values of the anatomic axes of the femur and tibia in relationship to the mechanical axis of the knee. The illustration shows that if the 95° condylar plate is placed parallel to the mechanical axis of the knee joint in the frontal plane, proper relationships between the anatomic femoral shaft axis and anatomic tibial shaft axis will be ensured. The tibial shaft axis is coaxial with the mechanical axis of the leg.

d The fragments of the distal femur fracture are traced on separate pieces of paper.

e The fragment containing the knee joint is placed coaxial with the mechanical axis of the knee such that the tibia is coaxial with the anatomic axis of the tibia.

Fig. 2.4

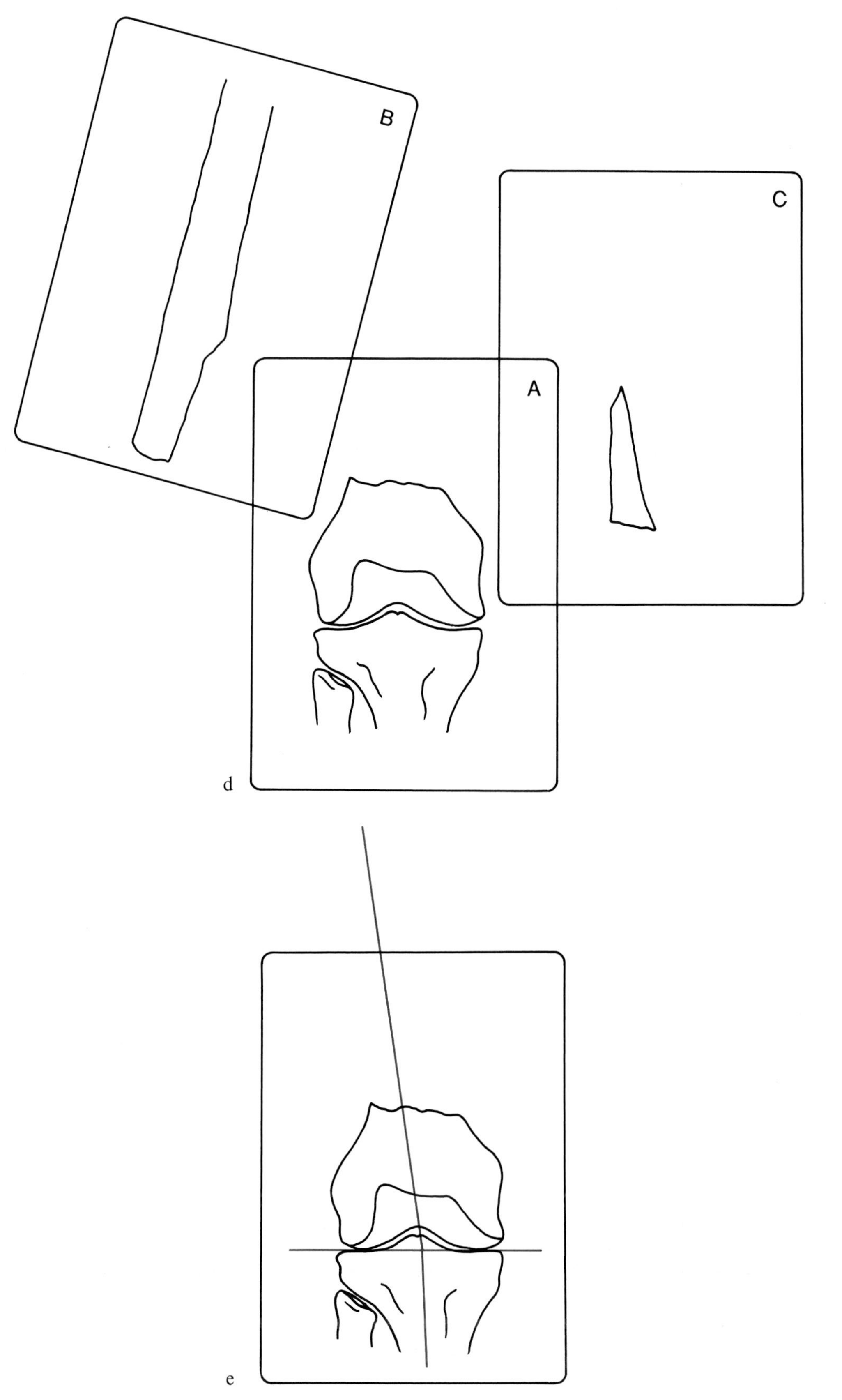

Fig. 2.4 (continued)

f The remaining tracings with the proximal fragment and the butterfly fragment of the femur are then reduced about the femoral shaft axis.

g With the femoral fractures reduced, the implant template is overlaid such that the blade lies parallel with the mechanical axis of the knee joint and the plate portion of the template adjacent to the femoral shaft. The proper length of implant may be selected and the number of screws and their function can be determined by the relationship of the plate to the reduced fracture on the drawing.

h The same steps may be carried out in the sagittal plane on the lateral view of the fracture to see the desired end result from the side.

Fig. 2.4

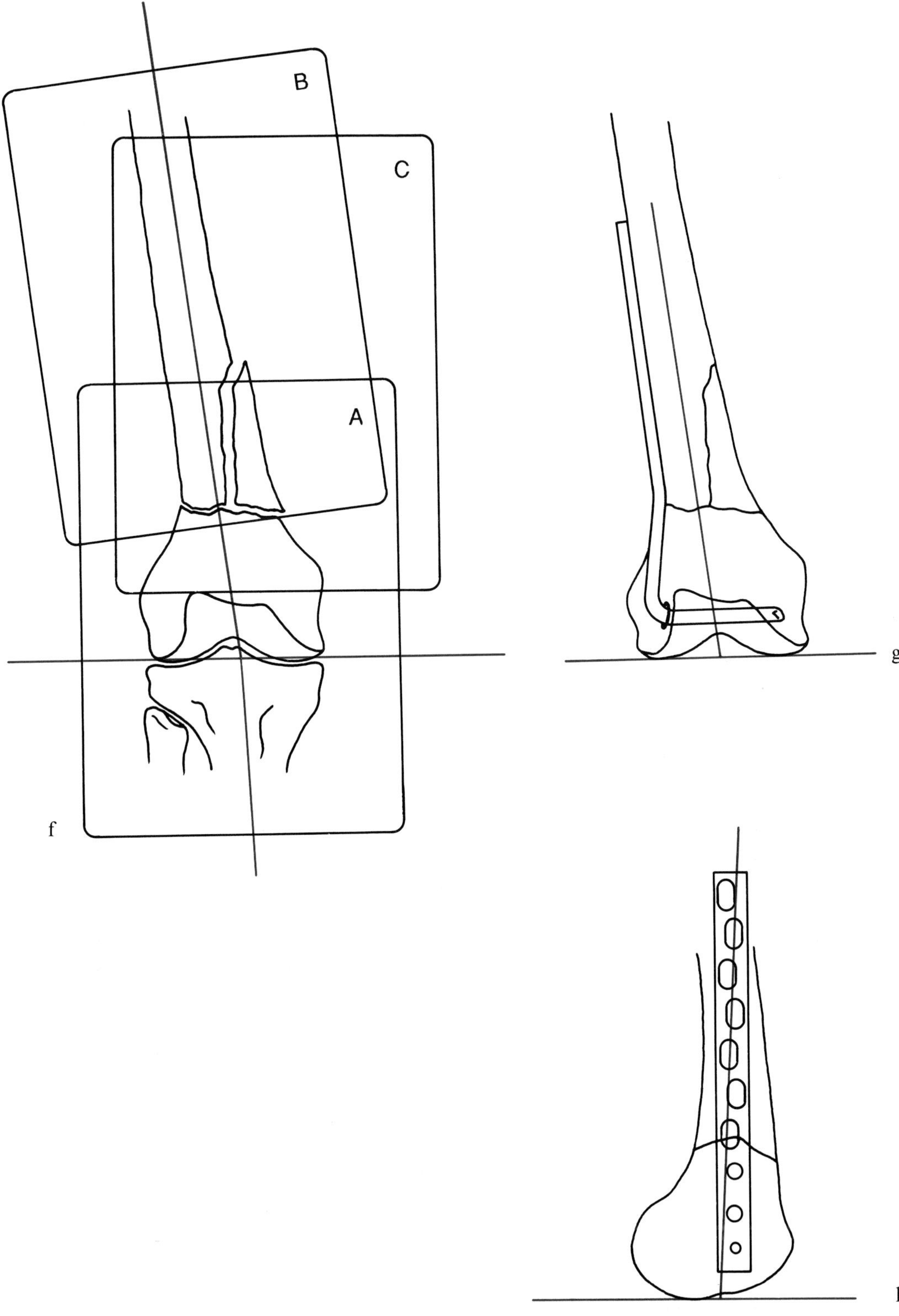

2.2 Principles of Reduction

A bone fractures when it fails under abnormal load. The damage is not confined to the bone but, to varying degrees, extends into the surrounding soft tissues. The primary requisite of reduction techniques is that they are gentle and atraumatic, and preserve the remaining vascularity.

2.2.1 What Reduction Must Achieve

In the *diaphysis* of a long bone, satisfactory reduction is obtained with the restoration of axial alignment in all three planes (frontal, sagittal, and horizontal). Displacements should be completely corrected in young adults and active individuals. Anatomic reduction of complex diaphyseal fragments should not be attempted where it would be at the expense of the vascularity of the bone.

The *metaphysis* has the same requirements as the diaphysis, but in addition, it frequently requires buttressing and cancellous bone grafting for support and to replace bone lost through impaction of the joint surface into the underlying cancellous bone.

The *epiphysis* is the articular segment of the bone and in this area absolute anatomic restoration is mandatory.

2.2.2 Types of Operative Reduction

2.2.2.1 Manual Reduction

Applicable for most simple fractures, the advantages of manual reduction are that it is quick and may restore some intrinsic stability. The disadvantages are that the clamp required to maintain reduction frequently interferes with the definitive fixation. Additionally, if the reduction is lost, it may not be reproduced by a second attempt. Resulting frustration may lead to a surgical struggle and turn the reduction into a traumatic maneuver.

Fig. 2.5

a A simple fracture of the mid-shaft of the femur. Holes 4.5 mm in diameter are made in the proximal and distal fragments such that they will not interfere with the definitive implant after reduction.

b With the femoral distractor attached, distraction of the fracture fragments is carried out. With distraction there is a tendency towards straightening of the femur and, if distraction forces are high, creating a deformity in the opposite direction from the distraction force – in this case a varus.

c The tendency towards straightening may be corrected by carrying out the distraction over a bolster. The bolster acts as a fulcrum to maintain the antecurvatum of the femur.

Fig. 2.5

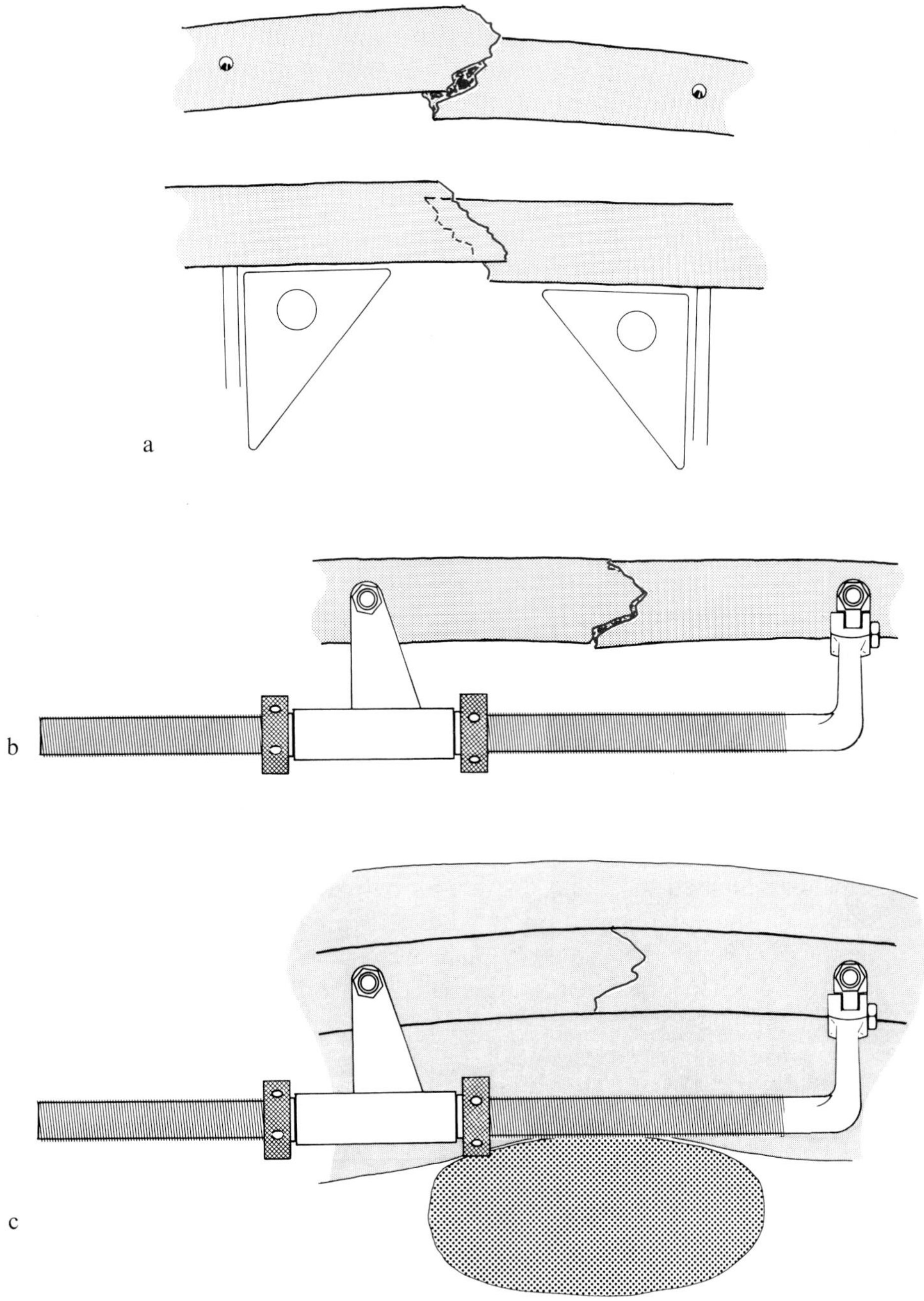

2.2.2.2 Mechanical Reduction

Reduction methods may be termed mechanical if they depend upon the use of distraction devices such as the fracture table, the large and small distractors, or the articulating tension device, or if the method involves the use of an implant which causes an "interference reduction" (e.g., intramedullary nail).

Fracture Table

This positions the patient so that an image intensifier can be used to control the reduction: it also maintains this position during fixation. Its main disadvantage is that the traction must be applied in a "linkage" system across at least one joint. The mobility of the limb is lost to the surgeon, and the flexibility of the surgical approach is frequently compromised.

Large and Small Distractors

These provide direct attachments to the proximal and distal main fragments which allow mobility of the fractured limb during the operative procedure. Angulation, displacement, and rotation may be corrected, and the device may then be used in compression to stabilize the fragments.

The main disadvantage of these devices is that their attachment directly to the bone requires additional holes. There is also a tendency to straighten a curved bone during the distraction procedure, and the eccentric force produced by the unilaterally mounted distractor may produce additional deformity (Fig. 2.5).

Articulated Tensioning Device

This may be used to obtain distraction by placing the hook of the device in an outward direction and attaching it to the bone in a semiclosed or closed position. The hook is placed against the end of a plate which has been attached to the opposite side of the fracture. On opening the articulated tensioning device, the hook pushes against the end of the plate, distracting the fracture fragments and facilitating reduction (Figs. 2.6, 2.7).

Fig. 2.6

a The articulated tensioning device in distraction mode. The plate is attached to the distal fragment by one or, after alignment in the sagittal plane has been obtained, two screws. An appropriate size bone-holding forceps is placed on the proximal side of the fracture holding the plate to the bone. Distraction is carried out. Comminution is reduced by means of the restored tension in the soft tissues.

b The comminuted fragments, in this case a lateral butterfly fragment, may be teased into final position with the use of a sharp hook.

c After the fracture fragments are reduced, coaptation of the fracture may be achieved by turning the articulated tensioning device into compression mode and making sure contact between the fracture fragments has been obtained. Caution must be exercised at this point, as too much tension on the plate will produce valgus deformity.

Fig. 2.6

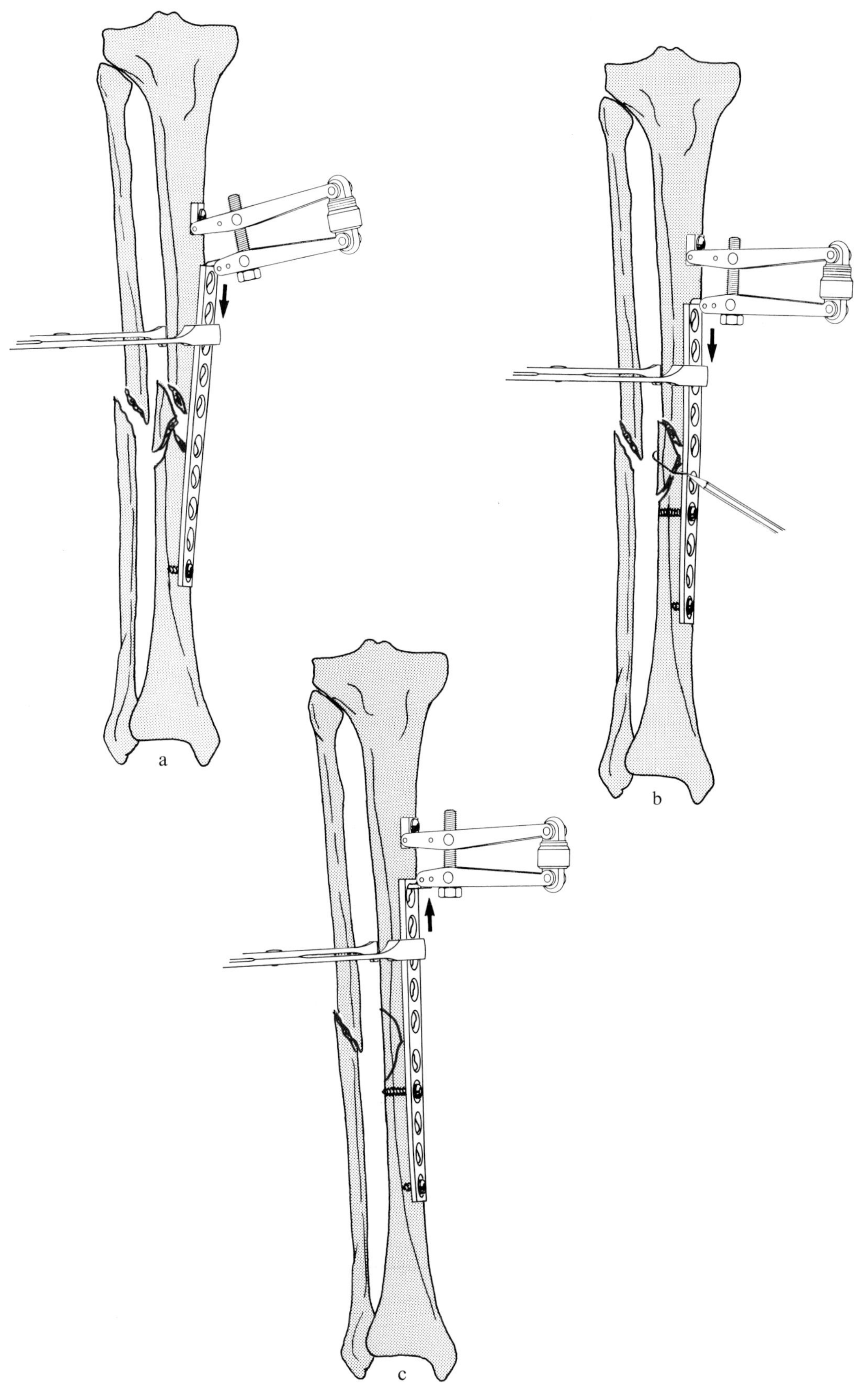

Fig. 2.7

a The same technique illustrated in Fig. 2.6, using an angled blade plate, may be employed in the proximal femur. The fracture is distracted with the articulated tensioning device off the end of the plate in distraction mode. A bone-holding forceps is used to hold the plate to the bone, in this case on the distal fragment.

b With distraction, the tendency for comminuted fragments to reduce is increased by restoring length. They may be teased into their final stage of reduction with a small instrument, and the leg may be maneuvered into a position that facilitates this reduction.

c, d Once the fragments have been reduced into the fracture gap, they are held in place with a pointed reduction forceps.

Fig. 2.7

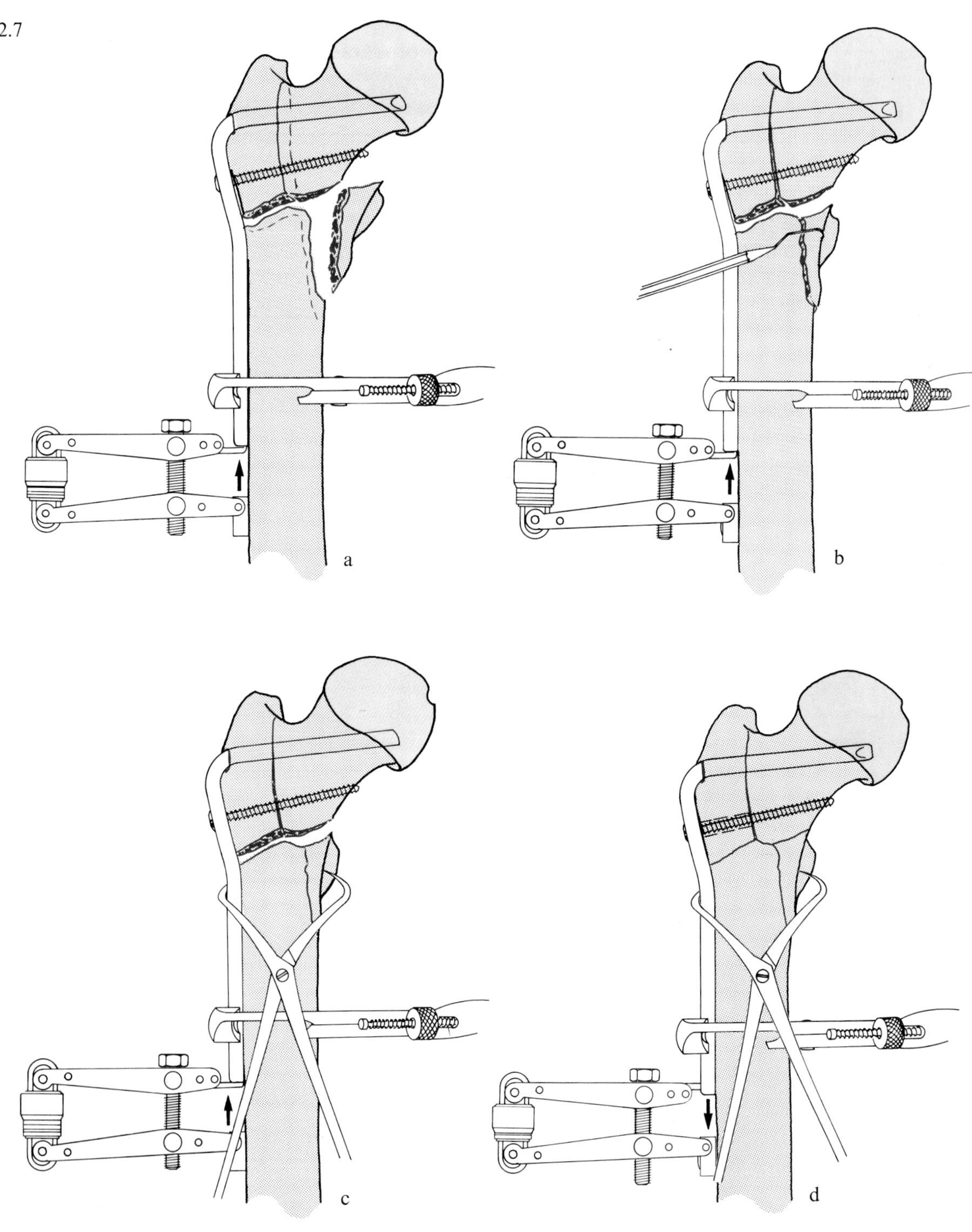

Interference Reduction

Reduction may be obtained with an implant through an interference mechanism. A simple example of this is the reduction achieved by an anatomically shaped intramedullary nail. As the nail crosses the fracture, with rotation controlled, the fracture is reduced by the interference fit.

A similar mechanism has been described by Weber, utilizing the "antiglide plate". The application of a properly contoured plate to one fragment of an oblique fracture results in interference between the plate and the displaced opposite fragment. As the plate pushes against the displaced bone, it forces the reduction along the oblique fracture surfaces (Fig. 2.8). This technique corrects small displacements and angulations, maintaining stability as the reduction occurs. The force required to reduce the fracture is concentrated at the location where it is most needed, and reduction is achieved because of the soft tissue attachments, not despite them. It requires careful preoperative planning.

2.2.3 Conclusion

The emphasis, in techniques of reduction, must be on the preservation of the viability of the soft tissues as well as of the bone. Mechanical reduction has the advantage, over manual reduction, of providing temporary or definitive stability as the reduction is accomplished.

Reference

Mast JW, Jakob R, Ganz R (1989) Planning and reduction technique in fracture surgery. Springer, Berlin Heidelberg New York

---

Fig. 2.8

a The use of an antiglide plate in an oblique fracture of the distal tibia. The plate should be precontoured from an X-ray of the opposite side; alternatively, the contour may be approximated by bending an arc with a radius of slightly less than 20 cm into the distal aspect of the plate after twisting the plate on its central axis, so that the plate exhibits about 25° of internal rotation distally.

b The plate is then attached to the fragment displaced away from the side of the bone to which the plate will be definitively fixed.

c The alignment of the plate with the distal fragment is corrected in the sagittal plane, and any rotational correction may be carried out at this time by the surgeon or the assistant. The next screw is then inserted.

d Finally a third screw is applied. As it is tightened, the plate, which has interfered with the proximal fragment in such a way as to cause it to reduce with the addition of each screw, brings about definitive repositioning. The principle of the antiglide plate was first described by Weber.

Fig. 2.8

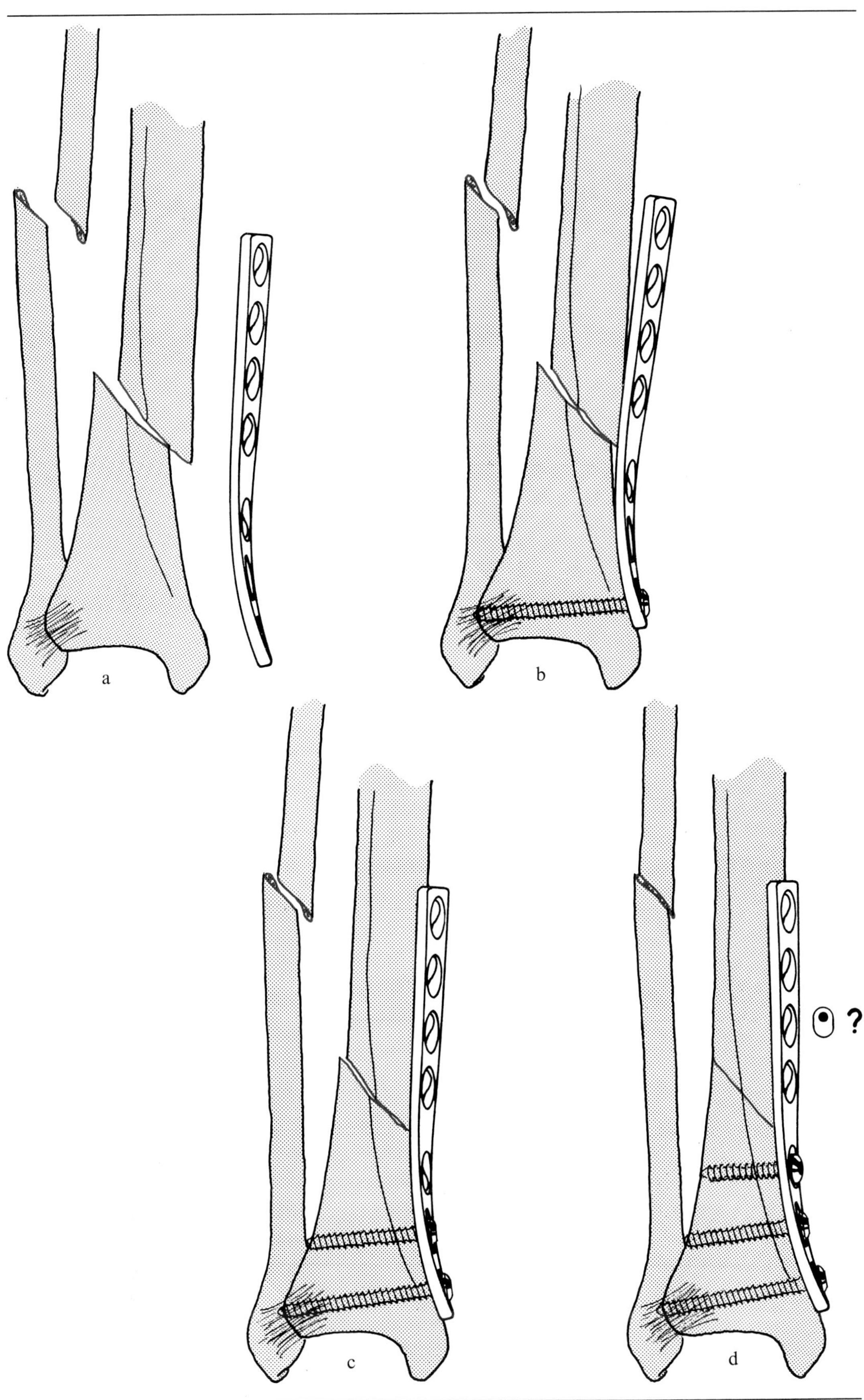

3 SCREWS AND PLATES AND THEIR APPLICATION

3.1 Screws

3.1.1 Function of Screws

Screws are used either to fasten plates or similar devices onto bone, or, as lag screws, to hold together fragments of bone.

3.1.2 Types of Screws

Screws are differentiated by: the manner in which they are inserted into bone, their function, their size, and the type of bone they are intended for. Thus we differentiate between self-tapping and non-self-tapping screws, lag screws, and large and small fragment cortical and cancellous screws.

One other major differentiation between screws is based on the manner in which they couple with a screwdriver. Thus screws may have a slot, a cruciate recess, a square, and so on. All but the smallest AO screws have a hexagonal recess and require a corresponding screwdriver with a hexagonal tip (Fig. 3.3). The screws couple securely with the screwdriver, which has completely obviated any screw holding devices on the screwdriver. This feature has proven itself to be of great advantage at the time of screw removal and insertion. At removal, once the tissue is cleared from the hexagonal recess in the screw head, the screwdriver can be easily inserted into the screw head and the screw turned without the screwdriver jumping out and stripping the recess. At insertion, the torque is transmitted evenly to the screw and there is no danger of tilting and losing control of screw direction or of stripping the recess. There is one further advantage of the secure coupling of the screw head with the screwdriver. At insertion, it is useful, and at times very necessary, to know the exact direction of a screw. By simply inserting the screwdriver into an AO screw the surgeon has an automatic guide to its direction.

3.1.2.1 Self-Tapping and Non-Self-Tapping Screws

Self-tapping screws (Fig. 3.1, right) are designed in such a way that once a pilot hole is drilled into bone they can be inserted by simply screwing them in. The pilot hole is somewhat larger than the core of the screw. Because the screw has to cut its own thread as it is inserted, it encounters considerable resistance, particularly in thick cortical bone. At times the resistance may be such that the torque required to drive the screw in is greater than the tolerance of the screw and the screw may break. In addition, the resistance to screw insertion may interfere with the accuracy of insertion, particularly if one is trying to insert the screw obliquely into bone to lag two fragments together. It used to be thought that self-tapping screws had a weaker hold in bone. Experimental investigation (Schatzker et al. 1975a–c) has shown that a self-tapping screw can be removed and reinserted without weakening its hold in bone provided it is carefully inserted. However, if inadvertently angled it will cut a new path and destroy the already cut thread, which is a disadvantage. Self-tapping screws should therefore not be used as lag screws.

Non-self-tapping screws (Fig. 3.1, left) require a predrilled pilot hole and then a careful cutting of their thread in cortical bone with a tap which corresponds exactly to the profile of the screw thread. Because the thread is cut with a tap the pilot hole corresponds in size almost to the core of the screw and the screw thread has a much deeper bite into the adjacent bone. There is much less heat generated when the screw is inserted because there is less resistance. The tap is designed in such a way that it is not only much sharper than the thread of a screw, but it also has a more efficient mechanism of clearing the bone debris, which therefore does not accumulate and clog its threads to obstruct its insertion. This allows one to work with much greater precision, particularly in thick cortical bone. The screws can be removed and reinserted with ease without the fear of inadvertently cutting a new channel, as a screw alone is not able to cut a channel in cortical bone. The screws are spun, therefore their core is perfectly straight and their surface is polished. Thus at the time of removal, fully threaded screws are easily removed. Recent investigative work has shown that in extremely thin layers of cortical bone, such as facial bones, self-tapping screws appear to have a better holding power than the non-self-tapping screws of corresponding size (Phillips and Rahn 1989). The non-self-tapping screw has clear superiority except in extremely thin cortical bone, cancellous bone, and in flat bones such as those of face, the skull, and the pelvis.

Fig. 3.1 Note the difference between the non-self-tapping screw (a) and the self-tapping screw. The pilot hole for the latter has to be larger (b) and the screw threads do not penetrate as deeply into the bone (c).

Fig. 3.1

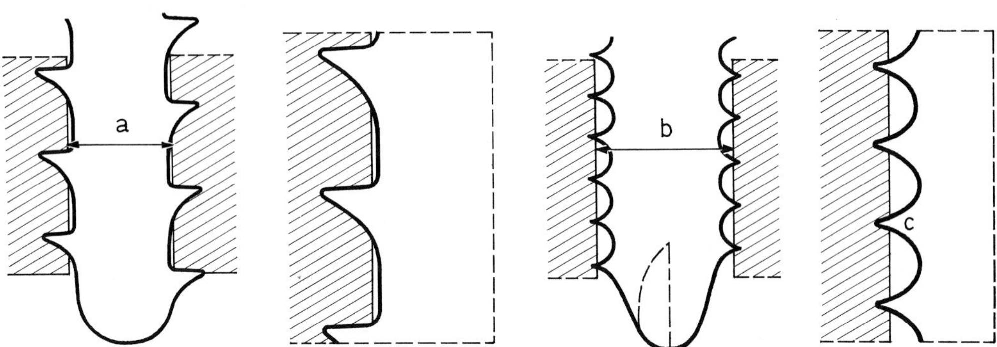

3.1.3 Cortex and Cancellous Bone Screws

3.1.3.1 Cortex Screws

Cortex screws (Fig. 3.2) are fully threaded. They are non-self-tapping so a tap is required to cut their thread before insertion. Since the holding power of a screw diminishes as the diameter of the screw approaches 40% of the diameter of the bone there are a number of different sizes of cortex screws available in the AO armamentarium to enable fixation of bones of different diameters. Each screw size has its corresponding drill bit and tap.

Fig. 3.2 The cortex screws.

I The 4.5-mm cortex screw.

a Fully threaded with a diameter of 4.5 mm and a 1.75-mm pitch.
b Screw head 8 mm in diameter with a 3.5-mm hexagonal recess.
c The core is 3 mm.
d The drill bit for the thread hole is 3.2 mm.
e The drill bit for the gliding hole is 4.5 mm.
f The tap has a diameter of 4.5 mm.

II The 3.5 mm cortex screw.

a Fully threaded with a diameter of 3.5 mm and a 1.25-mm pitch.
b Screw head 6 mm in diameter with a 2.5-mm hexagonal recess.
c The core is 2.4 mm.
d The drill bit for the thread hole is 2.5 mm.
e The drill bit for the gliding hole is 3.5 mm.
f The tap has a diameter of 3.5 mm.

III The 2.7-mm cortex screw.

a Fully threaded with a diameter of 2.7 mm and a 1.0-mm pitch.
b Screw head 5 mm in diameter with a 2.5-mm hexagonal recess.
c The core is 1.9 mm.
d The drill bit for the thread hole is 2.0 mm.
e The drill bit for the gliding hole is 2.7 mm.
f The tap has a diameter of 2.7 mm.

IV The 2.0-mm cortex screw.

a Fully threaded with a diameter of 2.0 mm and a 0.8-mm pitch.
b Screw head 4.0 mm in diameter with a 1.5-mm hexagonal recess.
c The core is 1.3 mm.
d The drill bit for the thread hole is 1.5 mm.
e The drill bit for the gliding hole is 2.0 mm.
f The tap has a diameter of 2.0 mm.

V The 1.5-mm cortex screw.

a Fully threaded with a diameter of 1.5 mm and a 0.6-mm pitch.
b Screw head 3 mm in diameter with a 1.5-mm hexagonal recess.
c The core is 1.0 mm.
d The drill bit for the thread hole is 1.1 mm.
e The drill bit for the gliding hole is 1.5 mm.
f The tap has a diameter of 1.5 mm.

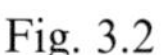

Fig. 3.2

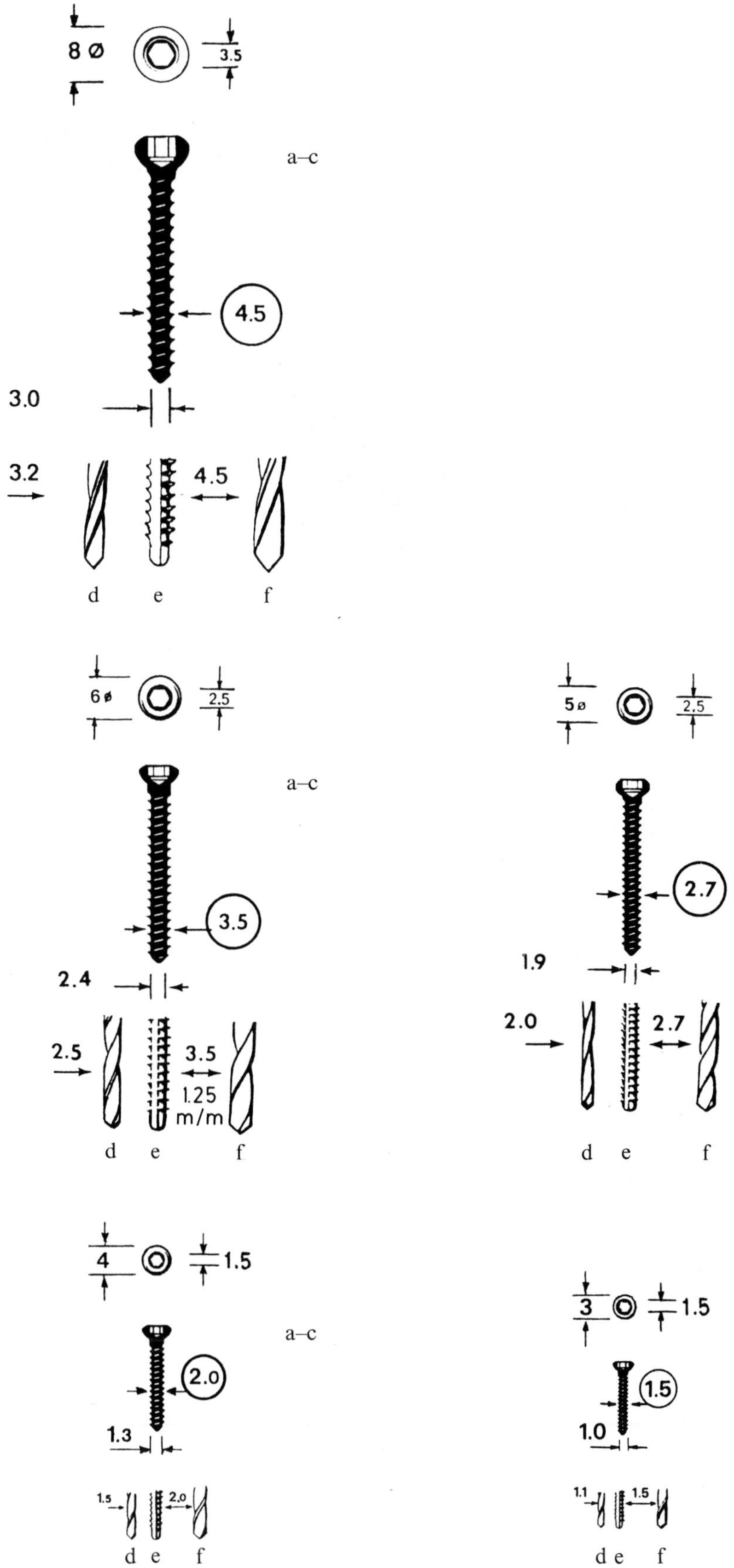

8 Ø 3.5
a–c
4.5
3.0
3.2 4.5
I
d e f

6 ø 2.5
a–c
3.5
2.4
2.5 3.5 1.25 m/m
II
d e f

4 1.5
a–c
2.0
1.3
1.5 2.0
III
d e f

5 ø 2.5
a–c
2.7
1.9
2.0 2.7
IV
d e f

3 1.5
a–c
1.5
1.0
1.1 1.5
V
d e f

Of particular note is the recently introduced AO 3.5-mm cortex screw. The pitch of this screw is different, as is the ratio of the outer diameter to the screw core. The core is larger (2.4 mm) than that of the corresponding cancellous bone screw (2.0 mm). The increase in the screw core thickness has increased the bending and torsional strength of this screw and has prevented shearing of the screws when used as load screws with the self-compressing DCPs.

3.1.3.2 Cancellous Bone Screws

Cancellous bone screws (Fig. 3.3) are characterized by a relatively thin core and a wide and deep thread. This increase in the ratio of the outer diameter to the core gives such a screw considerably increased holding power in fine trabecular bone, which characterizes metaphyseal and epiphyseal areas of bone. Cancellous bone screws are either fully or partially threaded. The fully threaded screws are used for fastening such devices as plates in metaphyseal and epiphyseal areas of bone. The partially threaded screws are used as lag screws. The cancellous bone screws differ not only in the number of threads but also in size. Thus there are the large 6.5-mm cancellous bone screws (Fig. 3.3a–c) and the fully and the partially threaded 4.0-mm small fragment cancellous bone screws (Fig. 3.3f). Cancellous bone screws are designed as non-self-tapping screws. Their thread must be tapped only in the near cortex. Tapping of the cancellous bone is unnecessary because the cancellous bone screw can easily cut a thread for itself, and its holding power is increased if its thread is not cut because it tends to compress the trabeculae together when it is driven in.

If there is a cortex opposite through which the cancellous bone screw can be inserted, the screw should also engage the far cortex since that significantly increases its hold in bone (approx. 6 times). In the metaphysis no tapping of the opposite cortex is required. If the far cortex is thick, as might be the case in a young individual, then the far cortex and the intervening cancellous bone may have to be tapped to facilitate the insertion of the screw.

To facilitate the insertion of cancellous bone screws acting as lag screws into fragments of bone, particularly during reconstructions of major epiphyseal or metaphyseal fractures such as the femoral condyles or the proximal tibia or for the fixation of subcapital fractures of the femur, the AO has recently introduced 3.5- and 6.5-mm cancellous bone screws

---

Fig. 3.3 The cancellous bone screws.

a–c The 6.5-mm cancellous bone screw with 8-mm spherical head and 3.5-mm hexagonal recess.

a Thread length 16 mm.

b Thread length 32 mm.

c Fully threaded.

All have a 6.5-mm diameter, 4.5-mm shaft and a 3.0-mm core. All require a 3.2-mm drill bit and a 6.5-mm tap.

d A 4.5-mm malleolar screw. Its thread has a diameter of 4.5 mm, it is partially threaded, has a trephine self-cutting tip, and a 3.0 mm core. It requires the 3.2-mm drill bit and 4.5-mm tap.

e Three sizes of serrated plastic washers for ligamentous avulsions and the 13-mm metal washers for cancellous bone screws.

f The small fragment cancellous bone screws: 4.0-mm cancellous bone screws with a 6-mm wide head with a 2.5-mm hexagonal recess. All have a core of 1.9 mm and a 1.75-mm pitch. All require a 2.5-mm drill bit and a tap for 4.0-mm cancellous bone screws.

Fig. 3.3

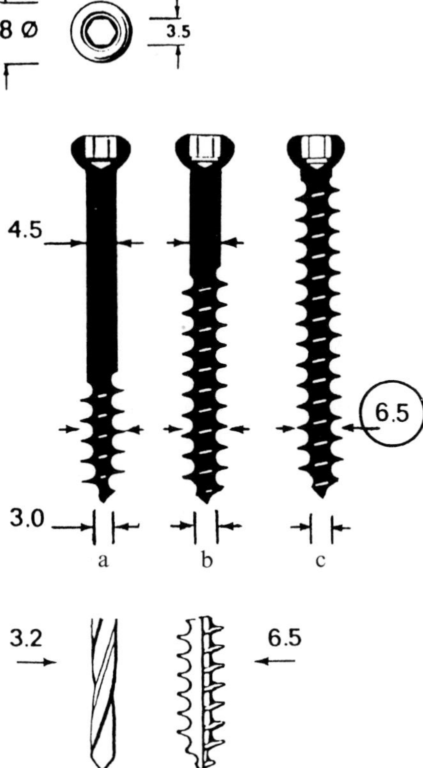

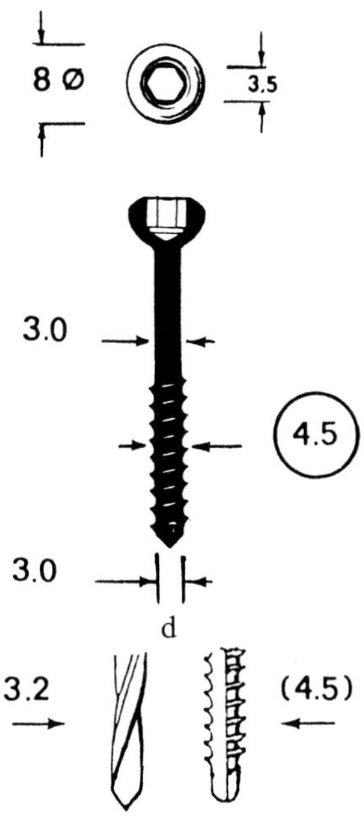

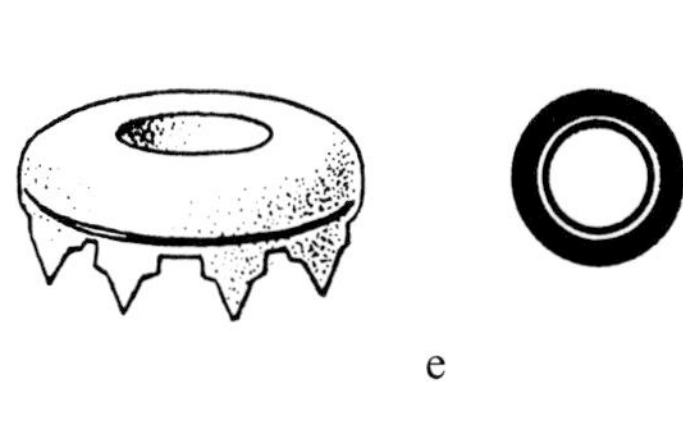

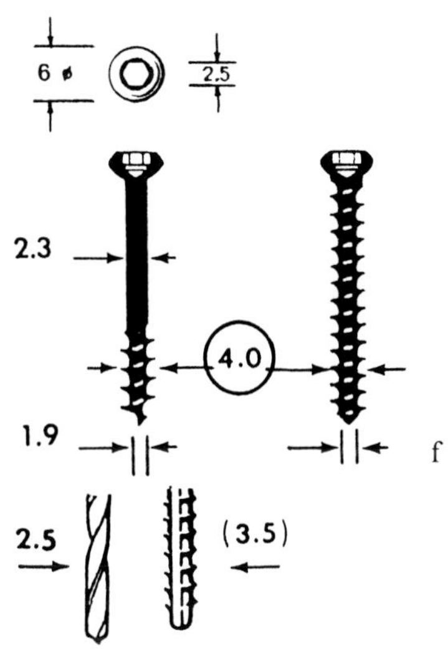

which are cannulated and can be inserted over Kirschner wires. (In the USA, the large cannulated cancellous bone screw has a thread diameter of 7 mm!)

Note: In very young individuals with very hard cancellous bone, difficulties may be encountered when inserting the 4.5-mm shaft of a 6.5-mm cancellous bone screw into a 3.2-mm pilot hole. In such cases, it may be helpful to enlarge that portion of the pilot hole to 4.5 mm.

3.1.3.3 Malleolar Screws

Malleolar screws (Fig. 3.3d) were originally designed for the fixation of the medial malleolus. They are partially threaded, have an outside diameter of 4.5 mm, have the same thread profile and pitch as the cortex screws, but have a trephine tip which allows them to cut their own path in cancellous bone. As partially threaded screws, they are a classical example of lag screws designed for the fixation of bone fragments. A thread can be precut for the malleolar screw with a 4.5-mm tap. The head is somewhat bulky – a potential disadvantage when wearing sports footwear but an advantage for easy localization at removal.

3.1.4 Techniques of Screw Fixation

In order to restore the ability of bone to support loads, its structural continuity must be restored. This can be done by the application of a plate to the bone once alignment is restored. As long as there is a gap between the fragments, however small, the load is transmitted via the plate from one fragment of bone to the next. The fracture surfaces by necessity will move in relation to each other and the plate will act as a load-bearing device. The stability of the fixation depends on the rigidity of the plate and the holding power of the screws. A fixation device which is subjected to full loads can fail due to mechanical overload or fatigue. Furthermore the stability so achieved is never absolute, no matter how rigid the plate. The most effective way of restoring structural continuity is to bring the fragments of bone not only into contact but also under compression. This permits direct transfer of load from one fragment of bone to the other, which diminishes the load borne by the fixation device, increases the stability of the fixation, and reduces corrosion. The most effective way to achieve compression between fragments of bone is by means of a lag screw.

Fig. 3.4 Summary of available screws, their corresponding drill bits and taps.

Fig. 3.4

TAP Ø	PILOT OR THREAD HOLE Ø		GLIDING HOLE Ø
1.5	1.1	1.5 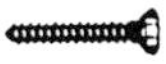	1.5
2.0	1.5	2.0 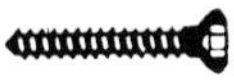	2.0
2.7	2.0	2.7 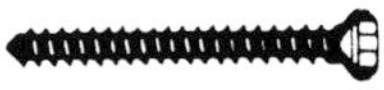	2.7
3.5/1.25mm	2.5	3.5 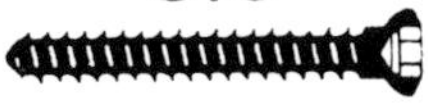	3.5
3.5/1.75mm	2.5	4.0 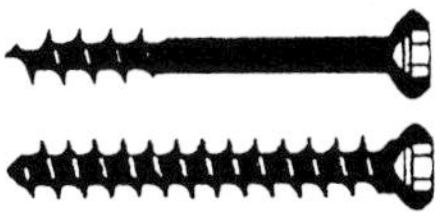	—
4.5	3.2	4.5 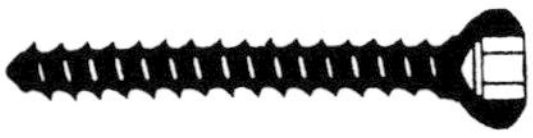	4.5
(4.5)	3.2	4.5 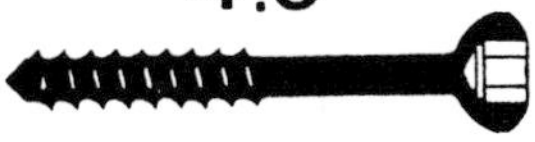	—
6.5	3.2	6.5 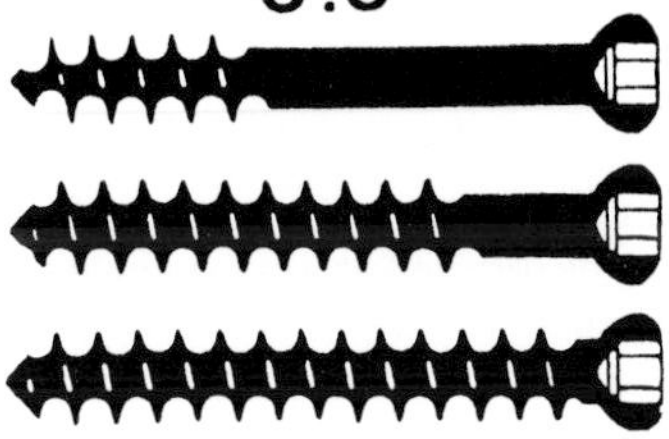	(4.5)

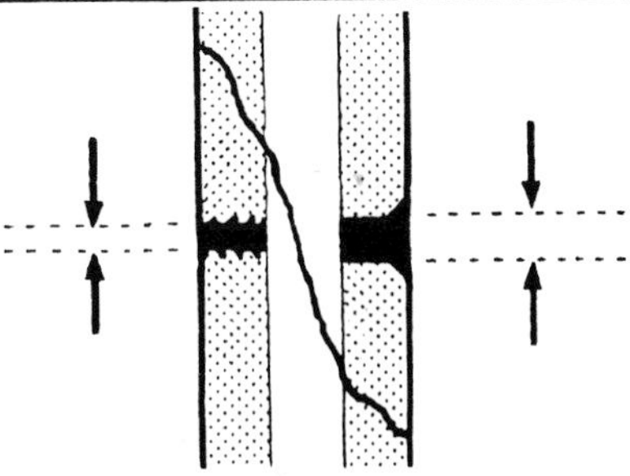

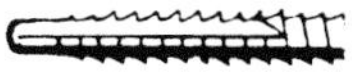

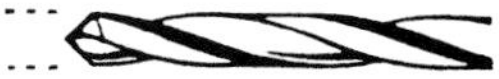

3.1.4.1 The Lag Screw

A lag screw is a screw whose thread takes purchase only in the far cortex. This means that the portion of the screw in the near cortex takes no purchase, either because the screw shank has no thread, or because the hole in the cortex is equal to or actually bigger than the outer diameter of the screw. Thus when a lag screw is tightened, it causes the two fragments of bone to be compressed (Fig. 3.5). The partially threaded screws, the malleolar screws and the large and small cancellous bone screws are lag screws designed for fixation of bone fragments by means of compression. The portion of the screw passing through the near cortex has no thread and hence will not engage in the near cortex, but the distal portion of the screw is threaded and will, therefore, engage the far cortex. As the screw is tightened, it will attempt to approximate the two fragments and interfragmental compression will be generated. This will be true as long as the screw thread does not cross the fracture line to engage in both fragments. If it does, as the screw is tightened it will fail to generate any compression at the fracture (Fig. 3.5c).

If a fully threaded screw is to function as a lag screw (Fig. 3.5b), the near cortex has to be overdrilled so that the hole in it is at least equal in size to the outer diameter of the screw thread. This hole is then called the *gliding hole*. The hole in the far cortex is drilled to the diameter of the pilot hole (its size is determined by the size of the core of the screw) and is then tapped with a tap which corresponds exactly to the thread of the screw. This hole now becomes the *thread hole*. If the gliding hole is in one fragment of bone and the thread hole in another, as the fully threaded screw is tightened, the fragments are squeezed together and interfragmental compression is generated.

The type of compression generated by a lag screw is referred to as static interfragmental compression. It is static because it does not change significantly with load. A lag screw is the most efficient way of achieving interfragmental compression and stability. It forms the basic building block of all stable fixation. It provides interfragmentary stability but does not provide a great deal of strength.

3.1.4.2 Technique of Lag Screw Fixation

In order to achieve maximal interfragmental compression, the lag screw must be inserted in the middle of the fragment equidistant from the fracture edges and directed at a right angle to the fracture plane. If the screw is not inserted perpendicular to the fracture plane, then as it is tightened a shearing force is introduced and the fragments will shift (Figs. 3.6, 3.7).

Fig. 3.5

a For a lag screw to compress two fragments, its thread must be engaged only in the far fragment.

b The cortex in the near fragment must be overdrilled in order to create a "gliding" or a clearance hole. This will ensure that the thread will take purchase only in the "thread hole" in the far cortex. Note also that for maximum compression the screw should be at 90° to the fracture line.

c If a screw thread engages both the near and the far cortex, then as it is tightened no compression is generated because the two cortices cannot come together.

In order to achieve maximal compression the lag screw must be inserted through the centre of both fragments and it must be directed at a right angle to the fracture plane.

Figs. 3.6, 3.7 If a lag screw is inserted at an angle other than 90° to the fracture plane, then as it is tightened it introduces a shearing moment and the fracture may displace.

Fig. 3.5

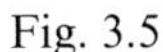

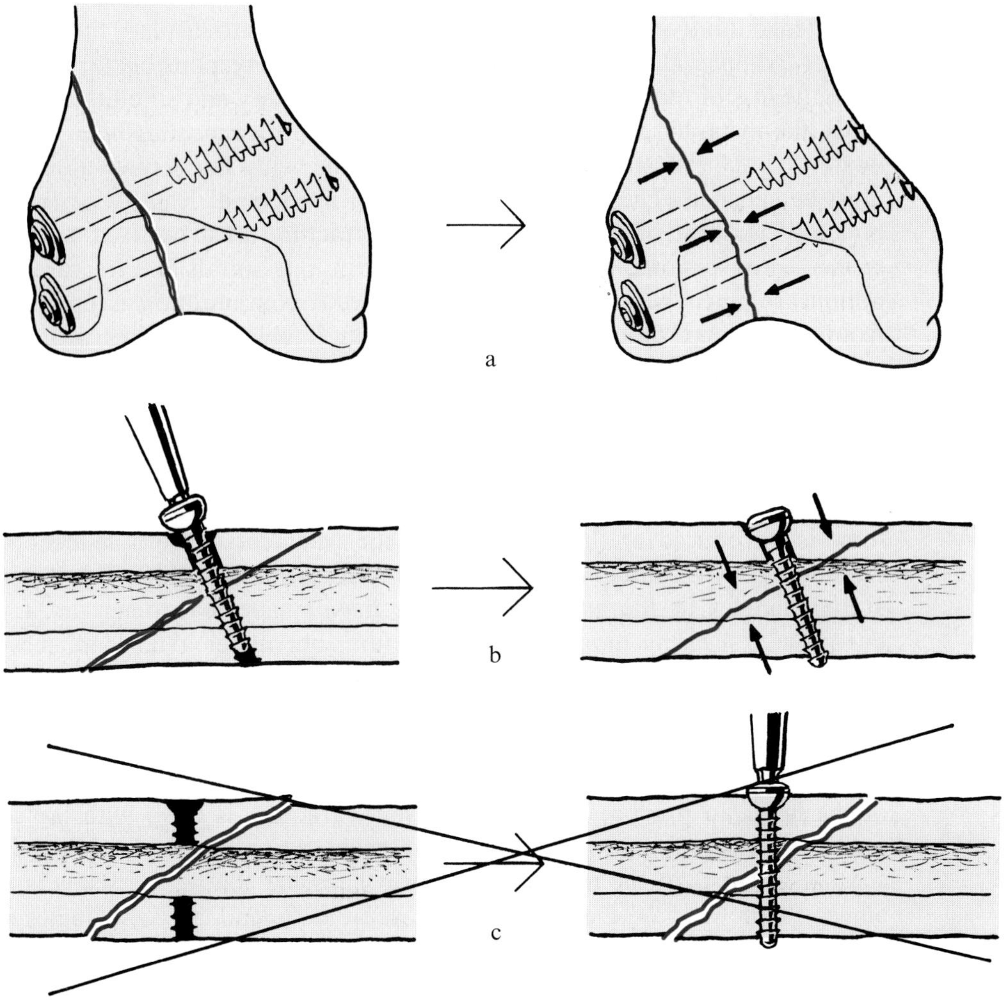

a

b

c

Fig. 3.6

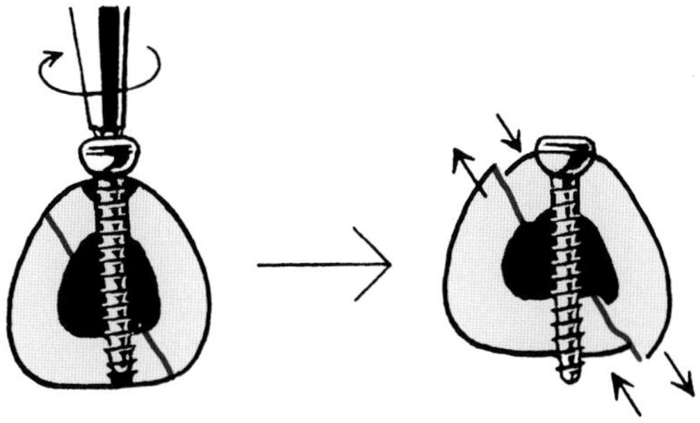

Fig. 3.7

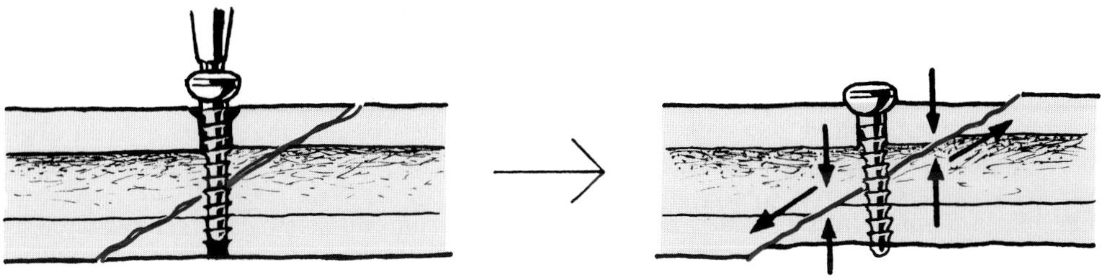

Similarly, if a screw is inserted at an acute angle to the fracture plane, then as it is tightened it introduces a shearing moment and tends to displace the fragments (Fig. 3.7). These fundamental errors in screw insertion are often responsible for the loss of reduction. With the loss of reduction, loss of structural continuity and stability are inevitable.

In the metaphyseal area, lag screw fixation with cancellous bone screws may be adequate. To achieve stability in diaphyseal bone with lag screws alone, two conditions must be satisfied. The length of the fracture must be at least twice the diameter of the bone at the point of the fracture, and the fracture must be fixed with at least two lag screws. Thus torsional fractures which result in long spirals and fractures without comminution are amenable to screw fixation alone. If comminution is present then lag screw fixation can and should be carried out, but it always requires protection by a plate (protection or neutralization plate, see p. 200) to prevent failure.

In assessing the stability achieved by means of lag screw fixation, we must consider firstly the direction in which a screw should be inserted in order *to generate optimal compression* and secondly the direction of insertion if the screw is *to withstand the forces tending to cause displacement* of the fragments. If the bone is loaded axially, a shearing force is introduced at the fracture and the fragments have a tendency to glide upon one another with consequent loss of reduction and stability (Fig. 3.8). If a screw is inserted at right angles to the axis of the bone, it will have a tendency as it is tightened to introduce a shearing moment at the fracture, but under axial load, it will prevent any tendency of the fragments to glide upon one another for displacement can occur only if the tip of the screw tears out of the thread hole or the screw head sinks through the gliding hole. Thus when securing a fracture with lag screws alone, ideally one screw should be at right angles to the fracture and a second at right angles to the long axis of the bone. In practice, when a long spiral fracture is fixed with lag screws, three or even four lag screws are used. The important parameter for stability, however, is the spacing rather than the number of screws. Thus the central lag screw is usually at right angles to the axis of the bone and those at each end at right angles to the fracture plane (Fig. 3.9).

Fig. 3.8 A lag screw inserted at right angles to the fracture plane provides maximum interfragmental compression but minimal axial stability. Under axial load, one fragment tends to glide on the other with loss of reduction and fixation. If a screw is inserted at right angles to the long axis of the bone, it provides maximum axial stability but tends to cause some dislocation of the fragments as it is tightened. Therefore, it is best to have one screw at right angles to the axis and the others at right angles to the fracture plane (see Fig. 3.9).

Fig. 3.9 In a spiral fracture which is fixed with more than two screws, the central screw is usually at right angles to the long axis of the bone and is thus able to prevent axial displacement. The other two screws will be at right angles to the spiral fracture plane and will ensure maximal compression.

Fig. 3.8

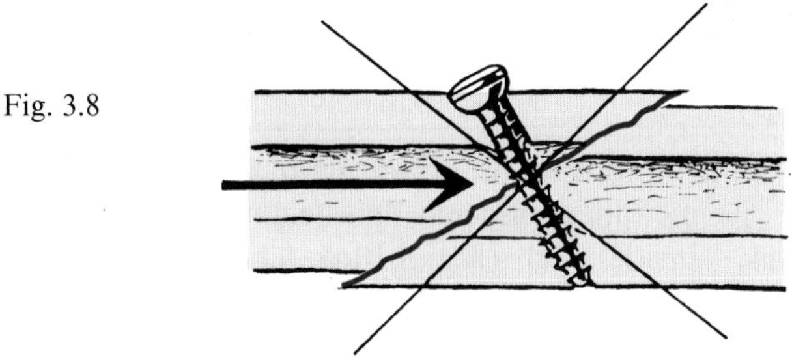

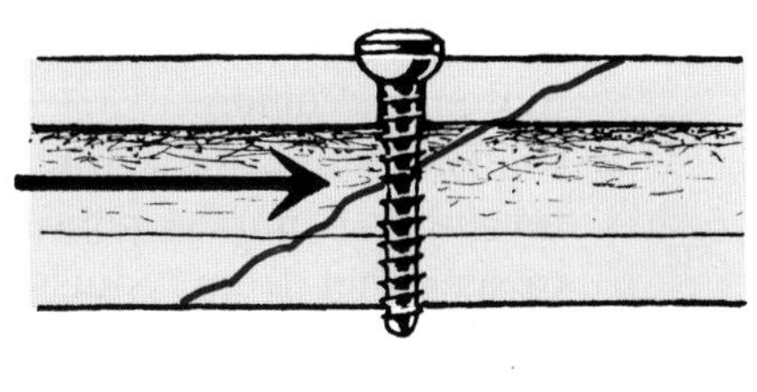

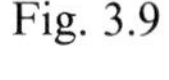

Fig. 3.9

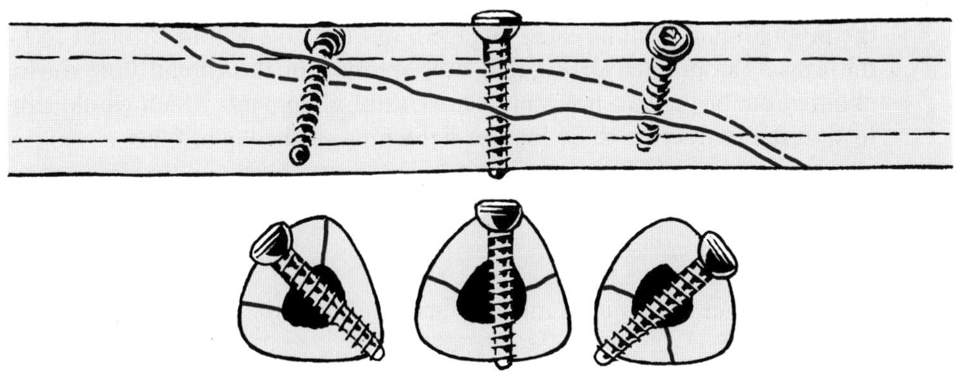

It is important to plan the internal fixation carefully prior to the reduction of a fracture. Reduction obscures such important guides to insertion of the lag screws as the direction of the fracture plane and the center of the two fragments. Once the fracture is reduced it becomes extremely difficult to aim with a drill bit exactly for the middle of the opposite cortex. It is far better to drill either the gliding hole or the thread hole prior to the reduction of the fragments. This technique results in the minimum stripping of the bone fragments (Fig. 3.10a, b) which preserves their blood supply, and encourages more rapid union.

The gliding hole for a 4.5-mm cortical screw can be drilled with the 4.5-mm drill bit either from the periosteal or from the medullary aspect. This technique is referred to as either from "outside in" or from "inside out" (Fig. 3.10a). The drill bit must be directed through the middle of the fragment and at right angles to the fracture plane. Similarly the thread hole can be drilled first ("thread hole first"). This is particularly important if the thread hole is to be drilled in the middle of the tip of a fragment which is completely obscured once the fracture is reduced. The thread hole is then pre-drilled from the medullary canal to the outside with the 3.2-mm drill bit. It is very important to drill the thread hole exactly in the direction the screw is to be inserted (Fig. 3.10b). If the thread hole is not drilled in the direction of the screw, the tip of the pointed guide will not stay engaged and the hole will be difficult to tap. Furthermore, the tip of the pointed drill guide must remain in the thread hole during drilling of the gliding hole or the two holes may end out of alignment, which would cause the fragments to shift and reduction to be lost on tightening of the lag screw.

Fig. 3.10

a, b The drilling of a gliding hole prior to the reduction either from the "outside in" (a) or from "inside out".

c The drilling of a thread hole prior to the reduction and the drilling of the gliding hole after reduction with the aid of the pointed drill guide.

Fig. 3.10

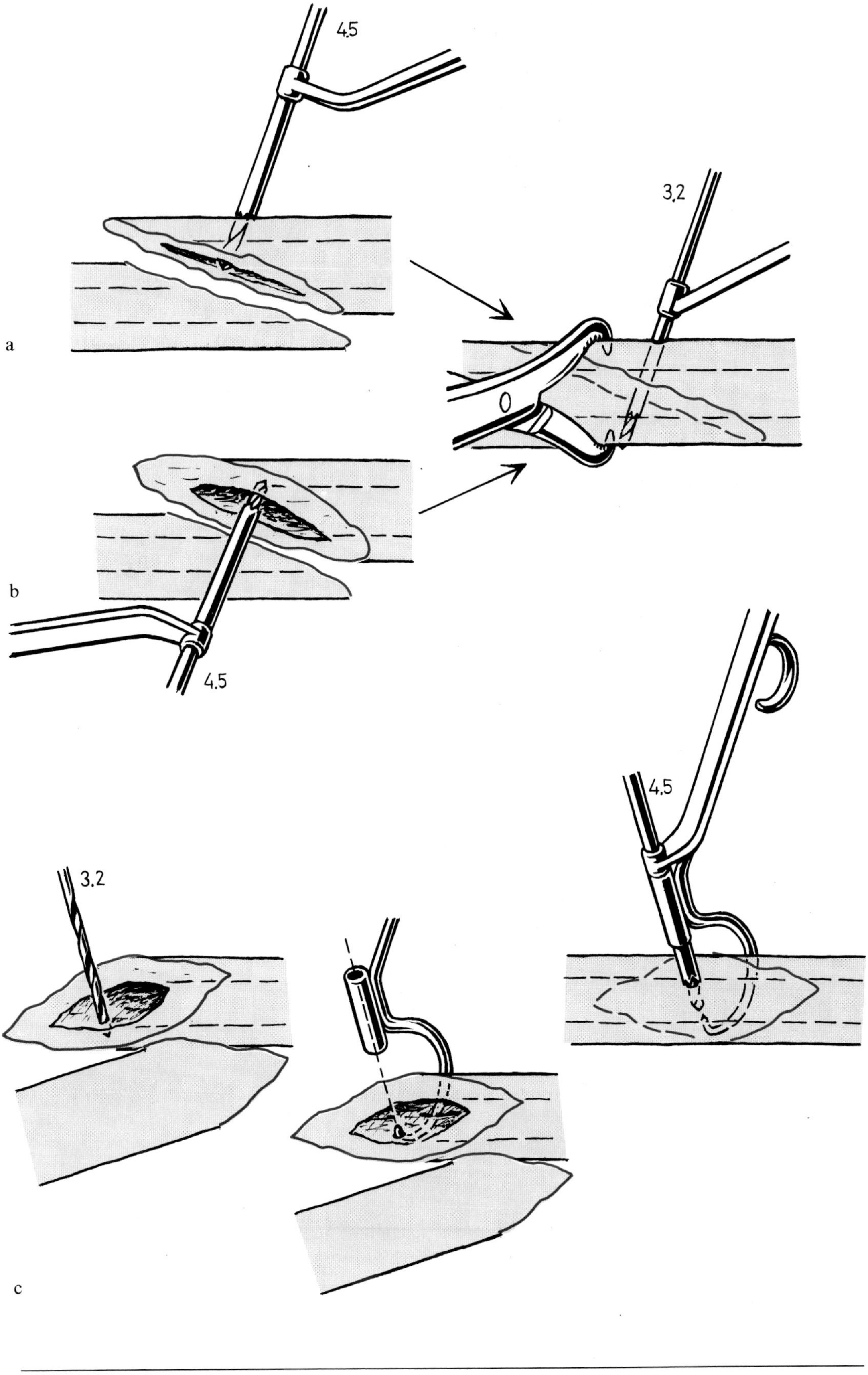

4.5

3.2

a

b

4.5

4.5

3.2

c

3.1.5 Indication for Lag Screw Fixation

As already indicated, whenever there are two fragments of bone whose size and geometry permit lag screw fixation then this technique should be used. Lag screws find their major application in the reconstruction of intra-articular epiphyseal and metaphyseal fractures (Fig. 3.11). The fractures in these areas are mostly the result of a shearing or cleaving force which results in fragments ideally suited for lag screw fixation. If there is an associated depression of the joint surface then lag screw fixation is used to hold the joint surface together under interfragmental compression once the depressed fragments have been elevated and the joint surface reduced (Fig. 3.12). An exception to this are fractures with such comminution that structural continuity cannot be restored by reduction because of substance loss. Lag screw fixation of these fractures would result in narrowing of the epiphysis and distortion of the joint (Fig. 3.13). Avulsion fractures are also ideally suited to lag screw fixation (Fig. 3.14).

In practice lag screw fixation alone is reserved for short tubular bones and for epiphyseal and metaphyseal fractures, for example, malleolar fractures. Although long spiral fractures of the tibia can be fixed with lag screws alone, this is no longer commonly practised due to the necessity to withhold weight-bearing, whereas when lag screw fixation is combined with a protection plate, some weight-bearing is possible. Bones such as the humerus and the femur are subjected to such great forces that lag screw fixation alone is not sufficiently strong and must be used in combination with a protection plate. The pattern of shaft fractures of the radius and ulna and the size of the fragments are such that lag screw fixation alone can never be employed.

Fig. 3.11 Lag screws find their major application in the reconstruction of intra-articular epiphyseal and of metaphyseal fractures.

a A 6.5-mm cancellous bone screw used for the fixation of a Volkmann's triangle (posterior lip) with the screw passing from front to back just above the ankle joint.

b Two 4.0-mm partially threaded small fragment cancellous bone screws used for fixation of the medial malleolus.

c A 4.0-mm partially threaded small fragment cancellous bone screw plus its 7.0-mm washer used for the fixation of the avulsed anterior syndesmotic ligament with its tubercular insertion (tubercle of Tillaux-Chaput).

d A 4.5-mm malleolar screw used for the fixation of an epiphyseal fracture separation of the distal tibia (Salter-Harris III). Line across fibula represents growth plate in a child.

e Two 4.0-mm partially threaded small fragment cancellous bone screws used for the fixation of a type A fracture of the medial malleolus.

f Two 4.0-mm partially threaded small fragment cancellous bone screws used for lag screw fixation of the epiphysis and of the condyle to the metaphysis of the distal humerus.

Fig. 3.11

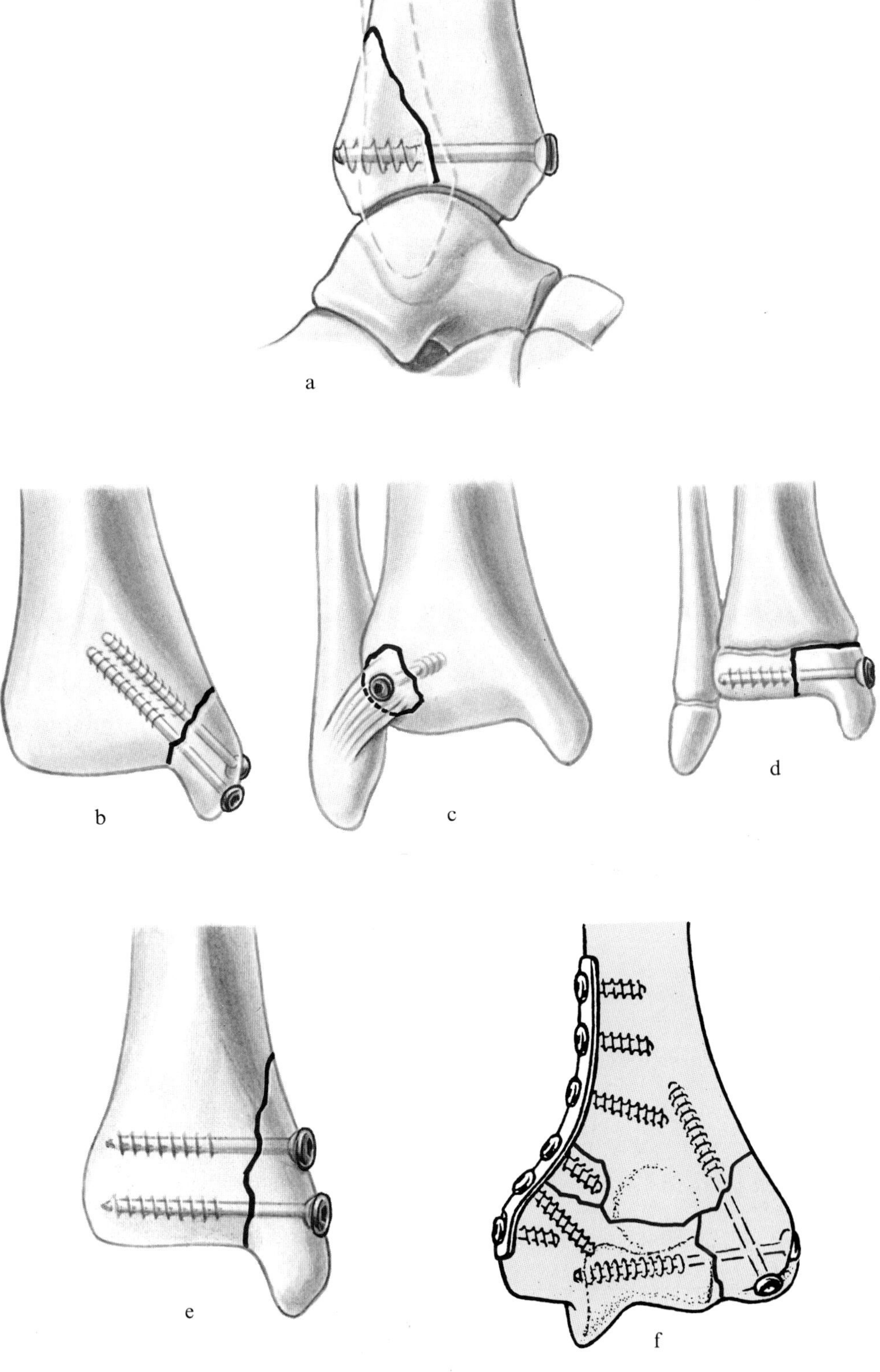

Fig. 3.12 If an intra-articular fracture is so complex that structural continuity cannot be restored, or if bone loss has occurred, one cannot attempt to achieve stability with a lag screw because this would lead to narrowing and distortion of the joint. Under these circumstances, stability is achieved by tapping all fragments and inserting a cortex screw which will ensure that the proper joint width is retained.

Fig. 3.13 Procedure in an impacted fracture of the lateral tibial plateau: apply very light compression! In addition, a buttress plate is required to prevent failure of the lateral cortex under load.

Fig. 3.12

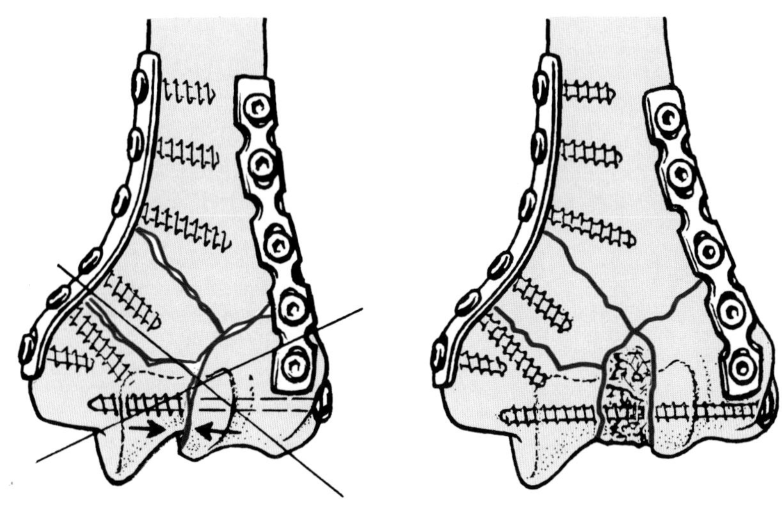

Fig. 3.13

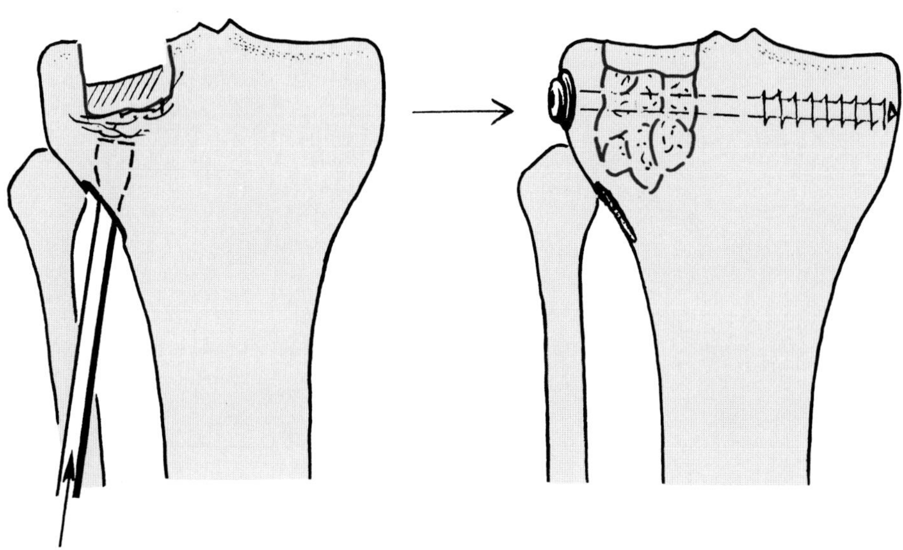

Fig. 3.14 Avulsion fractures are ideally suited for lag screw fixation.

a Because of persisting instability a fully threaded positioning screw has been inserted between the tibia and fibula with threads engaging both in the tibia and fibula to avoid compression! The two remaining screws are lag screws.

b, b′, c, c′ Good examples of lag screw fixation.

Fig. 3.14

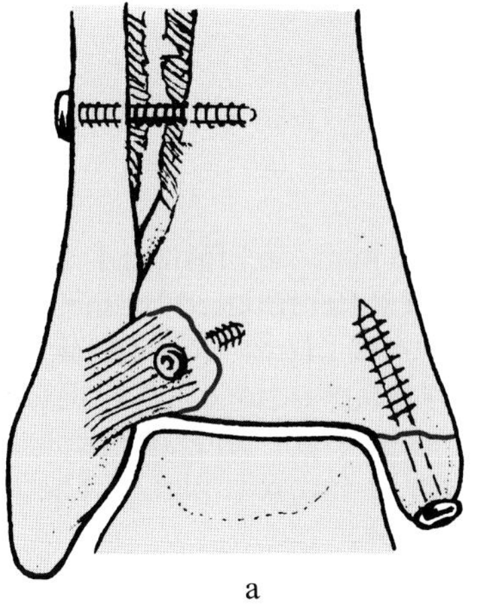

a

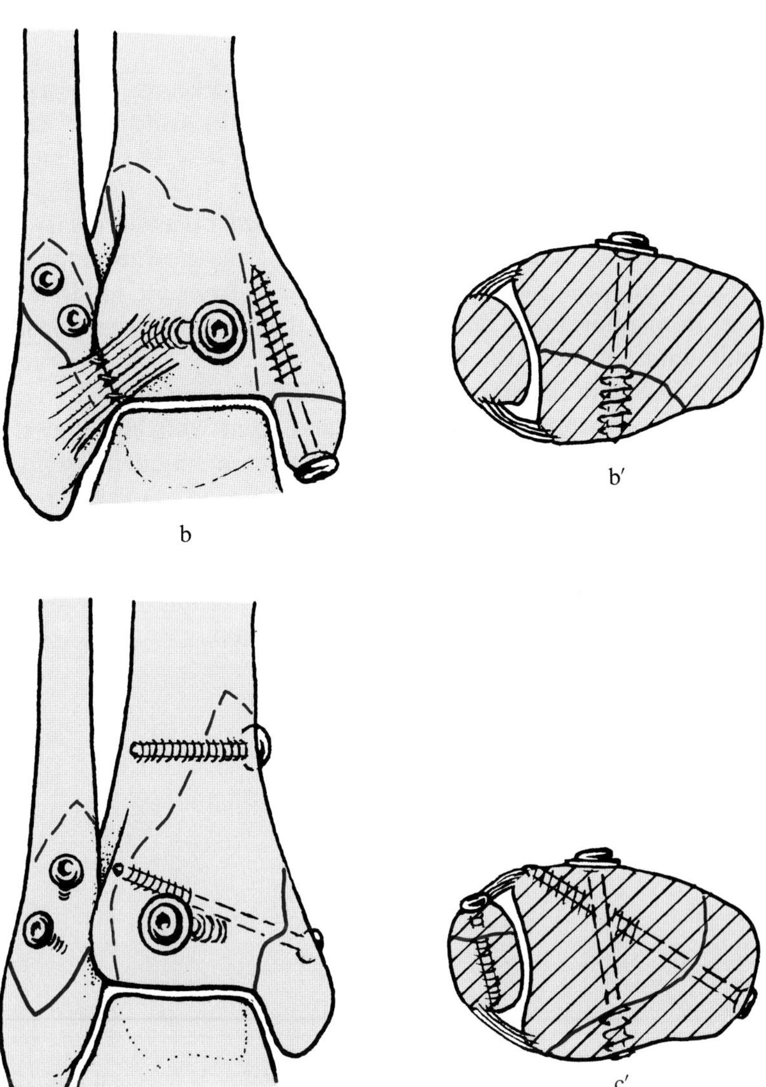

b

b′

c

c′

3.2 Plates

3.2.1 Function

Plates are devices which are fastened to bone for the purpose of providing fixation. They are principally differentiated by their function. Thus there are protection or neutralization plates, buttress plates, compression plates, and tension band plates. The shape of the plate is an adaptation of the plate to the local anatomy and does not denote any function. Thus straight and angled blade plates can function as protection plates, tension band plates or buttress plates. The name depends on the biomechanical function the plate is performing.

3.2.2 Protection or Neutralization Plates

Whenever the internal fixation of a diaphyseal fracture consists of a lag screw or screws in combination with a plate whose function is to protect the lag screw fixation, we refer to the plate as a protection or neutralization plate. Lag screw fixation alone is not able to withstand much loading. In order to allow patients early movement of the extremities after internal fixation as well as limited loading, it is necessary to protect most fracture zones fixed by lag screws with a plate. Such a plate protects the interfragmental compression achieved with the lag screw or screws from all torsional, bending and shearing forces. It is important to emphasize that the lag screw is responsible for interfragmentary stability and not the plate. A plate, even if it exerts axial compression, can never achieve the same degree of interfragmentary stability as a lag screw.

A wedge fracture is first reduced and fixed with lag screws (Fig. 3.15). A carefully contoured plate is then fixed to the two main fragments with a minimum of two to four screws. The type of plate (broad 4.5-mm or narrow 4.5-mm plate or the 3.5-mm plate) and the number of screws will depend on the bone being fixed and on the quality of the bone. A lag screw can also be inserted through the plate (Fig. 3.16). The combination of lag screws and a plate is the commonest type of internal fixation of diaphyseal fractures when screws and plates are used for their fixation.

Fig. 3.15 Note that in this wedge fracture, the primary stability is achieved with the lag screws and not the plate. A plate serves only to protect the lag screws.

Fig. 3.16 A lag screw can be inserted through the plate once axial compression has been generated. This greatly increases the stability of the fixation. (See also Fig. 3.39.)

Fig. 3.15

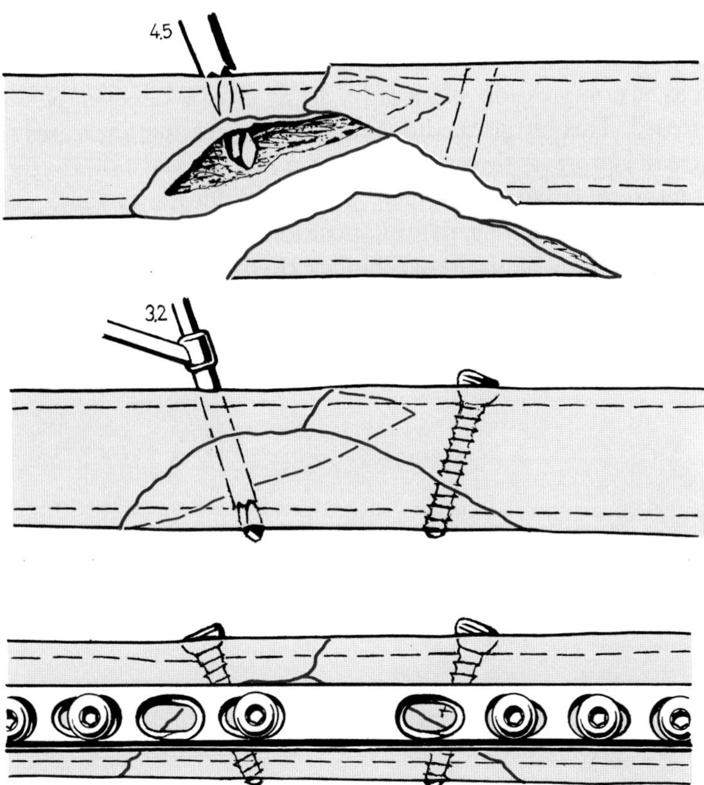

Fig. 3.16

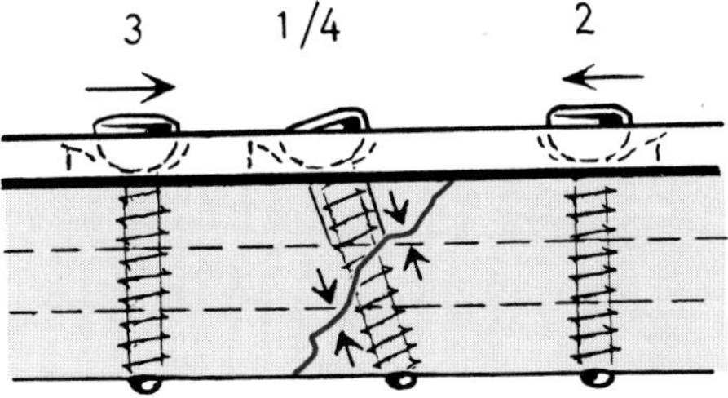

3.2.3 Special Protection or Neutralization Plates

It must be appreciated that a plate can at one time perform more than one function. Thus a protection or neutralization plate can, if the geometry of the fracture permits, serve as a compression plate (Fig. 3.17, left). Whenever possible an implant should be prestressed. This brings the bone under compression, increases the stability of the fixation, and greatly protects the implant from overload and failure. By virtue of its design, when the fracture is reduced, the DCP automatically exerts some axial compression even with the screws inserted in a neutral position. The plates must not only correspond to the bend in the shaft of the bone, but as the metaphyseal areas are approached, the plates must often follow a twist as well (Figs. 3.17, 3.18).

Fig. 3.17 A plate may have more than one function. This plate is acting not only as a protection plate but also as a compression plate.

In order that a DCP can serve as a neutralization plate, the plate must be contoured exactly and the screws must be inserted from the fracture towards the ends of the plate. As the neutral drill guide places the screws 0.1 mm away from the end of the DC slope they cause some axial compression.

Fig. 3.17

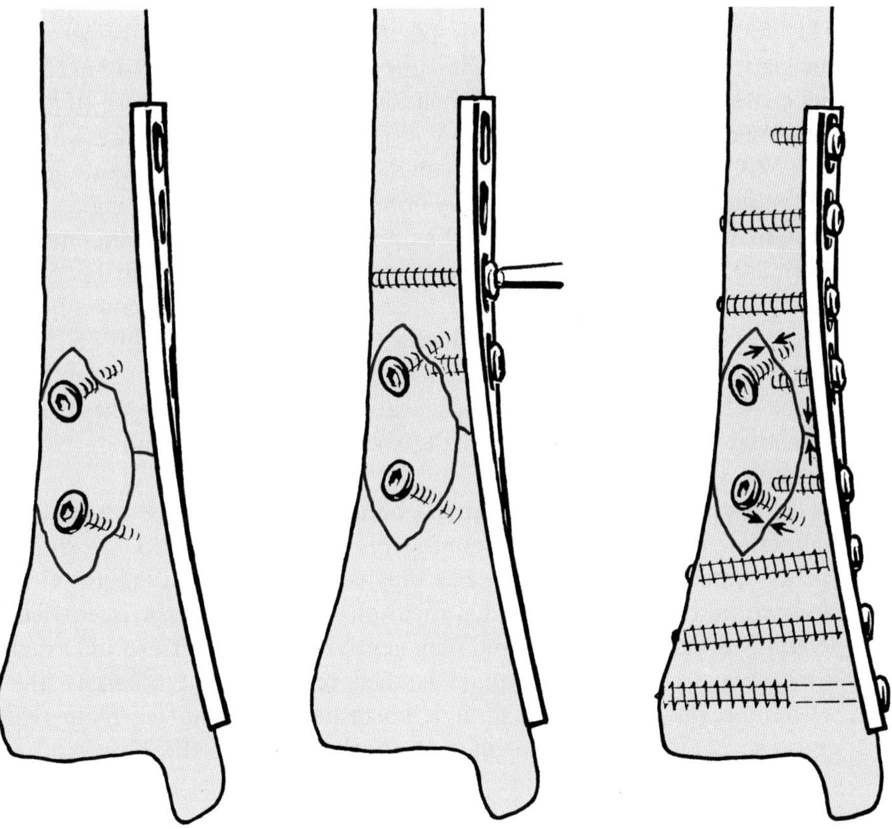

3.2.4 Contouring of Plates

Special contouring devices (Fig. 3.18) permit accurate and controlled shaping of the plates. The new shape is the result of plastic deformation and is permanent. With practice, the plates can be twisted at the time they are bent. This is accomplished by inserting the plate at an angle into the bending plier or press. Most of the time, however, the shaping of the plates is carried out using both the bending press or plier and the bending irons. Certain areas of bone, such as the pelvis around the acetabulum, the distal humerus, the mandible, etc., have extremely complex anatomy which makes the shaping of normal straight plates such as the DCP extremely difficult. To overcome these difficulties, the AO has developed *reconstruction plates*. Normal plates can be twisted and bent in the direction of their long axis, but they resist strongly any attempt to bend them in the direction of their short axis or width (Fig. 3.19). The design of the reconstruction plate is such that it permits bending about the PQ axis. The reconstruction plates are available in the 4.5-mm and 3.5-mm configurations. The design of these plates (Fig. 3.20a–d) is such that their contouring with the specially designed bending pliers and bending irons is simple and easy.

The contouring of any plates has been further facilitated by the design of the malleable templates. They come in different sizes to correspond to the different plates, such as the 4.5-mm or 3.5-mm plates, and they come in different lengths (Fig. 3.18a). They have been color coded for easy identification. Once reduction is carried out, the malleable template is laid on the bone and then gently shaped to correspond exactly to the underlying bone (Fig. 3.18b). The template is then removed and taken to the contouring device where the plate is shaped until it corresponds to the template (Fig. 3.18c, f). At the end, the contouring of the plate is checked against the bone and adjusted to make it perfect. In contouring a plate, care should be taken not to bend it back and forth because this weakens the plate.

Fig. 3.18 The contouring of plates.

Note that the plate is twisted with the bending irons and contoured with the bending press or plier.

a Colored malleable aluminum templates which correspond in size and shape to the plates.

b After the reduction of the fracture and fixation of the wedge fragment with lag screws, the template is placed on bone and carefully contoured. It will serve as a template for contouring of the plate.

c Twisting irons used to twist the plate. See also f.

d Hand-held bending pliers for contouring of the narrow DCPs. If a plate is inserted obliquely into the press, it can be bent and twisted at the same time.

e The bending press for the broad plates and a twisting iron shown in profile.

f, g The plate, once bent, is held in the bending press. It is then twisted with the twisting irons. After twisting the bend may have to be adjusted once again.

Fig. 3.18

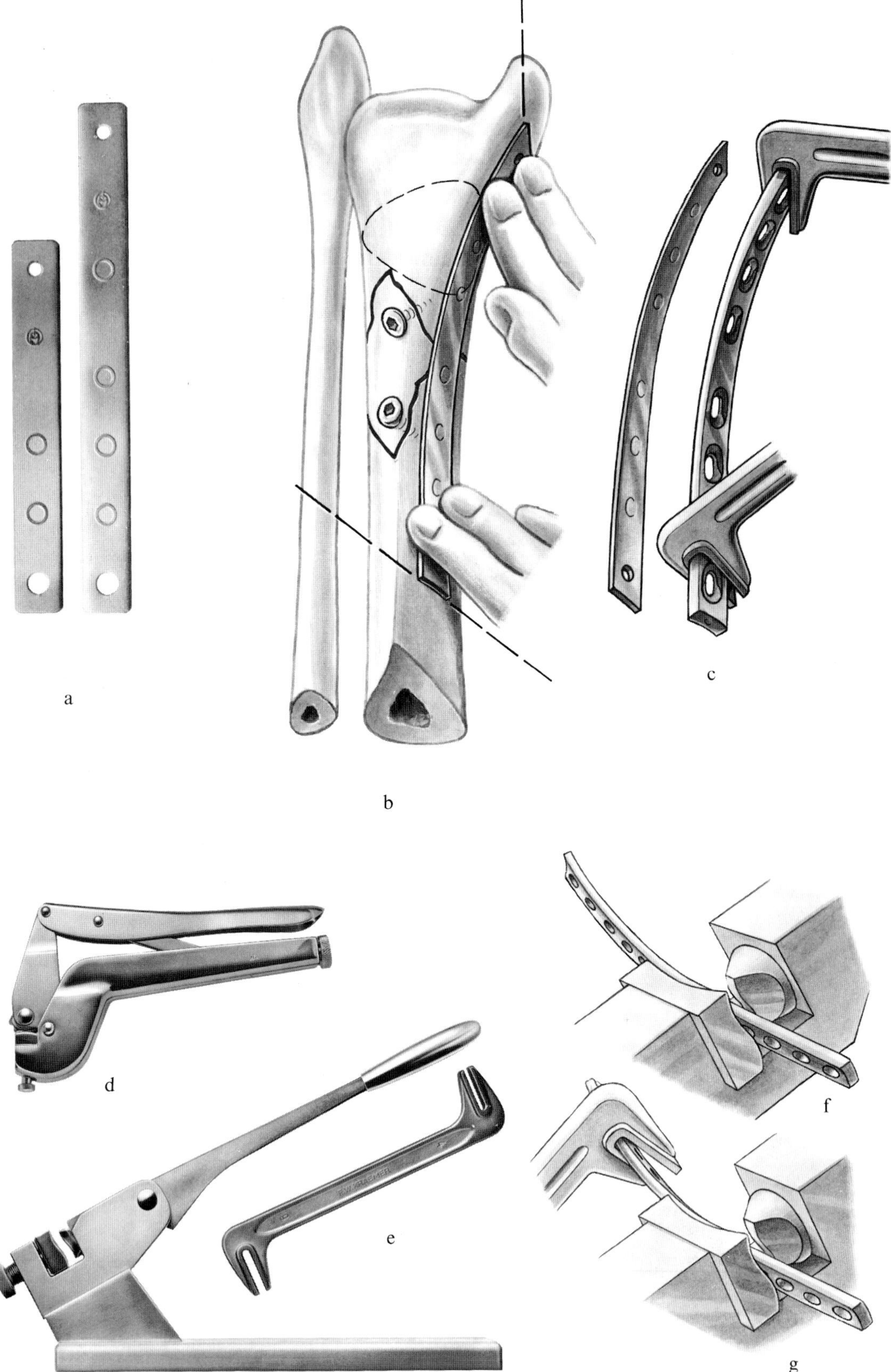

Fig. 3.19 A narrow or a broad DCP can be twisted about its XY axis and bent about its RS axis. It resists strongly any attempt to bend it about its PQ axis.

Fig. 3.20 The reconstruction plates and their contouring devices.

a The shape of both the 3.5-mm and the 4.5-mm reconstruction plates.

b The special twisting irons. They can also be used for bending of the plates about their PQ axis.

c Special bending pliers. With these the plates can be bent about their long XY and short PQ axes.

d The bending of the plates about their short PQ axis.

Fig. 3.19

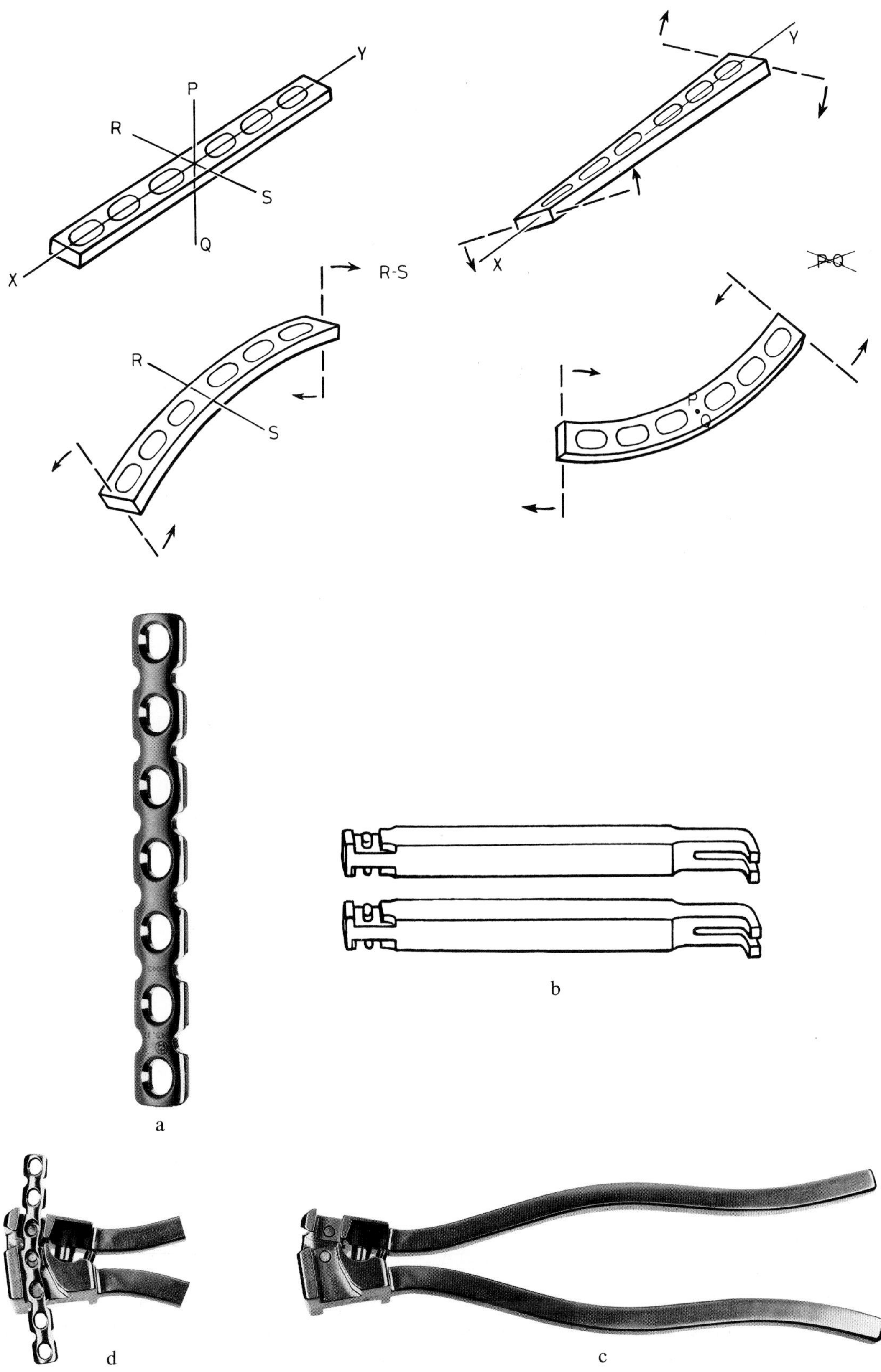

Fig. 3.20

a

b

d

c

3.2.5 Buttress Plate

One of the commonest applications of lag screw fixation is in the reconstruction of epiphyseal and metaphyseal fractures. Epiphyseal and metaphyseal areas of bone consist of large areas of cancellous bone surrounded by a thin shell of cortex. As a result of loading, they are also subjected to compressive and shearing forces. If the fracture is in the metaphysis and the cortical shell has been comminuted, the compressive forces tend to lead to an axial deviation or bending. Lag screw fixation cannot overcome these deforming forces of shear and bending. In order to prevent deformity, it is necessary to supplement the fixation with a supporting or a buttress plate. The function of the buttress plate is simply to prevent axial deformity as a result of shear or bending. Thus it must be applied to the area or cortex which has been broken and which is coming under load.

3.2.5.1 Technical Guidelines for the Application of a Buttress Plate

As the function of the buttress plate is to support, it must be firmly anchored to the main fragment but need not necessarily be fixed with screws to the fragment it is supporting. It must also correspond very accurately to the shape of the underlying cortex or a deformity could ensue. The order and manner in which the screws are inserted through a buttress plate are also important.

The screws must be inserted in such a way that under load there must be no shift in the position of the plate. Thus if the plate which is being used has oval holes (e.g. the DCP and LC-DCP the reconstruction plates or the semi-tubular or one-third tubular plates, etc.) then the screws fixing the plate to the shaft must be positioned in the screw holes of the plate close to the fracture (Fig. 3.21). In this position, as the load is applied, any tendency for the plate to shift is immediately arrested by the screws.

The recommended method of applying a buttress plate is first to contour it very accurately to the segment of bone and then begin its fixation to the bone in the middle of the plate and advance the insertion of screws in an orderly fashion one after another towards both ends of the plate.

Fig. 3.21 The principle of the buttress plate.

Whenever a screw is inserted through one end of an oval screw hole closest to the fracture it is in the "buttress mode". In the main fragment, the screws prevent any shift of the plate. The screws in the fragment which is being buttressed prevent any shift of the bone under the plate. This prevents any deformity under axial load. Begin the fixation of the plate to the bone in its middle and advance the insertion of screws in an orderly fashion one after another towards both ends of the plate.

a The buttressing of a tibial plateau.

b The buttressing of a pilon fracture.

Fig. 3.21

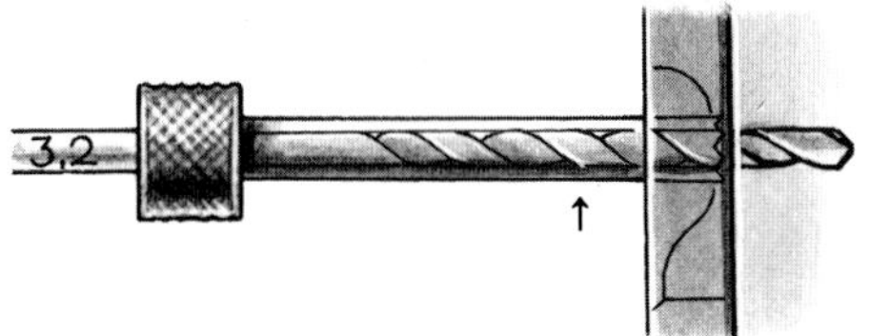

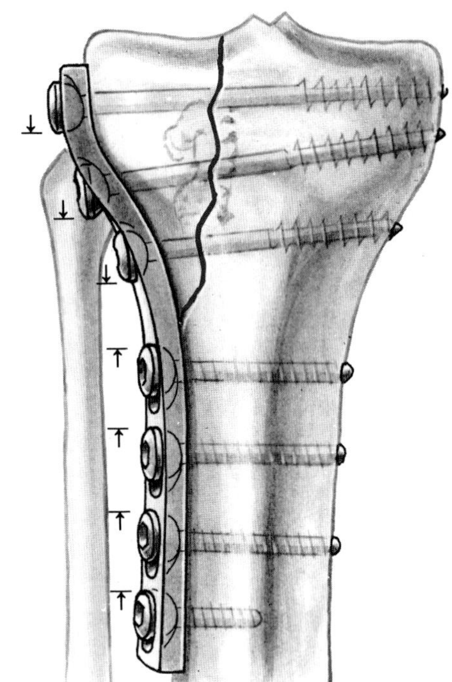
a

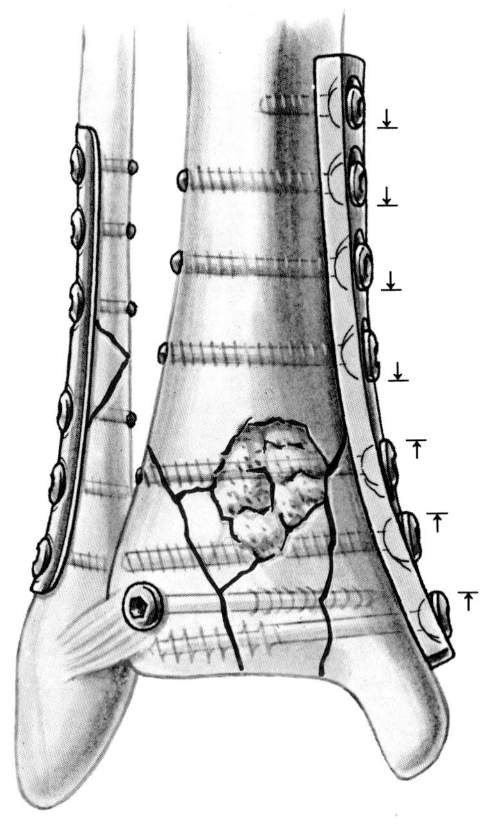
b

3.2.5.2 Plates of Special Design

Specially designed plates are used mainly in the metaphyseal areas of bone. As the ends of all long bones have very specialized shapes, the AO has designed a number of specialized plates to meet the anatomic and biomechanical requirements of these areas. It should be realized, however, that any plate that is carefully contoured to the shape of the bone can act as a buttress plate.

The "T plate" (Fig. 3.22) is used for the buttressing of the medial tibial plateau, the distal tibia, occasionally the medial distal femur, and the proximal humerus. It is a relatively thin plate which is not very strong. It is designed to buttress a thin cortex or prevent a defect in cancellous bone from collapsing, or, occasionally, for use as a tension band plate. If used in these areas and for the proper indications it will be found sufficiently strong.

The "T buttress plates" and their derivatives the "L buttress plates" which come with a right and a left offset, have a double bend to fit the lateral plateau of the tibia. Both the regular and the special T plates, as well as the L plates, have an oval hole. This has been designed to permit temporary fixation of the plate to the bone while still permitting some up and down adjustment. Once fixation is complete, the temporary screw can sometimes be removed and an oblique lag screw inserted to bring either a fracture or an osteotomy under interfragmental compression (Fig. 3.22). The "lateral tibial head plate" was designed as a buttress plate of the lateral tibial plateau (Fig. 3.22f, i).

Fig. 3.22 The different buttress plates for plateau fractures.

a A four-hole T plate.

b A T buttress plate.

c, d The L buttress plates (left and right).

e Note the double bend of the T and L buttress plates designed for the lateral plateau.

f, g Lateral tibial head plates available with five, seven and nine holes (left and right).

The T plate (a) fits the medial plateau better than (b).

Fig. 3.22

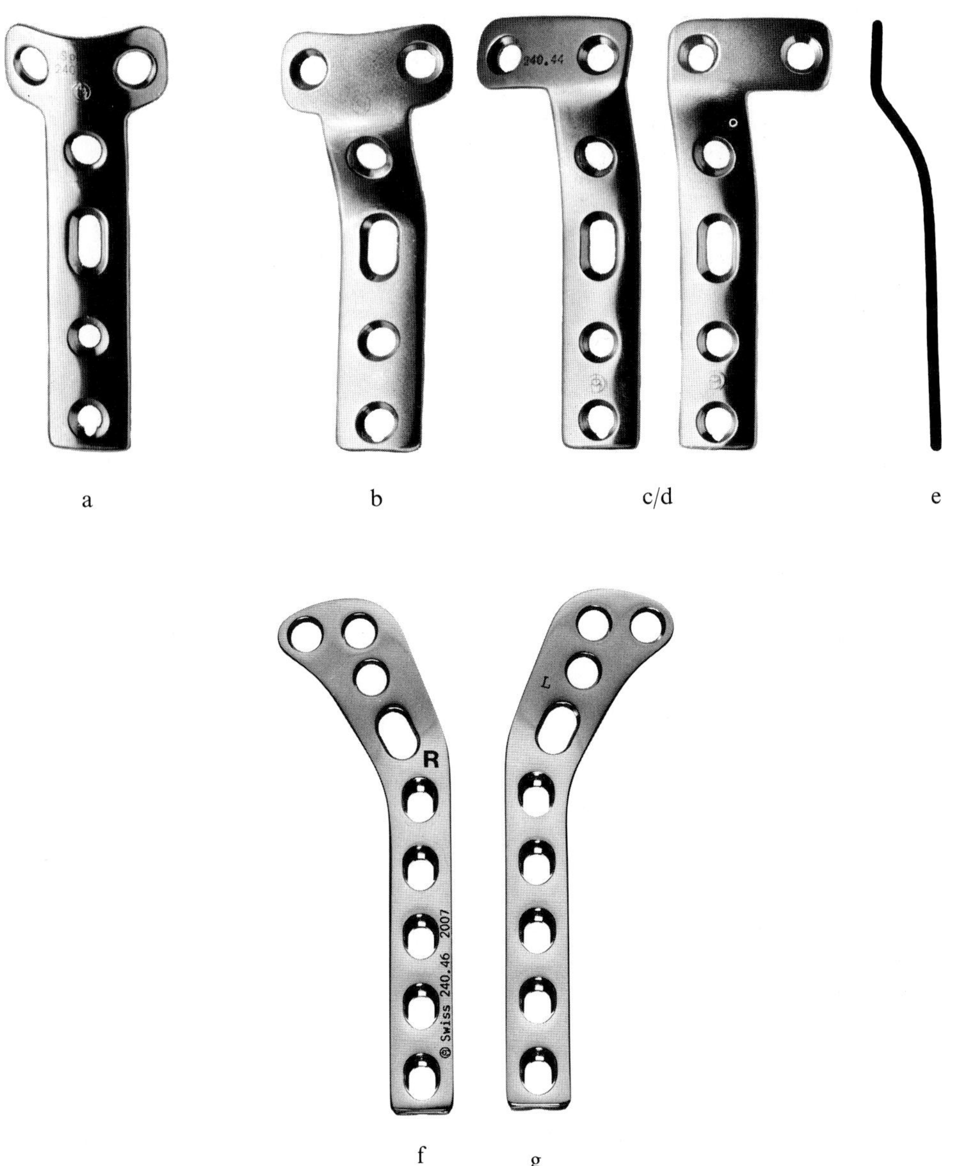

Fig. 3.22 The different buttress plates for plateau fractures (continued).

h, h′ The buttressing of the lateral plateau with an L plate.

i, i′ The buttressing of the medial plateau with a T plate.

j, j′ Lateral tibial head plate applied.

Fig. 3.22

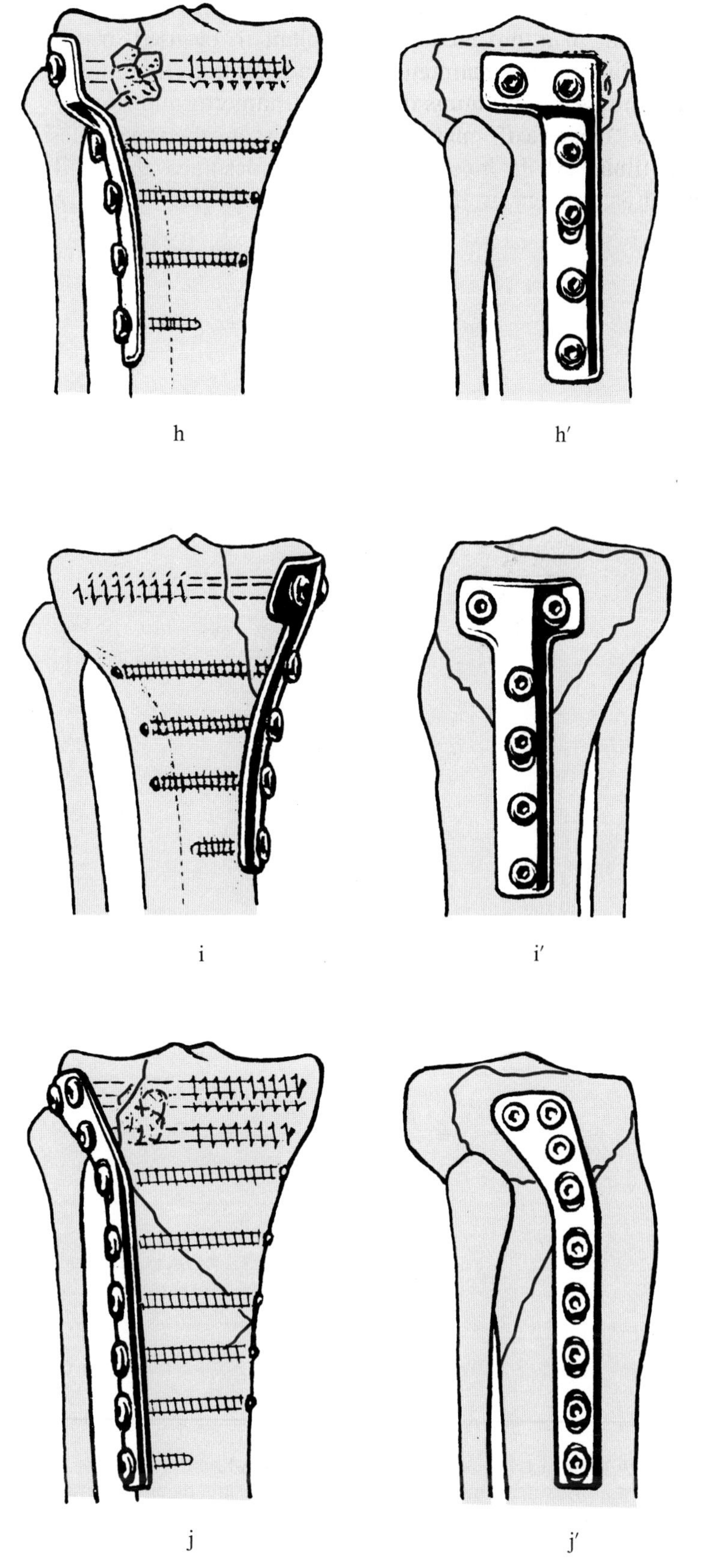

The "spoon plate" (Fig. 3.23) was initially designed as a buttress plate for pilon fractures with anterior crushing but a relatively intact posterior cortex. Experience has shown that it is too massive an implant to be used on the subcutaneous anterior crest of the tibia in the treatment of acute fractures. Its indication today is restricted mostly to metaphyseal nonunions of the distal humerus and tibia.

The "cloverleaf" plate (Fig. 3.24) is another plate designed for buttressing of the distal tibia. All its holes have been so designed that will take small fragment screws only. It is also very useful for fixation of fractures of the proximal humerus.

Fig. 3.23 The spoon plate is rarely used for the treatment of acute fractures as demonstrated in this illustration. It is used mainly to treat metaphyseal nonunions of the distal humerus and tibia.

Fig. 3.24 The "cloverleaf plate" is designed to buttress the distal tibia on its medial side.

Note: It takes small fragment screws in all holes.

Fig. 3.23

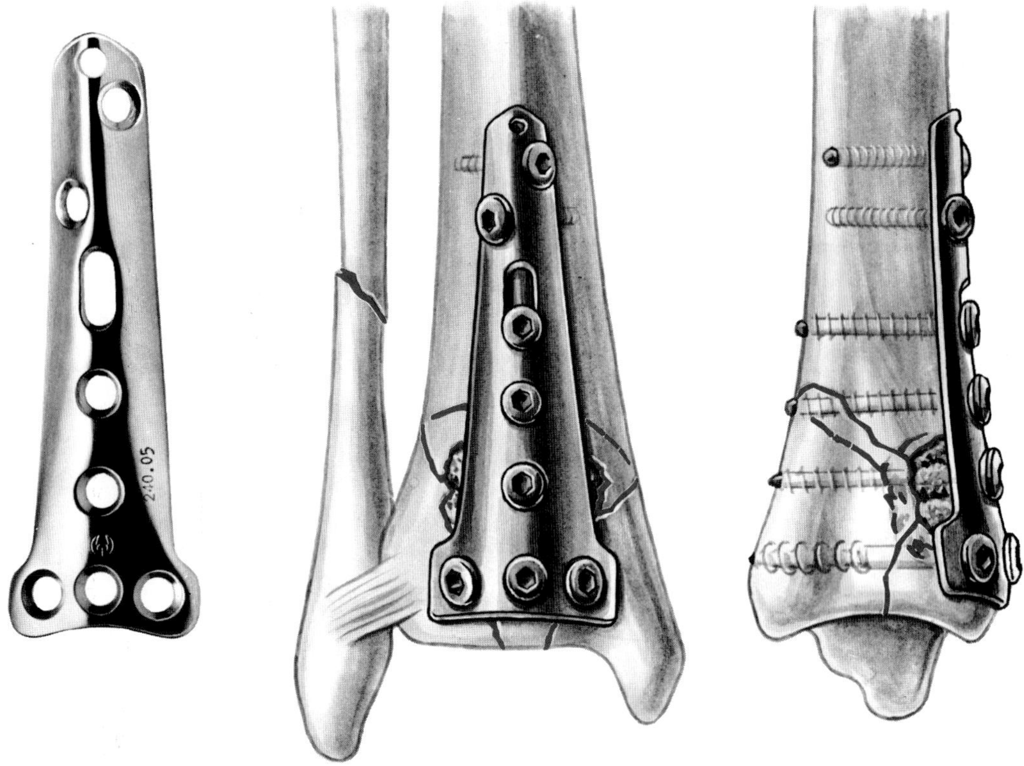

Fig. 3.24

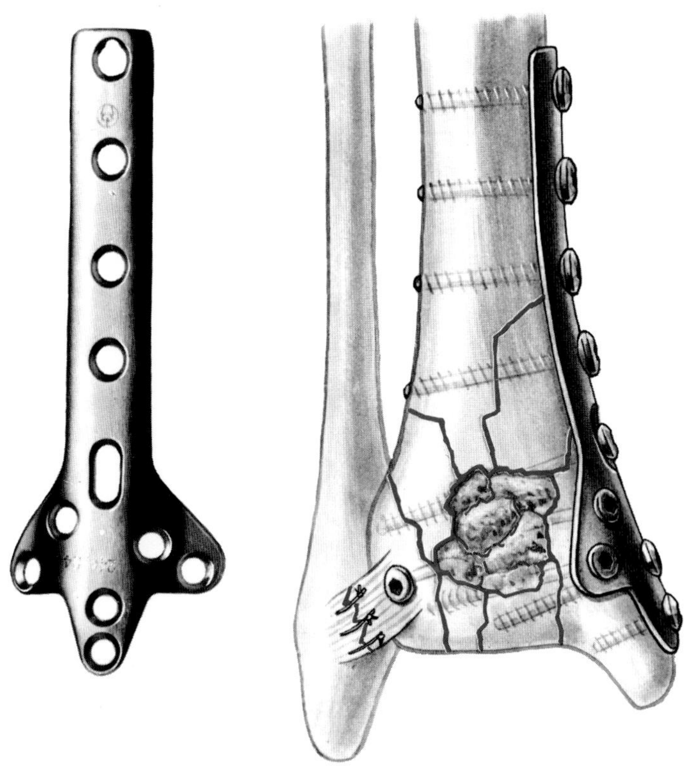

The "condylar buttress plates" (Fig. 3.25) have been designed to be used for C3.3 fractures of the distal femur. They come in a right and a left version. They are heavier and stronger than all other buttress plates since they have to withstand much greater forces.

There are also a number of plates which have been developed to be used with the small fragment screws, such as the plates for the distal radius and the many small T plates and L plates for the fixation of fractures of the distal radius and particularly of the hand and foot (Fig. 3.26).

Great care must be exercised when buttress plates are used in subcutaneous areas. Problems with wound healing have been encountered in such areas as the medial side of the distal tibia. The surgeon must, therefore, avoid putting these plates under badly contused skin flaps, and all incisions must be planned in such a way that they do not cross over plates.

Fig. 3.25 The condylar buttress plates for fixation of C3.3 supracondylar fractures of the femur. These plates come in a right and a left version and in different lengths.

Fig. 3.26 T plates designed to be used for the fixation of fresh fractures or osteotomies of the distal radius.

Fig. 3.25

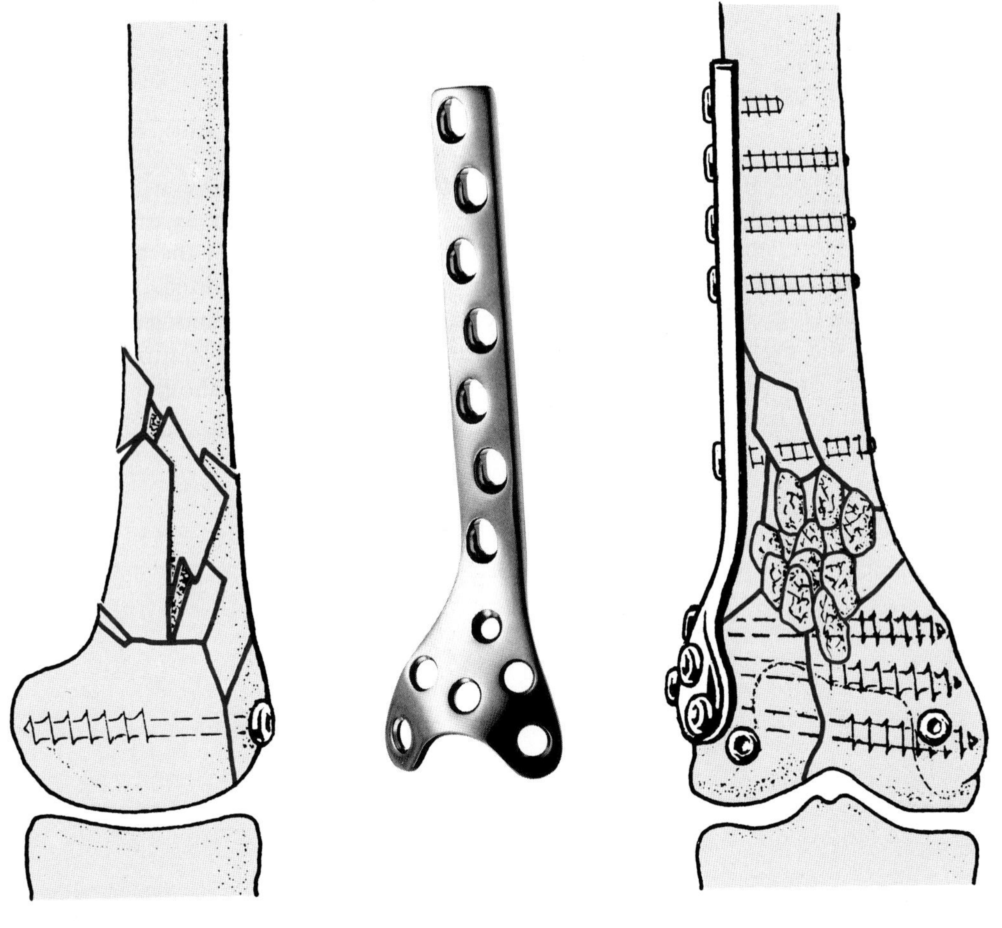

Fig. 3.26

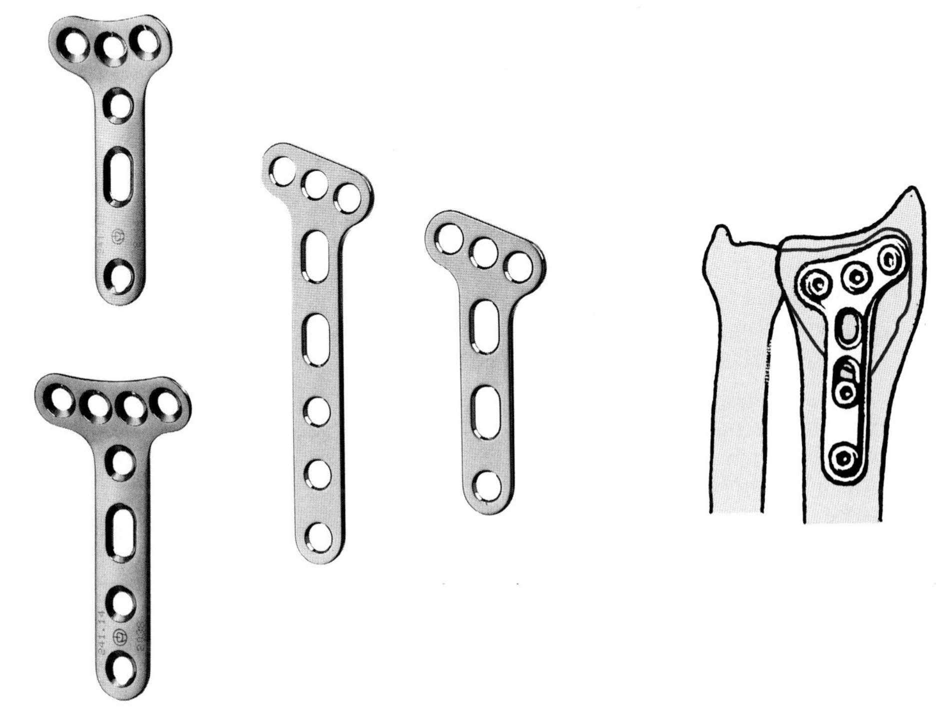

3.3 Axial Compression and the Compression and Tension Band Plates

3.3.1 Compression Plates

Transverse and short oblique fractures cannot be stabilized with lag screws but can be brought under compression with a plate. The plate acts as a static compression plate and exerts compression in the direction of the long axis of the bone. This can be accomplished either by taking advantage of the DCP holes alone or by adding the *tension device* (Fig. 3.27). It must be appreciated, as already emphasized, that the most efficient and the most stable means of achieving interfragmental compression is the lag screw. Therefore whenever possible, axial compression plates should also be combined with lag screw fixation (Fig. 3.16).

Fig. 3.27

a The articulated tension device with a pressure gauge and an excursion of 20 mm. The green indicates a compression of 30 kp and the red a compression of 120 kp.

Note: This tension device can also be used as a distractor. To be used in this mode its hook is turned over and the tension device is closed and fixed to bone so that the hook is against the end of the plate. As the tension device is then opened, it pushes against the plate which is fixed to the other main fragment. This produces distraction of the fracture and can be used to achieve indirect reduction of intermediate fragments by "ligamentotaxis".

b–d The use of the tension device to compress.

b Reduce the fracture and check the fit of the plate. Remove the plate and drill a 3.2-mm hole 1 cm from the fracture and measure its depth through the plate. Tap the hole and fix the plate to the bone with a 4.5-mm cortex screw of suitable length. Reduce the fracture and hold it reduced to the plate with a bone holding clamp.

c Engage the hook of the open tension device in the end hole of the plate and, using the tension device as a guide, drill a 3.2-mm hole. After measuring and tapping this hole, fix the tension device with a cortex screw to either one or both cortices depending on the quality of the bone. Osteoporotic bone requires fixation of the tension device to both cortices. With the articulated socket wrench (Kardan key), begin to tighten the screw of the tension device. This pulls on the plate and causes the fracture to be compressed.

d Once the tension device is fully tightened, the fracture is under maximal axial compression.

e, f Insertion of the remaining screws.

Fig. 3.27

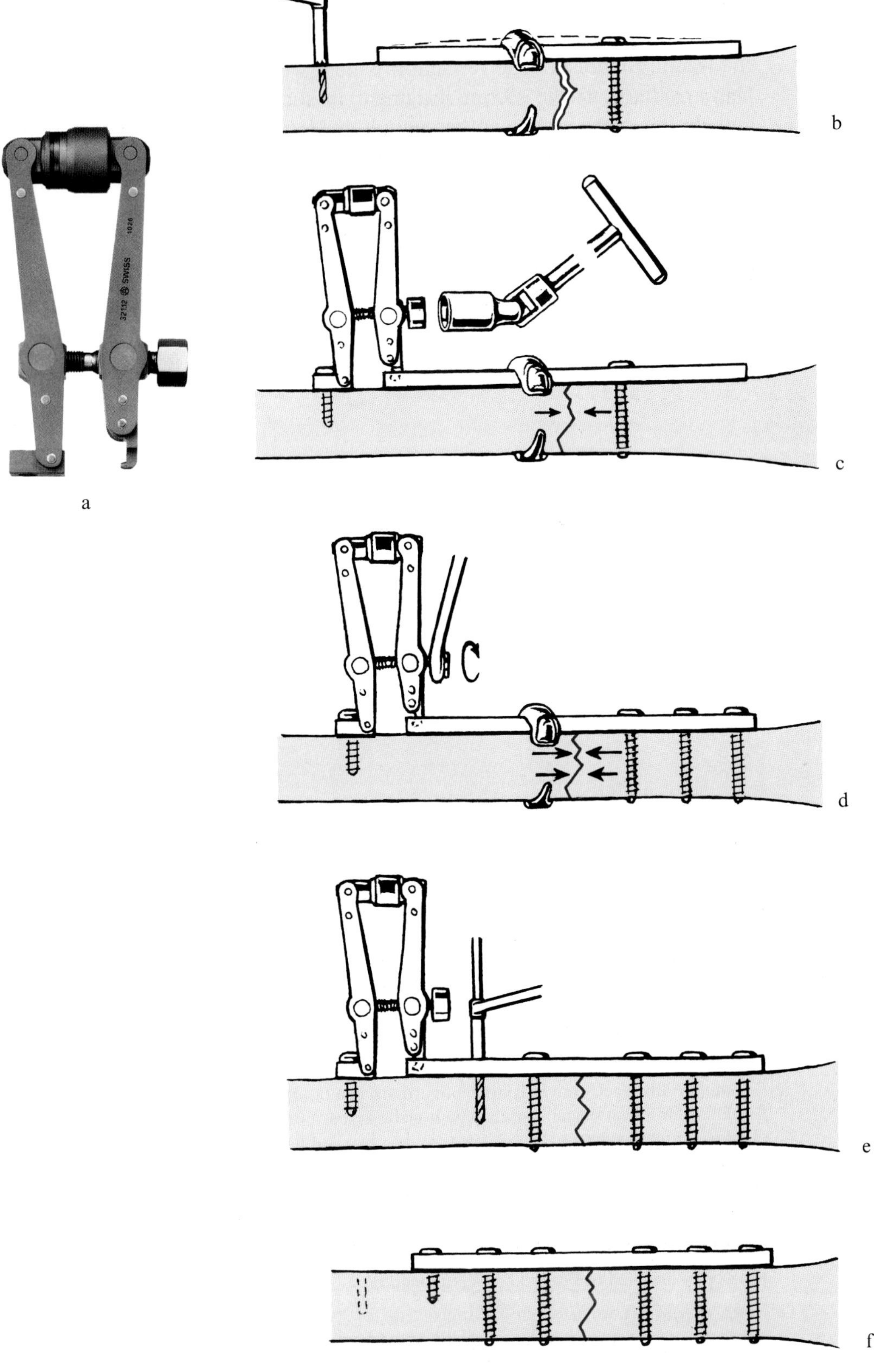

3.3.2 Technique of Achieving Axial Compression

The example of a transverse fracture in a straight segment of a diaphysis will help to explain axial interfragmental compression. A straight plate is fixed to one fragment and the fracture reduced. The reduction is held with a *reduction clamp* (Fig. 3.27). A *tension device* is fixed to the second fragment in such a way that its hook is engaged in the end of the plate and its other end is held to bone by a screw. If the spindle of the tension device is then tightened, the plate is brought under tension and the underlying bone under compression. If the bone is now carefully examined, two things will be noted. First, there is a gap in the fracture opposite the plate and second, the bone fragments deep to the plate have been impacted with the fracture line almost vanishing. This type of internal fixation was used by Schenk and Willenegger (1964) in their early experiments on primary bone healing. The contact of the cortices adjacent to the plate and the gap in the fracture opposite the plate in their work was also documented histologically as contact and gap healing (Fig. 3.28).

Fig. 3.28 Schematic representation of the healing of an osteotomy of a dog's radius under compression (drawn from histological material of Schenk).

a The cortex adjacent to the plate is in contact. There is no ingrowth of mesenchymal cells from either the periosteum or the endosteum. Note that there is a gap in the cortex opposite the plate.

b, b′ The bone ends in contact immediately adjacent to the plate show no changes within the first 3–4 weeks. Opposite the plate, the gap persists (b′).

c From the 4th week onwards, the bone ends in contact show active haversian remodeling. There is a proliferation of haversian canals which grow across both living and dead cortex bridging the osteotomy. This is contact healing.

d The gap in the cortex opposite the plate is invaded by blood vessels which appear within the first 8 days. These are accompanied by osteoblasts which deposit osteoid. This gives rise to bone lamellae which are oriented at 90° to the long axis.

From the 4th week onwards, these interfragmentary, transversely oriented lamellae of bone are replaced by axially oriented osteons. This is gap healing.

e High magnification of a remodeling osteon or "cutting cone" shows resorption and bone formation adjacent to one another. At the head are osteoclasts (1) which give rise to a resorption canal, which is then invaded by capillary sprouts (2). The circumferentially oriented osteoblasts (3) give rise to a new osteon (4).

Fig. 3.28

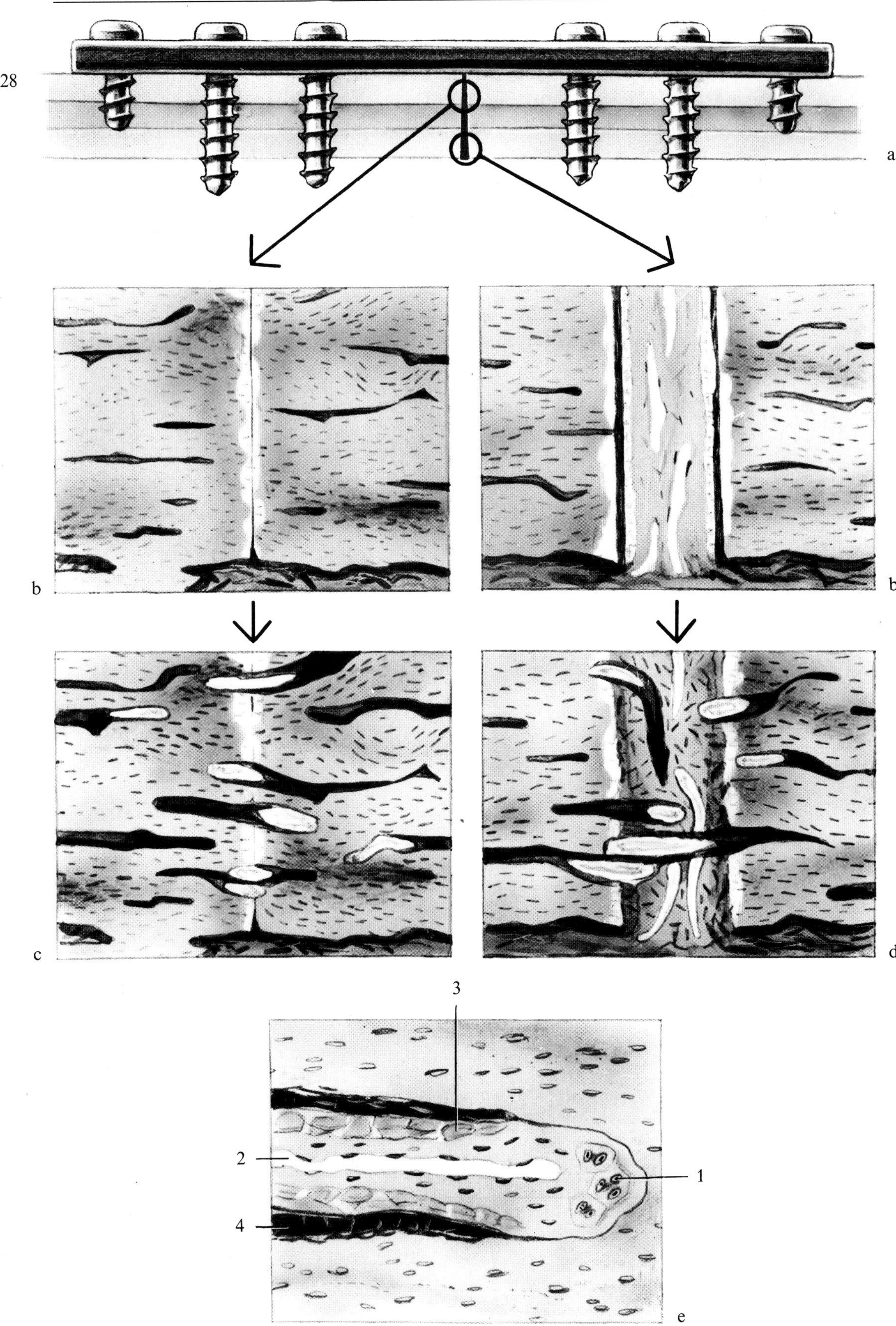

3.3.3 "Overbending" of Plates

To leave a gap in the opposite cortex is to decrease the stability of the fixation. This may result in micromovements with consequent bone resorption. Compression of the opposite cortex can be achieved by overbending the plate, which then, pressed against the bone, will act like a spring and close the gap in the opposite cortex (Fig. 3.29). Overbending can be used only when dealing with simple, two fragment fractures. In complex fractures, overbending will most often jeopardize reduction.

When short oblique fractures are fixed with compression plates using the tension device, the plate must be fixed first to the fragment which subtends an obtuse angle with the fracture plane under the plate (Fig. 3.30). When compression is then applied to the other fragment subtending an acute angle under the plate, this fragment glides under the plate and is pressed against the other fragment which, by virtue of its fixation to the plate, remains stable.

Fig. 3.29

a If a straight plate on a straight bone is placed under tension, only the cortex immediately adjacent to the plate comes under compression because the bone bends towards the plate. This results in a decrease of stability.

b After slight overbending of the plate in its middle, the plate is fixed to the bone with one screw approximately 1 cm away from the fracture line. The hook of the tension device is then hooked through the end hole of the plate and the tension device is fixed to the bone. This results in a slight gaping of the fracture below the plate but contact of one opposite cortex.

c As soon as the screw of the tension device is turned and tension is generated, the fracture surfaces begin to come under compression. As further tension is generated, the plate straightens out and both the plate and bone become straight. The whole fracture surface comes under compression and there is no longer any gaping at the fracture. Stability is greatly increased because of contact and prestress.

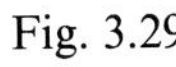
Fig. 3.29

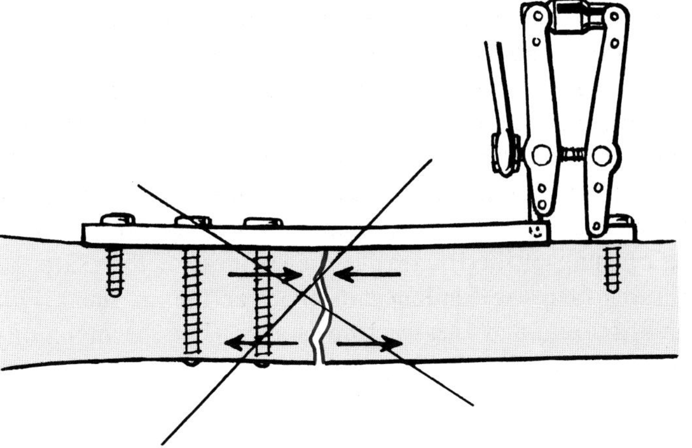
a

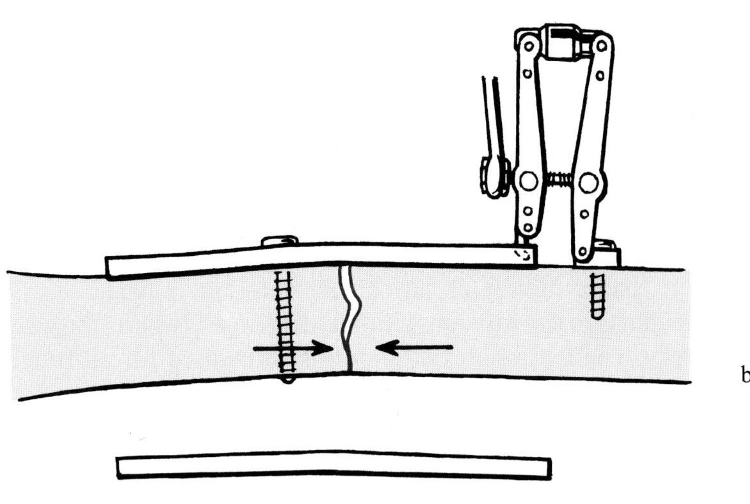
b

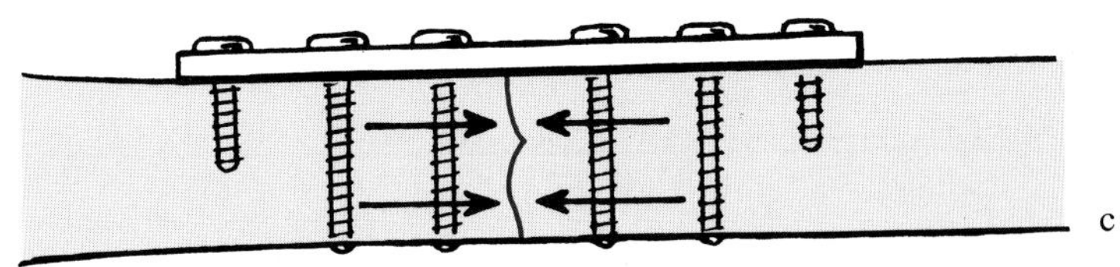
c

3.3.4 Combination of Compression Plate and Lag Screw

Biomechanical studies have shown that the bending and rotational stability of "axial compression fixation" of a transverse and particularly of a short oblique fracture can be greatly increased if a lag screw is inserted obliquely through the plate and across the fracture once axial compression has been generated. The increase in stability is due to the greater resistance of the fixation to torsional and bending forces. If there is a transverse or a short oblique fracture fixed with a compression plate, any force which tends to bend the bone and stretch the plate will increase the stability of the fixation (Fig. 3.30). If the force is directed, however, in the opposite direction, the only force resisting opening of the fracture is the stiffness of the plate. If there is a lag screw across the fracture, then the tendency of the fracture to open will be resisted by the screw. If the configuration of the fracture is such that the insertion of the screw will interfere with the position of the plate, then the plate should be applied and fixed to the bone as above. The lag screw should then be inserted across the fracture, outside the plate. It still greatly adds to the stability of the fixation even though it does not go through the plate. One should also remember that axial compression of an oblique fracture by a plate without an interfragmentary screw may cause the fragments to dislocate. The load must always be applied to the fragment with an acute angle next to the plate (Fig. 3.30a, b).

Most of the AO plates can be prestressed with the tension device. The broad and narrow DCPs as well as all the angled plates have a recess cut into the end hole which will receive the hook of the tension device. The tension device is, however, not necessary in all situations. Compression which can be generated with the self-compressing plates like the DCP and LC-DCP is usually sufficient. The tension device should be used, however, whenever the desired compression is greater than 100 kp or the gap to be closed is greater than 1 mm. This latter consideration is particularly important when dealing with pseudarthroses with or without deformity, where the use of the tension device is mandatory. The tension device should also be used for all fractures of the femur because of the high loads which must be resisted.

Fig. 3.30

a If a plate is fixed to the fragment which forms an acute angle with the fracture, then as axial compression is generated the fragments displace and reduction is lost.

b If, however, the plate is fixed to the fragment which forms an obtuse angle with the fracture, then as axial compression is generated the spike of the opposite fragment is driven against the plate, displacement is prevented, and

c Axial compression is achieved.

d To increase rotational stability and improve resistance to bending if a force is directed towards the plate, a lag screw should be inserted through the plate whenever possible to lag any short oblique or spiral fracture.

e, f The fixation is completed.

Fig. 3.30

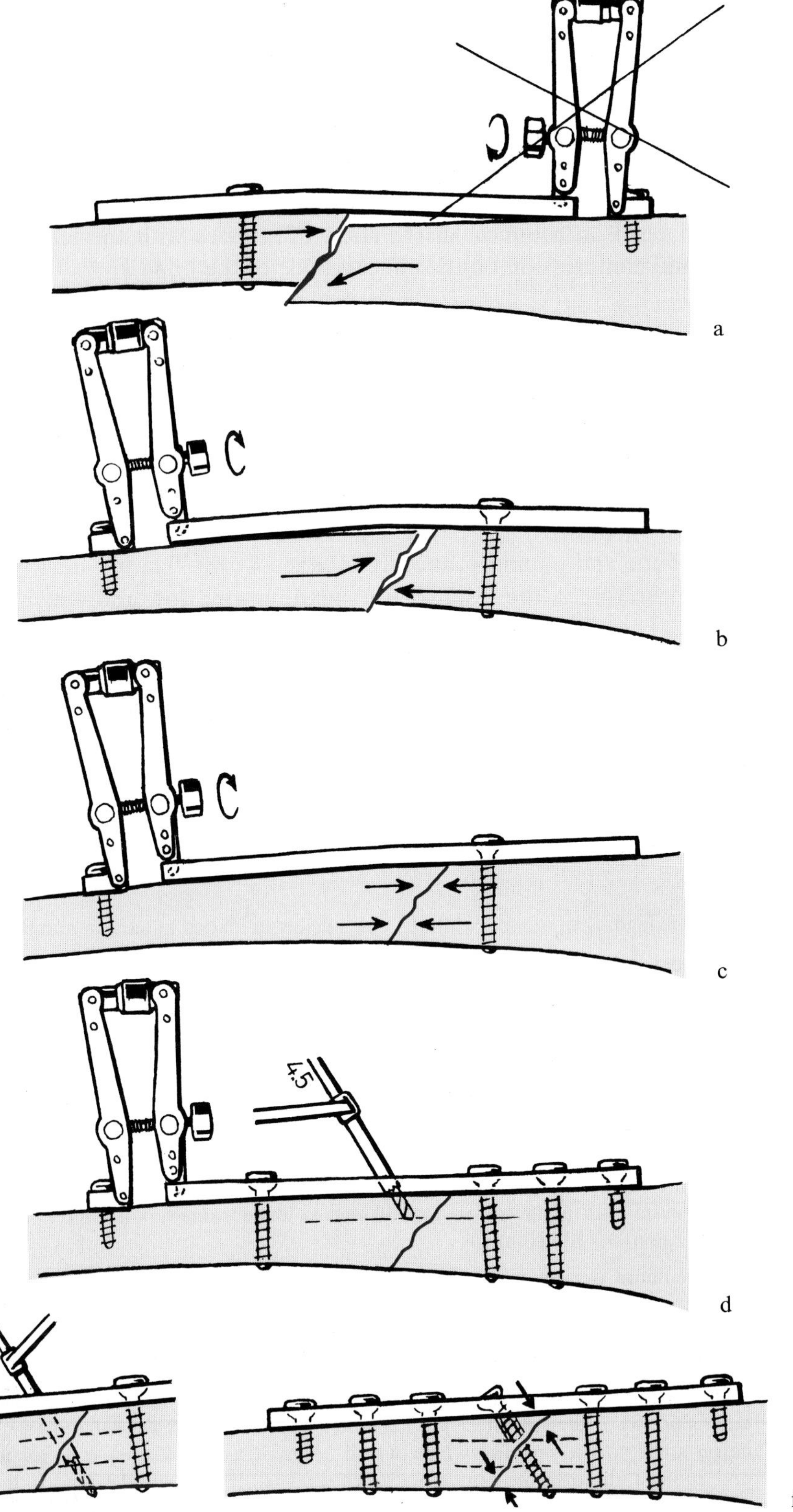

3.4 Dynamic Compression

3.4.1 The Eccentric Loading of Bones

Pauwels postulated that eccentrically loaded bones have one cortex loaded in tension and the other in compression (Fig. 3.31). This postulate has now been proven in vivo (Schatzker et al. 1980). The eccentrically loaded bone is subjected to bending stresses which result in a typical distribution of stresses with the tension coming on the convex side and compression on the concave side of the bone.

3.4.2 Tension Band Fixation

Pauwels (1935) borrowed from engineering the principle of tension band fixation and demonstrated its application in the internal fixation of eccentrically loaded bone (Fig. 3.31). In order to restore the load-bearing capacity of an eccentrically loaded fractured bone and minimize the forces borne by the fixation device it is necessary to absorb the tensile forces, the result of the bending moment, and convert them into compressive forces. This requires a tension band. A tension band is therefore a device which will exert a force equal in magnitude but opposite in direction to the bending force (Fig. 3.32). The tension band must be made of a material which resists tensile forces and which can be prestressed. The bone must be able to withstand compression. This means that the bone must not be comminuted either under or on the opposite side from the tension

---

Fig. 3.31

a Eccentric loading of a bone results in one side being loaded in tension and the other in compression.

b Unter an eccentric load, the gap will open first on the tension side.

c A plate applied to the tension side of bone will prevent the deformity. As load increases, the plate will be put under tension and the cortex opposite the plate will come under compression.

d If the plate is applied to the concave side which is under compression, under load the only resistance to deformity is the stiffness of the plate.

Fig. 3.32 Schematic drawing (after Pauwels) which illustrates the differences between load and stress and which demonstrates the principle of tension band fixation.

a If a column with a surface area of 10 cm^2 is loaded axially with 100 kp, it is subjected to pure axial compression $D = 10$ kp/cm^2.

b If the column is now subjected to eccentric loading, we have not only the axial compressive stresses but also additional bending stresses which give rise to further compressive stresses and tensile stresses. In our example, the resultant compressive stresses on the medial side D equal 110 kp/cm^2 and on the lateral side the tensile stresses Z equal 90 kp/cm^2.

c, d These bending stresses can be neutralized by a chain (or a wire) prestressed to exert a force equal and opposite to the weight. The chain then represents a tension band (c). The resultant compression corresponds to the pressure which would result if a second weight were placed on the opposite side and equidistant from the center of the column (d). Although the load is increased (200 kp), the total stress is reduced to a fifth ($D = 20$ kp/cm^2), because the bending stresses have been completely neutralized.

If we wish to use the tension band principle to achieve dynamically an increase in interfragmental compression, we must place the prestressed implant (wire or plate) wherever we have maximal tensile forces, i.e. furthest from the load axis.

Fig. 3.31

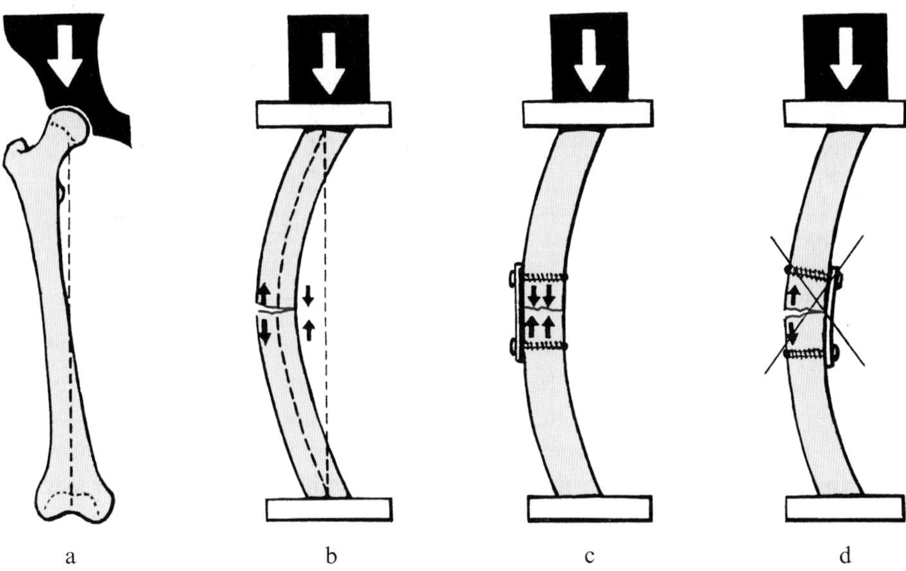

Fig. 3.32

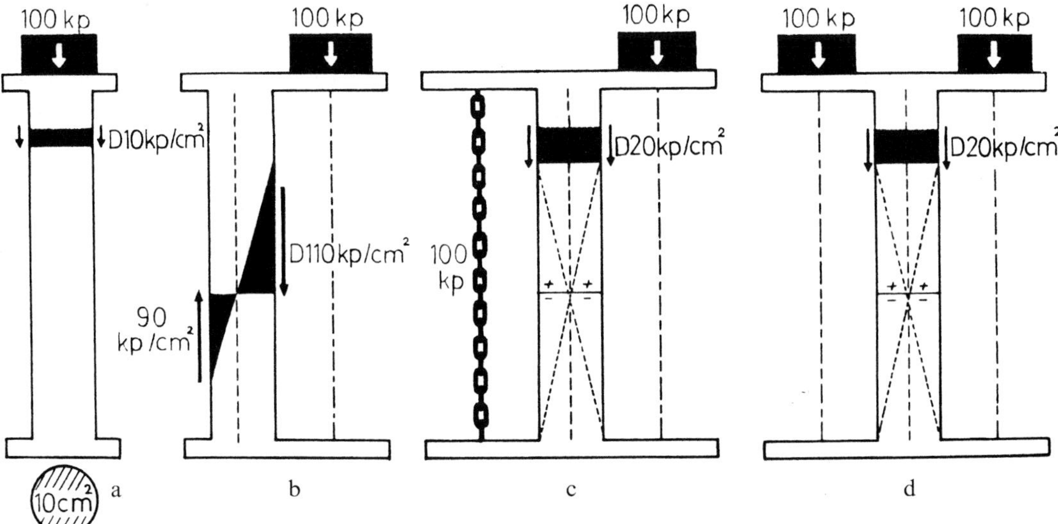

band. The prestressing of a plate (wire) in tension will result, as we have already learned, in axial compression of the bone. If such a bone is now subjected to eccentric loading, as for example the femur, the prestressing of the tension band plate will resist the tensile forces and convert them into compressive forces. This will result in a simultaneous increase and uniform distribution of compressive forces across the fracture. The dynamic component of the compression rises when the bone is loaded and is subjected to bending. The prestress in the tension band ensures that the bone remains loaded in compression even when the dynamic component of the loading is removed. Thus the fluctuations in the load are in magnitude and not in direction.

As already indicated, the prerequisites for tension band fixation are:

1. A plate or wire able to withstand the tensile forces
2. Bone which is able to withstand compression
3. An intact buttress of the opposite cortex

If the medial buttress (the opposite cortex) is deficient under load, the plate will be subjected to repetitive bending, will suffer fatigue and break.

Bones which are eccentrically loaded are the femur, the humerus, and the radius and ulna. Hence plates ideally should be applied to their tension side in order to function as tension band plates. In the femur, where the forces are enormous, the plate must be applied to the tension side. In the upper extremity, where the forces are much lower, this rule can be broken.

Pseudarthroses with deformity have a tension side and a compression side. Indeed, nature tells us which is which: the convex side is under tension and the concave side is under compression. This knowledge can be used when attempts are made to straighten deformities associated with pseudarthroses. If a plate is placed on the convex side of the deformity and is then placed under tension, it will function as a tension band. As the plate is progressively placed under greater and greater tension, the deformity will be gradually corrected until both the plate and the underlying segment of bone are perfectly straight. Such correction requires the use of the tension device. It cannot be carried out by making use of the loading principle of the self-compressing plates.

3.5 Bridging Plates

3.5.1 Bridge Plate

In order to maintain length and alignment a plate is occasionally used to bridge a badly comminuted segment of bone (Hierholzer). A plate is used in this manner when lag screw fixation of the individual fragments would result in their devitalization or when there is an actual gap and the plate is used to maintain the relative position of the fragments. This type of plate fixation is not stable: therefore every possible effort should be made to maintain all the soft tissue attachments and blood supply of the intervening comminuted fragments, since union will depend on the formation of a bridging callus rather than primary bone union. In these situations, techniques of indirect reduction are particularly useful. Both plate ends have to be solidly fixed to their corresponding part of the bone by three to four screws (Fig. 3.33a).

3.5.2 Wave Plate

A similar principle has been introduced by Weber with his "wave plate" (Wellenplatte). He deliberately bends the plate away from the nonunion (or comminuted area to be bridged) to leave some distance between bone cortex and plate (Fig. 3.33b) and inserts an autogenous cancellous graft between the bone cortex and plate. The three basic principles are described in Chap. 19 (legend to Fig. 19.33).

3.5.3 How Many Screws?

Experience has shown that to prevent mechanical failure of plate fixation, a certain number of screws is necessary to secure the plate to the bone. This varies from bone to bone and depends to some degree on the size and weight of the individual and the size and quality of the bone. In most individuals, the humerus requires six cortices of screw purchase on each side of the fracture, the radius and ulna five, the femur seven, and the tibia six. Osteoporosis, depending on its severity, will require a corresponding increase in the number of screws.

One should not feel compelled to fill every hole of the plate with screws. The failure of a plate does not depend on the presence or absence of a screw from a hole, but rather on the presence or absence of a bony defect a well as on its extent. The plate is more likely to fail if the bone defect is short as this results in considerable stress concentration. This is reflected by the stress concentration around a screw hole in the overlying plate. A plate will fail through a screw hole since it is the site of the stress concentration as well as the weakest portion of a plate. If the defect in the continuity of the bone is longer, the stresses are distributed over a longer segment and the stress per unit area is correspondingly lower. Thus bridge plating is likely to succeed if the defect is longer, particularly if it is filled with a number of viable bone fragments which will rapidly bridge with callus. If the defect is short, transverse, or oblique, failure is more likely, since there is not only a concentration of stresses but also a considerably longer healing time. Dead bone will not heal. Therefore if the fragments are small, it is best not to attempt screw fixation since it is likely to result in devitalization of the fragments, a delay in callus formation, and consequently failure.

Fig. 3.33

a A plate used to bridge a zone of comminution is called a bridge plate. It maintains length and rotational alignment by "splinting", a form of relative stability, rather than by providing absolute stability through compression. Union depends on the formation of callus.

b A wave plate (the principle is explained in Fig. 19.33).

Fig. 3.33

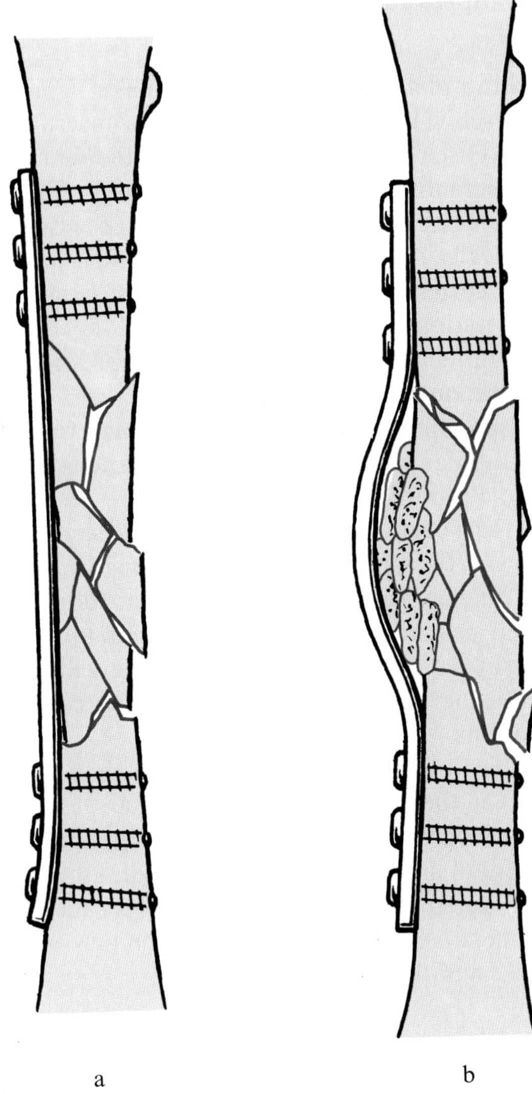

3.6 Self-Compressing Plates

3.6.1 Semi-Tubular, One-Third Tubular and Quarter-Tubular Plates, Dynamic Compression Plates

Self-compressing plates are plates which make it possible to achieve axial compression by combining screw hole geometry with screw insertion.

The first AO self-compressing plate was the semi-tubular plate (Fig. 3.34a). The oval holes and the eccentric placement of the screws accounted for its self-compressing property. To achieve axial compression by means of self-compressing plates, the fracture has to be anatomically reduced. The screws are then inserted eccentrically through the oval holes with the corresponding drill sleeve as far from the fracture as possible. This results in axial compression of the fracture (Fig. 3.34a–f). The 4.5-mm cortex screws are used with the semi-tubular plate. Similar axial compression can be achieved with the one-third tubular and the quarter-tubular plates. They are designed for use with smaller bones and the corresponding 3.5-mm and 2.7-mm small fragment screws.

The semi-tubular plate is only 1 mm thick and is easily deformable. It owes its rotational stability to its borders which "bite" into the underlying surface as the screws are tightened. It has been used on round bones such as the radius or on crests like the anterior crest of the tibia and only as a tension band plate, as its greatest strength is in tension. The chief indications for the semi-tubular plates were therefore fractures of the radius and proximal ulna, particularly comminuted fractures of the olecranon, and boot-top fractures of the distal tibia. Today, the semi-tubular plate has few uses. It remains useful as a tension band in the open book injury of the pelvis and as a buttress plate in some situations.

The one-third tubular plates are useful in the treatment of lateral malleolar fractures and fractures of the metacarpals and metatarsals. The quarter-tubular plates together with the small T plates and L plates are used in hand surgery.

Despite careful use, there have been many failures with the semi-tubular plates particularly in comminuted areas of the long bones because the plates fatigued and broke. They have been almost completely replaced by the new generation of self-compressing plates, the 4.5- and 3.5-mm DCPs.

Fig. 3.34

a The semi-tubular plate.

b The one-third tubular plate.

c The quarter-tubular plate.

d–f The compression of a transverse fracture of the fibula with a one-third tubular plate.

d A 2.5-mm drill hole is made in one fragment, 1 cm from the fracture. The depth is measured through the plate, the hole is tapped with a 3.5-mm cortex tap and a 3.5-mm cortex screw is inserted but not completely tightened. The fracture is now reduced and held reduced with the bone clamp. With a hook, traction is applied to the plate and using the 3.5/2.5-mm drill sleeve, a 2.5-mm hole is drilled eccentrically through the plate as far from the fracture as the hole allows.

e The depth is measured, the hole is tapped and the second 3.5-mm cortex screw is inserted. As the screw head engages the plate, it is pushed towards the fracture together with the bone fragment which generates axial interfragmental compression.

f The alternate tightening of the first and the second screw will result in axial compression and stable fixation. The remaining screws are inserted in the neutral position through the center of the oval holes.

Fig. 3.34

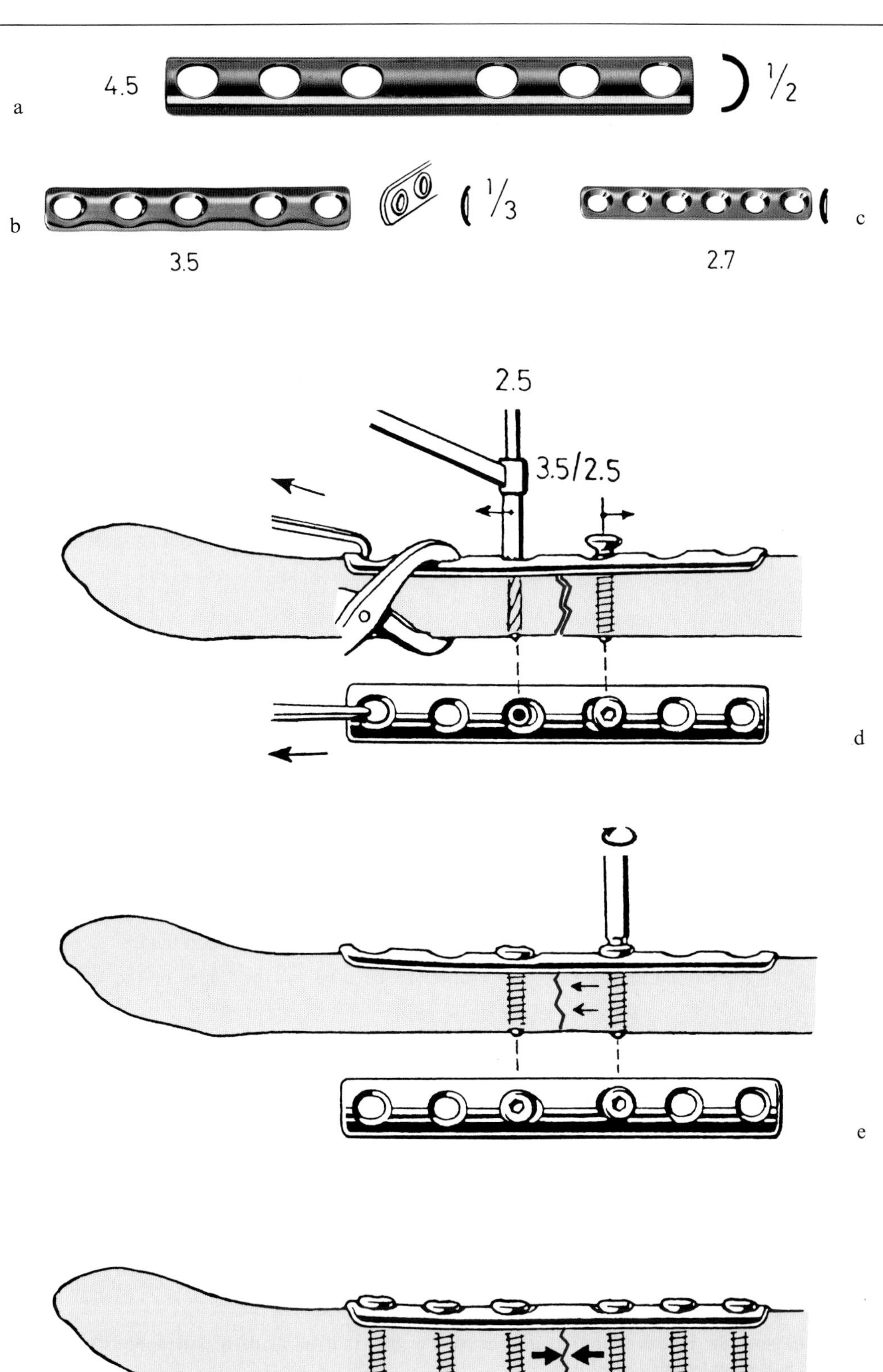

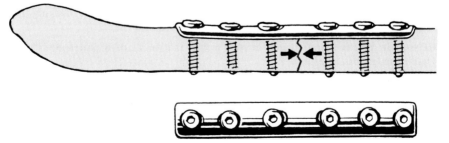

The DCP (Fig. 3.35) represents a significant improvement on the round hole plates. It is a self-compressing plate due to the special geometry of the screw hole. This screw hole geometry makes it possible to achieve axial compression without the use of a tension device, and the screws can be angled in any direction. This plate is adaptable to many different internal fixation situations and can be used as a static compression plate, a dynamic compression plate, a neutralization plate and a buttress plate. Both the narrow and the broad DCPs are considerably stronger than the semi-tubular plates and plate failures have become rare.

Axial compression results from an interplay between screw hole geometry and eccentric placement of the screw in the screw hole. The screw hole is a combination of an inclined and a horizontal cylinder which permits the downward and horizontal movement of a sphere, the screw head. Sideways movement of the screw head is impossible. The aim is to position the screw head at the intersection of the inclined and downward cylinder. At this point the screw head has a spherical contact in the screw hole which results in maximum stability without completely blocking the horizontal movement of the screw (Fig. 3.36).

Fig. 3.35

a The broad DCP (plate and its profile) to be used on the humerus and femur.

b The narrow DCP (plate and its profile) to be used on the bones of the forearm, on the tibia and on the pelvis.

c The 3.5-mm DCP (plate and its profile) to be used with 3.5-mm cortex screws. It should be used on the radius and ulna.

d The 2.7-mm DCP (plate and its profile) to be used with 2.7-mm cortex screws.

Fig. 3.36 The screw hole and the spherical gliding principle.

a A sphere (the screw head) glides down an inclined cylinder (the screw hole). This combination of downward and horizontal movement of the screw causes a horizontal movement of the underlying bone with respect to the stationary plate. A sideways movement is impossible. The aim is to position the screw head at the intersection of the inclined and horizontal cylinder. At this point, the screw head has a spherical contact in the screw hole, which results in maximum stability without blocking the horizontal movement of the screw towards the fracture.

b The screw hole is manufactured in such a way that in shape it corresponds to the scheme of the two half-cylinders described in a.

c Here we see the exact representation of the shape of the screw hole. The inclined half-cylinder is for self-compression or self-loading and the horizontal cylinder is to prevent blocking or obstructing the screw in its horizontal path. This guarantees that only compression will be exerted at the fracture.

d Schematic representation of the sloped gliding hole and its corresponding spherical screw head. We see in the left portion of the screw hole the inclined load plane and on the right, the horizontal sliding plane.

Fig. 3.35

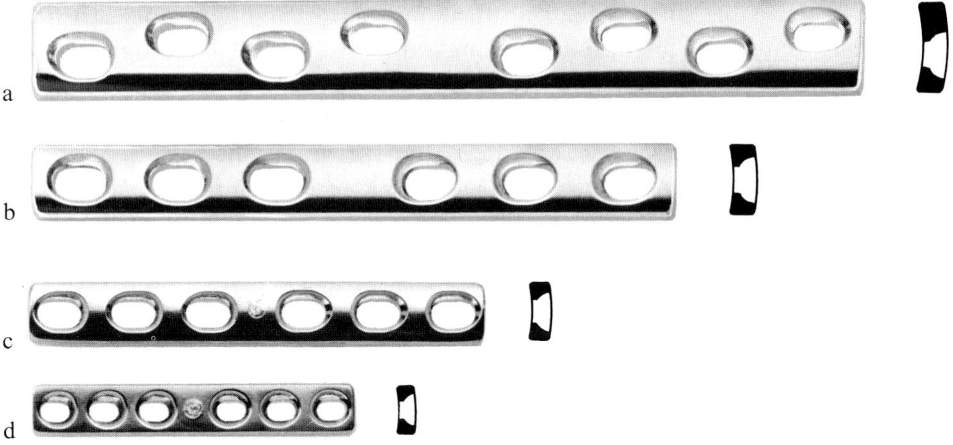

Fig. 3.36

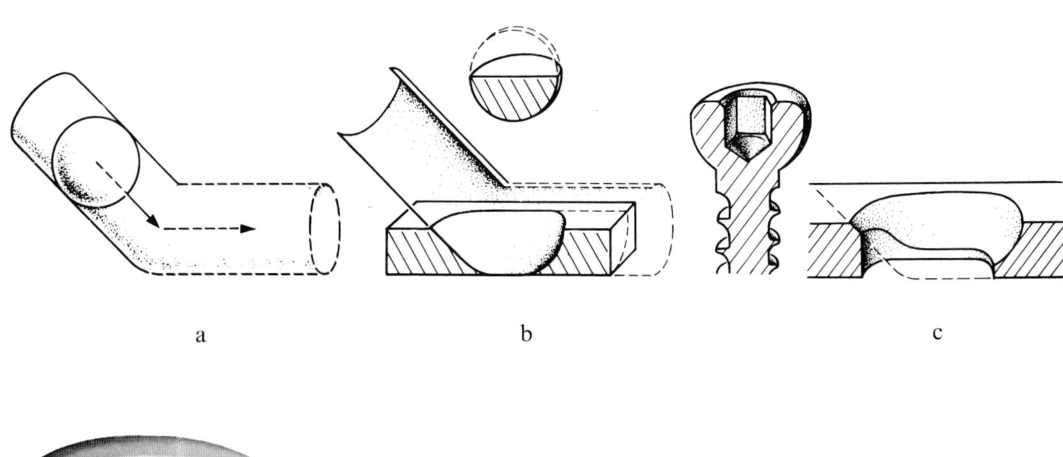

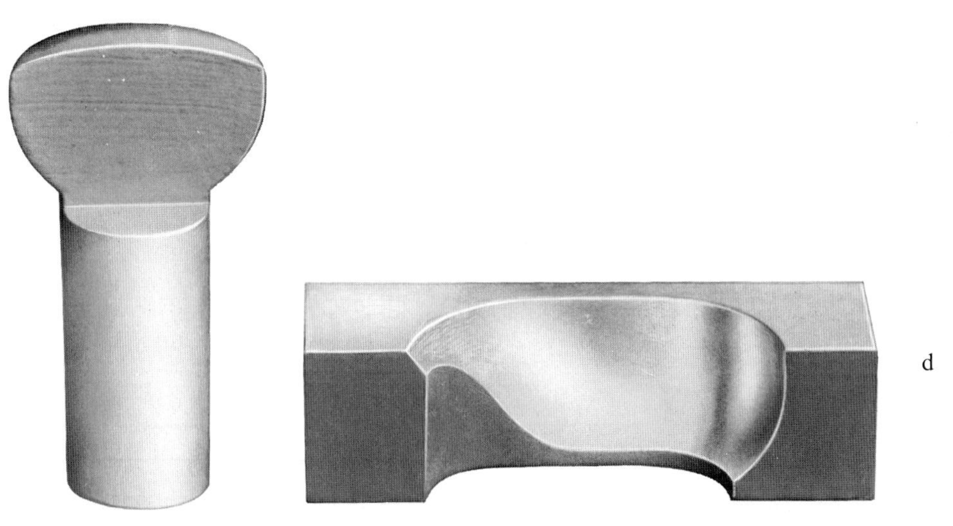

The DCPs require the use of two drill guides. The neutral drill guide (green) (Fig. 3.37a) has a central hole for the drill bit. It allows the screw to be inserted in the neutral position, that is, at the intersection of the two cylinders which make up the screw hole. In this neutral position, the drill guide results in a 0.1-mm loading, so that even when inserted in the neutral position and fully tightened, the screws cause a slight degree of axial compression.

The load guide (gold in color) (Fig. 3.37b) has an eccentric hole for the drill bit, which must be inserted away from the fracture. This results in the load screw being inserted initially 1.0 mm away from the neutral position in the screw hole. When the screw is tightened, its head slides downwards along the inclined plane of the cylinder as well as horizontally towards the fracture. As the horizontal displacement is resisted by the bone, the horizontal movement results in axial compression of the bone and tension in the plate. Following an anatomic reduction of the fracture with fragment contact, insertion of one screw in the load position results in an axial compression of 50–80 kp. In order to increase the load, that is increase the impaction of the fragments, more than one load screw can be inserted, although that is rarely necessary. The first load screw must then be slightly loosened before the second screw is completely tightened. When a substantial load is required, such as in the femur or with pseudarthroses, the tension device should be used first.

If the DCP is used as a buttress plate, the 3.2-mm drill sleeve should be used as a drill guide with the sleeve pressed in the screw hole towards the fracture (Fig. 3.21a, b). Since the outer diameter of the sleeve is 4.5 mm, the hole is drilled in such a position that when the screw is tightened, its head will be pressed against the plate in the locking position.

As already indicated, the shape of the screw head and of the screw hole in the DCP permits the angulation of screws in all directions. This allows a much better adaptation of the screw direction to the particular anatomy of the fracture (Fig. 3.38). It also greatly facilitates the insertion of an oblique lag screw across the plate. It must be stressed again and again that whenever possible, the stability of the internal fixation should be enhanced by the insertion of an oblique lag screw through the plate across the main fracture line. This applies when the plate is being used as a neutralization plate, but even more so if it is used as a compression plate. It is relatively easy to carry out this principle when dealing with oblique fractures, but it is also recommended in the fixation of transverse fractures in large bones like the femur and tibia if these are fixed with plates.

Fig. 3.37 The drill guides for the DCP.

a Neutral drill guide (green). It places screw 0.1 mm from end of slope, inducing some axial compression.

b Load drill guide (gold). It places screw 1 mm from end of slope.

Fig. 3.38 The interplay between the spherical screw head and the geometry of the screw hole permits the angulation of the screws in all directions (maximum 25° longitudinally, 7° sideways).

Fig. 3.37

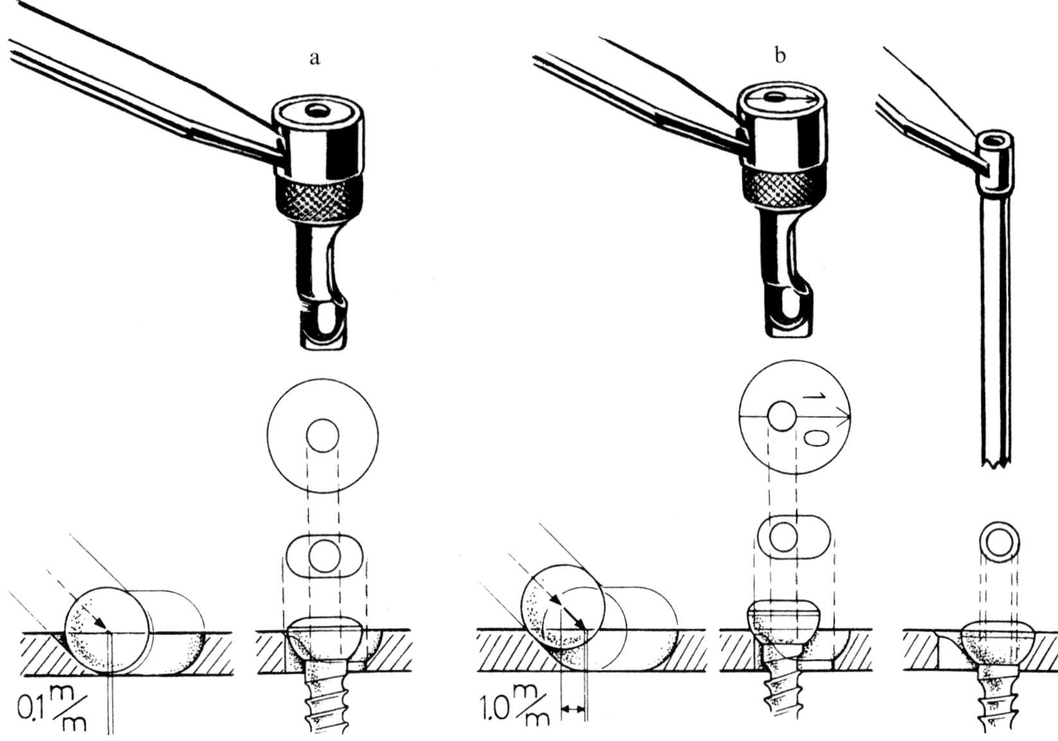

Fig. 3.38

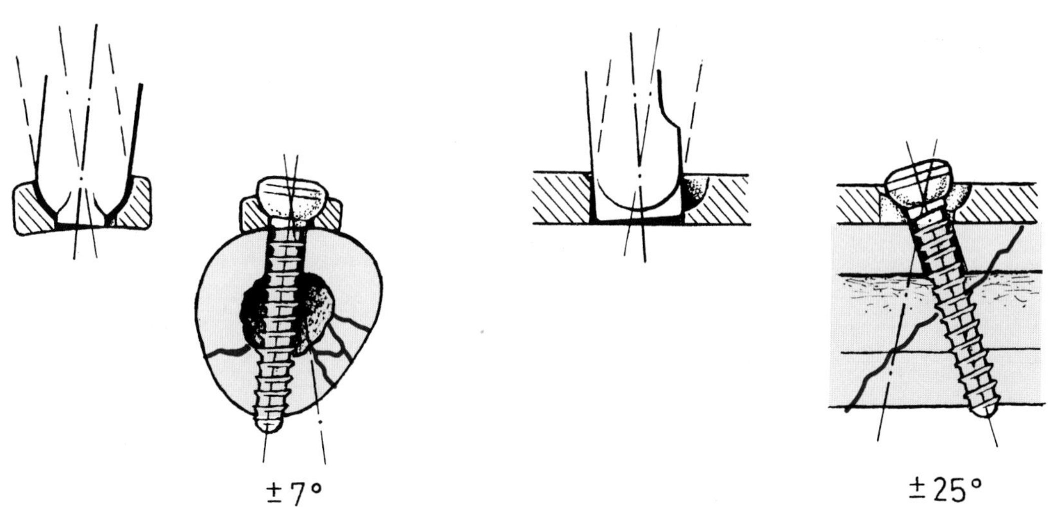

There are two options available to the surgeon when he comes to insert the lag screw through the plate across the fracture. He can either carry out the reduction and axial compression and then drill the gliding hole and thread hole of the lag screw (Fig. 3.30) or he can drill the gliding hole before the reduction is carried out. The latter is the preferred method of proceeding and consists of six steps (Fig. 3.39):

1. Drill the gliding hole with the 4.5-mm drill bit in the fragment which subtends an acute angle with the fracture plane (Fig. 3.39a).
2. Reduce the fracture and insert the 3.2-mm drill sleeve through the plate into the predrilled gliding hole (Fig. 3.39b).
3. Fix the plate with one screw in neutral position to the opposite fragment which subtends an obtuse angle (Fig. 3.39b).
4. Now insert one screw in the load position in the fragment which contains the gliding hole. Tightening this screw generates axial compression (Fig. 3.39c, d).
5. Drill the thread hole for the lag screw, measure the length and insert the screw (Fig. 3.39e).
6. Add the remaining plate screws in a neutral position as required (Fig. 3.39f).

There are fracture situations where the important interfragmentary lag screw cannot be inserted across the plate (see Sect. 3.3.4), but should still be inserted across the fracture.

The "anatomy" of the DCP allows the surgeon to also carry out compression fixation of a segmental fracture with each fracture line being placed separately under axial compression.

Fig. 3.39 Axial compression fixation of a short oblique fracture with a DCP (maximum angulation 25° longitudinally, 7° sideways).

a First drill the gliding hole with the 4.5-mm drill bit.

b Reduce the fracture. Insert the 3.2-mm drill sleeve (3.5/4.5) through the plate into the predrilled gliding hole and fix the plate with one screw in a neutral position to the opposite fragment which subtends an obtuse angle with the fracture plane. Before drilling the 3.5-mm hole, the plate is drawn (see arrow!) towards the fragment so that the 4.5-mm drill guide buttresses against the slope of the plate hole!

c, d Insert one screw in the load position into the other fragment. As the screw is tightened, axial compression is generated.

e Drill the thread hole for the lag screw. Measure, tap and insert the lag screw.

f Insert the remaining screws in the neutral position.

Fig. 3.39

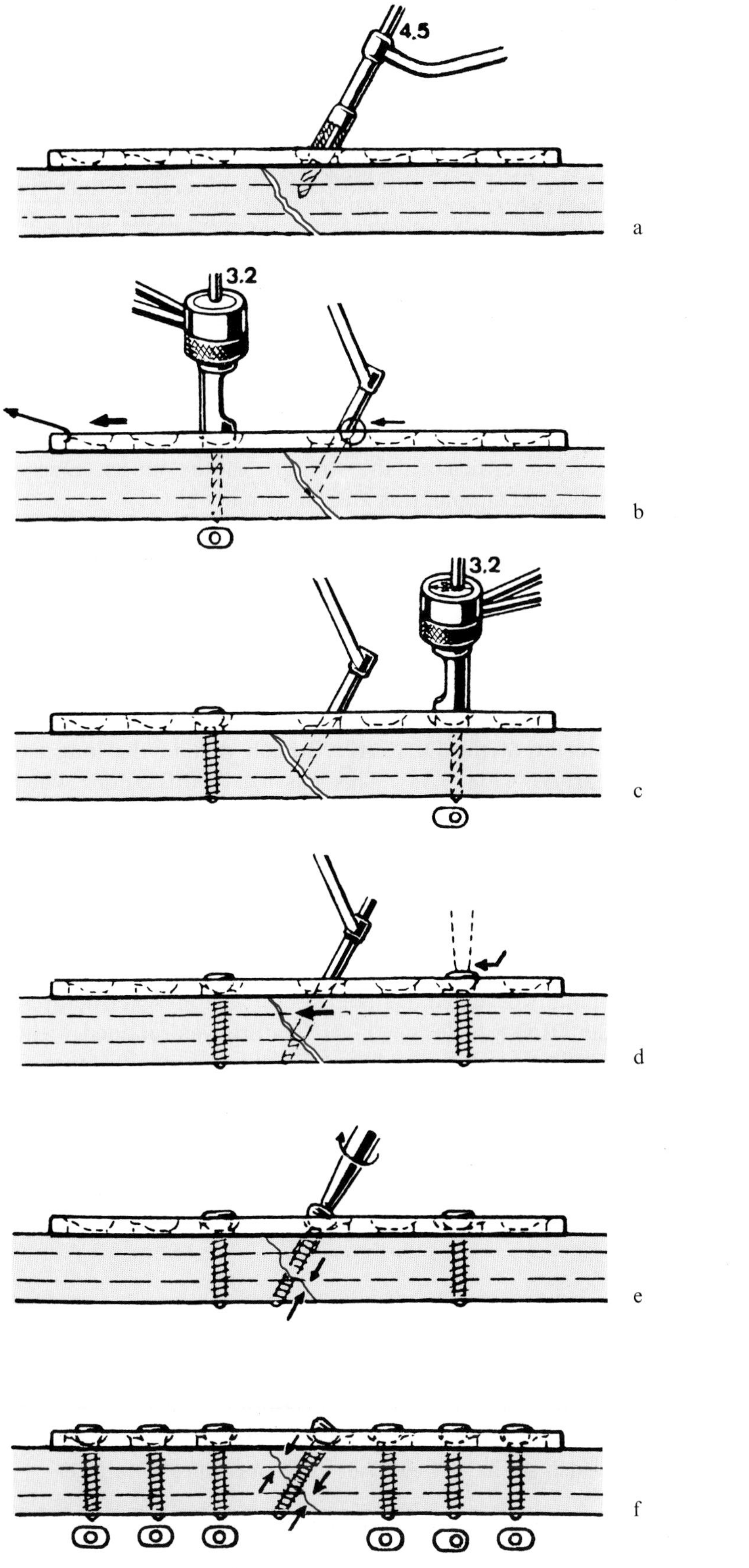

3.6.2 Limited Contact DCP (LC-DCP)

3.6.2.1 Shortcomings of the DCP

Flat Undersurface

The DCP has not only proved itself more versatile than the round hole plate, but also ensured the elimination of the inconsistencies in achieving successful axial loading which were seen with the round hole plate (Galeazzi et al.). Although the DCP has withstood the test of time, over the years certain shortcomings have become apparent.

The extensive contact of the undersurface of the plate with bone leads to major interference with periosteal blood supply. This has been shown to be the main reason for plate induced osteoporosis (Gautier). The potential danger of such necrosis is the possible formation of a sequestrum underneath the plate. There is also the possibility of a significant mechanical problem. The bone underneath the plate and immediately adjacent to the fracture is critical to the strength of the union. Due to the interference with the periosteal blood supply, this area heals more slowly.

Because of the circumscribed lack of or delayed cortical healing, at the time of plate removal from the tension side of the bone, there is a notch in the bone, which is no longer protected by the plate. This notch behaves as a stress riser and may induce or facilitate a refracture.

Inclination

The geometry of the DCP hole is such that in the long axis, a screw cannot be tilted more than 25° (Fig. 3.38). This has led to difficulties whenever attempts are made to lag short oblique fractures through the plate, and has resulted in less than optimal interfragmental compression.

Distribution of Plate Holes

The conventional round hole plates had an extended middle segment without holes. They were originally designed to stabilize short diaphyseal fractures, particularly of the forearm. When the DCP was designed, this feature was retained without any particular rationale. This middle segment has led to difficulties when a fracture with a zone of fragmentation has to be stabilized. Once the position of the plate is chosen and the first hole drilled, because of the middle segment it becomes impossible to shift the plate in the long axis of the bone. The drill hole in bone will not fit the plate holes even if the new position of the plate suits the overall fixation better. Under these circumstances, the only solution for the surgeon is a longer plate.

Fragile Lining

Plates with a rectangular cross section provoke the formation of a comparatively thin bony wall along the length of the plate. These longitudinal ridges add to the strength of the bone when the plates are removed. If the ridges so formed are thin they are easily nicked at the time of the plate removal. This not only renders the bone less strong, but may also act as a stress riser and contribute to failure.

3.6.2.2 Solutions to the Problems of the DCP

Structured Undersurface

Improved Circulation: Extensive animal studies have shown that grooves in the undersurface of plates significantly improve the blood supply of plated bony segments (Joerger). To be effective such grooves must be of adequate depth and width. As a corollary to the improvement in the periosteal blood supply and cortical blood supply, the osteoporosis which was said to have been the result of the so-called "stress shielding" has disappeared. This plate related osteoporosis has been shown conclusively to be the result of the initial vascular insult and consequent avascular necrosis which then provoked corresponding florid bone remodelling.

Callus Bridge: As already alluded to above, a closely applied plate results in avascular necrosis of the underlying cortex and delayed healing of the superficial layers of bone immediately adjacent to the fracture. When the plate is removed, this small gap can serve as a stress riser and weaken the bone. If a plate is contoured in such a way that a gap (a wave, Fig. 3.33b) is created between the plate and the bone adjacent to the fracture, the circulation is not affected to the same degree and a small bridge of callus develops in this "critical zone" which greatly adds to the strength of the bone. Grooves in the undersurface of the plate act in a similar way and allow for the formation of a small amount of callus in the most critical area. Experiments with grooved plates used to stabilize osteotomies in sheep and dogs have shown a marked increase in the strength of the fracture area as early as three months after surgery.

Undercut Screw Holes

Each screw hole has been fitted out with oblique undercuts at both ends (Fig. 3.40Ac). This allows a screw to be tilted up to 40° in each direction of the long axis of the bone. This has greatly eased the passing of lag screws through the plate, particularly when lagging short oblique fractures. In addition, it has contributed to a significant reduction in the contact area of the plate with bone.

Uniform Spacing of Screw Holes

The uniform spacing of screw holes and the elimination of the middle segment allows for easy shifting of the plates in the long axis as well as easy changes in the plate length (Fig. 3.40Aa, b).

Trapezoid Cross Section

The trapezoid cross section of the plate with the smaller surface in contact with the bone has resulted in the formation of lower and broader ridges of bone along the length of the plate than those previously observed with the plates with rectangular cross section. Such ridges are less likely to be injured at the time of plate removal (Fig. 3.40Ad).

Additional New Compressing Principle

The basic spherical gliding principle of the screw within the screw hole of the DCP has been preserved, but the screw hole has been redesigned so that this feature is present at both ends of the hole. This improves the versatility of the plate when complex fractures are being fixed.

The Avoidance of Bone Damage and Improvement in Compression

Whenever a lag screw is passed through a DCP screw hole to lag a fracture, it is subjected to a translational force which tends to shift the screw head towards the buttress position as the screw is tightened. This may give rise to one of two complications:

1. Either the screw head or thread may abut against the inner wall of the plate hole. Because of friction this may significantly reduce axial compression. It may also damage the plate or the screw.
2. The thread of the screw may bite on one side into the wall of the gliding hole, which may reduce the lag effect by as much as 37% (Klaue).

The use of an elongated and undercut screw hole together with a newly designed partially threaded cortex screw whose shaft diameter equals the outer diameter of the screw thread avoids these complications.

Titanium

This is known to be biologically exceptionally inert and therefore it is well tolerated as an implant material. Commercially pure titanium avoids any potentially toxic components such as vanadium. The mechanical limitations of pure titanium are well known. New technical advances, however, in the way titanium is treated have made it possible now for titanium to reach 90% of the strength of the stainless steel used for implants. Thus titanium appears to be the best metal from the point of view of tissue tolerance and avoidance of low grade immunological complications.

Fig. 3.40 A The LC-DCP.

a The surface of the plate.

b The undersurface of the plate.

c Note the oblique undercuts at both ends of each screw hole. This permits a tilting of the screw of 40° maximum in each direction in the long axis of the bone.

d Note the trapezoid cross section of the plate and the undercuts between the screw holes.

The different undercuts greatly reduce the contact area between the plate and the bone.

Fig. 3.40 B Technical characteristics of the LC-DCP.

a The LC-DCP screw hole acts in a similar way as does that of the DCP: the position of the screw is neutral, i.e. at the intersection of the inclined cylinder with the horizontal cylinder.

b The use of the load guide results in a maximal compressive displacement of 1.0 mm.

c Detail of the construction of the screw hole composed of three cylinders meeting at obtuse angles.

d The inclined cylinder of one side and the horizontal one within the plate hole with more marked undercut.

e The screw with spherical undersurface always provides a congruent fit between screw head and plate hole. The plate hole with two symmetrically opposed inclined compression slides.

f The universal plate drill guide used for neutral positioning of the screw. When the universal plate drill guide is pressed down the screw head is positioned onto the horizontal cylinder (neutral buttress position).

g The universal plate drill guide used for load positioning of the screw. When the universal plate drill guide is not pressed down, the screw head is positioned onto the inclined cylinder (variable degree of loading, max. 1.0 mm).

Fig. 3.40 A

Fig. 3.40 B

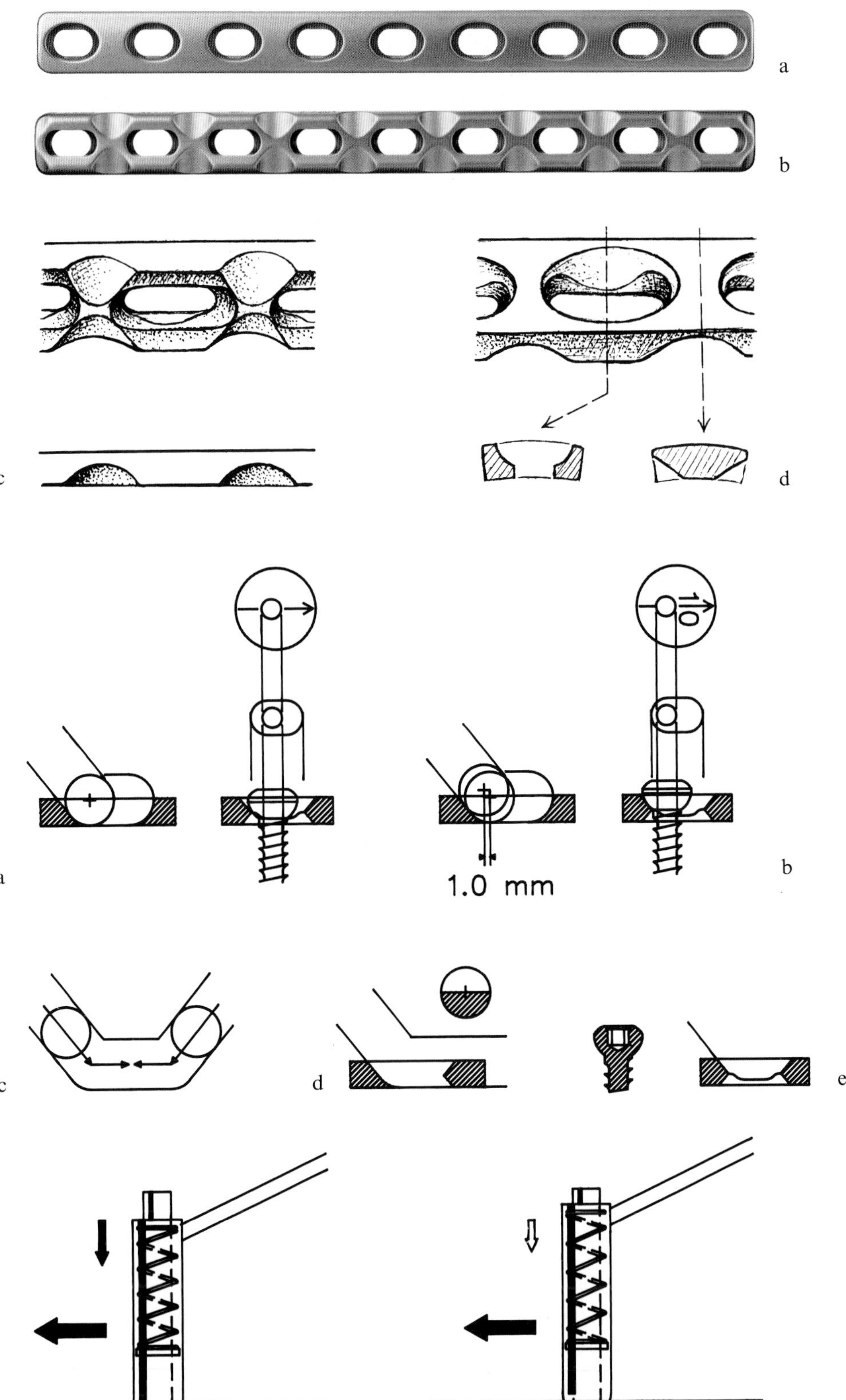

3.6.2.3 Clinical Application of the LC-DCP

Conventional Use

The LC-DCP may be used in exactly the same way as the DCP. For the experienced surgeon there are additional features which provide a definite improvement in plate function.

The plate must be used with the new LC-DCP drill guide. The old DCP drill guide should *not* be used. In order to avoid confusion the handle of the new LC-DCP drill guide is shaped like the plate. A neutral and a load guide are provided within the same instrument. The arrow of the neutral as well as of the load guide must always point in the direction of the fracture plane to be compressed. The new smooth-shaft lag screw with its improved efficiency and increased strength should always be used to generate compression either in the load position or as a lag screw.

Additional Possibilities

The screw hole of the LC-DCP is the same as the screw hole of the DCU (dynamic compression unit). This screw hole imparts tremendous versatility to the plate:

- It allows a lag screw to be inclined in an arc of 80° in the long axis of the plate.
- It is symmetrical and provides additional compression by taking advantage of the force vector directed towards the fracture line which has been created when the screw head hits the horizontal extension of the screw hole.

Using the neutral LC-DCP drill guide, screws can be inserted in the buttress position. To achieve this, the neutral drill guide is used with the arrow pointing away from the fracture line.

The grooves reduce the stiffness of the plate between the screw holes. This has resulted in a more even distribution of the stiffness of the plate and has made it easier to shape the plate by allowing bending between the screw holes.

All these additional features of the LC-DCP are provided without requiring specific changes in the application technique.

Fig. 3.40C Clinical use of the universal plate drill guide.

a The universal plate drill guide allows for tilting in a plane perpendicular to the long axis of the plate. It limits the sideways tilting to a maximum of 7°.

b The universal plate drill guide allows for longitudinal tilting of 40°.

c The shaft screw. The thread is 4.5 mm/3 mm wide, the shaft corresponds to the outer diameter of the thread. This screw offers advantages when used as lag screw and when used as axial compression screw (improved stiffness and strength).

Fig. 3.40D The equal distance between the screw holes allows easy shifting of the plate at surgery.

Fig. 3.40C

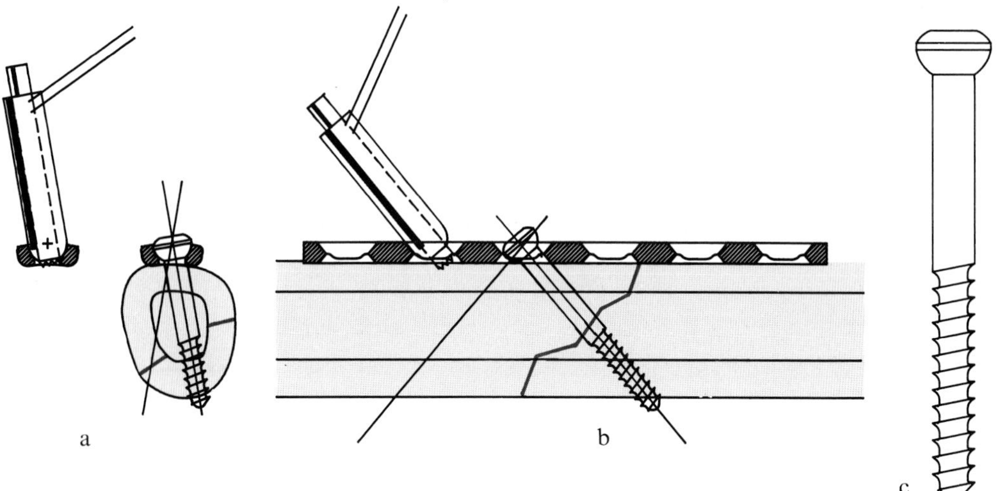

Fig. 3.40D

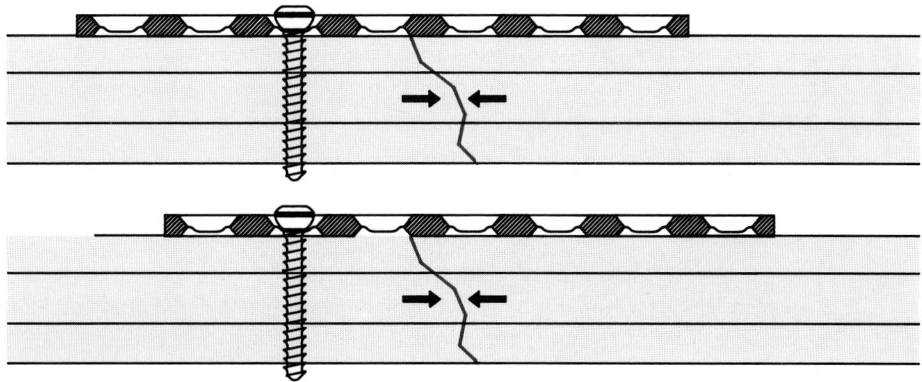

Fig. 3.40E Universal drill guide and drill sleeve for 4.5-mm and 3.5-mm cortex screws.

a The 4.5-mm system.

b The 3.5-mm system.

Fig. 3.40F Double drill guide for the 4.5-mm and 3.5-mm cortex screws.

Each guide is provided with two inserts, one (green) guiding the drill bit to the neutral position, the other one (yellow) to the load position (1.0 mm).

a The 4.5-mm drill guide viewed from above. Both drill guides are provided with arrows. These should always point to the fracture or osteotomy.

b View from below. The undercuts should remind the user that this drill guide should be used with the LC-DCP.

c The 3.5-mm drill guide viewed from above.

Fig. 3.40 E

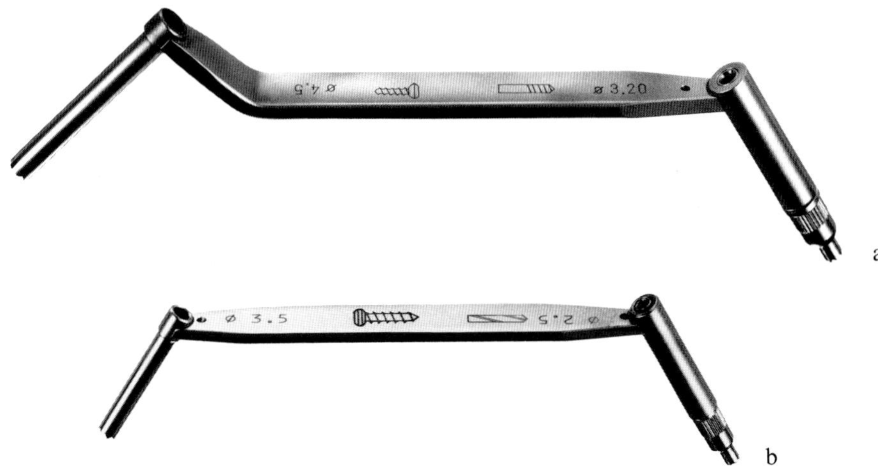

Fig. 3.40 F

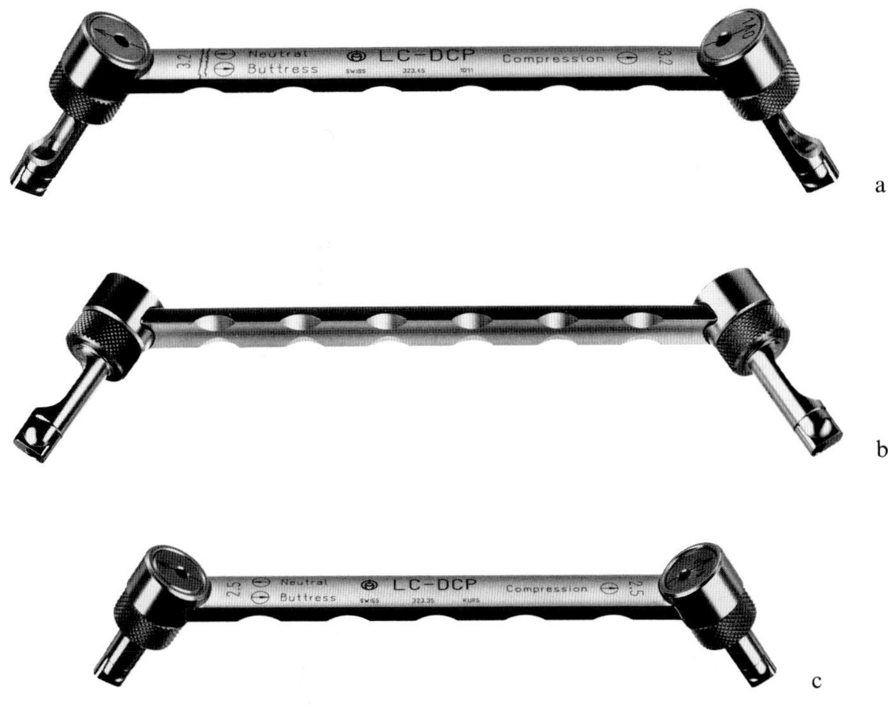

Fig. 3.40G The application of the LC-DCP in steps, procedure 1.

a Initially the fracture is bridged by the plate. Using the neutral drill guide, the first screw is applied to the fragment, which forms an obtuse angle with the fracture near the plate. The resulting space between fracture plane and plate undersurface guides the opposite fragment towards the plate. The arrow of the neutral drill guide points towards the fracture. The screw is seated at the neutral position far from the fracture.

b After adaptation of the fragments, a screw hole for axial compression is drilled in the fragment, which forms an acute angle near the plate. Here the load guide is used. Once again the arrow points towards the fracture line to be compressed. At this position, a shaft screw will be inserted with optimized rigidity and strength (compared with the standard 4.5-mm cortex screw) for axial compression. The same procedure is therefore used as for application of a lag screw. A gliding (4.5-mm) hole and a threaded (3.2-mm) hole are drilled.

c Using the universal plate drill guide, the threaded (3.2-mm) hole for the lag screw is drilled. It is subsequently overdrilled (4.5 mm) in the near cortex to create a gliding hole. As for any other application where a drill bit is used in an inclined position, the three-fluted drill bit positions the drill hole more precisely than the conventional two-fluted drill bit.

d The lag screw and the remaining screws are inserted.

e Completion of the internal fixation. Some short screws are used if the bone is strong. In porotic and/or small bones, long screws and/or a longer plate may be chosen.

Fig. 3.40 G

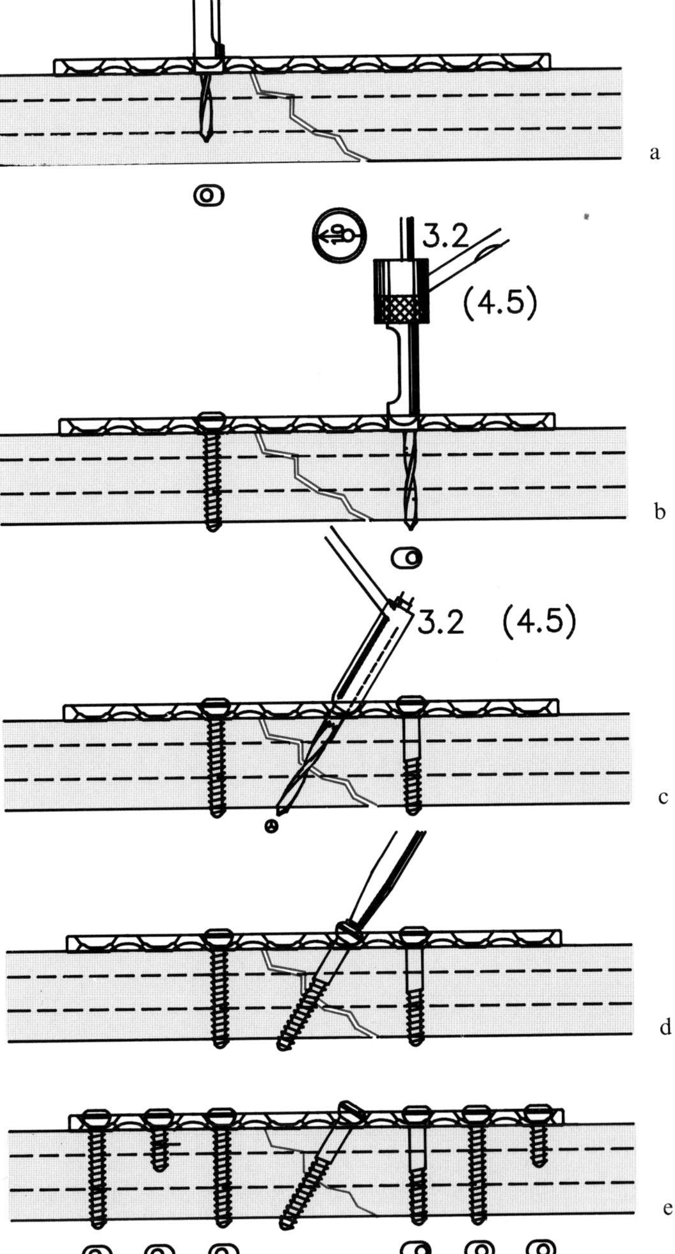

Fig. 3.40 H The application of the LC-DCP in steps, procedure 2.

a Using the 4.5-mm sleeve connected to the universal plate drill guide, the gliding hole is drilled for the lagged plate screw.

b The fracture is then bridged by the plate whereby the tightly inserted universal plate drill guide assures perfect alignment. Using the neutral drill guide, the first screw is inserted into the fragment, which forms an obtuse angle near the plate. The resulting space between fracture plane and plate undersurface guides the opposite fragment towards the plate.

c With the load drill guide, a screw hole for axial compression is inserted into the fragment which forms an acute angle near the plate. Here a shaft screw is used.

d After perfect reduction of the fragments, the lag screw is inserted by drilling the thread hole in the opposite cortex, cutting the thread etc.

e The subsequent screws are then inserted. Here again the length and the number of screws chosen varies according to the quality and geometry of the bone and to the pattern of the fracture.

Fig. 3.40 H

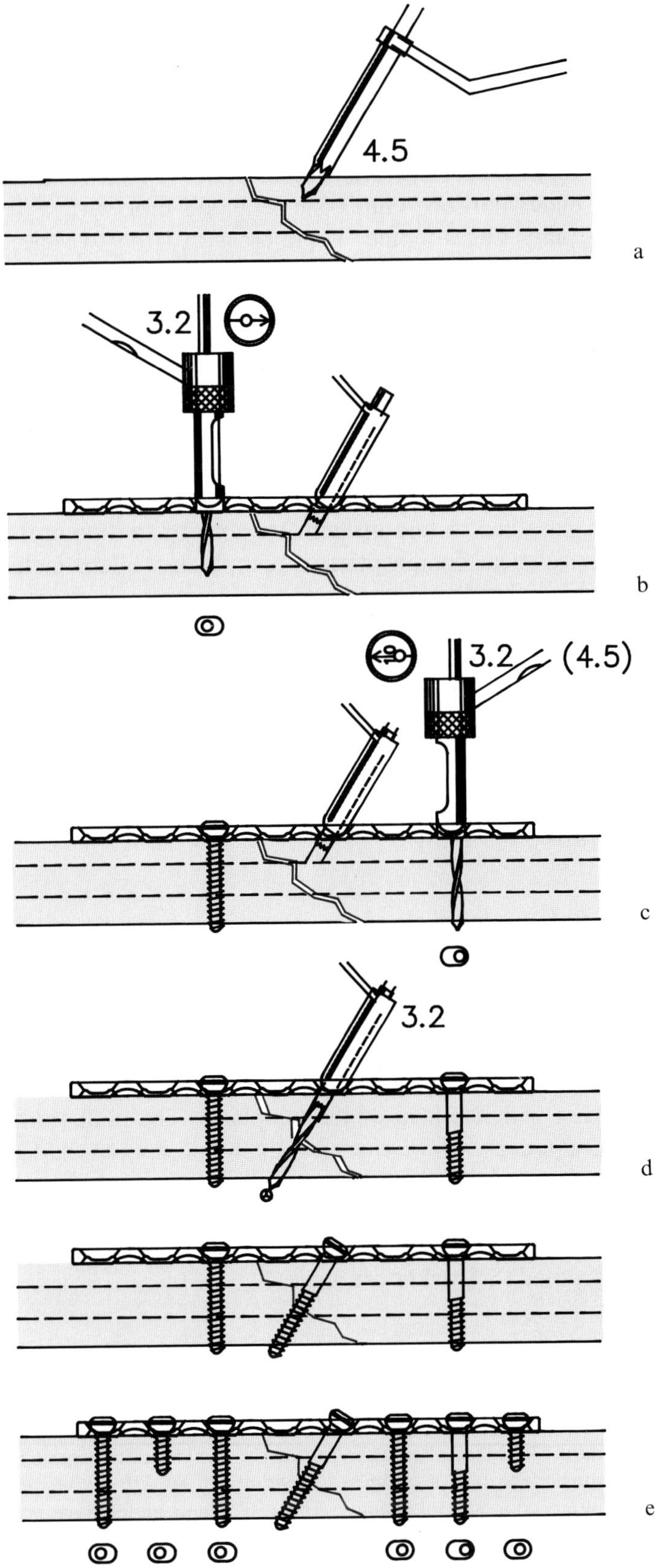

4.5

a

3.2

b

3.2 (4.5)

c

3.2

d

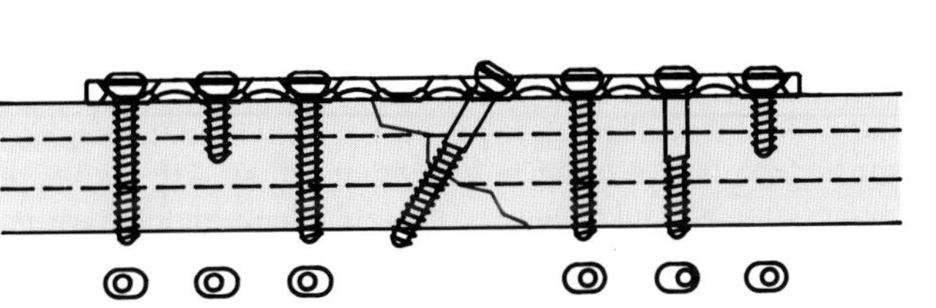

e

3.7 Angled Plates

3.7.1 General Principles

In 1959, the AO developed the angled plates (Fig. 3.41 A, B). The "U" profile was chosen for the blade portion, and a single blade unit with a fixed angle between the blade and the plate was adopted in preference to the two-piece variable angle devices. The advantage of the fixed angle is the increased strength and the increased corrosion resistance of the implant. The disadvantage is the increased difficulty of insertion. In the proximal femur the blade has to be inserted in the middle of the femoral neck and at a predetermined angle to the shaft axis. In addition, the plate portion of the angled blade plate has to be inserted so that it will line up with the axis of the shaft at the end of the procedure (Fig. 3.44d, d′). In the distal femur the blade has to line up with the joint axis and with the inclination of the patellofemoral joint and be inserted exactly into the middle of the anterior half of the femoral condyles at a predetermined distance from the joint, and the plate has to line up with the axis of the femoral shaft (Fig. 3.46a, b). Because of these technical complexities, a preoperative plan, including a preoperative drawing, is essential so that the operation can follow it step by step. The surgeon must also exercise great care at the time of surgery and pay particular attention to anatomic landmarks, position, and inclination of the implants in order to follow the preoperative plan. This usually ensures that at the end of the procedure everything fits and that the desired end result is achieved.

3.7.2 Preoperative Planning

An X-ray of the normal side is required in order to have a template on which to plan the procedure. For the proximal femur, the X-ray must be taken with the hip in 15°–20° internal rotation to correct for anteversion. For the distal femur, accurate anteroposterior and lateral X-rays centered on the joint are necessary. The outlines of the proximal or the distal femur are drawn in, as are all the fracture lines. The fracture pattern determines the steps of the internal fixation as well as the choice of plate. The selected plate is drawn in with the help of the templates. The plan should include the order in which the different steps will be carried out, should denote the function of the different screws, should indicate if a gliding hole or a thread hole needs to be predrilled before the reduction is carried out, and whether a bone graft is necessary. All the guide wires which are necessary to execute the procedure must also be shown and their function and inclination carefully noted (Schatzker rationale).

Fig. 3.41 A The 130° angle plates.

a The standard 130° blade plates used for the fixation of intertrochanteric and occasionally for subtrochanteric fractures. The blades come in lengths of 50, 60, 70, 80, 90, 100 and 110 mm. Intermediate sizes can be obtained on special request. The 130° blade plates have been replaced almost entirely by the DHS.

b U profile of the blade.

c The longer 130° angle plates with four, six and nine holes.

Fig. 3.41 A

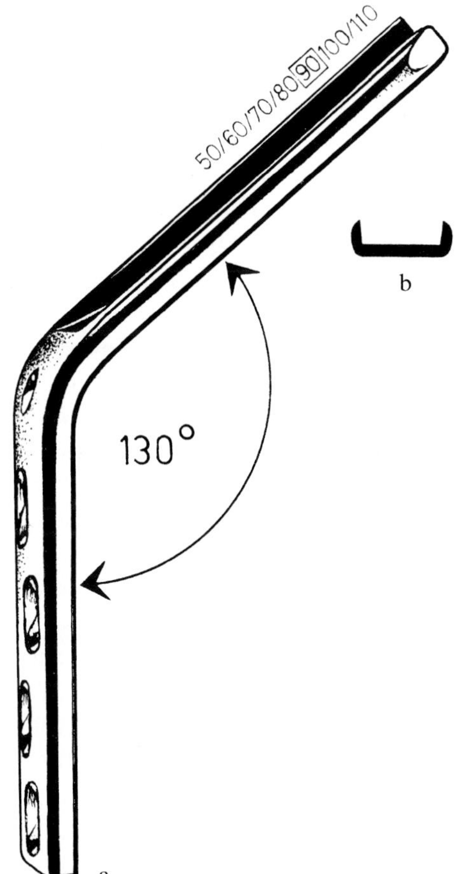

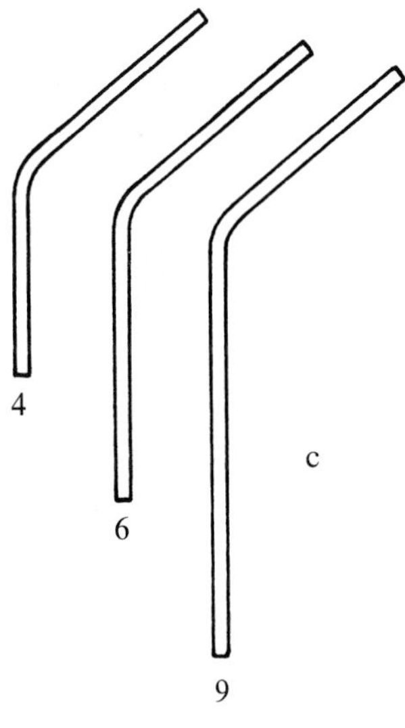

These working drawings are necessary before any surgical procedure is embarked upon. They are of particular importance before corrective osteotomies, because they are the only way the surgeon can check preoperatively the result of the osteotomy as well as his three-dimensional concept of the procedure.

3.7.3 Implants and Instruments

A number of specialized instruments have been developed which greatly facilitate the exact execution of the operation in accordance with the preoperative plan. Neither an X-ray nor an image intensifier is a substitute for a three-dimensional concept of the local anatomy, nor will they serve as a guide to the correct insertion of the guide wires. Correct insertion is based on the anatomic landmarks and on the particular device employed for fixation. The X-ray or the image intensifier are, however useful to verify the definitive insertion of the seating chisel or of the specialized guide wire for the dynamic hip or condylar screw. An X-ray is also useful as a permanent intra-operative record of the position of the guide wires and of all the internal devices as well as of the position of an osteotomy if one is being carried out.

3.7.4 The Angled Plates for the Proximal and Distal Femur

Initially the AO developed the 130° plate (Fig. 3.41 A) for use in the proximal femur and the condylar blade plate (Fig. 3.41 B) for use in the distal femur. With time it became evident that the condylar plate could also be used for the treatment of certain intertrochanteric and subtrochanteric fractures of the proximal femur. Following further modifications and refinements, the AO has developed the dynamic hip screw (DHS) and the dynamic condylar screw (DCS). These two have almost replaced the "U" profile angled blade plates in the treatment of fractures, but the latter continue to be used in reconstructive surgery such as osteotomies. The original fixed angle devices are described in detail because all the specific features, indications and anatomic considerations apply in exactly the same way to the DHS and to the DCS which will be described later.

The 130° angled plate has a blade with a U profile (Fig. 3.41 A). The plate portion comes in varying lengths depending on the particular fracture to be fixed. Thus the four- or six-hole plates are used for most intertrochanteric fractures, and the longer plates (9–12 holes) for subtrochanteric fractures.

The condylar plate (Fig. 3.41 B) has a fixed angle of 95° between its blade and plate portion. The shortest plate available has five holes. The length to be used will vary with the fracture pattern. The shortest blade is 50 cm, and the length of the blade chosen will depend on the size of the femur and whether the plate is being used in the distal or proximal femur.

Fig. 3.41 B The condylar plate.

a The most commonly used condylar plate has five holes. The two holes next to the blade take cancellous bone screws; the other three take cortex screws. The blades come in varying lengths of 50, 60, 70 and 80 mm. The 70-mm blade is the one most commonly used in the proximal femur and the 50-mm blade is the one most commonly used in the distal femur.

b The U profile of the blade.

c The 7-, 9- and 12-hole condylar plates for the fixation of longer fractures.

Fig. 3.41 B

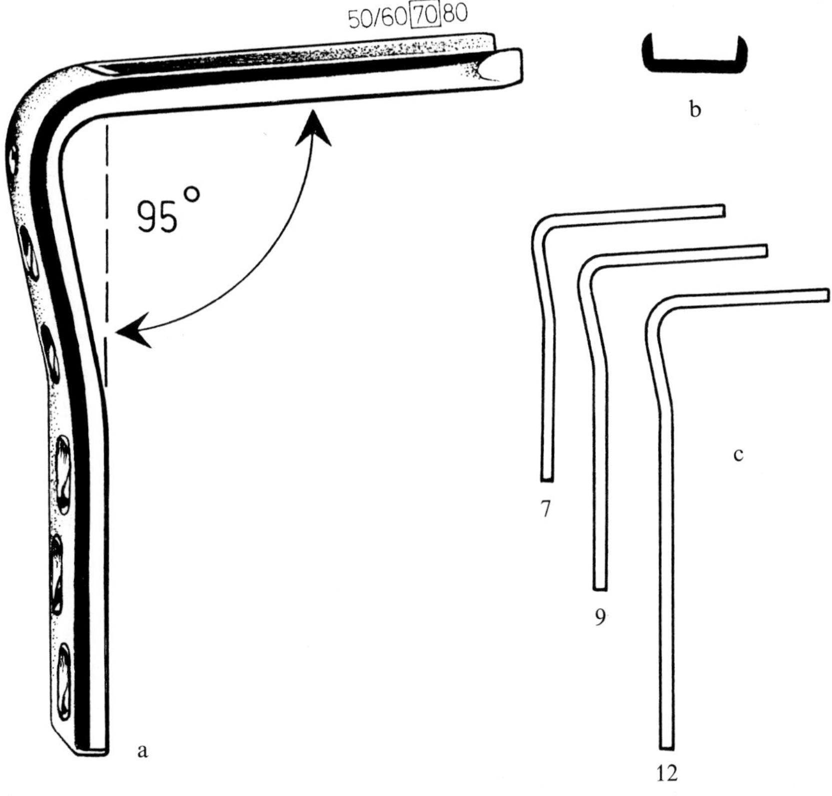

3.7.5 The Position of the Blades Within the Proximal Femur

In considering which is the best position for the blades of the angled blade plates within the proximal femur, it is important to note the trabecular orientation and distribution of bone. There is a zone within the head where the tension and compression trabeculae intersect. This is the only area which is filled with bone and the only one to offer resistance and purchase (Fig. 3.42). It is best to insert the blades in the frontal plane in such a way that they are just below the point of trabecular intersection and in the sagittal plane in the center of the neck and not aimed anteriorly and posteriorly. When correctly inserted, the condylar plate should pass about 10 mm below the superior cortex of the neck and the blade of the 130° plate should be about 6–8 mm above the calcar. The neck at the base is almost rectangular, and within the bone there is not enough room to pass these devices any closer to the bone than indicated (Fig. 3.42). If one attempts to pass the blades closer to the bone they either deflect and take a wrong path or bind or break the bone.

Fig. 3.42A Note the tip of the blade of the 130° angled plate in the lower half of the femoral head and note that the blade passes 6–8 mm above the calcar. The blade enters through the lateral cortex at a point approximately 3 cm distal to the rough line of the greater trochanter.

Fig. 3.42B Ideal position of the condylar plate in the proximal femur.

Note the tip of the blade in the lower half of the femoral head. The blade passes below the superior cortex of the neck. A cortical screw has been used to fix the plate to the calcar.

Fig. 3.42 A

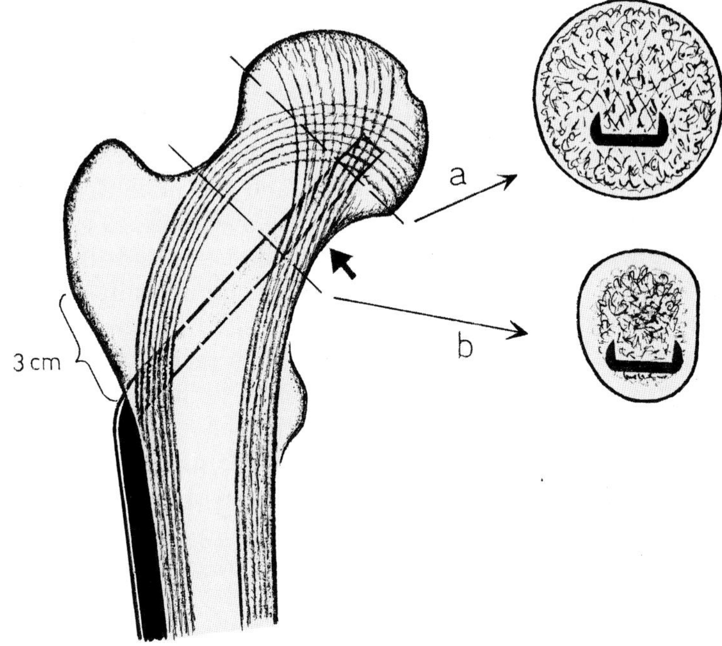

Fig. 3.42 B

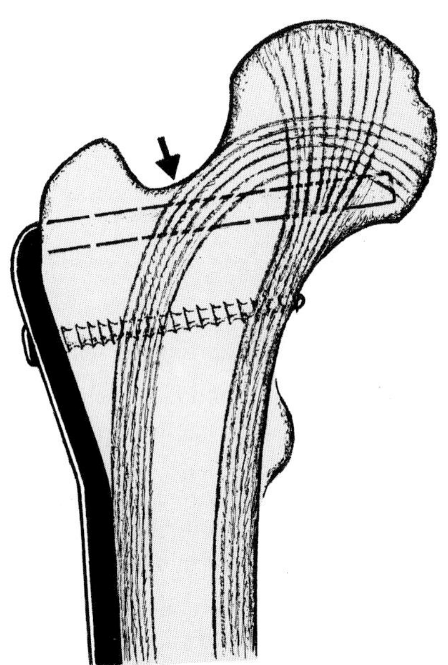

3.7.6 The Instruments

Before an angled blade plate can be inserted into bone, a channel must be drilled and precut with the U-profile seating chisel (Fig. 3.43a, b). The sides of the tip of the seating chisel have been ground to converge slightly, which enhances the centering of the seating chisel within the neck. The tip has also been ground in such a way that when it is inserted obliquely into the neck, it will not bite into the calcar.

The fixed angle between the blade and the plate does cause some initial difficulty, but with preoperative planning this can be overcome, as can the insertion of these devices into bone with the help of Kirschner guide wires and the available aiming devices such as the triangular angle guides (Fig. 3.43h) and the condylar blade guide (Fig. 3.43g).

The seating chisel guide (Fig. 3.43c) is used to determine the rotation of the seating chisel about its long axis. It is slid over the seating chisel, and in the internal fixation of the proximal or distal femur, the aim is to have the flap in line with the long axis of the femur. The angle between the flap and the body of the seating chisel can be set with the aid of the condylar or an angle guide, but the angle between the seating chisel and the bone, that is, the inclination of the seating chisel, is determined with the aid of the condylar guide or an angle guide and is indicated with a Kirschner wire guide. This is a more accurate method of determining the inclination than setting the angle of the seating chisel guide (Fig. 3.44b, b′).

During insertion the rotation of the seating chisel about its long axis is controlled with the slotted hammer (Fig. 3.44d, d′) which is also used for hammering the seating chisel out of bone after its insertion.

Fig. 3.43 Instrumentation.

a The seating chisel used for cutting the seat for the blade in the proximal and distal femur.

b The U profile which corresponds to the profile of the blade of the angled plates.

c The seating chisel guide is used to determine the rotation of the seating chisel about its long axis. It is slid over the seating chisel. In internal fixation of the proximal and distal femur, the flap of the seating chisel guide must be in line with the long axis of the femur. The angle between the flap and the body of the seating chisel guide may be set with the aid of the condylar blade guide or the triangular guide and may be maintained by tightening the screw with a screwdriver.

d During insertion, the rotation of the seating chisel is controlled with the slotted hammer. The slotted hammer serves also for removal of the seating chisel and for the hammering out of the blade holder with a plate.

e The plate holder is used for insertion and removal of plates. The plate should be so fastened in the plate holder that the long handle is always in line with the blade of the angled plate.

f The impactor is used to drive the last 5 mm of the blade into the bone.

g The condylar blade guide subtends an angle of 85° (for its use see Fig. 3.44b′).

h The triangular angle guide with a 50° angle. When applied to the lateral cortex of the femur, its lateral edge, when projected, will subtend an angle of 130° with the femoral shaft.

i The triple drill guide has a fixed angle of 130° and can simplify the insertion of the 130° angled plates. It can also be slid over the bottom of the condylar guide. Its removable guide is slid over either a 3.2-mm drill guide or a 3-mm Kirschner wire which is previously inserted in line with the neck axis and serves as the directional guide for the triple drill guide (for use see Fig. 3.44a′).

j The router is used for conversion of a 4.5-mm drill hole into a slit.

Fig. 3.43

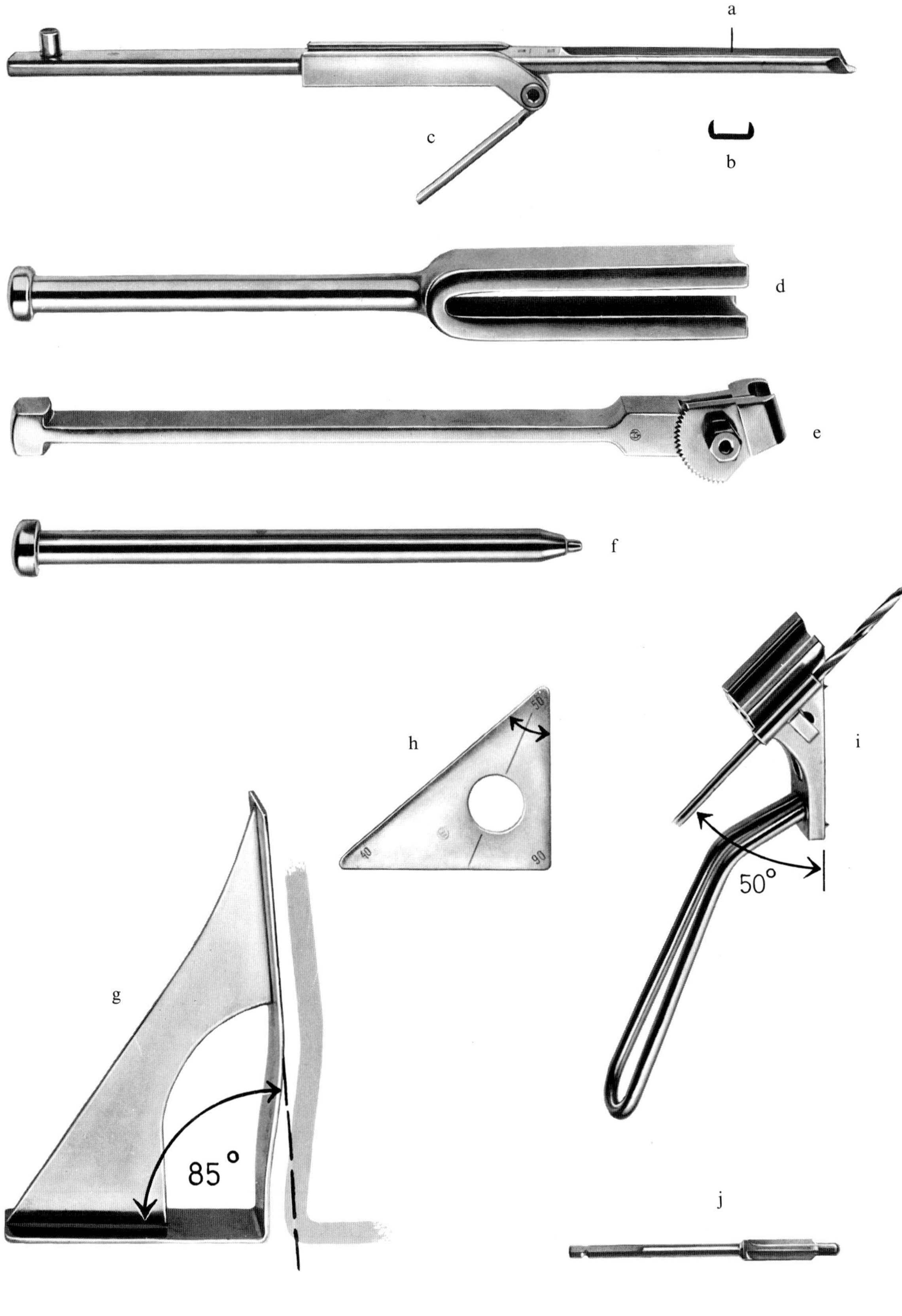

The plate holder (Fig. 3.43e) is used for the insertion and removal of angled plates. It is very important at insertion to adjust the holder so that the handle is perfectly in line with the blade. If there is any angulation, the blade can be easily guided into the bone out of alignment with the precut channel, causing a lot of problems. Once inserted into bone, the plates are driven in the last few millimeters with the impactor.

3.7.7 Proximal Femur: Preparation of the Seat for the Blade

Once the position of the blade is determined on the preoperative drawing, the surgeon will know the exact position the seating chisel should occupy in bone. As indicated, the direction for the seating chisel is given by the correctly inserted guide wires (Fig. 3.44a, b, b′). The position of the definitive guide wire is determined from its relation to the local anatomy and to other guide wires and from the angle it subtends with the bony axes. A seating chisel can only be inserted into bone with the aid of the definitive guide wire. Once inserted, its position can be verified radiologically. It is much more important to develop a three-dimensional concept of the local anatomy of the bone and to understand the relationship of the devices to the bone than to try to insert them into bone with radiological control. This also applies to the insertion of guide wires. In order to insert the fixed angle devices correctly into bone, four points must be observed: the axis of the femoral neck; the angle between the blade and the femoral shaft axis; the point of entry of the blade into bone; and finally the rotation of the seating chisel about its long axis.

The guide to the axis of the femoral neck is the guide wire, which is inserted anteriorly in line with the axis of the neck. This often requires opening of the capsule anteriorly. This guide wire must pass below the anterior ridge which runs along the front in the intertrochanteric area or the wire will be deflected anteriorly and give a false direction (Fig. 3.44a). This guide wire ensures the correct centering of the seating chisel in line with the neck axis.

The angle between the blade and the femoral shaft axis: This depends on which angled blade plate is being used and whether an attempt is being made to change the

---

Fig. 3.44 How to determine the position of the blade in the proximal femur.

a The neck axis. A Kirschner wire is inserted low down along the anterior aspect of the neck below the ridge and is driven into the head.

a′ The preparation of the hole for the insertion has been made easier by the development of the triple-angle guide (1). Insert through the removable guide (2) either a 3.2-mm drill bit (3) or a 3.0-mm Kirschner wire. As soon as this drill bit or Kirschner wire comes to lie 8–10 mm above the calcar and in line with the neck axis one can drill the first anterior 4.5-mm drill hole to a depth of 4–6 cm. Leave the drill bit in the bone (4) and use another 4.5-mm drill bit to drill the remaining two holes. Remove the triple-angle guide and the drill bit and enlarge the drill holes (5) with the router (6) in order to convert the three holes to a slit (7). Bevel the hole distally (8) for a few millimeters to receive the shoulder of the angled plate. This will prevent the shattering of the lateral cortex.

b When inserting the 130° angled plate, use the triangular angle guide with the 50° angle, place it along the lateral cortex of the femur and drive a Kirschner wire into the greater trochanter which is parallel to the first Kirschner wire and parallel to the upper edge of the triangular guide.

b′ For the insertion of the condylar plate, the condylar plate guide is placed along the lateral cortex. A second Kirschner wire is inserted parallel to the first Kirschner wire in the axial view and parallel with the upper edge of the condylar plate guide in the Al view. It is driven into the greater trochanter above the planned point of entry.

Fig. 3.44

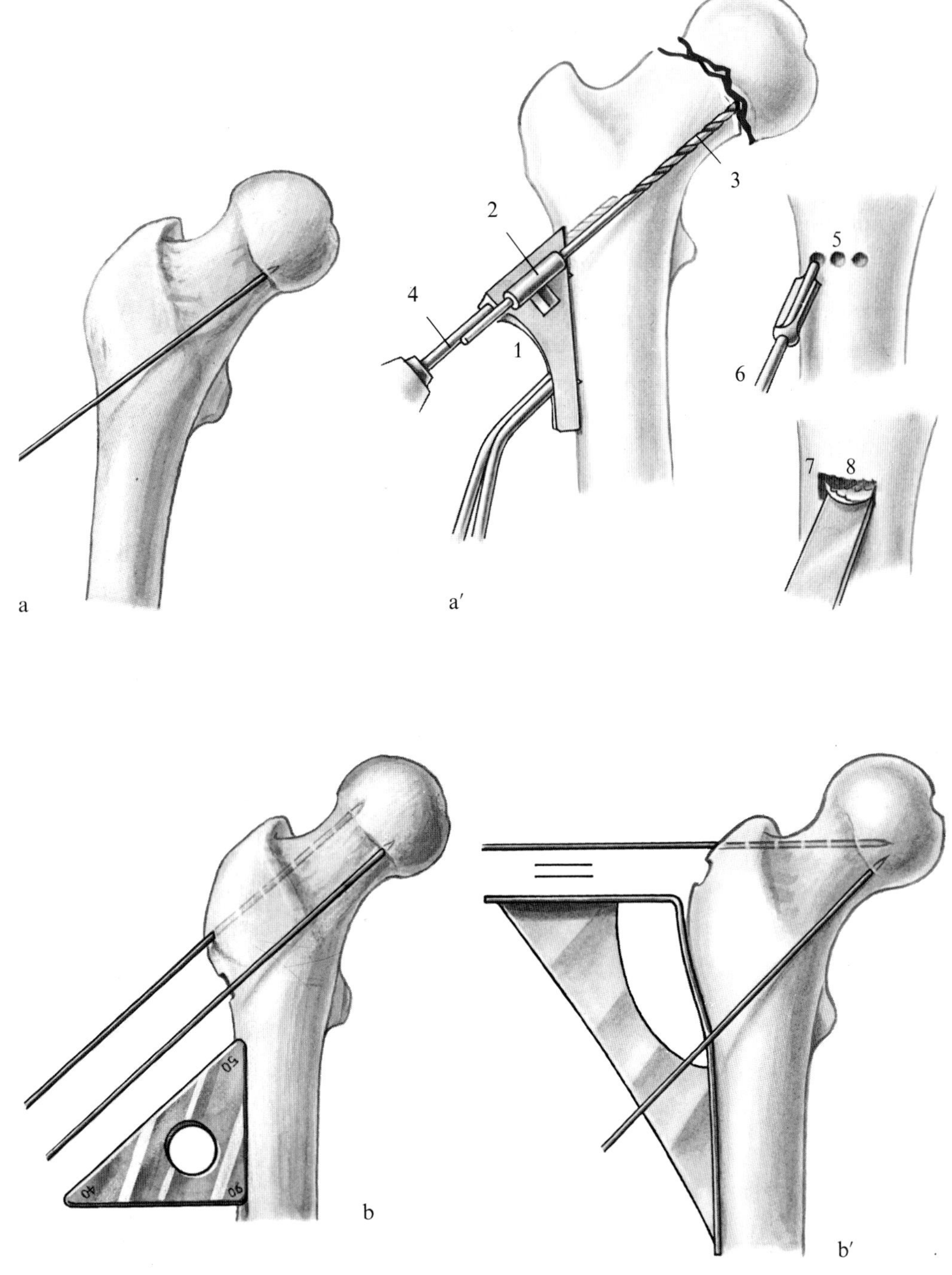

neck shaft angle as might be the case in a corrective osteotomy. If the plate being inserted is the condylar plate, the condylar guide with an angle of 95° is used as the guide to its insertion. The condylar guide is brought up to and along the lateral cortex of the femoral shaft and a Kirschner wire is inserted into the tip of the greater trochanter parallel to the top of the condylar guide (Fig. 3.44b′). This guide wire (in the axial view) must also be parallel to the guide wire indicating the neck axis (a). This guide wire (b′) now becomes the definitive guide wire for the insertion of the seating chisel. If the 130° blade plate is being inserted, then the 50° triangular guide is used and the steps repeated as above (Fig. 3.44b).

The point of entry is determined first on the preoperative drawing from the position of the specific implants in bone. It is best to relate it to the rough line on the greater trochanter which can easily be found at the time of surgery. If the plate is being inserted through the trochanter, as for instance the condylar plate, then the point of entry must be in the anterior half of the greater trochanter (Fig. 3.44c′) to make certain that the seating chisel will come in line with the axis of the neck. This is because the greater trochanter flares posteriorly at an angle of 30°–40°. If we are inserting a 130° device through the lateral cortex of the shaft, it must be inserted through the center of the lateral cortex (Fig. 3.47c). If the opening is made in error posteriorly then the seating chisel is deflected anteriorly. If the opening is too far to the front then the seating chisel is deflected posteriorly as it enters the neck and head. If an error is made in choosing the entry point, it will not be possible to correct the malalignment of the implant in bone until the point of entry is corrected.

In order to open the femur correctly and prevent any straying in position or direction, we prefer to predrill the cortex. The entry for the seating chisel is therefore predrilled with a 4.5-mm drill bit, enlarged with a router and completed with an osteotome. The cortex must be beveled to receive the shoulder of the angled plate.

The rotation of the blade about its long axis: In carrying out an open reduction of a fracture, the aim is to reconstruct the normal anatomy and return the bone to its prefracture configuration. This means that the plate must come to lie in line with the shaft. This alignment is determined with the aid of the seating chisel guide in making sure that its flap lines up with the long axis of the femur (Fig. 3.44d, d′). In carrying out corrective osteotomies, it is sometimes desirable to achieve either an extension or a flexion of the proximal fragment. This would determine the angle between the seating chisel guide and the shaft at the time of the insertion of the seating chisel into bone.

Fig. 3.44 How to determine the position of the blade in the proximal femur (continued).

c The point of entry for the 130° angled plate is directly in the middle of the lateral cortex.

c′ The point of entry in the greater trochanter is in the anterior half of its lateral bulge.

d′ The rotation of the blade about its long axis: Insert the seating chisel guide over the seating chisel. Set the angle between the flat of the guide and the seating chisel (85° for condylar plates and 50° for the 130° angle plates). With the slotted hammer rotate the seating chisel about its long axis till the flap of the seating chisel guide comes to lie in line with the long axis of the femur. Hammer in the seating chisel parallel to its guide wire.

Fig. 3.44

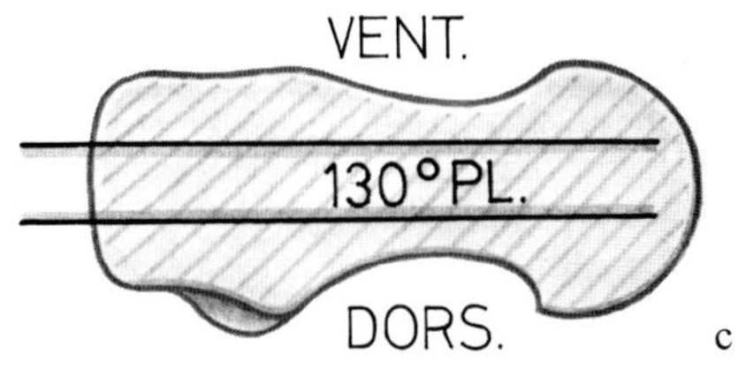

c

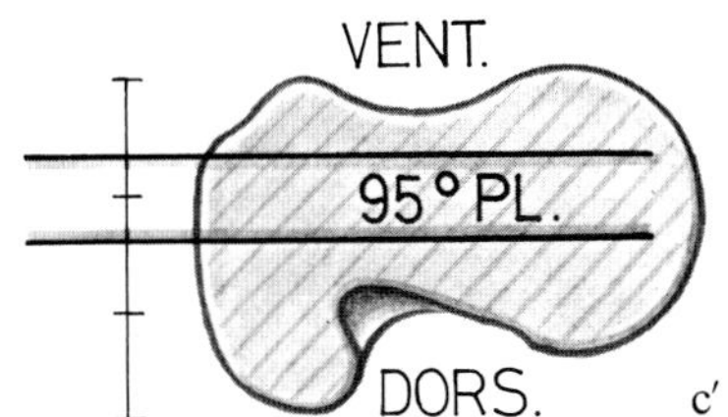

c′

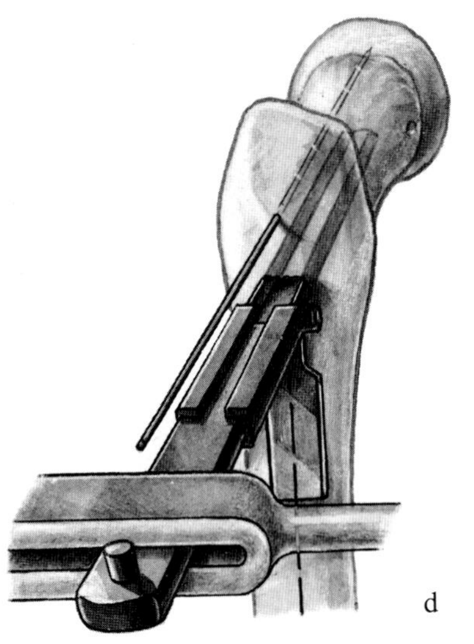
d

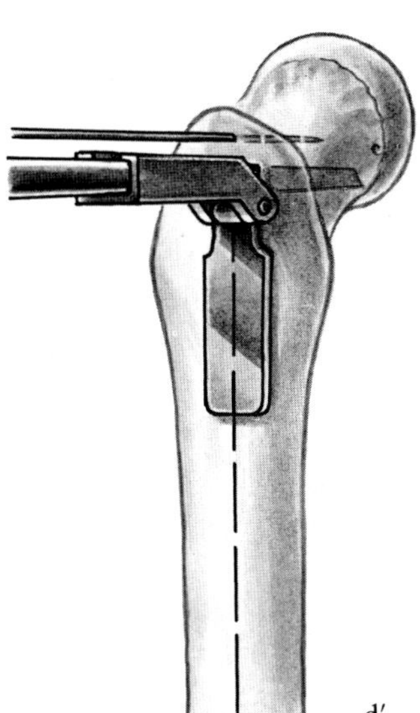
d′

3.7.8 Insertion of the Plates into the Proximal Femur

Once the seating chisel is inserted, the position should be checked radiologically. This determines not only the position but also whether the length chosen on the preoperative plan still applies. A slight alteration in the rotation of the limb can change the length of the blade by as much as 10 mm. Once all the determinations are complete and if no alteration is necessary, the seating chisel is removed by hammering it out with the slotted hammer. The chosen plate is then inserted into the plate holder and the blade is pushed by hand into the precut channel. The blade should encounter little resistance and light hammer blows should be more than enough to drive it into bone. If greater resistance is encountered, the blade may have strayed from the precut course. If that happens, remove the blade, recut the channel and reinsert the blade. When the plate is about 5 mm from the bone, remove the plate holder and seat the plate with the impactor. The above applies to all angled blade plates regardless of their angle.

The blade alone does not secure a very strong hold in bone. It must be stabilized, whenever possible, with at least one screw. This applies to the proximal and distal femur. Thus when the condylar plate is inserted into the proximal femur, it is secured with one or two cortex screws passed through the most proximal two holes of the plate into the calcar. If the holes for these screws are drilled with the 3.2-mm drill bit, the drill bit will strike the endosteal aspect of the calcar obliquely, and be deflected up the neck where it may break. To prevent this complication, overdrill the outer cortex with a 4.5-mm drill bit. This allows the insertion of the 3.2-mm drill sleeve through the hole almost to the calcar. The drill sleeve will now guide the drill bit and prevent its deviation and the calcar will be drilled without difficulty (Fig. 3.45). This technique is necessary only if the drill bit strikes the bone at an oblique angle. It is not necessary in the distal or proximal femur if a 130° plate is being anchored.

The insertion technique described makes use of the local anatomy of the bone, which provides the landmarks for the insertion of the guide wires and eventually of the seating chisel. This is very important because sometimes the fracture may be so complex that it is necessary to insert the angled plate into the proximal fragment prior to the reduction of the fracture. The landmarks which must be identified and exposed are: the anterior aspect of the neck and the anterior half of the femoral head; the rough line; and the superior cortex of the neck.

Fig. 3.45 Insertion of the condylar plate into the proximal femur.

a Determination of the neck axis and the blade direction.

b In order to triangulate the fixation of the condylar plate in the proximal femur, insert a cortex screw as a lag screw into the calcar. Drill first with a 4.5-mm drill bit to a depth of about 4 cm. Aim at right angles to the plate and slightly distally away from the blade.

c Insert the 3.2-mm drill sleeve. This will guide the 3.2-mm drill bit and will prevent it from gliding along the calcar, which will also prevent the breaking of the drill bit. Drill the calcar, determine the screw length, tap the thread and insert the corresponding cortex screw.

d Fix the plate. Often a second lag screw can be inserted into the proximal fragment. The importance of a medial buttress is discussed in Chap. 12.

Fig. 3.45

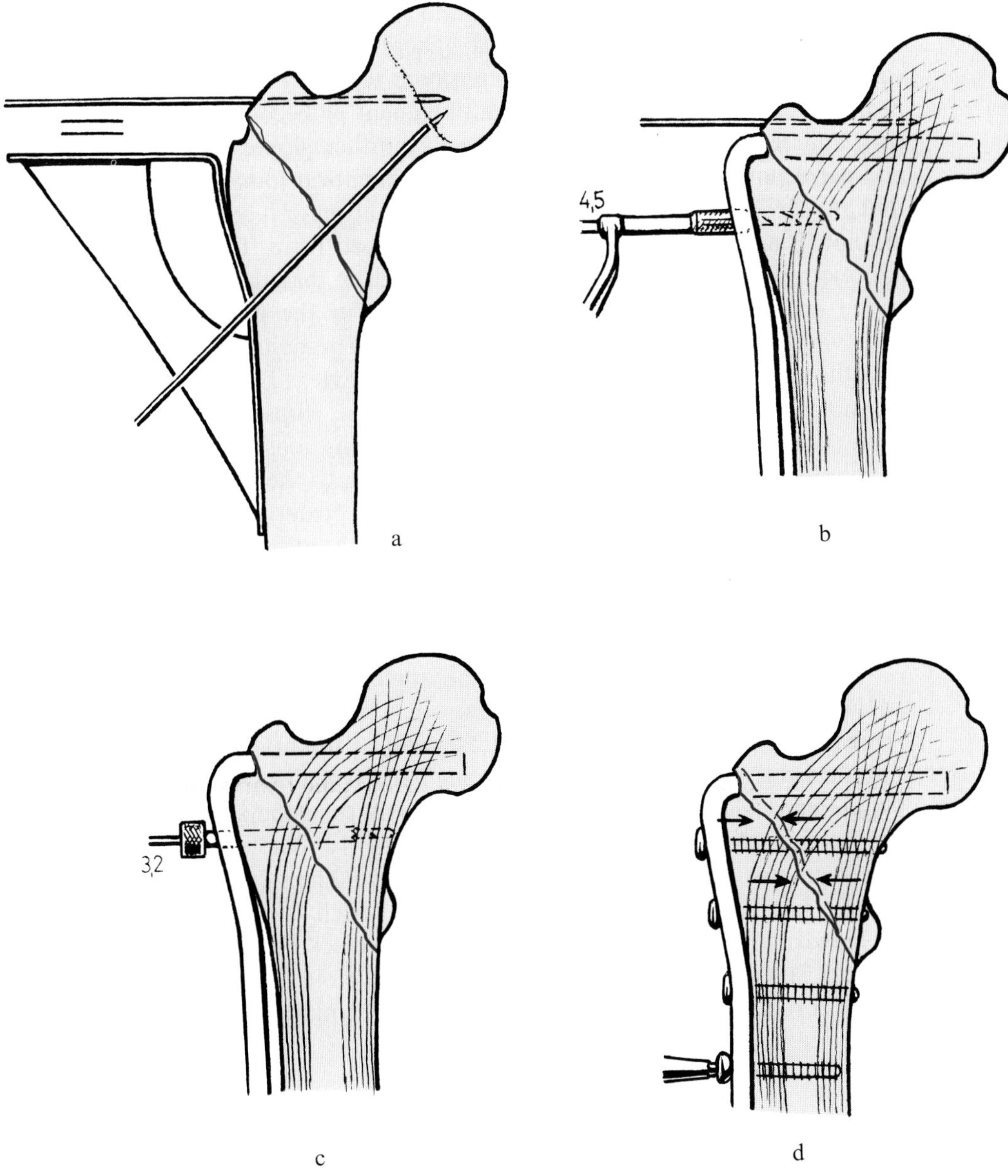

3.7.9 Insertion of the Plates into the Distal Femur

The surgical anatomy of the distal femur is complex and can present serious problems to the unwary surgeon. When viewed in cross section, the shape resembles a trapezoid with the medial side inclined about 25° and the lateral about 10° (Fig. 3.47b). The posterior diameter is longer than the anterior. Therefore a plate which appears to be just the right length on an anteroposterior X-ray is too long and will penetrate the cortex and protrude deep to the medial collateral ligament or become subcutaneous. This can cause pain and restrict movement. The anterior surface slopes downwards to the medial side and corresponds in inclination to the patellofemoral joint. Care must be taken therefore that any device inserted is parallel to this inclination or it could end up in the patellofemoral joint. Finally, when the distal femur is viewed from the side and the posterior cortex is projected as a line distally, it becomes evident that the condyles appear to have been added on posteriorly to the shaft. Therefore for the purpose of internal fixation, any plate which is inserted into the epiphysis and is to line up with the shaft must be inserted into the middle of the anterior half of the condyles. The circumference of the condyles resembles an ellipse. The longest diameter of the ellipse represents the longest diameter of the femoral condyles and is at 90° to the long axis of the shaft. Therefore in order to choose the entry point of any angled device into the distal femur, identify the longest diameter and divide it into an anterior and a posterior half. Choose the midpoint of the anterior half at a point 1.5 or 2 cm from the distal joint surface and through this point drop a perpendicular to the longest diameter of the condylar ellipse. This point is the correct entry point and the perpendicular will denote the alignment of the plate, which will line up with the long axis of the shaft (Fig. 3.50).

The condylar blade plate subtends an angle of 95°. When the blade is inserted parallel to the joint surface the plate will line up with the shaft and the physiological angle between the shaft and the knee joint axis will be maintained (Fig. 3.46a). It is important that the distal femoral fragment not be medialized or displaced anteriorly. This will happen if the angled blade is inserted more posteriorly than the anterior half since the condyles are significantly larger posteriorly than anteriorly! The medialization and anterior displacement not only disturb the loading of the knee, but also make reduction of the fracture impossible and result in instability which can lead to failure of the fixation. The predrilling and the use of the seating chisel is as for the proximal femur (see Sect. 3.7.7). One should never attempt to correct the medialization by osteotomizing the lateral cortex to facilitate deeper seating of the plate. This may lead to complete loss of fixation in the distal fragment!

Fig. 3.46 Insertion of the condylar plate into the distal femur (without an intercondylar fracture).

a In the frontal plane, the blade lies parallel to the knee joint axis and the plate lies along the lateral cortex of the shaft.

b Location of the entry point in the sagittal plane. When the posterior cortex of the shaft is projected distally as a line, it divides the epiphysis into an anterior and a posterior half. The condyles appear as if they were tacked on posteriorly to the shaft. Note that the longest diameter AC is at 90° to the axis of the shaft. The window W for the condylar plate is in the middle of the anterior half BC and 1.5–2.0 cm from the distal end of the femur.

c, c′, c″ Placement of three Kirschner wires and introduction of the seating chisel parallel to the third Kirschner wire which in the frontal plane is parallel to wire 1 and in the sagittal plane to wire 2. (See also Fig. 3.47a, b.)

Fig. 3.46

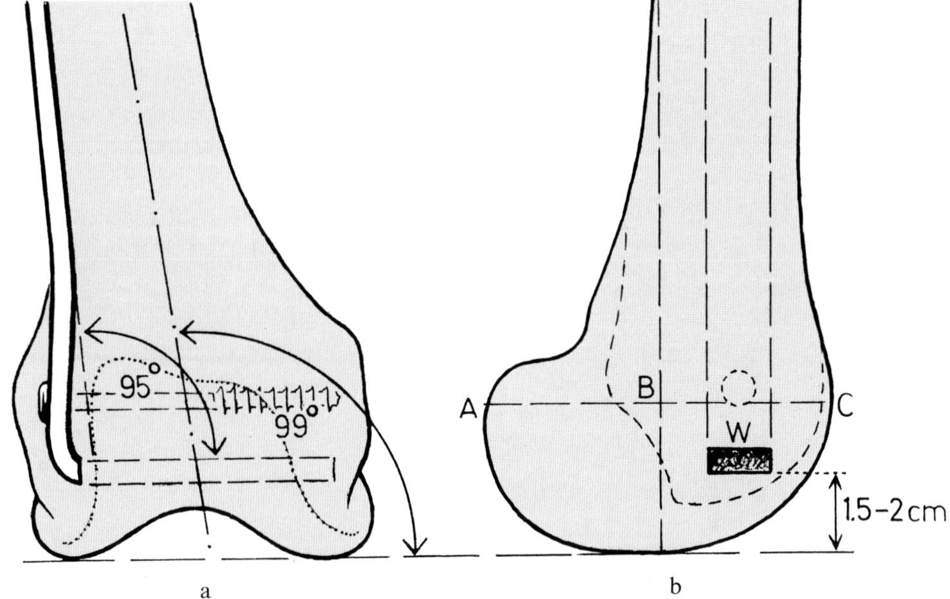

a b

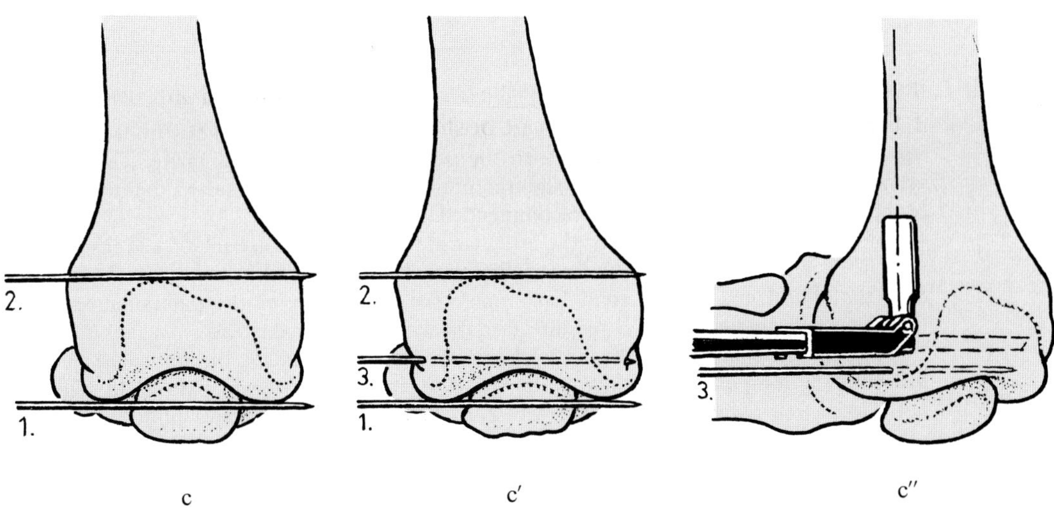

c c′ c″

Fig. 3.47 Insertion of the condylar plate into the distal femur in the presence of a Y fracture.

a The condylar fragments are reduced and fixed with two large cancellous bone screws. These must be carefully positioned not to interfere with the position of the condylar plate. These screws stabilize the vertical intercondylar component of the fracture. They are usually inserted slightly proximal to the entry of the blade. The use of washers is recommended.

After reduction and fixation of the articular block, bend the knee to 90° and insert the first Kirschner wire (1 or 1 a) which marks the knee joint axis. The second Kirschner wire (2) is inserted anteriorly over the lateral and medial condyle to mark the inclination of the patellofemoral joint. These two Kirschner wires indicate the desired direction for wire 3 and for the blade.

A third Kirschner wire (3) is now driven in 1 cm proximal to the joint, the entry point being in line with the long axis of the femur. Its direction in the AP view is parallel to Kirschner wire 1 and in the axial view parallel to Kirschner wire 2. It will serve as the definitive guide for the seating chisel.

The point of entry is prepared by first drilling three holes with the 4.5-mm drill bits and then enlarging the holes with the router. The window is then beveled by the chisel to accommodate the bend of the plate. The seating chisel is then driven in. The assistant must apply firm counter-pressure against the medial condyle while the seating chisel is being driven in. The seating chisel guide must be in line with the shaft axis. If the bone is very hard, the path for the seating chisel should be predrilled with the 3.2-mm drill bit by making three or four holes parallel to Kirschner wire 3.

When determining the length of the blade, one must keep in mind that the distal femur is a rhomboid and that the medial wall is inclined at a 25° angle. Thus a blade which on an AP X-ray appears to be just the right length would be too long and would protrude medially. The correct length is 15–20 mm less. Once these holes are drilled, the length of the blade can be verified with a depth gauge.

b Insert the blade of the correct length. Reduce the plate to the lateral cortex of the shaft and secure the plate with two more large cancellous bone screws in the distal fragment. This adds rotational stability to the plate.

c Fix the articulated tension device to the femoral shaft and apply axial tension – then fix the plate to the proximal fragment.

Fig. 3.47

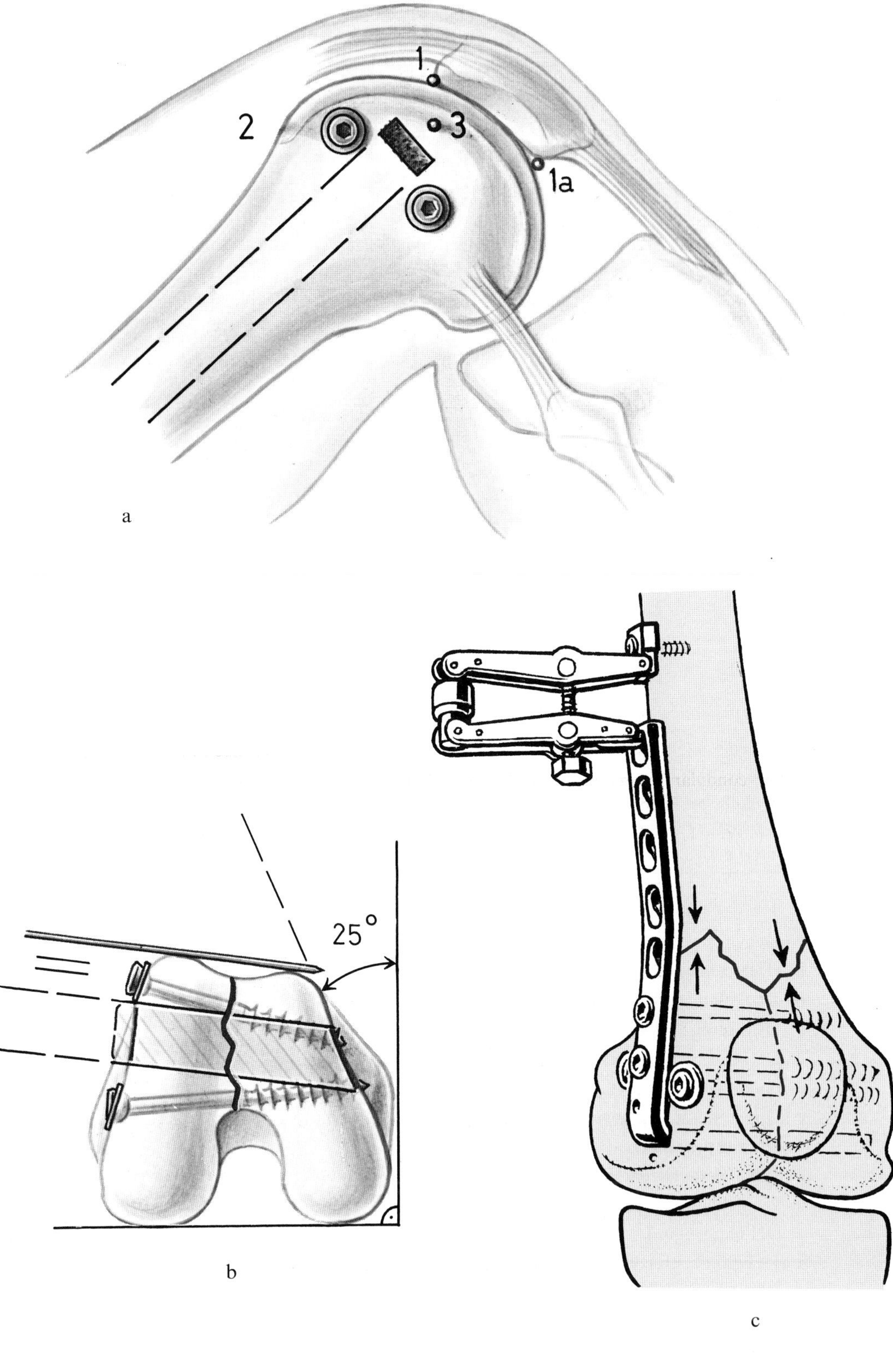

3.8 The Dynamic Hip Screw (DHS) and Dynamic Condylar Screw (DCS)

Recent refinements have led to the development of first the dynamic hip screw and more recently the dynamic condylar screw (Fig. 3.48). The DHS finds its indications in fractures of the 31 A1, A2 and A3 type. The technical steps to be taken are described in the legends to Fig. 3.49. In A2 and A3 fractures, with a mobile trochanteric fragment, there is a tendency for these fragments to dislocate laterally. To prevent upward and posterior displacement of the greater trochanter it can be fixed with a tension band wire passed around the insertion of the abductors and the most proximal plate screw.

The DCS — primarily designed for distal femur fractures and intercondylar fractures — has found increasing application in certain intertrochanteric and particularly in very proximal subtrochanteric fractures. Although more resistant to fatigue fracture than the 95° condylar blade plate because of its increased thickness, the DC is not a panacea to be used indiscriminately. Fatigue fractures have occurred when biomechanical considerations were ignored.

Fig. 3.48 The dynamic hip screw (DHS) and the dynamic condylar screw (DCS).

- a DHS plate, 135°, four holes.
- a′ DHS screw (65–115 mm).
- b DCS plate, 95°, eight holes.
- b′ DCS screw (50–115 mm).
- c DHS/DCS compression screw.
- d Guide pin with threaded tip.
- e Direct measuring device.
- f DHS triple reamer.
- g Tap and short centering sleeve for tap.
- h Wrench and long centering sleeve for wrench.
- i DHS angle guide.
- i′ T-Handle with coupling for use with angle guide.
- j DCS triple reamer.
- k Coupling screw.
- l Guide shaft.
- m Impactor with plastic tip.
- n Coupling screw for DHS/DCS screw removal.

Fig. 3.48

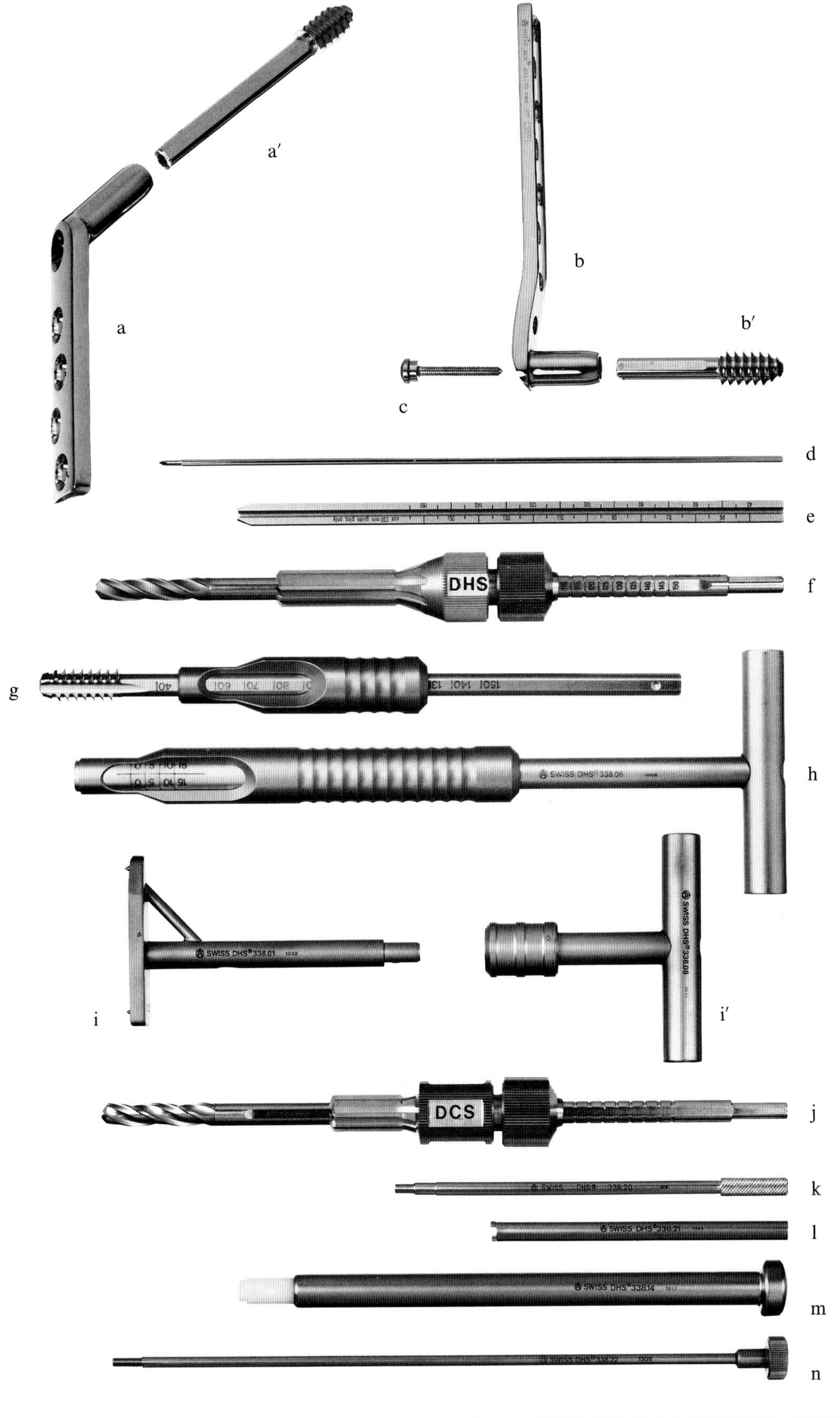
a′
a
b
b′
c
d
e
DHS
f
g
h
SWISS DHS® 338.06
i
SWISS DHS® 338.01
i′
SWISS DHS® 338.08
DCS
j
k
l
m
n

Fig. 3.49 Application of the dynamic hip screw.

a The patient lies supine. Use of the fracture table is optional, of the image intensifier desirable. Reduce the fracture. Secure preliminary fixation of the fracture with Kirschner wires. The position of these wires should not interfere with the subsequent positioning of the DHS screw and the DHS plate. To determine femoral neck anteversion, a Kirschner wire is passed over the front of the femoral neck. Use the appropriate DHS angle guide with the T handle and hammer the Kirschner wire gently into the head.

b The DHS angle guide is placed against the middle of the femoral shaft (see b′), and positioned so that the guide tube points to the center of the femoral head. Open the lateral cortex with 2-mm drill bit. Insert the guide pin into the center of the femoral head and advance it to the subchondral bone. The pin should remain in place throughout the procedure. Threaded ends help to secure it in bone and prevent it from sliding out. The guide pin should lie in the middle of the femoral neck, in both the AP and axial views. Check the guide wire placement. If its position is not perfect, it must be changed before proceeding further.

c Slide the direct measuring device over the guide pin and read off directly the length of the pin within the bone (e.g. 105 mm). Remove the additional anterior frontal Kirschner wire.

d The three elements of the DHS triple reamer are designed to prevent wrong assembly. The triple reamer itself is marked DHS and therefore should not be confused with the DCS reamer.

The drill hole should end 10 mm short of the subchondral bone plate. Set reamer to correct depth (e.g. $105-10=95$ mm) and ream the hole. The DHS triple reamer provides three functions in one operation: reaming for the screw; for the plate barrel; and for the plate barrel junction. Reamer depth is adjustable in 5-mm increments.

e If the guide wire is inadvertently withdrawn with the DHS triple reamer, it must be immediately reinserted, since otherwise there is considerable risk of placing the screw in a wrong direction, away from the original bore hole, especially in porotic bone. Correct repositioning of the guide pin is easy with the short centering sleeve and a DHS screw inserted backwards in the sleeve as a guide.

f In hard cancellous bone, the thread should be precut with a tap. Use the shorter of the two centering sleeves with the tap.

g To insert the screw into bone, one must assemble the coupling screw, the guide shaft and the hip screw. To do this, insert the coupling screw through the hollow guide shaft in to the hip screw. The ridge and slot between the guide shaft and the screw must interdigitate. The wrench is first inserted into the longer centering sleeve. The assembled coupling screw, guide shaft and selected screw are then inserted into the wrench and this whole assembly is then slid over the guide pin and the centering sleeve is introduced into the predrilled hole. By turning the wrench, the screw is driven into the femoral neck until the zero mark on the wrench reaches the lateral cortex. This means that with this selected length of the screw, the tip of the screw is 10 mm from the joint. In osteoporotic bone, the screw can be inserted 5 mm deeper. The T handle of the wrench must be parallel to the femoral shaft at the end of the screw insertion, otherwise the DHS plate will not lie in line with the shaft (see g′).

h The wrench with centering sleeve is removed and the DHS plate is slid onto the assembly and the coupling screw and guide shaft are removed.

Fig. 3.49

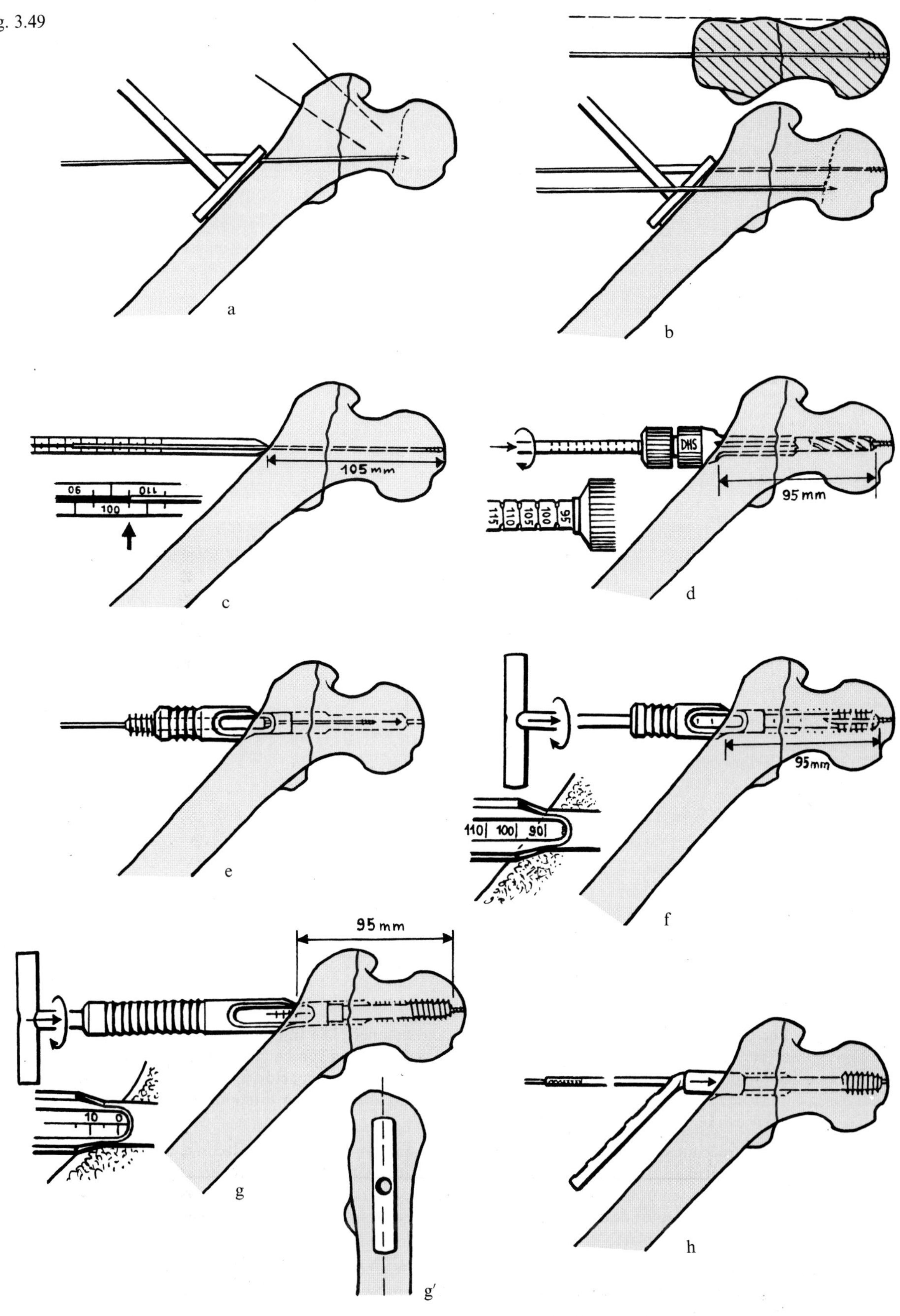

b′
a
b
105 mm
90
110
100
c
DHS
95 mm
115
110
105
100
95
d
e
95mm
110
100
90
f
95 mm
10
0
g
g′
h

Fig. 3.49 Application of the dynamic hip screw (continued).

i With the impactor, the plate is seated against the cortex of the femur.

j, k The plate is then fixed to the shaft in the usual manner. The fracture must now be impacted. Traction of the fracture table should be released first. The impaction can be achieved either with the compression screw or by delivering a few blows with the help of the impactor against the plate and shaft. Care must be taken when using the compression screw, particularly in osteoporotic bone, because the DHS-screw can be inadvertently pulled out of the head.

l In subtrochanteric fractures, the proximal fragment can very often be secured with an additional screw across the plate. No attempts should be made to fix the lesser trochanter with a screw through the plate. The lesser trochanter lies posteriorly. If medial continuity has to be restored including the lesser trochanter, this must be done by inserting a lag screw from anterolateral to posteromedial at approximately a 45° angle to the plate.

m Implant removal. After removal of the DHS plate, the wrench is placed over the DHS screw and the long coupling screw is screwed into the DHS screw, which allows traction to be exerted whilst turning the screw counter-clockwise.

Fig. 3.49

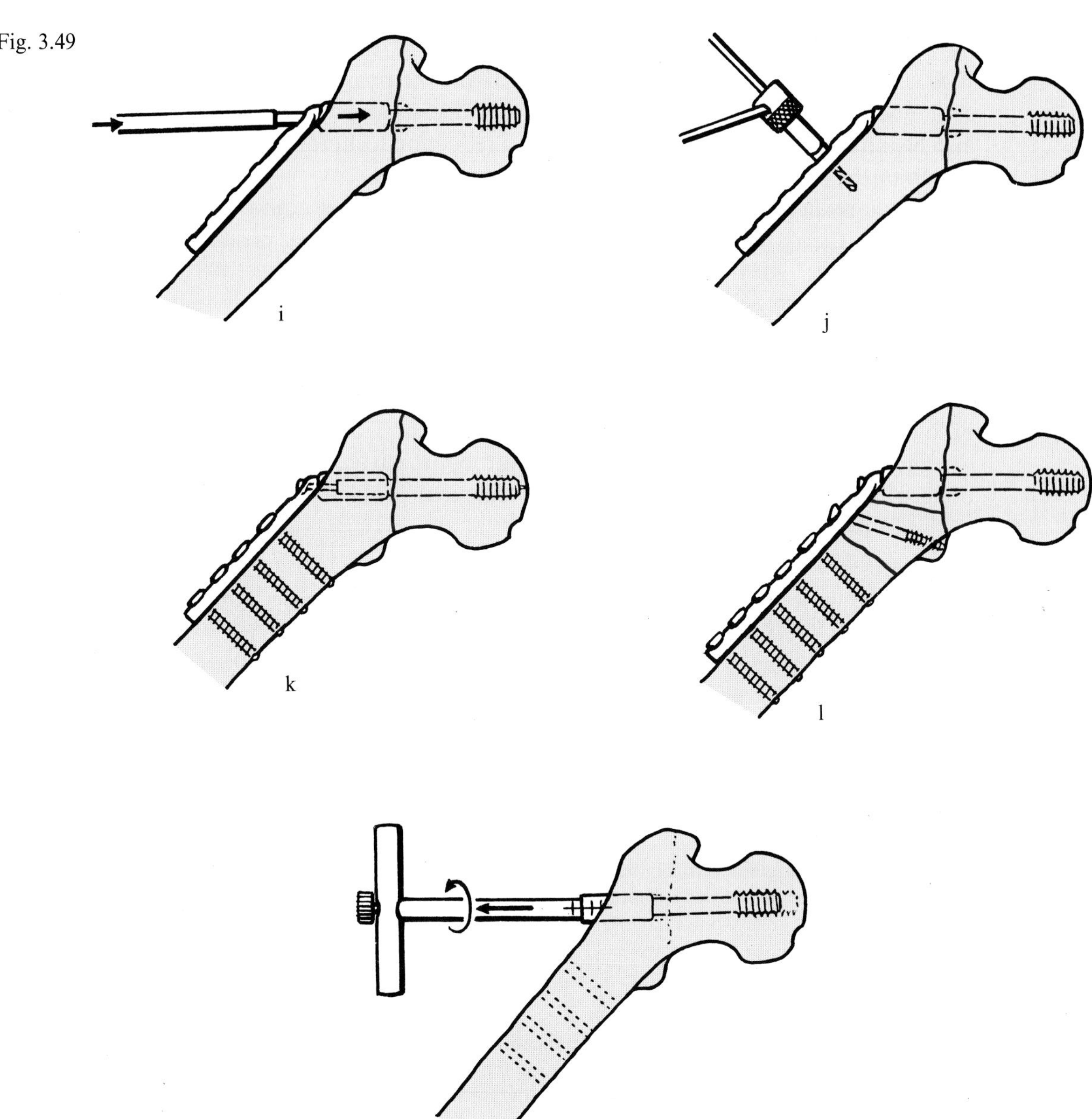

A per- or subtrochanteric fracture with no medial support may still lead to implant failure when fixed with the DCS if healing is significantly delayed. Care has to be taken to either reconstitute the medial support or to induce early periosseous bone formation by a medial cancellous onlay graft. Application of the DCS is described in detail in Fig. 3.50 for the distal femur and in Fig. 3.51 for the proximal femur for per- and subtrochanteric fractures. A rapid medial bony bridge in severely comminuted fractures can also be induced by resorting to the "indirect reduction techniques" with meticulous preservation of the blood supply to the bony fragments.

Valgus reduction in inter- and pertrochanteric fractures admittedly may increase the stability of the reduction but at the price of a marked valgus position of the knee and a very unphysiological weight-bearing axis of the leg.

It should be stressed that the DHS and the DCS used proximally need careful placement of the screw in the neck, but both implants are more forgiving in terms of axial alignment of the side plate to the shaft than the blade plates.

For several reasons the dynamic condylar screw is becoming more popular in fixation of low, supracondylar fractures and for intercondylar T and Y fractures.

The introduction of the seating chisel into bone, particularly into very hard cancellous bone of young adults, can pose serious technical problems. At times the resistance in

---

Fig. 3.50 Insertion of the DCS into the distal femur in the case of a 33-C1 fracture (Y fracture).

a Reduction of the articular fracture and preliminary fixation with Kirschner wires. Care has to be taken that these wires should not interfere with the subsequent positioning of the DCS screw and DCS plate.

b The location of the entry point of the guide pin for the condylar screw. Determine the longest AP diameter of the lateral condyle 2 cm proximal from the most distal joint surface. The entry point is in the middle of the anterior half of this AP diameter or at two-thirds of the longest diameter of the lateral condyle, perpendicular to the shaft axis.

c The articular fracture is now stabilized by replacing the Kirschner wires by cancellous lag screws. An alternative is to use the large cannulated cancellous bone screws and leave the Kirschner wires in place until the screws are inserted.

d The direction of the guide pin for the condylar screw has to be determined from two crucial Kirschner wires. The first one is inserted to mark the knee joint axis along the two condyles. This will indicate the position of the guide pin in the frontal plane (AP view). The second must indicate the slope of the patellofemoral joint (axial view).

e The correctly placed guide pin with the threaded tip is now inserted in such a way that in the AP view it is parallel to the first Kirschner wire indicating the knee joint axis and in the axial view it is parallel to the second Kirschner wire indicating the slopes between the two condyles, that is, the direction of the patellofemoral joint. The guide pin should be inserted as far as but not through the medial cortex. It should penetrate it only when there is severe osteoporosis.

f The guide pin is placed.

g The direct measuring device is slid over the guide pin and the length of the portion in bone can be read off directly on the measuring device (e.g. 80 mm).

If the position of the guide pin, checked with an image intensifier or X-ray, is found to reach the medial cortex, 10 mm must be subtracted from the measured length or the DCS would penetrate the medial cortex of the anterior half of the condyles, which is narrower than the posterior half. Thus if on X-ray the wire is seen to reach the medial cortex and the portion in bone measures 80 mm, 10 mm must be subtracted and the triple reamer set to a depth of 70 mm. The depth of the reamer is adjustable in 5-mm increments.

h The three elements of the DCS reamer are assembled, passed over the guide pin and the drill hole is made.

i If the guide pin is inadvertently withdrawn together with the DCS reamer, it must be immediately reinserted. Otherwise, there is a considerable risk of placing the screw in the wrong direction, away from the original bore hole, especially in porotic bone. It is easily repositioned by using the short centering sleeve and a DCS screw inserted backwards in the sleeve as a guide.

Fig. 3.50

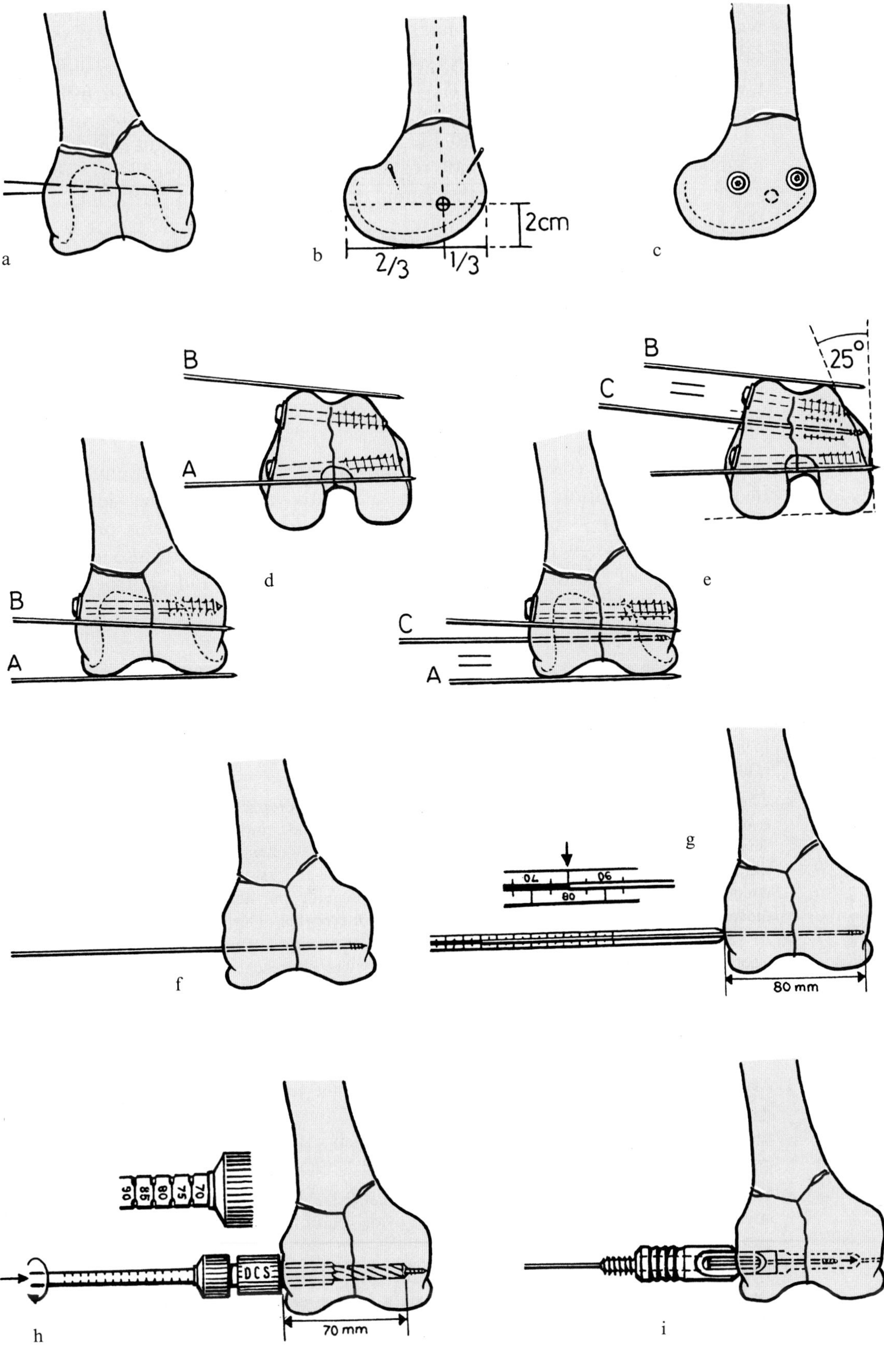

the distal femur can be such that despite predrilling of the path for the seating chisel, when the surgeon attempts to hammer it into bone, the internally fixed distal femur falls apart with loss of fixation of all the lag screws. Also the insertion of the seating chisel parallel to a guide wire is difficult particularly if one is not accustomed to the technique. This can occur even if the guide wire is correctly inserted.

These difficulties have led to the development of an implant which is inserted over a guide wire and which does not require any hammering (Fig. 3.50). The path for the guide wire is predrilled with the 2-mm drill bit. Seen from the front, it is parallel to the knee axis and in the axial view – with the knee bent 90° – it is parallel to the slope from the medial to the lateral condyle, indicated by the ventral Kirschner wire. The position of the guide wire can be checked radiologically before insertion of the device. Thus if the guide wire is in the right position, the correct orientation of the implant is guaranteed. If the guide wire is not correctly placed, a repositioning of the guide wire is a much simpler task than the changing of the position of the seating chisel.

Mistakes

A condylar screw (the same holds true for the blade of the condylar plate) inserted in a "valgus position" will force the knee into varus when the side plate is fixed to the femoral shaft – conversely, when inserted in varus, a valgus position of the knee will result. Any screw (or blade!) inserted too far dorsally will cause anterior and medial displacement of the distal fragment. Precise positioning and control of the guide wire is crucial!

Fig. 3.50 Insertion of the DCS into the distal femur in the case of a 33-C1 fracture (continued).

j In hard cancellous bone, one should precut the screw thread with the tap. The short centering sleeve is used to guide the tap.

k Choose a screw 5 mm shorter than the reamed hole. To prepare the condylar screw for insertion, the coupling screw is inserted through the hollow guide shaft and is screwed in to the condylar screw. The ridge and the slot between the guide shaft and the screw must interdigitate. Slide the longer of the two centering sleeves over the wrench and insert the assembled guide shaft and screw into the wrench. The whole assembly is now slid over the guide pin and the centering sleeve is pushed into the prereamed hole to seat snugly against the bone cortex. The insertion of the screw is now begun by turning the wrench clockwise. Make sure that the screw advances in the centering sleeve. Continue inserting the screw until the 5-mm mark on the wrench reaches the lateral cortex. This means that the threaded tip of the screw lies close to the medial wall of the distal femur while the rear end of the screw is 5 mm deep to the lateral cortex. Ensure that the last turn is stopped so that the handle of the wrench is in line with the femoral axis (k′). In osteoporotic bone the screw may be driven in to the 10 mm mark.

l After removal of the wrench and the centering sleeve, the appropriate DCS plate is slid over the coupling screw and over the inserted screw.

m With the impactor, the side plate is seated against the shaft of the femur. The plate is locked to the condylar screw with the compression screw.

n Two cancellous screws are then inserted into the distal condylar complex across the plate to increase interfragmentary compression fixation and provide rotational stability for the implant in the distal fragment.

o The articulated tension device is fixed to the proximal end of the side plate first in traction mode for indirect reduction and then to achieve axial compression of the transverse fracture plane and achieve additional stability.

p Implant removal: After removal of the DCS plate, the wrench is placed over the DCS screw and the long coupling screw is fixed to the DCS. This allows traction to be exerted while unscrewing the DCS.

Fig. 3.50

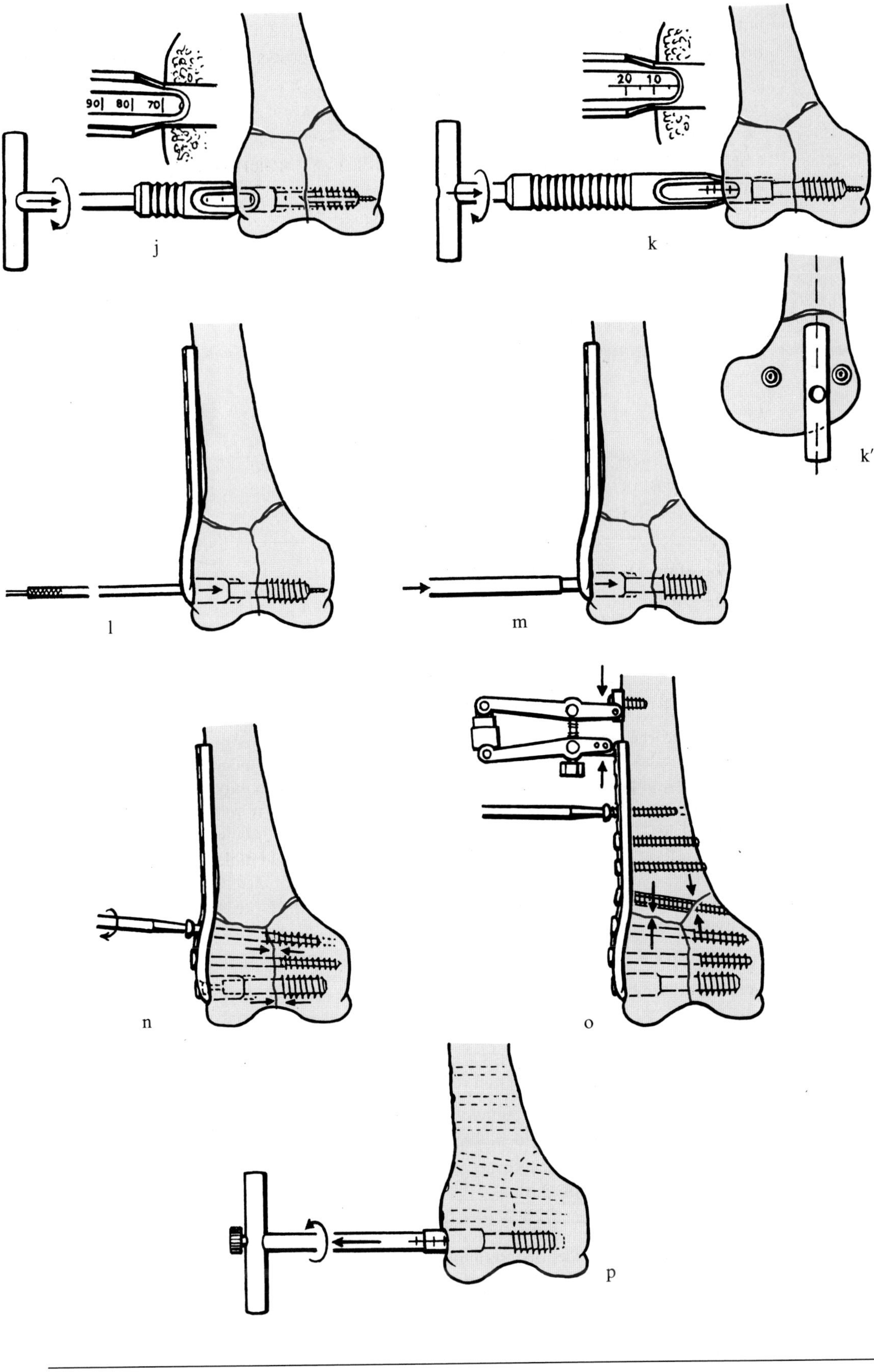

j

k

k′

l

m

n

o

p

Fig. 3.51 Insertion of the DCS into the proximal femur.

a With the patient in a supine position, a long lateral incision is made, reflecting vastus lateralis anteriorly. If necessary the insertion of vastus lateralis at the rough line is partly cut, leaving about 1 cm of the tendinous insertion for subsequent suture. The femoral neck anteversion is determined with a ventral Kirschner wire which is gently hammered into the head. To find the correct direction for the guide pin, use the condylar blade guide which subtends an angle of 85°. The actual placing of the guide pin is related to the AP diameter of the trochanter. Note that the greater trochanter is eccentric in its relation to the femoral neck and that the junction of its anterior and middle thirds (a′) marks the middle of the neck. This will mark the point of entry of the guide pin. Note also that when inserted into the neck the pin should lie not less than 1 cm from the superior cortex. This can be checked with the X-ray. The guide pin has to be introduced in such a way that it is parallel to the axis of the femoral neck considering its anteversion (axial view) and parallel to the condylar guide (AP view). The guide pin is inserted until its tip lies about 2 cm short of the articular surface in the lower half of the femoral head.

b After checking the correct positioning of the guide pin with X-ray, the length within bone is measured directly with the measuring device.

c The DCS triple reamer is set to the same length, passed over the guide pin and the hole is drilled.

d In relatively hard bone, the thread of the DCS should be cut with a tap. If the guide pin should inadvertently be withdrawn, the same trick as used distally (Fig. 3.50i) can be applied for its reinsertion. It is recommended to stabilize the proximal fragment during taping and also during insertion of the screw with a bone-holding clamp. The DCS is inserted using the longer of the two centering sleeves. In osteoporotic bone, the screw is advanced 5 mm further, cutting its own way in the bone.

e At the end of insertion, the T handle of the wrench must be parallel to the femoral shaft to allow the plate barrel to be slid over the screw shaft and then come to lie in line with the femoral shaft.

f–h The plate is seated against the cortex with the impactor. To increase the stability of the device in the proximal fragment, the plate should be fixed to the calcar with at least one screw. Drill a 4.5-mm hole in the lateral cortex through the most proximal screw hole and insert the 3.2-mm drill sleeve. This will stop the 3.2-mm drill bit from gliding along the calcar while you are drilling a 3.2-mm hole in it. After measuring the depth and tapping, insert the appropriate cortex screw.

Once the fracture is reduced, the plate is fixed to the shaft. Where possible apply lag screws for additional compression of fracture areas. Remember, however, that anatomic reduction must not be achieved at the expense of vascular supply to the fragments. Quite often the bridging mode of plate application is advisable, as is indirect reduction! (See Chap. 2.)

Fig. 3.51

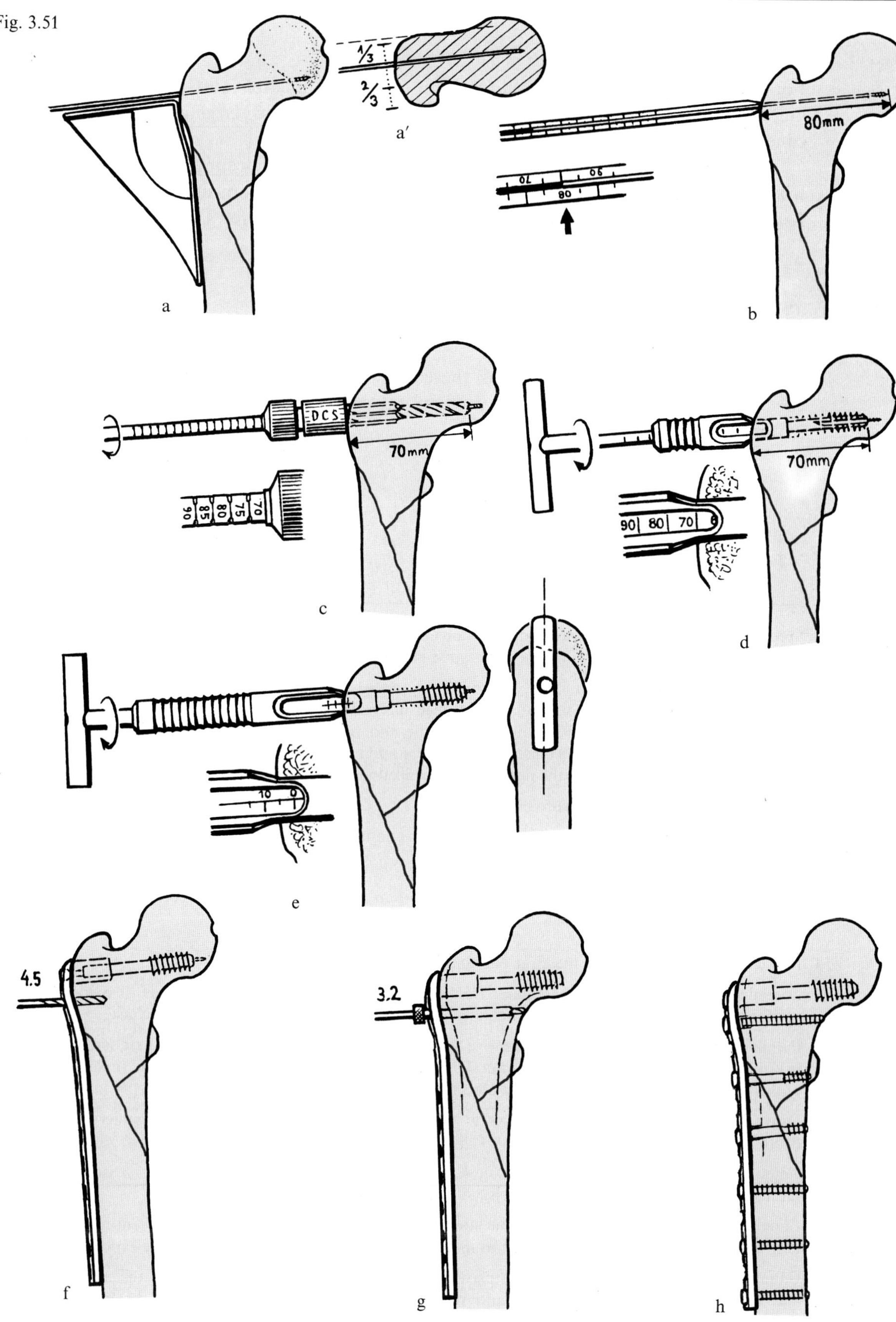

1/3
2/3
a'
80mm
70
80
90
a
b
DCS
70mm
90
85
80
75
70
c
70mm
90
80
70
0
d
10
0
e
4.5
f
3.2
g
h

3.9 Cannulated Cancellous Bone Screws

For precise placement of cancellous bone screws in metaphyseal and epiphyseal sites, guidance by a guide wire may be advantageous. To this end, large and small cannulated cancellous bone screws are available.

Very often, Kirschner wires used for temporary fixation occupy just the very position where a cancellous bone screw would have its optimal biomechanical effect. If such Kirschner wires can be used as guide wires for cannulated screws, the problem is solved.

3.9.1 The Large Cannulated Cancellous Bone Screws

The primary indication for the use of these screws is compression fixation in the metaphyseal region of large bones, such as the femoral neck, the femoral condyles and the tibial plateau and other such sites.

Fig. 3.52 Specifications of the large cannulated cancellous bone screws.
2.1-mm cannulation to accommodate a threaded guide wire of 2 mm.

Thread diameter: There is a slight difference in thread diameter between the USA/Canada and the rest of the world. In the USA/Canada, the thread has a diameter of 7 mm, which is thought to provide extra holding power. It should be noted that the end holes of the DCP as well as of the LC-DCP and other plates do not accept these screws. The standard large cannulated cancellous bone screw has an identical thread diameter to the normal large cancellous bone screw, i.e. 6.5 mm.

Continuous 4.5-mm shaft and core diameter.

Noncutting tip. Ensures accurate screw placement as defined by the path of the guide wire.

Reverse cutting flute. Facilitates screw removal particularly in dense bone.

Standard AO/ASIF screw design. Low profile 8.00-mm head, large hexagonal recess and buttress thread profile.

Fig. 3.53 Instrumentation for use with the large cannulated cancellous bone screws.

a, a′ Threaded guide wire, 2.0 mm. Maintains fracture reduction throughout the procedure. Provides a precise path for controlled drilling, tapping and screw insertion. Threaded tip maximizes purchase.

b, b′ Parallel guide. Triangle-patterned guide wire holes ensure parallel placement of up to three screws, resulting in optimal fracture stability and impaction. Diamond-patterned positioning holes permit precise placement of the parallel guide prior to guide wire placement for screws.

c, c′ Direct measuring device. Determines screw length based on direct measurement of guide wire insertion depth.

d, d′ Cannulated drill bit, 4.5 mm; drill sleeve, 4.5 mm. Permits drilling without loss of provisional stability. Drill sleeve protects surrounding soft tissue during drilling.

e, e′ Cannulated tap. Allows tapping of the lateral cortex or, in dense bone, over the entire nonthreaded length of the guide wire. It is calibrated to indicate insertion depth, to minimize X-ray exposure.

f, f′ Cannulated hexagonal screwdriver. It provides excellent torque transfer between the surgeon's hand and the screw, for ease of insertion and removal. Based on standard design of the large hexagonal screwdriver. Accommodates holding sleeve for large screwdriver.

Fig. 3.53

Fig. 3.52

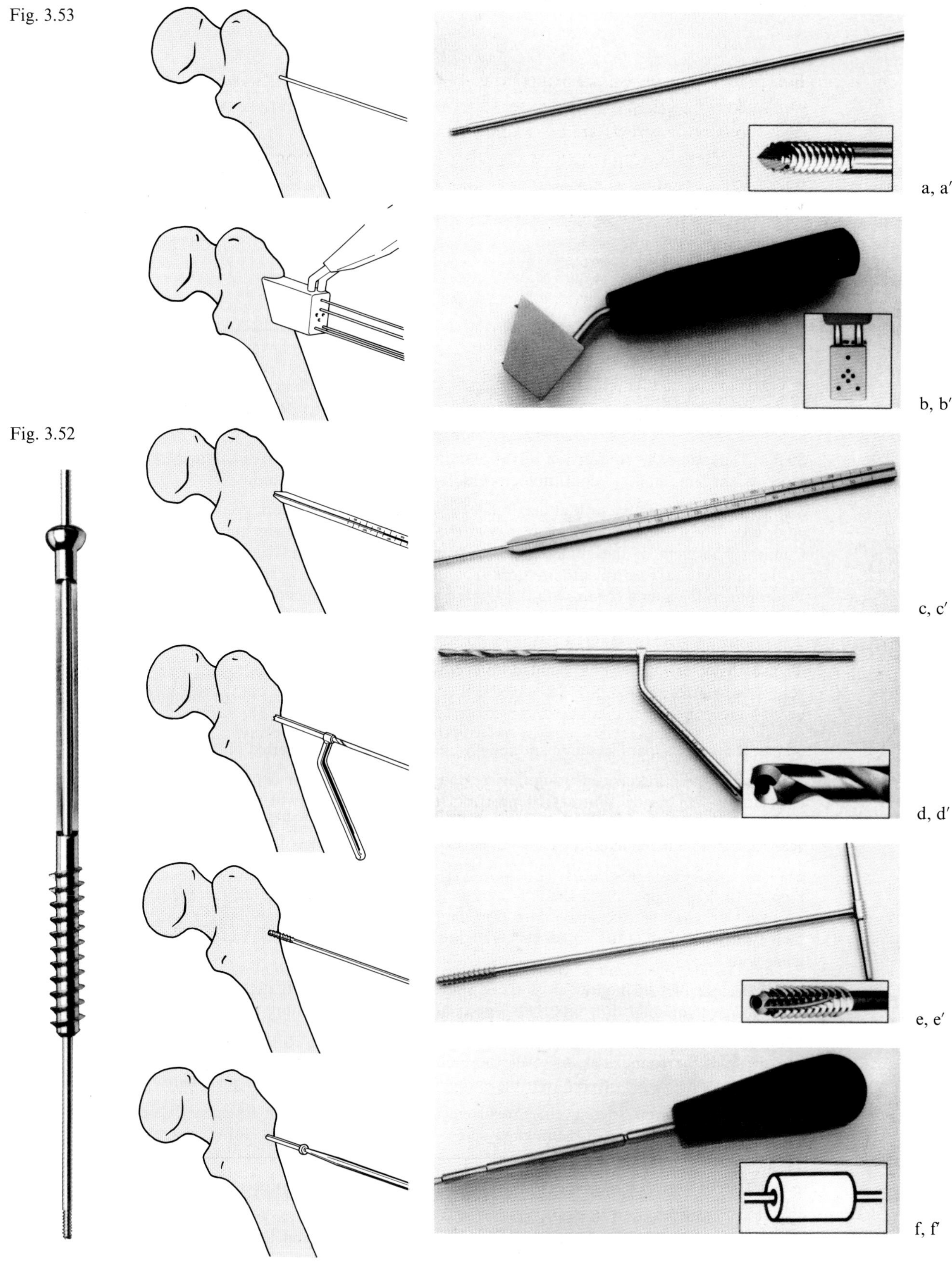

Fig. 3.54 Technique for insertion of large cannulated cancellous bone screws.

In the management of femoral neck fractures, the parallel guide is used to position three parallel wires. For independent screw fixation, place a 2.0-mm threaded guide wire and proceed to step h.

Step a: Determine the anteversion of the femoral neck by placing a threaded guide wire on the anterior aspect of the femoral neck; confirm the position with image intensification.

Step b: While running the drill at maximum rpm to minimize deflection, gradually advance a positioning guide wire. The telescoping wire guide may be used to direct the guide wire and further minimize deflection. Confirm placement of the guide wire under image intensification. The guide wire should be parallel to the anteversion wire (placed in step a) in the AP and axial views. Remove the anteversion wire. Predrilling of the lateral cortex with the 2.0-mm drill bit is recommended in dense bone.

Step c: Place the parallel guide over the positioning guide wire through one of the central diamond-patterned positioning holes. The parallel guide's position may be adjusted by replacing it over the positioning guide wire through one of the adjacent positioning holes.

Step d: Insert a guide wire into the subchondral bone of the femoral head through each of the outer triangle-patterned placement holes.

Step e: Remove the parallel guide and the positioning guide wire (inserted in step b).

Step f: Using the direct measuring device, determine the insertion depth of the three guide wires. To calculate drilling depth, subtract 10 mm from this reading; this will prevent penetration of the joint. To calculate screw length, subtract 5 mm from the original reading; this will compensate for the 5-mm screw head, which remains outside of the near cortex. Example: if the direct measuring device reads 105 mm, drilling depth is 95 mm and screw length is 100 mm.

Step g: In dense bone, place the 4.5-mm cannulated drill bit and the drill sleeve over the guide wire. To avoid drilling over the guide wire threads, drill to the depth determined in step f, and confirm by image intensification. Care must be taken not to direct the drill bit, but rather to let it follow the guide wire.

Note: Because of their hollow cross section and long length, cannulated drill bits are more susceptible to breakage than solid drill bits. Use less axial force, avoid bending and advance the drill bit slowly to minimize the possibility of breakage.

Step h: Pass the cannulated tap over the guide wire and tap the near cortex. In dense metaphyseal bone, it may be necessary to tap over the entire nonthreaded length of the guide wire.

Step i: Select a screw so that the thread engages only the opposite fragment. Using the cannulated screwdriver, insert the large cannulated screw over the guide wire. Confirm fracture impaction with image intensification.

Note: The washer for large cancellous bone screws may be used to prevent the screw head from sinking into the near cortex.

Step j: Remove and discard the guide wire. Repeat screw insertion technique (steps f–i) for remaining screws.

Important: To prevent loss of reduction, drill, tap and insert each screw before proceeding to the next.

Fig. 3.54

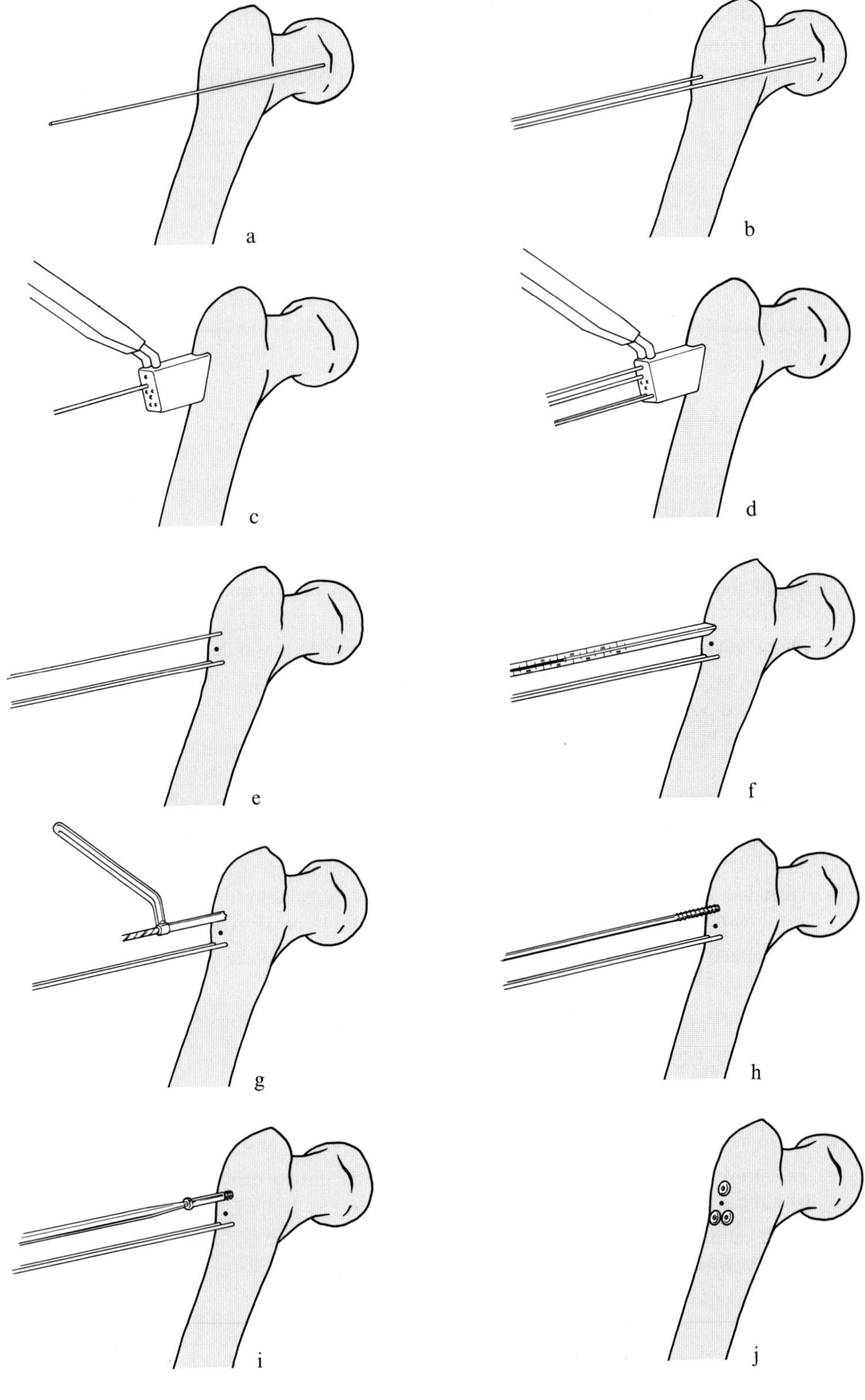

3.9.2 The Small Cannulated Cancellous Bone Screw

The small cannulated cancellous bone screw (3.5 mm) is indicated in the metaphysis of long bones, such as the distal radius, the distal humerus and, particularly, distal and proximal tibia, but also in the small carpal bones such as the scaphoid.

Fig. 3.55 Specifications of the small cannulated cancellous bone screw.

Thread diameter 3.5 mm, pitch 1.25 mm, for good purchase and effective interfragmentary compression.

Continuous 2.5-mm shaft/core diameter, for strength and elimination of stress concentration at the shaft/core junction.

Cannulation 1.35 mm. Accommodates guides wires of 1.25-mm diameter with threaded tip.

Tapered tip. Minimizes fragment displacement during insertion.

Reverse cutting flute for easy screw removal.
Length h. From 10 mm to 50 mm in 2-mm increments, either partially or fully threaded.

Fig. 3.56 Instrumentation for use with the small cannulated cancellous bone screw.

a Threaded guide wire, 1.25 mm. The threaded trocar tip allows insertion of guide wire without high axial force, thus preventing displacement of small fragments.

b Threaded telescopic drill guide with stop. Allows precise setting to a predetermined depth, in order to prevent overdrilling. Includes 3.5-mm and 2.7-mm insert sleeves.

c Cannulated drill bit, 2.7 mm with long quick coupling end. Works with the drill guide with stop: 1.35-mm cannulation permits drilling over the guide wire.

d Direct measuring device. Provides direct reading of preset drilling depth and guide wire insertion depth.

e Small cannulated countersink, with quick coupling, cuts a recess for the screw head. Quick-connects to tap handle.

f Small cannulated tap. Allows precise tapping of near cortex and dense metaphyseal bone. Quick-connects to tap handle.

g Tap sleeve. Protects soft tissue during tapping and during drilling of a gliding hole in the near cortex with the 3.5-mm cannulated drill bit.

h Small cannulated hexagonal screwdriver. Fully cannulated for insertion of the small cannulated screw over the guide wire. Accommodates a holding sleeve.

i Small hexagonal screwdriver shaft. With quick coupling end.

j Cannulated drill bit, 3.5 mm. For drilling a gliding hole in the near cortex.

k Stylet. For cleaning cannulated instrumentation.

l Small drill sleeve, 1.25 mm/2.7 mm diameter.

m Screw forceps.

n Clip of washers.

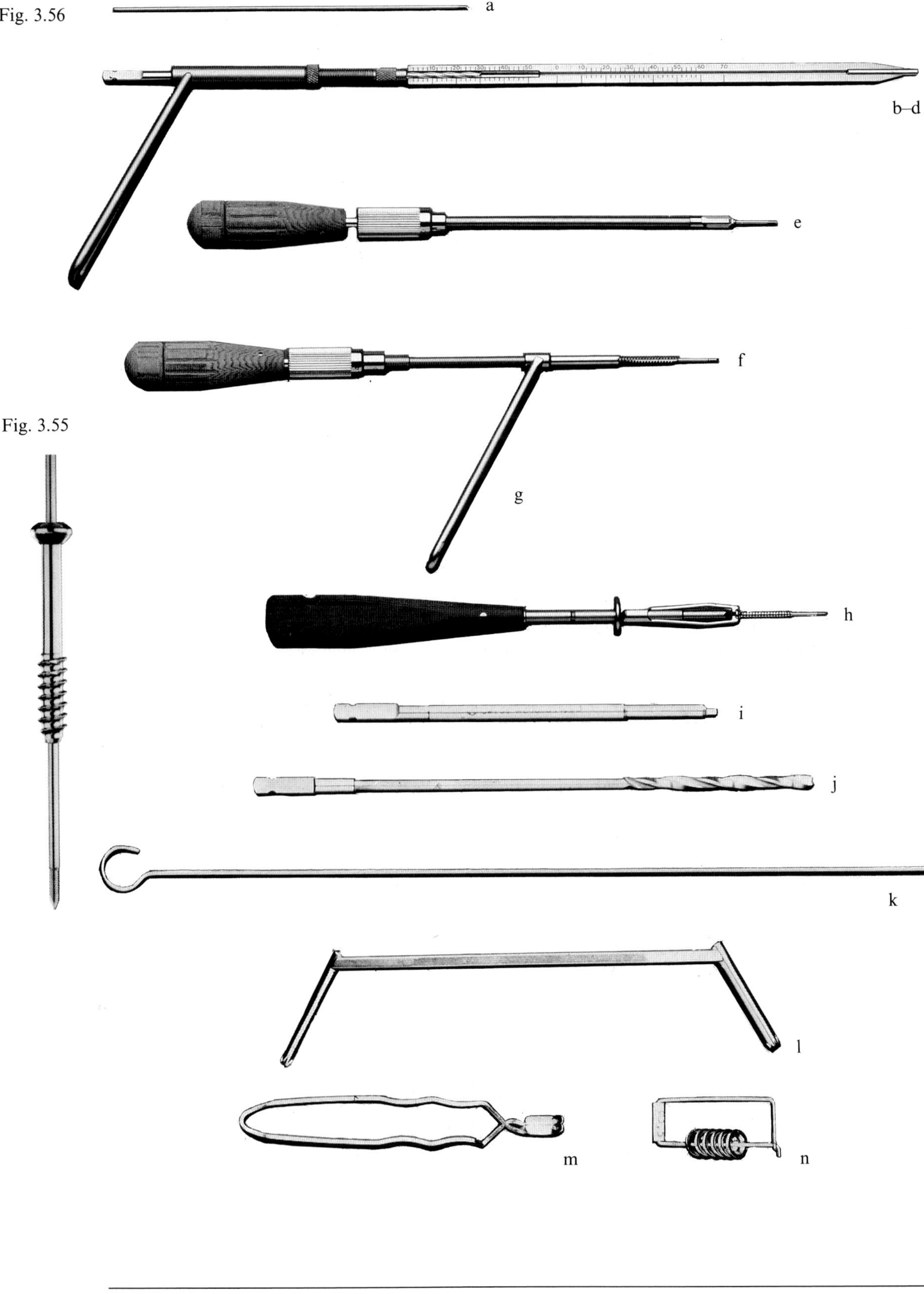

Fig. 3.56

Fig. 3.55

Fig. 3.57 Technique for insertion of small cannulated cancellous bone screws.

Basically the insertion of the Kirschner wire should be followed directly by insertion of the screw over the guide wire. As soon as there is any resistance in the cortex to be penetrated, this cortex should be opened by a cannulated drill bit (3.5 mm) for a few millimeters and then the screw inserted. In very hard bone (particularly in the cancellous metaphysis or epiphysis of children), tapping part or even all the way may be necessary. Then steps a–f as depicted should be followed.

Step a: After reducing the fragments, insert a 1.25-mm threaded guide wire using the small air drill and the small drill sleeve. The guide wire should cross the fracture line and penetrate the far cortex. It is critical to confirm guide wire positioning in three views under image intensification. Remove the drill sleeve. To prevent rotation of the fragment, place a second guide wire parallel to the first, following the same procedure.

Step b: To determine guide wire insertion depth, slide the tapered end of the direct measuring device over the guide wire. To determine drilling depth subtract 5 mm* from this reading; this will prevent penetration of the far cortex.

*Note: Always consider the specific indication when calculating drilling depth; use 5 mm as a guideline only.

Step c: Insert the 2.7-mm cannulated drill bit into the drill guide with stop until the quick coupling end of the bit rests on the drill guide. Insert the drill bit into the nontapered end of the direct measuring device, and loosen the knurled nut on the drill guide with stop. Rotate the threaded end of the drill guide with stop until drill bit length corresponds to drilling depth. Tighten the knurled nut.

Step d: Place the drilling assembly over the threaded guide wire. Drill until the quick coupling end of the drill bit contacts the drill guide with stop.

Note: If the fracture pattern necessitates insertion of a fully threaded screw, drill a gliding hole in the near cortex before proceeding to step e. Use the drill guide with stop, with the 3.5-mm insert sleeve, and the 3.5-mm cannulated drill bit.

Step e: Tap the near cortex using the tapping assembly. In dense metaphyseal bone, tap over the entire nonthreaded length of the guide wire.

Step f: Select a small cannulated bone screw of the same length as the depth drilled. Using the small cannulated screwdriver, insert the screw over the guide wire. Remove and discard the guide wire. Repeat the procedure for additional screws.

Fig. 3.57

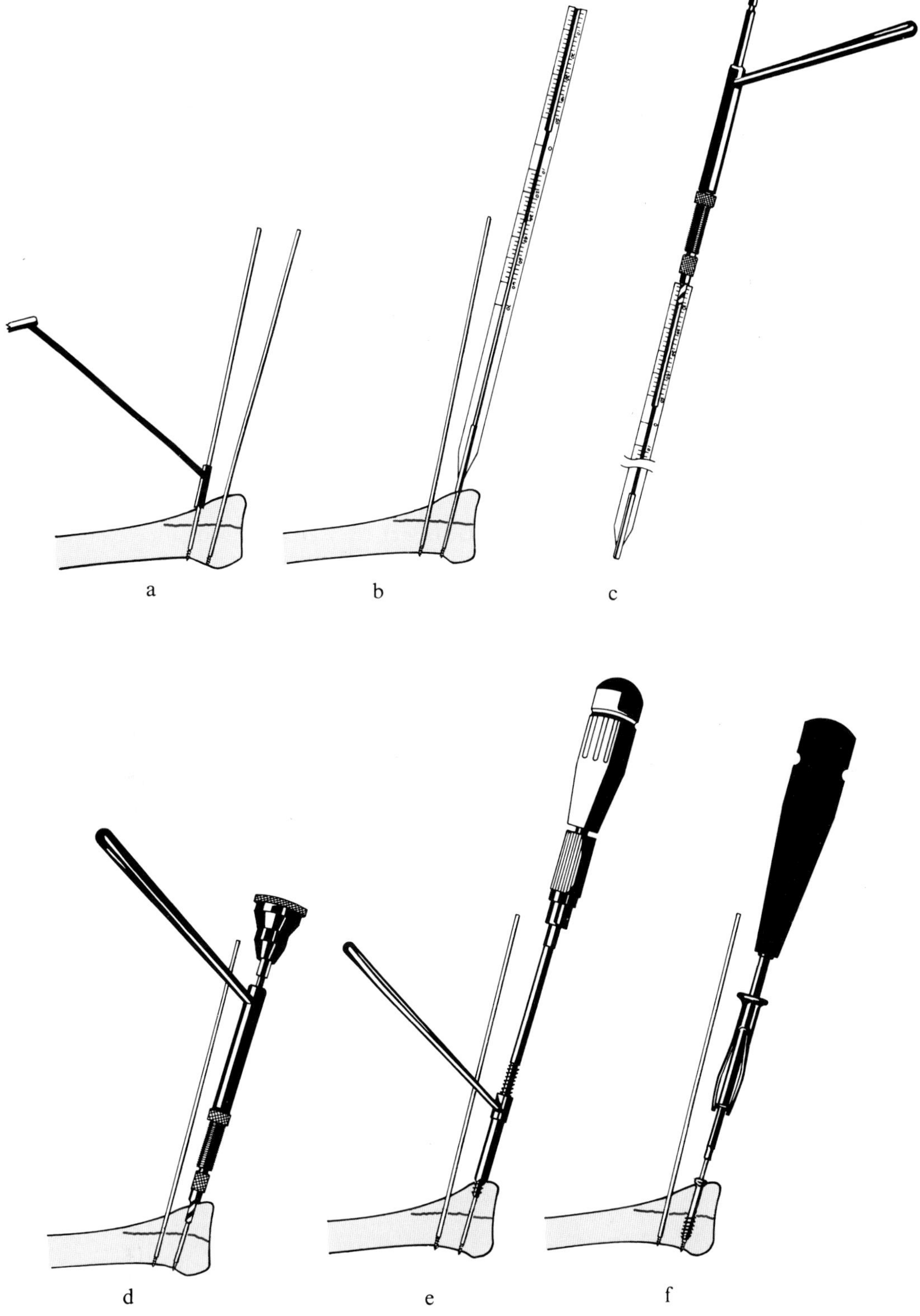

References

Allgöwer M, Matter P, Perren SM, Rüedi T (1973) The dynamic compression plate. Springer, Berlin Heidelberg New York

Ansell RH, Scales JT (1968) A study of some factors which affect the strength of screws and their insertion and holding power in bone. J Biomechanics 1:279–302

Charnley J (1953) Compression arthrodesis. Livingstone, Edinburgh

Danis R (1947) Theorie et pratique de l'ostéosynthèse. Masson, Paris

Gozna ER, Harrington IJ (1982) Biomechanics of musculoskeletal injury. Williams and Wilkins, Baltimore London

Key JA (1932) Positive pressure in arthrodesis for tuberculosis of the knee joint. South Med J 25:909–915

Müller ME, Allgöwer M, Schneider R, Willegger W (1979) Manual of internal fixation, 2nd edn. Springer, Berlin Heidelberg New York

Pauwels F (1935) Der Schenkelhalsbruch, ein mechanisches Problem. Enke, Stuttgart

Phillips JH, Rahn BA (1989) Comparison of compression and torque measurements of self-tapping and pre-tapped screws. Plast Reconstruct Surg 83:447–4556

Regazzoni P, Rüedi T, Winquist R, Allgöwer M (1985) The dynamic hip screw implant system. Springer, Berlin Heidelberg New York

Schatzker J, Sanderson R, Murnaghan P (1975a) The holding power of orthopaedic screws in vivo. Clin Orthop 108:115–126

Schatzker J, Horn JG, Sumner-Smith G (1975b) The effects of movement on the holding power of screws in bone. Clin Orthop 111:257–263

Schatzker J, Horn JG, Sumner-Smith G (1975c) The reaction of cortical bone to compression by screw threads. Clin Orthop 111:263–265

Schatzker J, Manley PA, Sumner-Smith G (1980) In vivo strain gauge study of bone response to loading with and without internal fixation. In: Uhthoff H (ed) Current concepts of internal fixation of fractures. Springer, Berlin Heidelberg New York, pp 306–314

Schenk R, Willenegger H (1964) Histologie der primären Knochenheilung. Langenbecks Arch Klin Chir 308:440–452

4 MEDULLARY NAILING OF FEMUR AND TIBIA

4.1 Intramedullary Nailing

The biomechanical principles of intramedullary splinting were established by the intramedullary nailing technique introduced by Küntscher in 1940. Splinting provides only relative stability with no interfragmentary compression. In stable fractures, however, it permits early weight-bearing, which produces axial compression between the two main fracture fragments. The intramedullary nail is a load-sharing device which permits load-bearing across the fracture site. Active functional after-treatment is therefore possible in most cases. In the early 1950s, Küntscher also introduced intramedullary reaming. This permitted the use of nails which more accurately fit the diaphyseal portion of the medullary canal and has led to improved fixation. Küntscher's concept of the "detensor" (1969) was the predecessor of the current concepts of interlocking, which considerably extend the indications for intramedullary nailing. At present we distinguish between the conventional and the interlocking techniques.

4.1.1 Indications for Intramedullary Nailing

For anatomic, biological, and technical reasons, intramedullary nailing has as yet not proved suitable for diaphyseal fractures in the upper extremity. AO/ASIF has therefore limited intramedullary nailing to shaft fractures of the femur and tibia.

Because of possible damage to the growth plate, the use of intramedullary nailing in children is not advocated. In children with severe multiple trauma, intramedullary nailing of the femur may be indicated exceptionally as a life-saving procedure only. In severe open fractures, especially of the tibia, increased risk of infection limits the indications for intramedullary nailing in combination with reaming. Unreamed nailing in combination with interlocking may be considered as an alternative.

We distinguish between good and extended indications for nailing. Transverse and short oblique midshaft fractures of the femur and tibia are considered good indications, for which conventional nailing is the method of choice. This method is also suitable for the treatment of delayed union and pseudarthrosis in the same anatomic areas.

Fractures in the transitional zones, segmental and comminuted fractures require interlocking or other methods of fixation. Dynamic locking at only one end of the nail improves rotational stability and still permits axial compression on weight-bearing. Static locking at both ends of the nail provides optimum control of rotation and length, but weight-bearing may be hazardous until the fracture is bridged and the nail is "dynamized" by removal of the relevant locking bolts. Postoperative treatment depends upon the axial and rotational stability achieved by internal fixation.

4.1.2 Open Versus Closed Intramedullary Nailing

In the open nailing technique, the fracture is exposed and reduced under direct visual control. In the closed technique, a fracture table or distractor is used for fracture reduction. An image intensifier controls reaming and nailing. The closed nailing technique minimizes damage to soft tissues and to the periosteal and muscular blood supply, and minimizes blood loss. For these reasons, it is the preferred method; it is, however, technically demanding. The extent of reaming depends upon the fracture pattern and the localization of the fracture.

4.2 AO/ASIF Implants for Intramedullary Nailing

4.2.1 Design History of the AO/ASIF Intramedullary Nail

AO/ASIF originally developed a thin-walled flexible and partly slotted femoral intramedullary nail with a cloverleaf cross section and a slight curvature of the axis. The slot was placed on the convex side. More than 600000 nails of this design have been distributed, and most of them have been implanted. In 1987, the new universal femoral nail was introduced. It was developed after wide clinical experience with the old, partly slotted nail[1] to introduce an efficient locking system (Fig. 4.1) and give a better anatomic fit.

The original AO tibial nail was developed as a result of the observation that with a flexible nail, the axial curvature of the medullary canal can be disregarded. However, the need for rotational stability soon led to the development of Herzog's bend, an angle formed near the proximal end of the nail (Fig. 4.2). The idea of locking to prevent rotation of the nail about its longitudinal axis and to stabilize the short distal fragments was already instrumental in the early AO/ASIF tibial nails. They had two oval slots facing medially and laterally to allow insertion of ledge wires. Rotation of short proximal fragments was prevented by cortex screws introduced across the proximal end of the tibial nail. The earlier editions of this manual contain a detailed description of the old tibial nail, which is still available, and of the surgical technique for its use.

In 1987–1988, AO/ASIF developed a new universal tibial nail. Computer tomography and a number of anatomical specimens were used to determine the best form to match the average medullary canal. The elastic and plastic deformation of tibial intramedullary

[1] From 1980 to the end of 1988, more than 3300 clinical cases of the use of AO/ASIF intramedullary nails were documented at the computer data base of the AO Documentation Centre in Berne, Switzerland.

Fig. 4.1 AO/ASIF universal femoral nail.
a Anteroposterior view.
b Mediolateral view.

Fig. 4.2 AO/ASIF tibial nail. The nail's characteristic feature is Herzog's bend near its proximal end.

Fig. 4.3 AO/ASIF universal tibial nail.
a Anteroposterior view, showing the characteristic anteroposterior locking hole on the distal side.
b Mediolateral view, showing the five characteristic mediolateral locking holes.

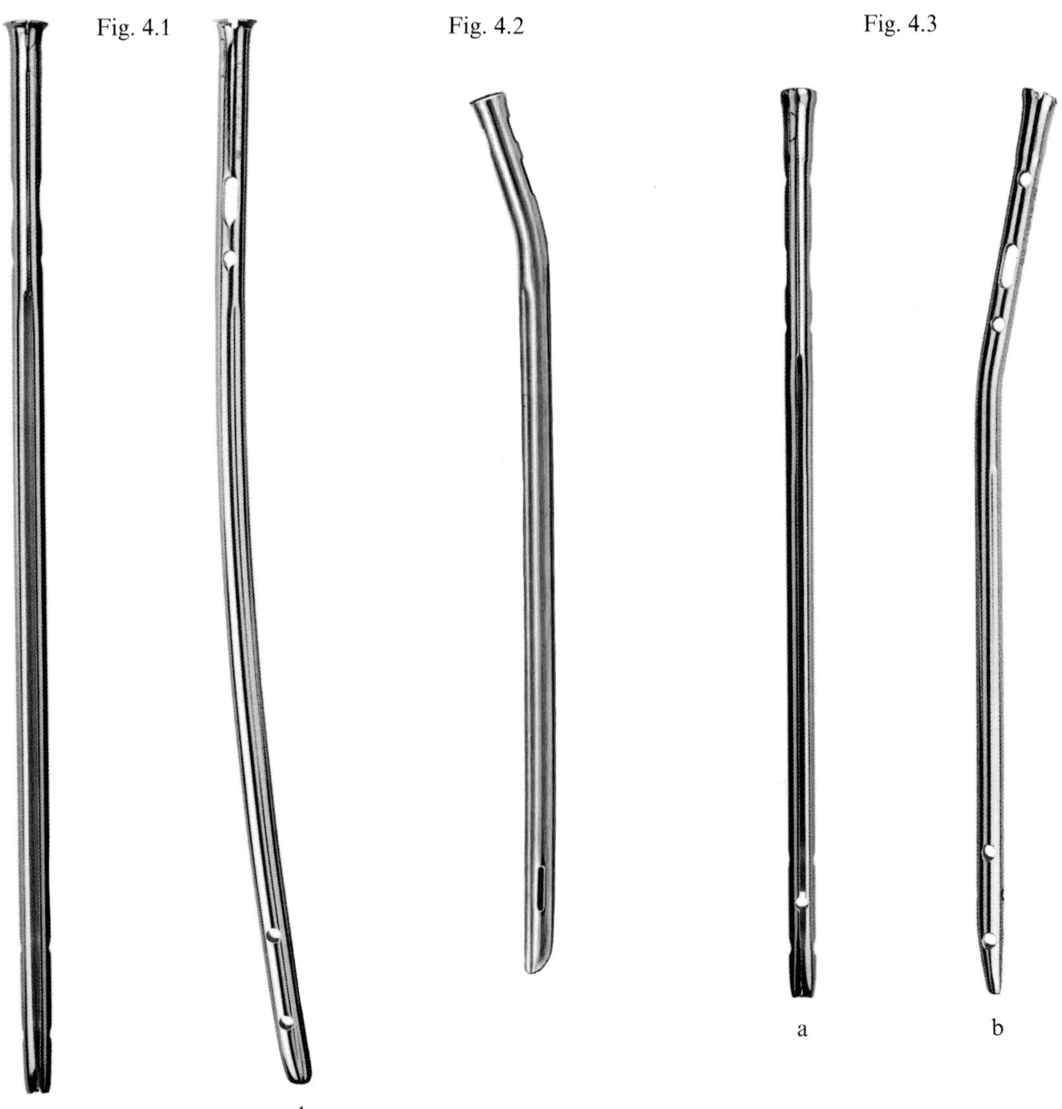

Fig. 4.1 Fig. 4.2 Fig. 4.3

nails, and the observation of stress distribution in the cortical bone during insertion showed that the anatomic position for the AO/ASIF bend is at two-thirds of the length, the proximal third being smoothly bent to an angle of 11° (Heini 1987; Heini et al. 1987) (Fig. 4.3).

4.2.2 The AO/ASIF Universal Femoral Nail

The universal femoral nail developed by AO/ASIF is a tube with a cloverleaf cross section and a longitudinal slot. The nail's characteristic features are essential for its functional reliability (Fig. 4.4).

Its 1.2-mm-thick wall, its diameter, and the longitudinal slot give the nail a certain flexibility under bending and torsion. At the same time they provide the necessary strength under functional stress.

The continuous longitudinal slot prevents a concentration of stress at the upper end of the slot, particularly under torsion, and promotes an even distribution of stress over its full length.

The nail's conical proximal end has an internal thread which provides secure fixing of the threaded conical bolt for attaching the insertion handle for the insertion and removal of the nail. The dovetail ("keystone") slot closes the tube and prevents flaring on insertion of the threaded conical bolt. Positioning grooves precisely align the insertion handle with the nail.

The nail has a curvature corresponding to the average anatomic curvature of the femur (1500 mm radius).

For locking, the femoral nail has two locking holes at the proximal and the distal end. These are accessible from both medially and laterally. One of the holes at the proximal end is slotted to allow dynamic locking. The circular holes for static locking measure 5 mm.

Fig. 4.4 Characteristic features of the universal femoral nail.

a The nail's 1.2-mm-thick walls help ensure stiffness.

b The continuous longitudinal slot prevents stress concentration at the proximal end.

c The conical thread provides secure fixing of the threaded conical bolt used for attaching the insertion and extraction handle.

d The dovetail slot prevents flaring of the tube and reduces torsional deformation of the nail.

e The positioning grooves ensure exact alignment of the insertion handle in predetermined positions.

f The nail axis has a 1500-mm radius of curvature. This is similar to the average anatomic curvature of the femur.

g Two distal locking holes, 5 mm in diameter.

h Locking hole for dynamic locking.

i Locking hole for static locking. The two locking holes (h) and (i) can be used in a flexible manner, depending upon the surgical objectives.

k Cloverleaf cross section.

Fig. 4.4

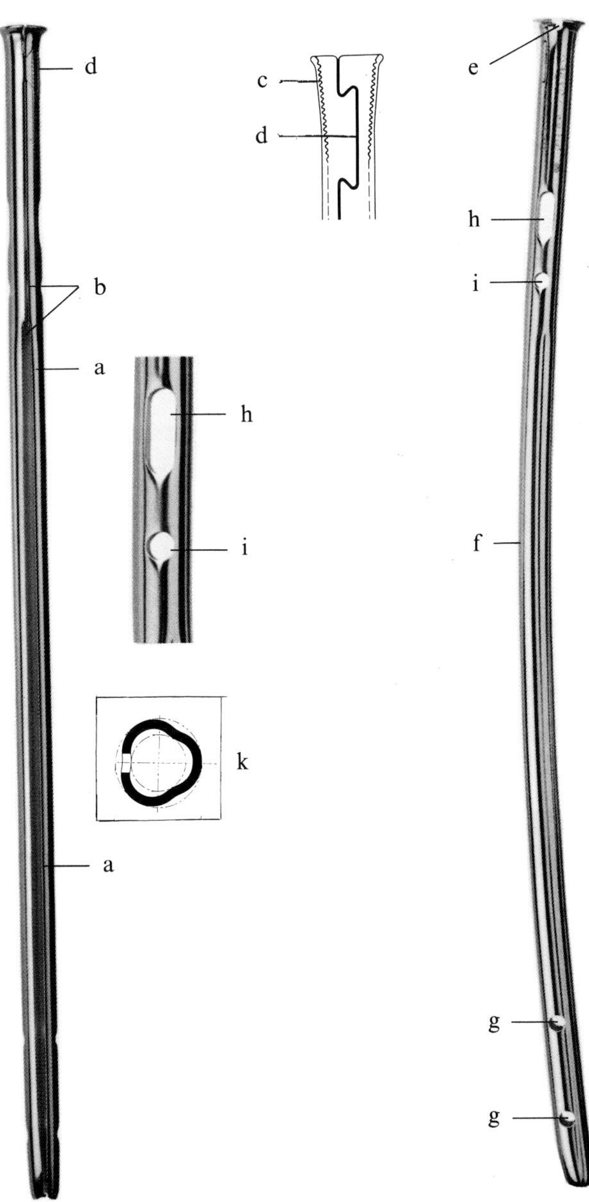

4.2.3 AO/ASIF Universal Tibial Nail

The universal tibial nail is a tube with a cloverleaf cross-section and a longitudinal slot. Its characteristic elements are practically the same as those of the universal femoral nail (Fig. 4.5).

Its 1.2-mm-thick wall gives the nail both the requisite strength and reasonable flexibility (see Perren 1987). A continuous longitudinal slot on the dorsal side prevents stress concentrations, particularly under torsion, and promotes an even distribution of stress over the length of the nail (Mathys 1987). The internal thread at the conical proximal end firmly fixes the threaded conical bolt for securing the handle for insertion and removal. The proximally located dovetail slot closes the tube and prevents flaring at insertion of the conical bolt.

Positioning grooves at the end of the nail align the insertion handle with the nail. The proximal beveled end reduces pressure between the edge of the nail and the patellar ligament.

The tapered tip is designed for safe insertion. It slides in smoothly along the dorsal wall of the medullary canal. This minimizes the risk of injury to the dorsal wall of the bone and prevents the nail from becoming jammed (Fig. 4.41).

The AO/ASIF bend in the nail takes into account the anatomic angle of about 11° formed by the axis of the access canal and that of the medullary canal.

In some 50% of all cases, the nail is used without locking. But for extended indications, the locking technique may be necessary. For this purpose, the universal tibial nail has three holes for mediolateral access at its proximal end. The middle hole is slotted for dynamic locking, the other two, 5 mm in diameter, for static locking.

At the distal end, there are again three holes, two for mediolateral access and the middle one for anterior access. This hole is used if medial soft tissue cover is inadequate or if the proximal mediolateral hole is too close to the fracture site.

Fig. 4.5 Characteristic features of the universal tibial nail.

a 1.2-mm-thick-walls.

b Continuous longitudinal slot on the dorsal side.

c Conical thread.

d Dovetail slot.

e Positioning grooves.

f Beveled end.

g Specially tapered tip.

h AO/ASIF bend.

i Dynamic locking hole.

k Proximal static locking holes, 5 mm in diameter.

l Distal mediolateral locking holes.

m Distal anteroposterior locking hole.

Fig. 4.5

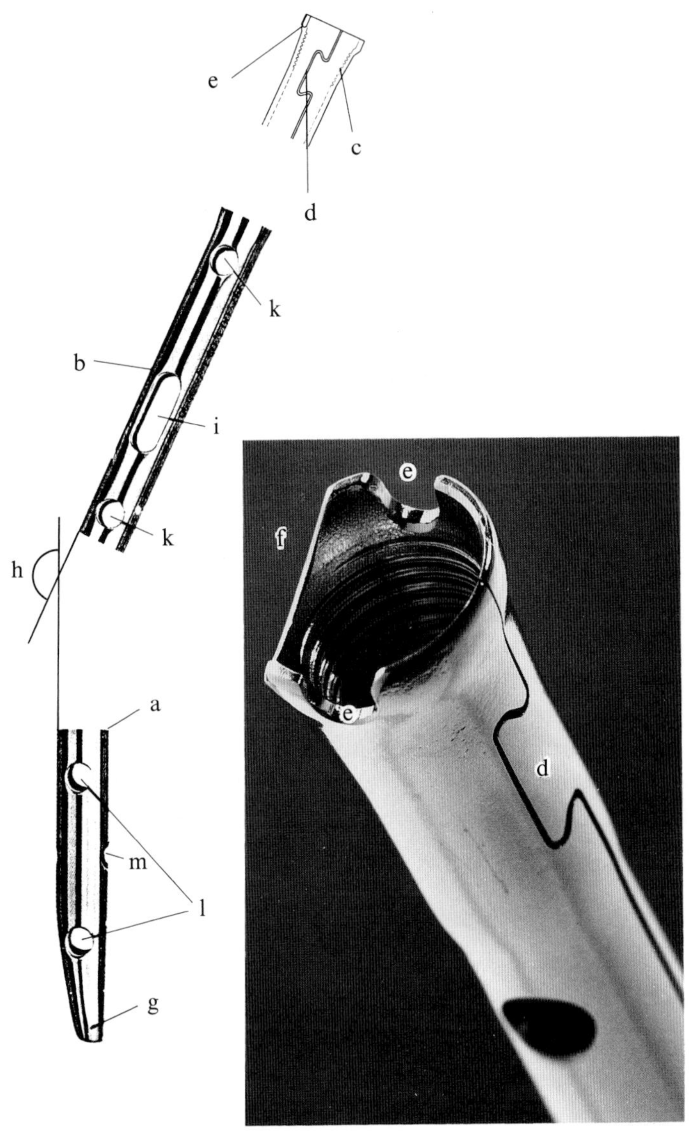

4.2.4 The Locking Bolt (Fig. 4.6)

The locking bolt has an outer diameter of 4.9 mm and a core diameter of 4.3 mm. This ensures adequate static and dynamic strength.

The flat screw thread runs along the entire length and prevents accidental loosening by slight oversize of the core. The self-tapping trocar tip permits insertion of the locking bolt after only one drilling process with the 4.0-mm drill bit. This reduces the number of steps, avoids potential problems with tapping and renders the locking procedure much easier.

4.3 AO/ASIF Instruments for Intramedullary Nailing

4.3.1 Instruments for Reaming the Medullary Canal

The recommended operating technique is based on Küntscher's work (1952) with reaming of the medullary canal. As the medullary canal is not cylindrical but has an hourglass shape, reaming was introduced to adapt the bone to the nail providing a large contact area between bone and nail.

To open the medullary canal of the tibia an awl is used (Fig. 4.7a). It is available in two sizes, large and small.

For the femur the same awl has also been recommended. To provide a more precise access at the piriform fossa we now use the cannulated cutter (Fig. 4.7b) in conjunction with the centering pin (Fig. 4.7c). For insertion, the centering pin is fixed to the universal chuck (Fig. 4.8) and then the cannulated cutter is slipped over the centering pin and fixed.

Fig. 4.6 Locking bolt.

a Slight oversize of core exerts radial preload and helps in preventing accidental loosening.

b Self-tapping trocar tip reduces operating time. When selecting the appropriate length with the depth gauge, always add 2 mm!

Fig. 4.7 Instruments for opening the medullary canal.

a Small awl.

b Cannulated cutter.

c Centering pin.

Fig. 4.8 Universal chuck with T handle.

Fig. 4.6

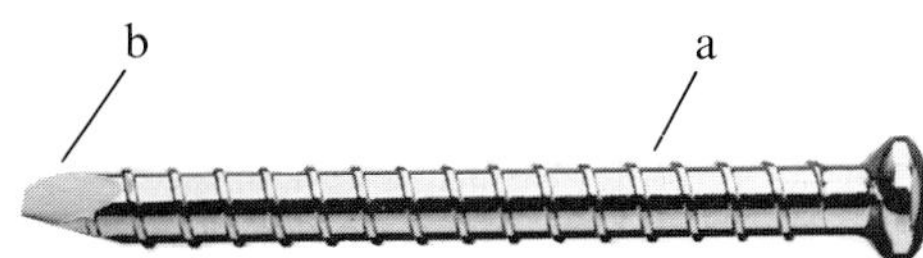

Fig. 4.7

a

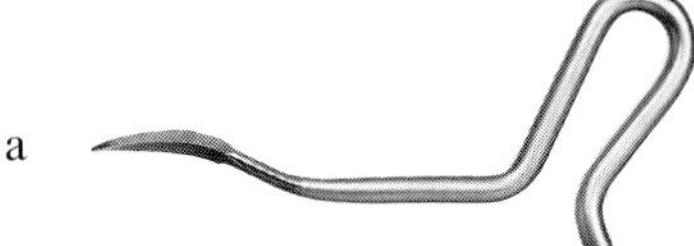

b

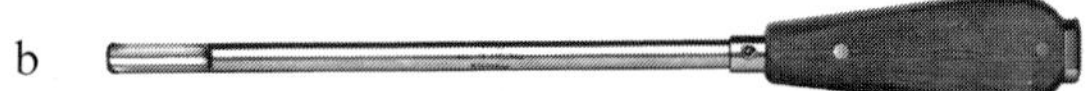

c

Fig. 4.8

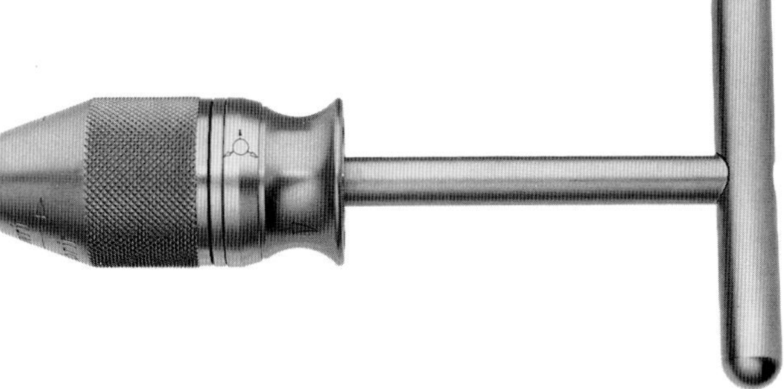

The most important guide is the 3-mm thick reaming rod with the offset ball tip (Fig. 4.9a). The ball prevents the reamer from traveling beyond its end and allows withdrawal of a jammed reamer. Distal to the ball, the tip of the reaming rod is slightly bent. This facilitates positioning as the rod passes along the medullary canal. Rotation of the reaming rod makes picking up axially displaced fragments easier. A holding forceps (Fig. 4.9b) is used to hold the reaming rod. It replaces the earlier holding device (Fig. 4.9c).

In case the reaming rod encounters resistance when introduced, for example in a pseudarthrosis, the instrument set includes hand reamers with diameters from 6 mm to 8 mm (Fig. 4.9d) for opening up the medullary canal. To protect the soft tissue, a tissue protector according to Böhler is used (Fig. 4.9e).

Further reaming equipment is illustrated in Fig. 4.10.

Fig. 4.9 Instruments for reaming the medullary canal I.

- a Reaming rod, 3 mm outer diameter × 950 mm long with offset ball tip.
- b Holding forceps.
- c Holder (now replaced by holding forceps).
- d Hand reamers.
- e Tissue protector (according to Böhler).

Fig. 4.10 Instruments for reaming the medullary canal II.

- a Universal drill with right-angled drive and a working speed of about 350 rpm.
- b Flexible shaft, 9 mm outer diameter with fixed front-cutting reamer.
- c Flexible shaft, 8 mm outer diameter for reamers up to 12.5 mm in diameter.
- d Flexible shaft for 13–19 mm diameter reamers.
- e Medullary reamers, 9.5–12.5 mm diameter, in 0.5-mm steps.
- f Medullary reamers, 13.0–19.0 mm diameter.
- g Air jet (not to be sterilized!).
- h Air tube.
- i Medullary tube for exchanging reaming rod for guide rod.

The flexible shafts permit a maximum reaming depth of 440 mm. The air jet and tube (g, h) are used for cleaning the inside of the reamers and flexible shafts.

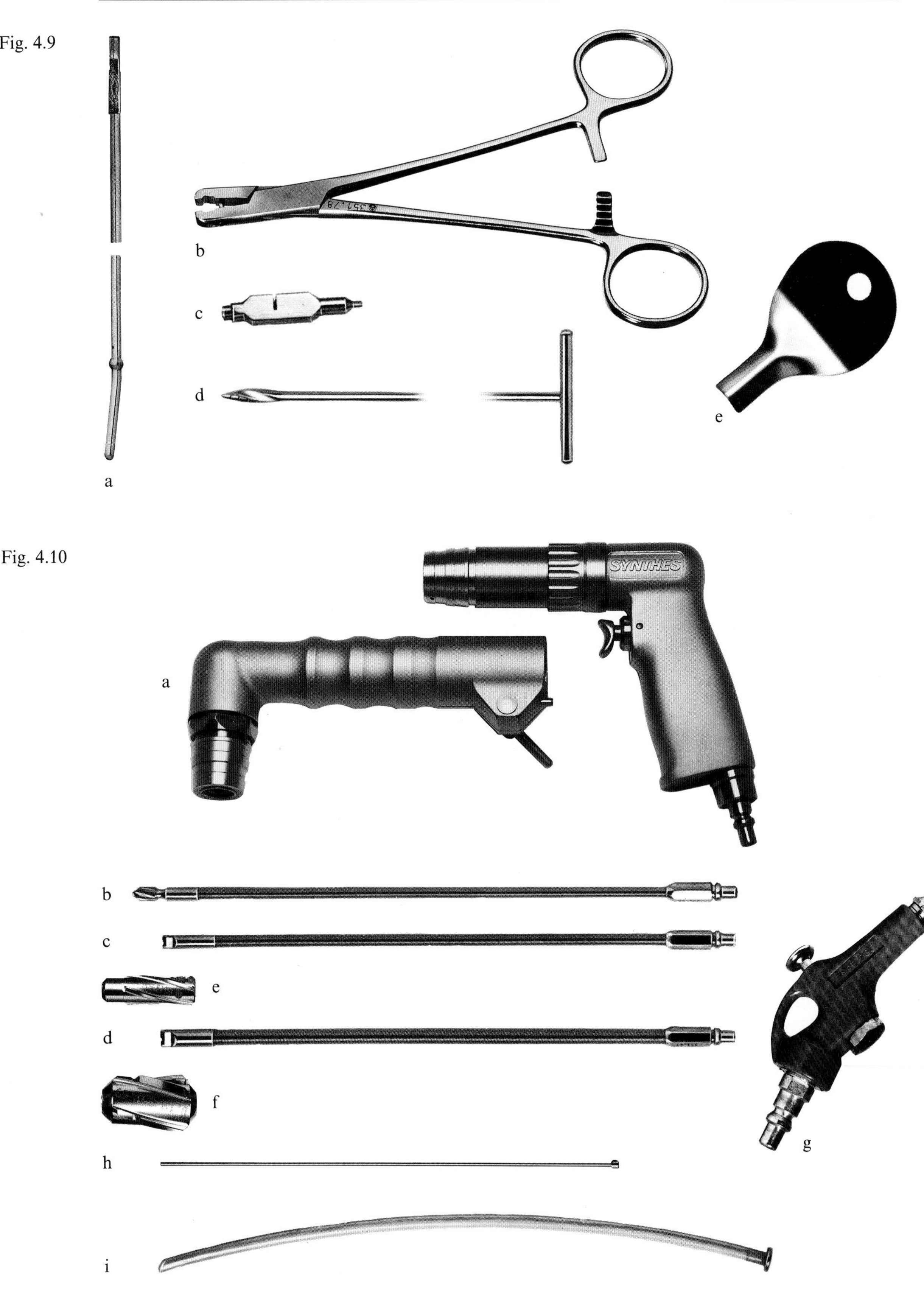
Fig. 4.9
a
b
c
d
e
Fig. 4.10
SYNTHES
a
b
c
e
d
f
g
h
i

4.3.2 Instruments for Inserting Universal Intramedullary Nails

For both femoral and tibial nails the guide rod is the most important instrument. Originally a 4-mm guide rod (Fig. 4.11a) was used for the femoral nail and the earlier generation of AO/ASIF tibial nails. For the somewhat stiffer universal tibial nail, a more flexible 3-mm guide rod (Fig. 4.11b) is mandatory. This rod is flattened at both ends to prevent the passage of reamers. The 4 mm guide rod is still recommended for femoral nails.

The instruments necessary for inserting femoral nails are shown in Fig. 4.12.

The markings on the insertion handles, on the threaded conical bolts and on the nuts have recently changed. Earlier instruments were marked "9 to 12", "12 to 16" and "16 to 19" mm; the new ones are marked "9–12", "13–16" and "17–19" (see Fig. 4.12).

To prepare the universal femoral nail for insertion, proceed as follows:

Screw the threaded conical bolt by hand into the nail, then slide the insertion handle over it until its cams engage in the positioning grooves at the end of the intramedullary nail. Tighten the conical bolt lightly either by hand or by means of the socket wrench. Attach the locking nut to the conical bolt and tighten it with the pin wrench. Screw the ram guide to the end of the conical bolt (Fig. 4.13).

Use the ram to drive in the nail over the guide rod (Fig. 4.13). To prevent the guide rod backing out, use the guide rod retainer.

Figure 4.14 shows the instruments used for inserting tibial nails.

To prepare the universal tibial nail for insertion, proceed as follows:

Fit the insertion handle on the nail, screw the conical bolt through the insertion handle into the nail, and lightly tighten the bolt with the combination wrench. Note that the conical bolt for the tibia fits through the handle only from the proximal side.

Set the locking nut on the free end of the conical bolt and tighten securely with the socket wrench. Check that the cams of the insertion handle engage properly in the positioning grooves at the end of the nail; the handle should point medially. Then screw on and tighten the curved driving piece firmly with the driving head fitted and tightened by the pin wrench (Fig. 4.15).

For both the femur and the tibia, the insertion handle and the intramedullary nail form a firmly connected entity that reliably transfers any force required and is easy to use (Fig. 4.16).

To disentangle the insertion handle, conical bolt and nail, use the open-end or socket wrench to release the conical bolt. To do so, hold the insertion handle firmly and slacken the locking nut about half a turn. This ensures that there is little or no force applied to the nail and prevents its deformation and thus jamming of the conical bolt (Fig. 4.17).

For both femur and tibia, extract the nail with the ram guide fitted with the flexible grip. Use the ram guide to guide the ram and strike the ram against the grip's metal head (Fig. 4.16).

Fig. 4.11 Guide rods.

a Guide rods, 3 mm in diameter, for tibial nailing. To prevent use of the guide rod for reaming, its flattened ends do not accept reamers.

b The 4-mm guide rod is still recommended in femoral nailing.

Fig. 4.11

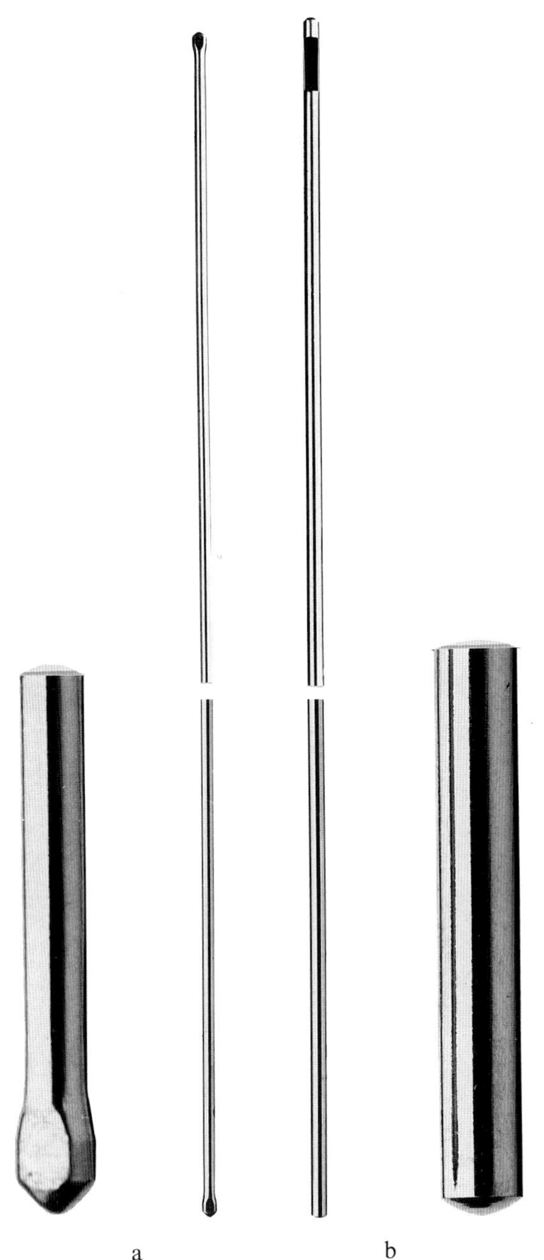

Fig. 4.12 Instruments for inserting femoral nails.

a Insertion handle for 9–12 mm outer diameter universal femoral nail, threaded conical bolt, and locking nut.

b As (a), but for 13–16 mm nails.

c As (a), but for 17–19 mm nails.

d Ram guide. This is screwed to the free end of the threaded conical bolt.

e Ram (about 1.5 kg), cannulated to slide on the guide tube.

f Guide rod retainer. Inserted in the guide tube, the guide rod retainer prevents the guide rod backing out due to inertia.

g Pin wrench, used for tightening the locking nut on the threaded conical bolt.

h Socket wrench.

i Combination wrench.

k Flexible grip, used for holding the ram guide and for extracting the nail.

l Gauge (autoclavable), used for control of diameter of medullary nails and reamers.

Fig. 4.13 Assembly with guide tube and ram for inserting the femoral nail.

a Insertion handle.

b Threaded conical bolt inserted in the universal femoral nail.

c Locking nut.

d Ram guide.

e Ram.

f Flexible grip.

g Guide rod retainer.

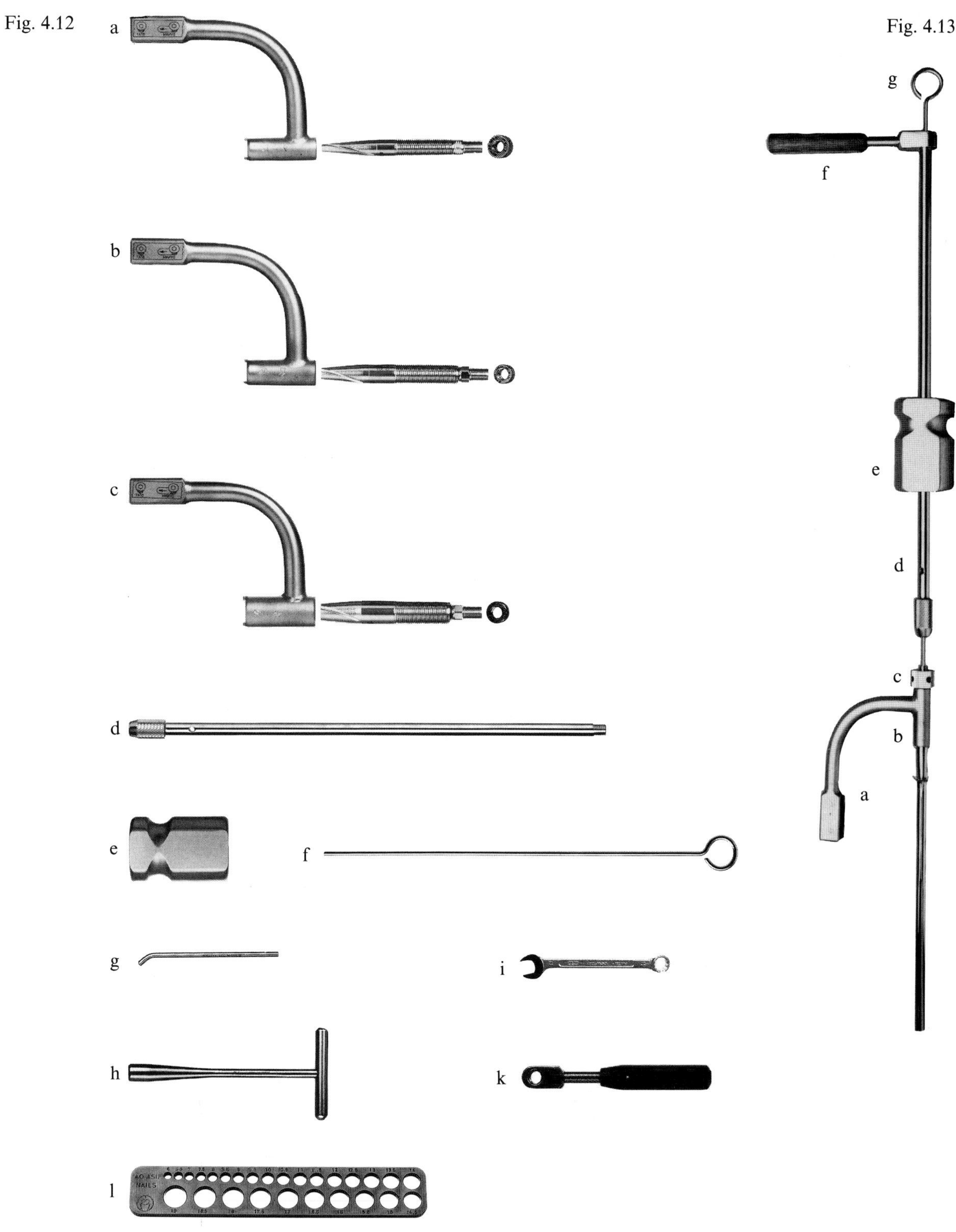

Fig. 4.12

Fig. 4.13

Fig. 4.14 Instruments for inserting the tibial nail.

- a Insertion handle for 10–14 mm outer diameter tibial nail, threaded conical bolt and locking nut.
- b Ram guide.
- c Flexible grip.
- d Curved driving piece.
- e Driving head.
- f Ram.
- g Pin wrench.
- h Combination wrench.
- i Socket wrench.
- k Gauge (autoclavable).
- l Guide rod retainer.

Fig. 4.15 Assembly with ram guide and ram for inserting the tibial nail.

- A Standard assembly with driving head for insertion by hammer.
- B Alternative assembly with ram guide for insertion by ram.
- a Insertion handle for tibial nails. For greater clarity, the position of the handle is shown turned through 90°, parallel with the plane of the illustration. Properly oriented, the bend of the curved driving piece is perpendicular to the plane of the illustration, i.e. mediolateral.
- b Threaded conical bolt.
- c Locking nut.
- d Curved driving piece.
- e Driving head.
- f Ram guide.
- g Ram.
- h Guide rod.

Fig. 4.14

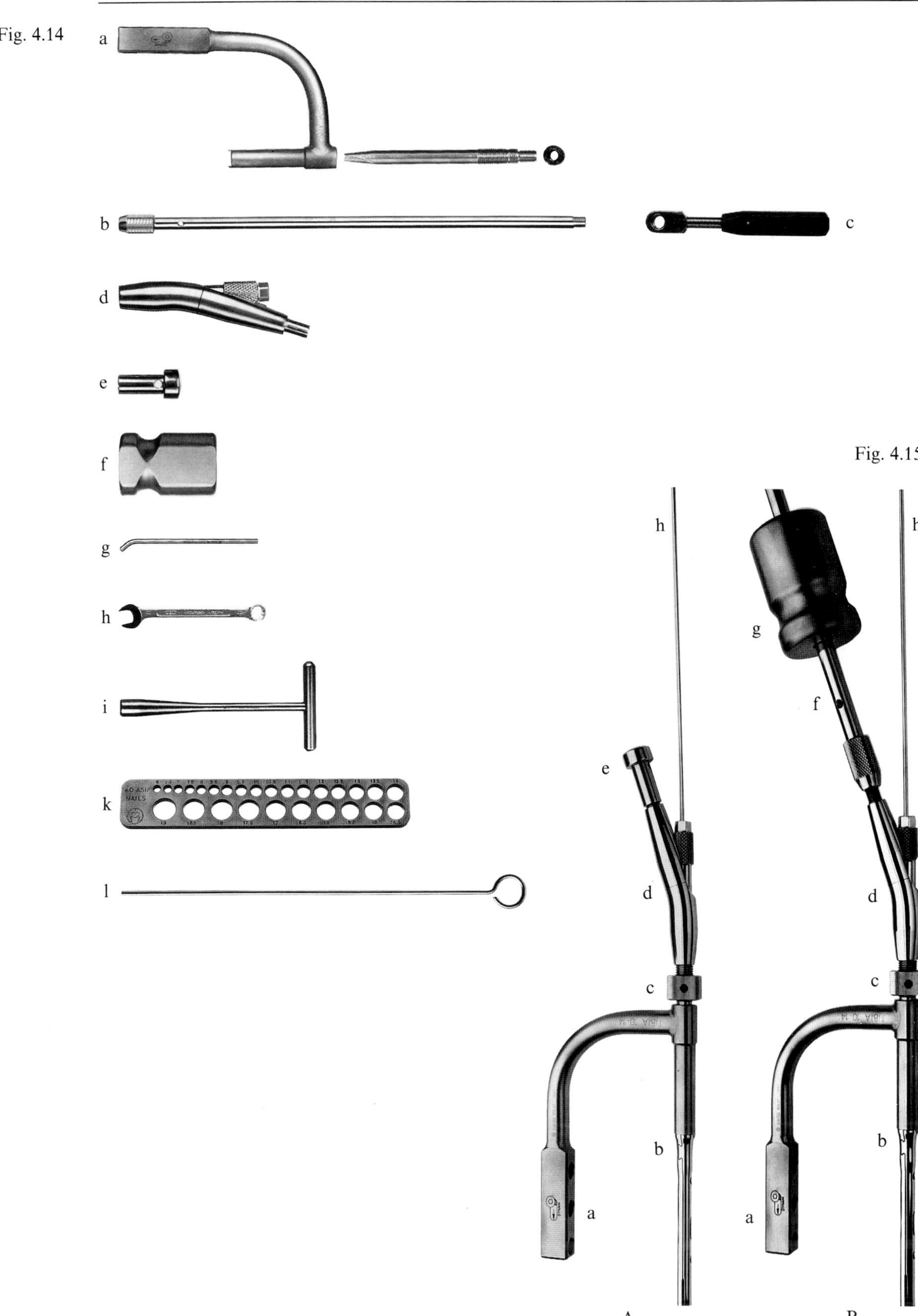

Fig. 4.15

Fig. 4.16 Universal femoral and tibial nails with insertion handle attached.

a Universal tibial nail with insertion handle.

b Universal femoral nail with insertion handle for 13–16 mm nails.

Note: The threaded conical bolt for tibial nails does not fit femoral nails and their insertion handles.

Fig. 4.17 Unscrewing the threaded conical bolt.

a If the insertion handle is not held by hand when the conical bolt is unscrewed, the torque M applied by the wrench is transmitted through the nail to the bone. The bone has to resist with the reactive moment M_r. This action causes the nail to deform in V_1 and V_2. Thereby the conical bolt is jammed.

b The proper way to release the conical bolt is to hold the handle firmly to neutralize the torque M as it is applied. The positioning grooves G permit the direct transmission to the handle of the reactive moment M_r in the plane of the entry aperture of the nail. As a result, the nail is not subjected to stress and there is no deformation.

c If the conical bolt jams, grip the proximal nail end with the locking plier and use the combination wrench to slacken the bolt.

Fig. 4.16

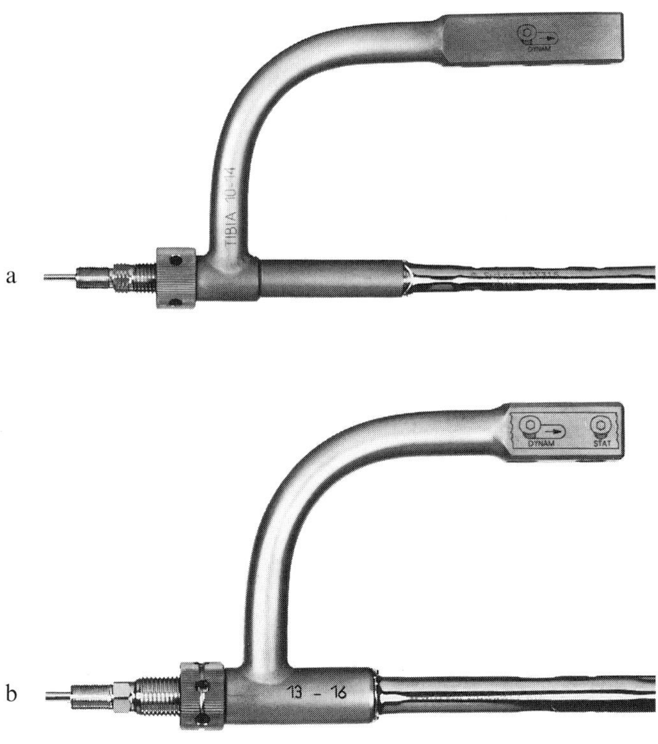

Fig. 4.17

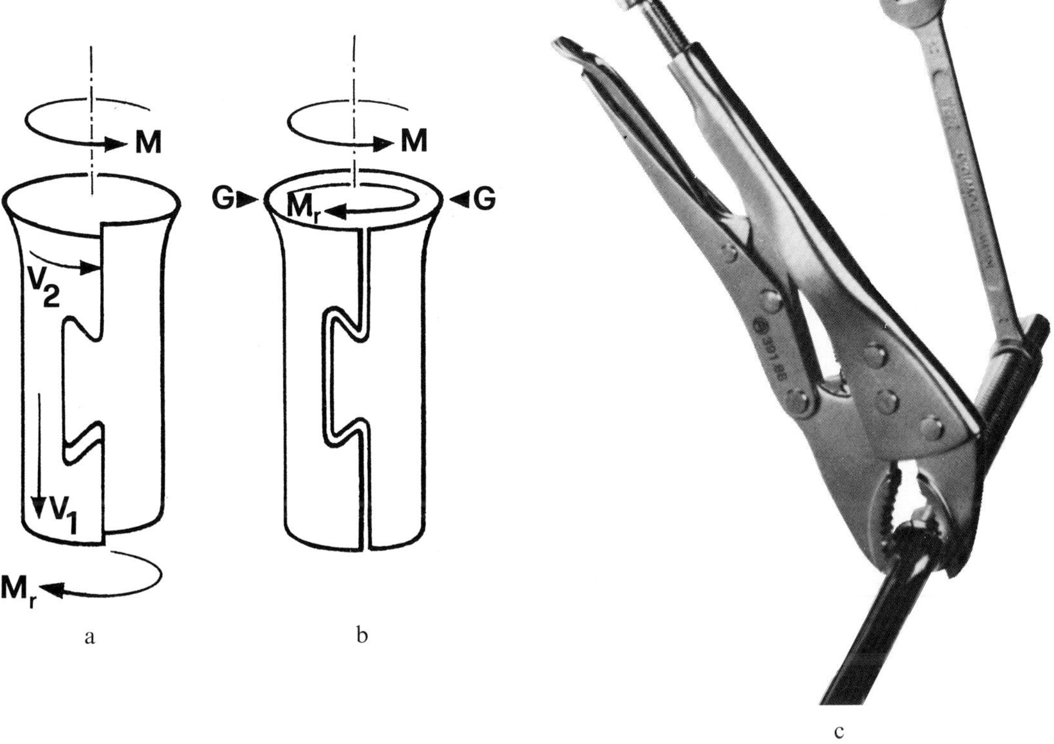

4.3.3 Locking Instruments for Femoral and Tibial Intramedullary Nails

Locking requires instruments to locate the locking holes. Proximal locking is very simple, because the insertion handle serves as the aiming device. Apart from slight differences in the shape of the insertion handles, there is no difference between locking procedures on the femur and the tibia (Fig. 4.18).

Distal locking is impossible without an x-ray image intensifier. The nail's deformation due to bending and torsion during insertion makes accurate positioning in the distal region using mechanical aiming devices impossible. The instruments necessary for distal locking are shown in Figs. 4.19–4.21.

The 3.2- and 4.5-mm drill bits are necessary only if 4.5-mm shaft screws are used. For some time, the AO used these drill bits to prepare the seat for these screws used for interlocking – a procedure which is not recommended any more and should only be considered if there is no locking bolt available.

Fig. 4.18 Using the insertion handle as a guide for proximal locking of AO/ASIF universal nails.

A Proximal locking of the universal femoral nail. The insertion handle has two aiming holes.

a Assembly with inserted drill sleeve and trocar. For proximal locking, the insertion handle remains attached to the nail and acts as the aiming device. It has a distal hole for locating the static locking hole in the nail, and a proximal slotted hole for dynamic locking.

b Use the proximal hole in the handle for dynamic locking. Insert the trocar and tissue protector sleeve, and advance them to the bone surface.

c Use the distal hole in the handle for static locking. The procedure is the same as for dynamic locking.

B Proximal locking of the universal tibial nail. The insertion handle has three aiming holes to permit some variation in positioning the locking bolts. Otherwise, the technique is similar to femoral proximal locking.

a Assembly with drill sleeve and trocar inserted.

b Use the proximal hole for static locking.

c Use the middle hole for dynamic locking.

d The distal hole is also used for static locking.

Fig. 4.18

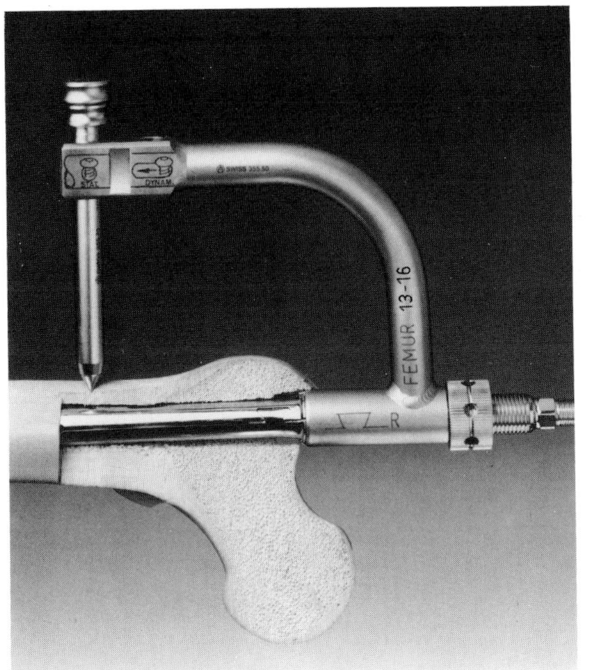

a

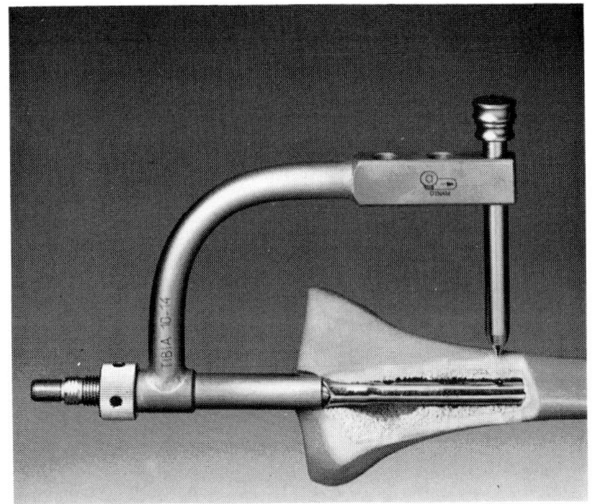

a

b c

A

b c d

B

Fig. 4.19 Instruments for distal locking.

a 4.0-mm diameter drill bit on 4.5-mm diameter shaft. The 4.5-mm shaft ensures accurate guidance of the drill bit in the 4.5-mm inner diameter drilling sleeve.

b Hexagonal screwdriver for AO screws, for tightening fixation and locking bolts, and for adjusting the direction finder on the aiming device. The holding sleeve for screws many be fitted on the screwdriver and can be used for removal of screws.

c Depth gauge for locking bolts. Due to the shape of the locking bolt's head and tip, add at least 2 mm to the measured length to obtain the correct length of bolt.

d Distal aiming device, with direction finder and aiming trocar.

e Self-cutting fixation bolts for femoral and tibial nailing, in connection with distal aiming device.

f 8-mm and 4.5-mm diameter tissue protection sleeves.

g Trocar.

Fig. 4.19

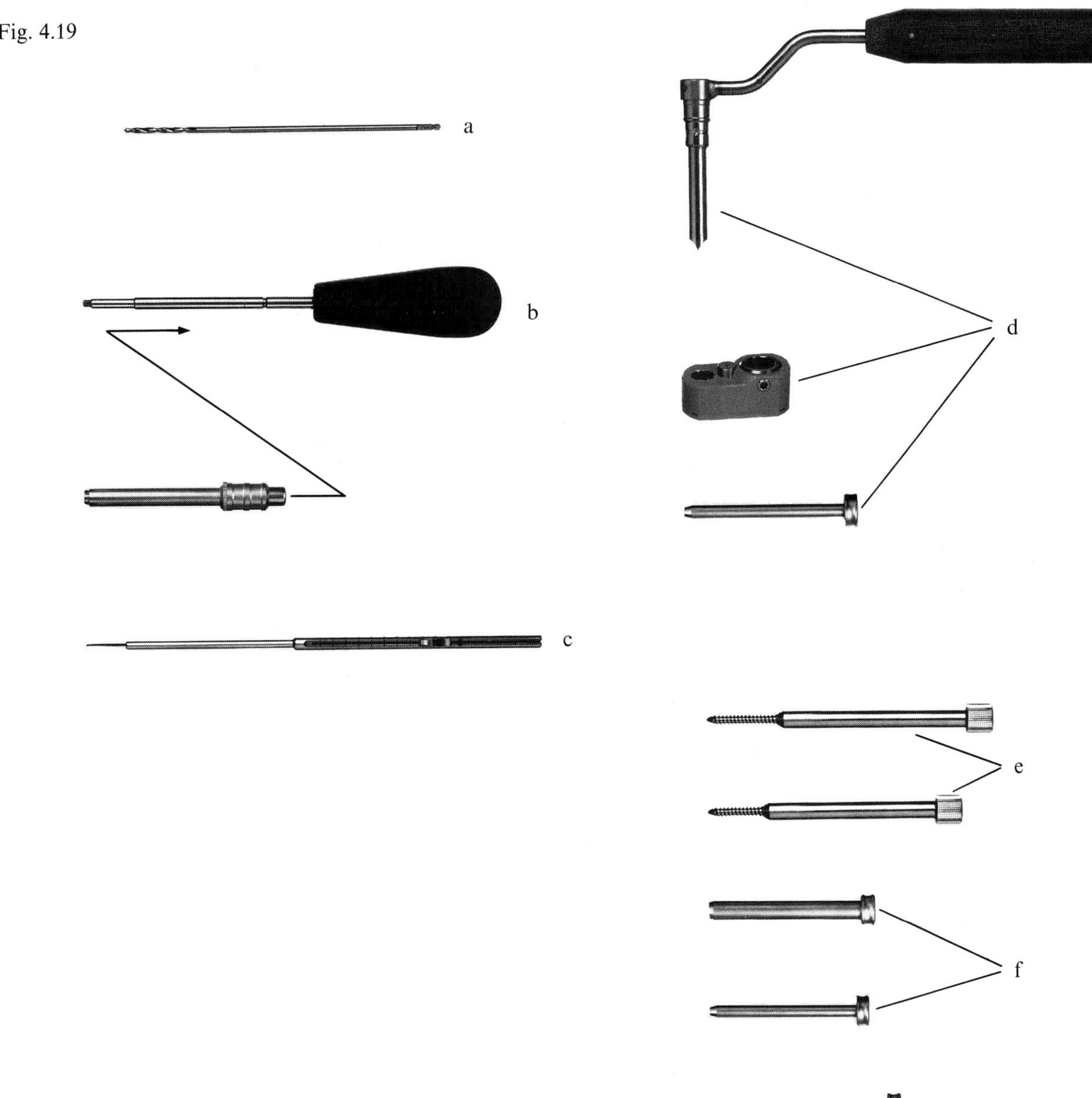

Fig. 4.20 Distal aiming device.

a The aiming device is a handle with inserts. It has a removable

b Direction finder, of fiber-reinforced phenolic resin.

c The handle with inserts and assembled direction finder.

d The metal edges permit the alignment of the direction finder parallel to the nail's axis.

e The insert may be a trocar, an aiming trocar or a protection sleeve.

Fig. 4.21 Direction finder on the distal aiming device.

a The direction finder has a metal dot and two metal rings. With the dot centered in the two concentric circles, the direction finder's axis is parallel to the image intensifier's beam when the source is placed near the leg. The direction finder is adjusted to compensate a divergence of 4° of the beam.

b The aiming trocar also has a metal dot. This permits centering the trocar exactly in the locking hole.

c The metal bars help in locating the second locking hole when the aiming device is exactly centered and fixed in the first locking hole. Turn the direction finder until the metal bars are parallel to the nail's axis (c); the positioning hole (d) is then automatically aligned with the second locking hole, which may not appear as a circle on image intensifier monitor.

d The positioning hole (d) is the same distance from the axis of the aiming device as the two locking holes in the nail. This facilitates location of the second locking hole.

Fig. 4.20

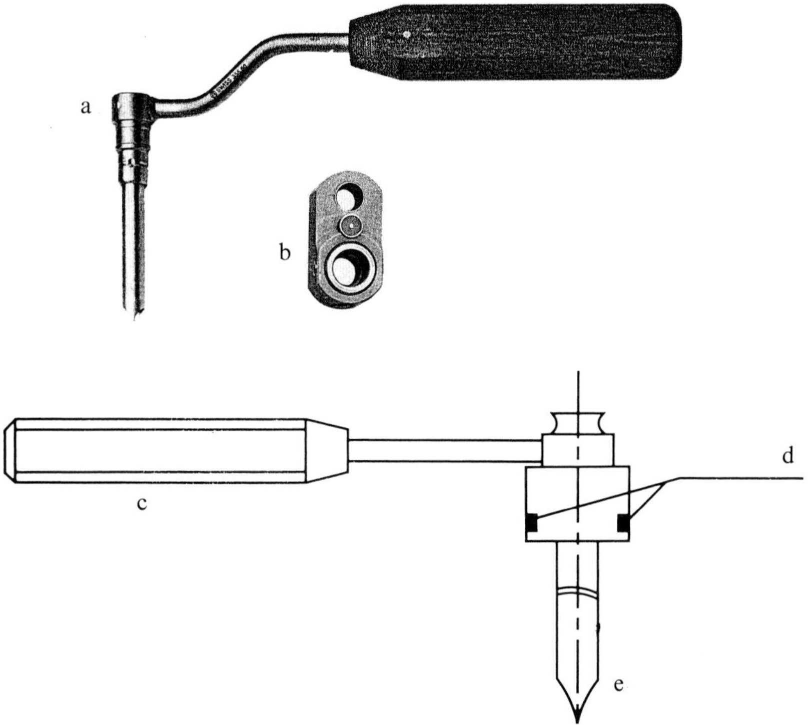

Fig. 4.21

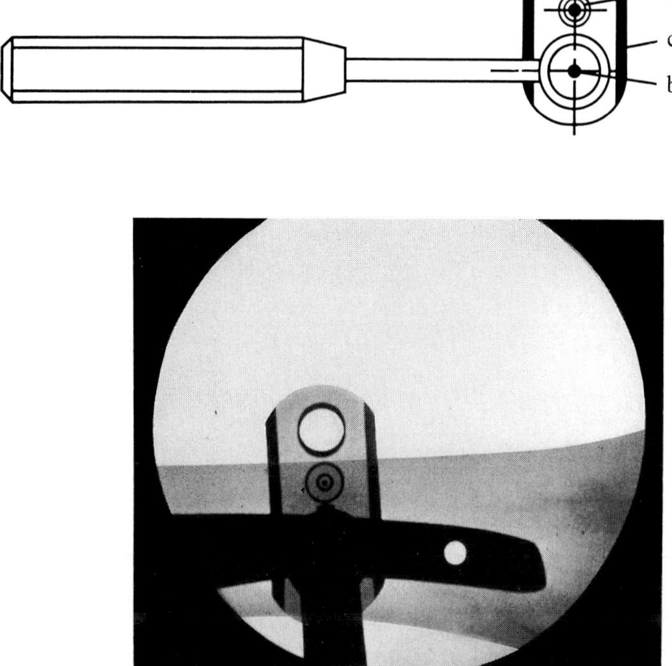

4.3.4 The Large Distractor

The distractor is used temporarily for gentle open or closed reduction of fractured long bones, pelvis and acetabulum. In many cases it makes the relatively difficult task of positioning the patient on a fracture table unnecessary. The large distractor will also facilitate the reduction of complex articular fractures.

The femoral distractor was originally developed from the Harrington distractor and proved invaluable for many years (M.E. Müller et al. 1977; Fig. 4.22). In 1988 an improved model of the large femoral distractor was introduced, which greatly increased its adaptability (Fig. 4.23). At its proximal end, the distractor has a sleeve-holding bracket. Each joint of the distractor can be released and fixed separately. Used in conjunction with the distal carriage, it permits movement about several axes and in several planes. This makes the distractor readily adaptable for coping with awkward positioning problems (Fig. 4.24).

For the closed reduction of fractures prior to intramedullary nailing, additional aiming devices are necessary (Figs. 4.25, 4.26).

Fig. 4.22 Distractor (large, simple model).

a Threaded rod.

b Distal carriage.

c, d Locking nuts.

e Fixation nut.

f, f′ Schanzscrew-holding sleeve.

Fig. 4.23 Distractor (large, for three-dimensional application).

a Proximal and distal Schanz screws are used for attaching the distractor to the fragments.

b Distal carriage and

c Proximal sleeve-holding bracket permit movement about several axes and in several planes.

d Locking nuts secure the parts, 14 mm inner diameter.

e Threaded rod.

f Schanzscrew-holding sleeve fixes the Schanz screws to the distractor.

Fig. 4.22

Fig. 4.23

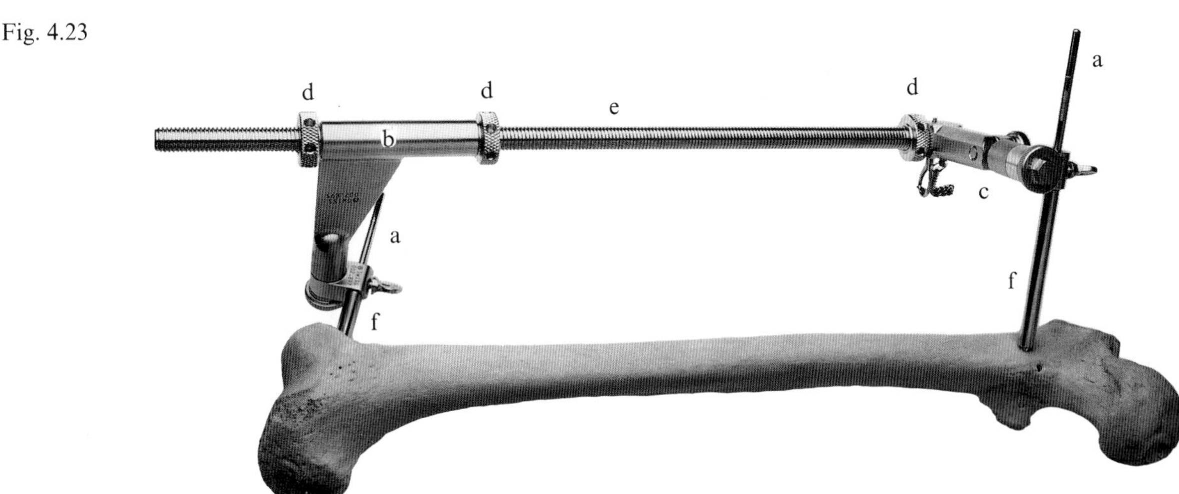

Fig. 4.24 Joints of the distractor.

a The modified large distractor permits movement about several axes and in several planes.

b Distal carriage.

c Proximal sleeve-holding bracket.

Fig. 4.25 Additional aiming equipment in conjunction with femoral nailing.

a The curved aiming attachment fits on the insertion handle for AO/ASIF universal nails.

b The curved aiming attachment (*3*) is designed to prevent the Schanz screw (*4*) touching the intramedullary nail, represented in the figure by the manipulation nail (*1*).

c For femoral nailing, open the bone from the piriform fossa and ream to 10 mm. Then set a manipulation nail (*1*) in position. Fit the curved aiming attachment (*3*) on the insertion handle (*2*) and insert the proximal Schanz screw perpendicular to the universal nail's axis (*4*). Distally, fix the distractor to the femur by a Schanz screw parallel to the axis of the knee joint. Then proceed with reduction, ream the cavity and drive in the nail (see Sect. 4.4).

Fig. 4.24

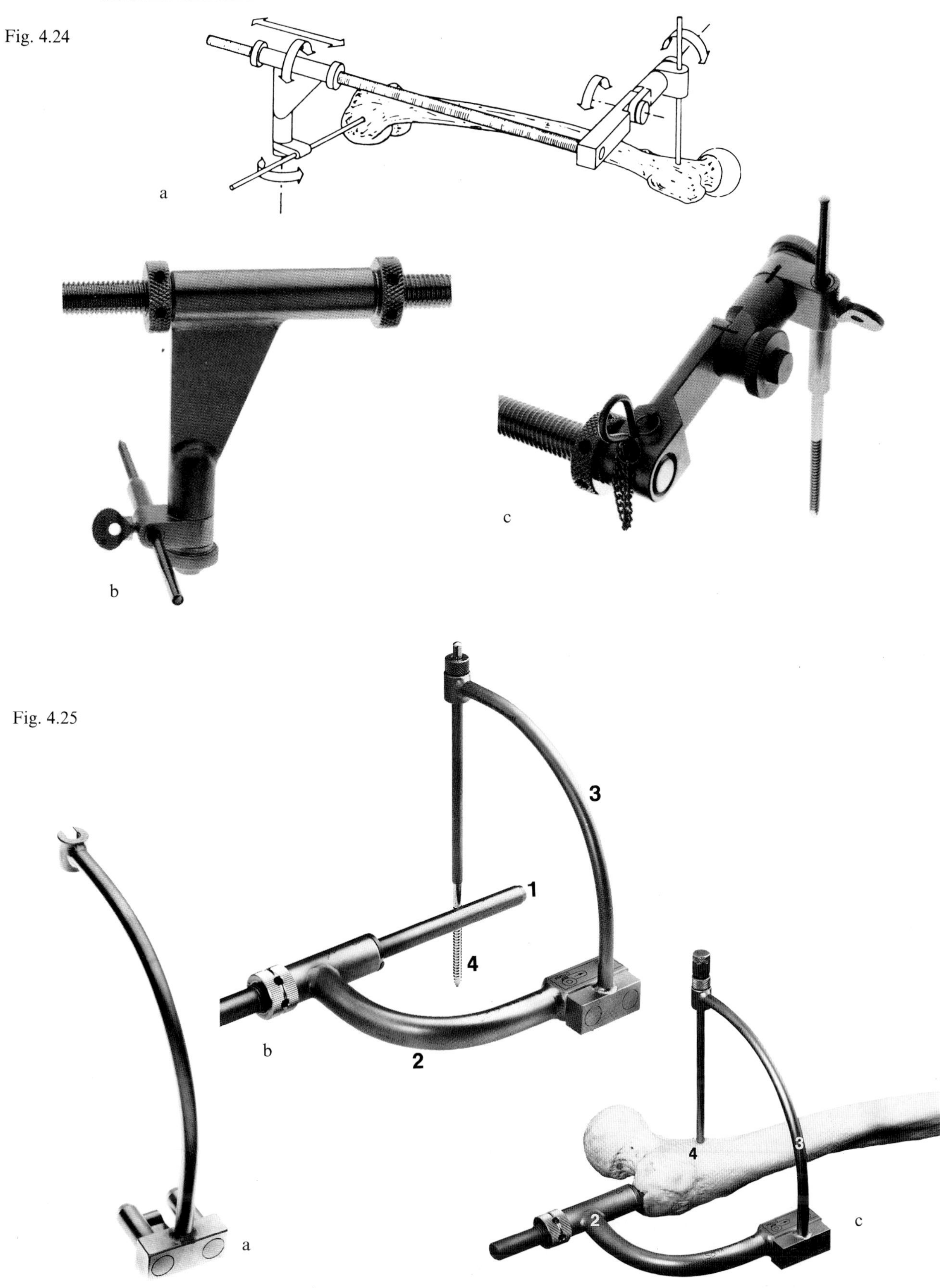

Fig. 4.26 Positioning of a Schanz screw in the proximal femur.

a The insertion handle is fixed firmly on the manipulation nail. The cut c–c is shown in b.

b The anatomical situation of the cut c–c shows the optimal positioning of the Schanz screw avoiding the arteria and vena femoralis and the nervus ischiadicus. (The description follows Faure and Merloz 1987).

1 Femur (Trochanter minor); *2* M. tensor fasciae latae; *3* M. vastus lateralis; *4* M. vastus intermedius; *5* M. vastus medialis; *6* M. rectus femoris; *7* M. sartorius; *8* M. iliopsoas; *9* M. pectineus; *10* M. adductor longus; *11* M. adductor brevis; *12* M. adductor magnus; *13* M. gracilis; *14* M. semitendinosus; *15* M. semimembranosus; *16* M. biceps femoris; *17* M. gluteus maximus; *18* A. and V. femoralis; *19* A. and V. profunda femoris; *20* V. saphena magna; *21* N. ischiadicus.

Fig. 4.26

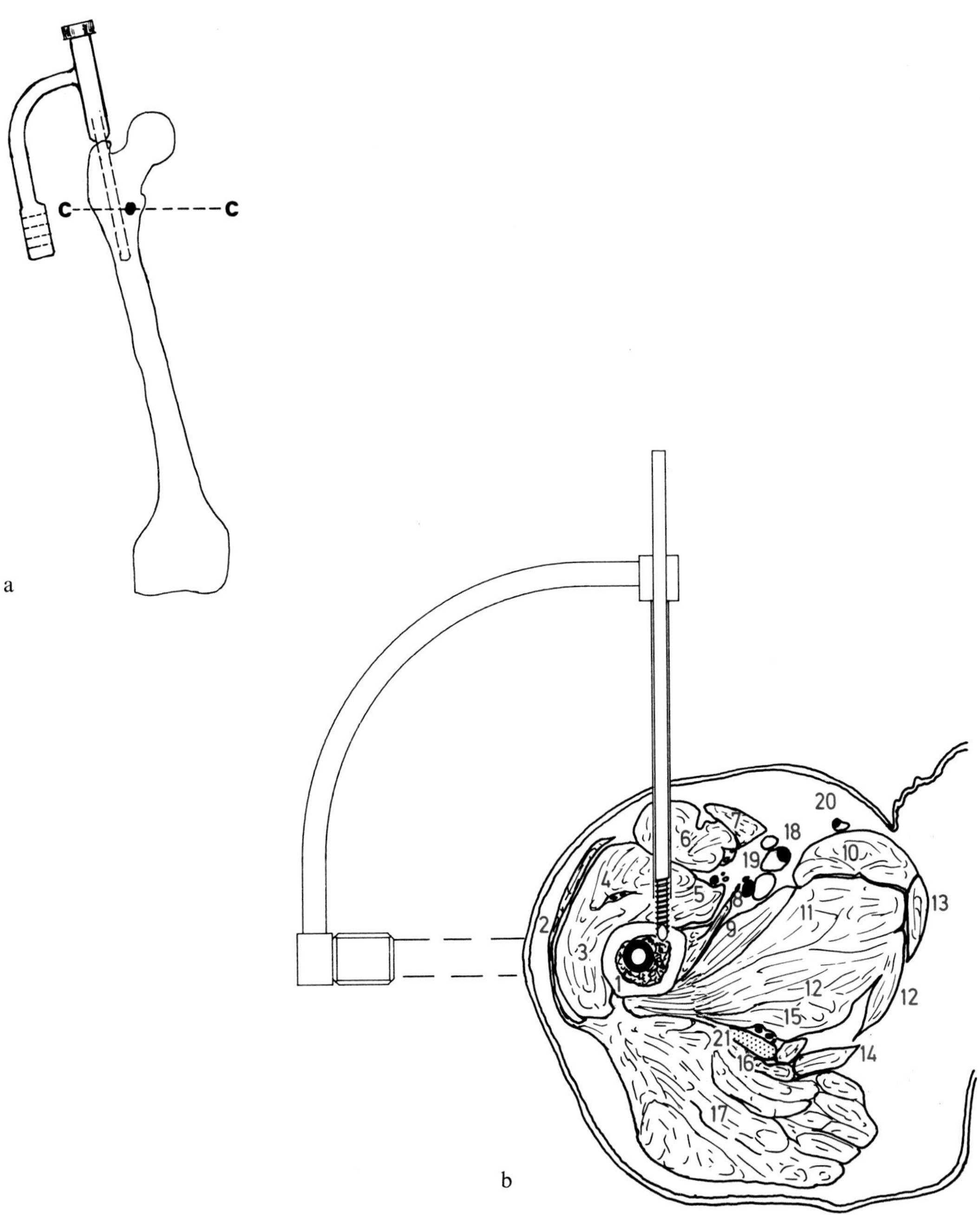

4.4 Intramedullary Nailing Technique for Closed Fractures of the Femur

4.4.1 Anatomic Considerations

In intramedullary nailing of the femur, the choice of the correct point of insertion is particularly important. The point of insertion in the technique used for many years with the conventional AO/ASIF femoral intramedullary nail was immediately lateral and ventral from the tip of the greater trochanter (Müller et al. 1977). This occasionally led to an undesirable thinning of the medial cortex and not infrequently to valgus bending of the nail.

With the development of the universal femoral nail, the earlier point of entry was no longer suitable because of the nail's stiffness and curvature, since it would not allow reaming along the bone axis and caused the nail to twist during insertion. This necessitated locating the point of insertion in the prolongation of the medullary canal – the piriform fossa (Fig. 4.27; Zuber et al. 1988).

Fig. 4.27 Point of insertion recommended since 1988 for AO/ASIF universal femoral nail.

a Current approach with the cannulated cutter over the centering pin, recommended since 1988. The detail shows the centering pin in the tip of the cannulated cutter.

b Anterior aspect.

c Superior aspect. The point of insertion is located in the piriform fossa, i.e. further medially than in the conventional technique.

Fig. 4.27

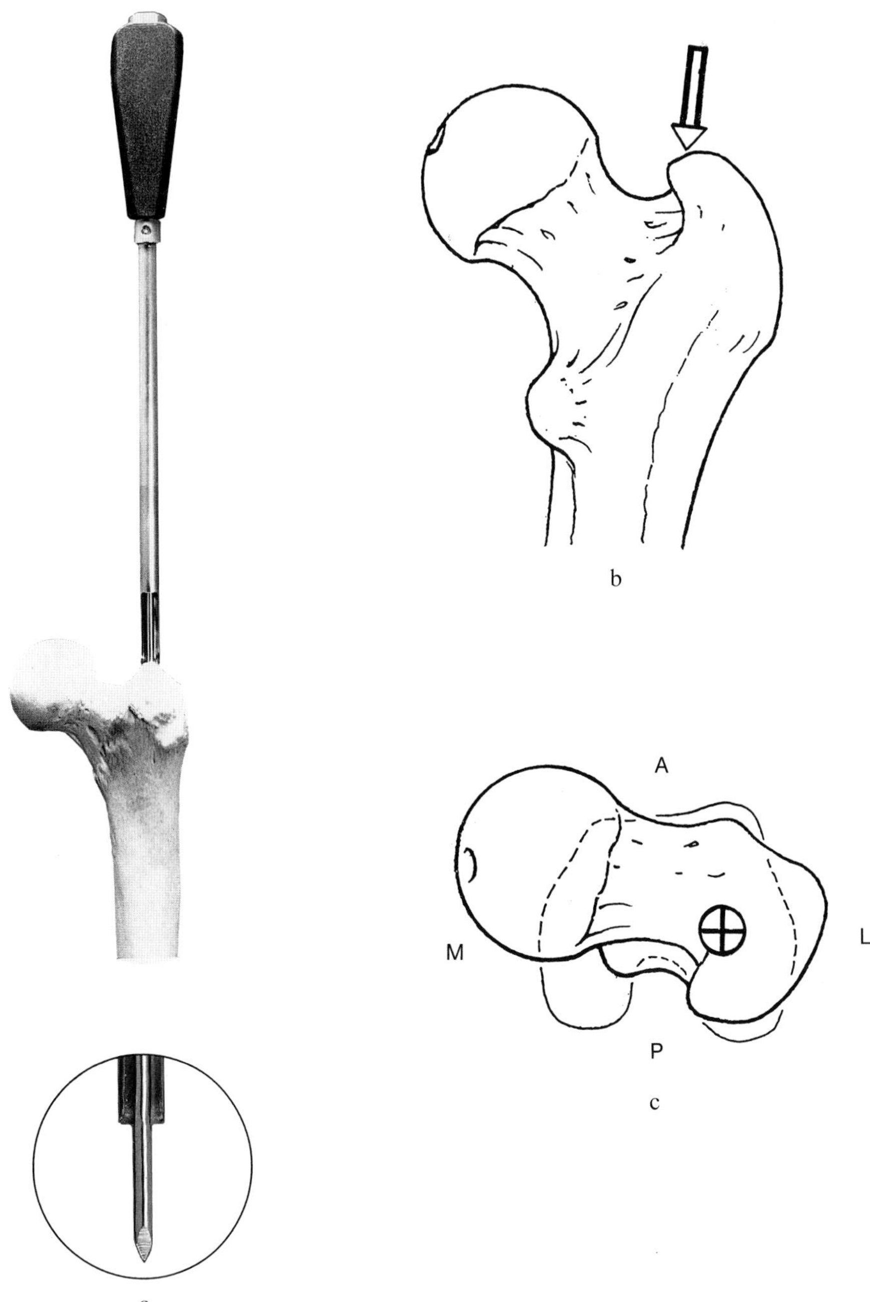

4.4.2 Preoperative Positioning of the Patient

The fracture may be reduced by open or closed technique. Closed reduction, with the patient positioned on a fracture table, is the preferred method (Figs. 4.28, 4.29). For this, an image intensifier is necessary. Alternatively the large distractor may be used, eliminating the need for a fracture table (Figs. 4.30, 4.31). It simplifies reduction, particularly in patients with multiple trauma.

Fig. 4.28 Lateral positioning on a fracture table. For lateral positioning, use a fracture table with long cantilever extensions. Place the patient in a lateral decubitus position, with the pelvis held exactly vertical by pelvic supports on both sides of the table. The perineum rests on a well-padded perineal post. In male patients, check that the genitals are freely mobile.

Fig. 4.29 Supine positioning on a fracture table. In supine positioning on a fracture table, the leg of the injured femur is allowed to hang with the knee flexed at 90°. The patient's pelvis should lie flat on the table to ensure the correct rotational alignment of the femur. Rotation cannot be corrected. If possible, slightly adduct the injured leg at the hip.

Fig. 4.30 Lateral positioning on a standard table. On a standard table, place the patient in a lateral position; a vacuum mattress may be helpful. Flex the injured leg forward at about 45°, with the knee bent at 90° and the foot placed on the uninjured leg. Use a distractor for reduction.

Fig. 4.31 Supine positioning on a standard table. In supine positioning on a standard table, slightly abduct the uninjured leg in a lateral direction and adduct the injured leg. Use a distractor for reduction.

Fig. 4.28

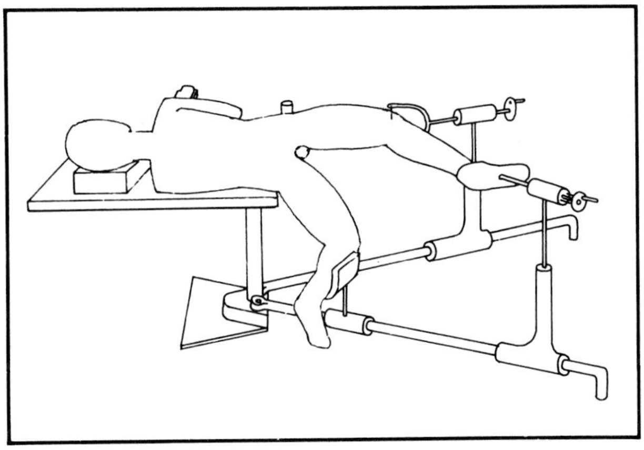

Fig. 4.29

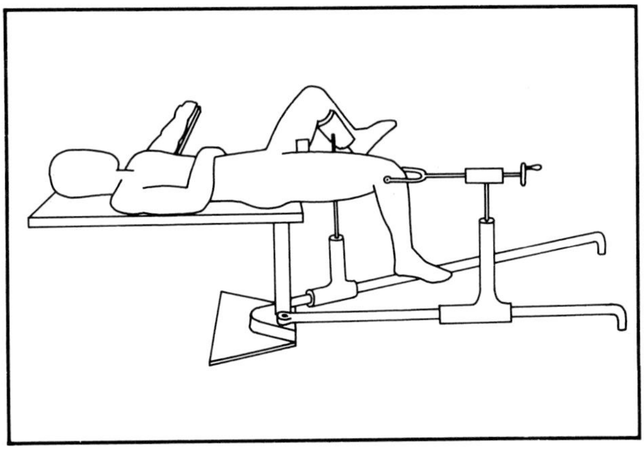

Fig. 4.30

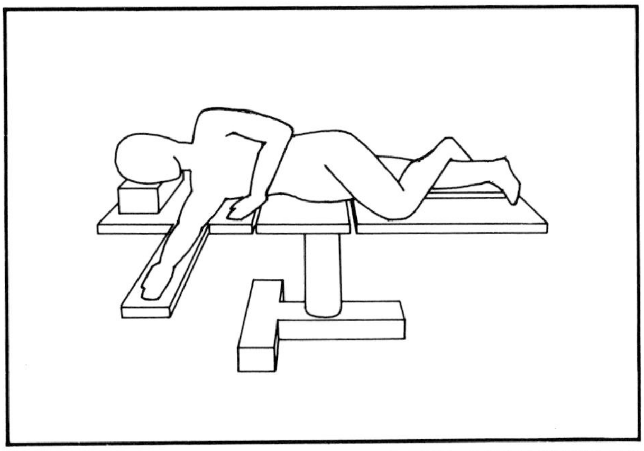

Fig. 4.31

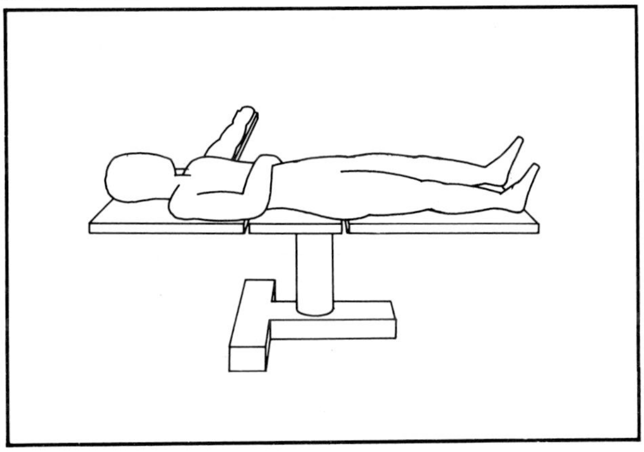

4.4.3 Choice of Nail Length

To determine the approximate length of nail before surgery, measure the distance from the tip of the greater trochanter to the intra-articular space of the knee on the patient's uninjured side and subtract 20–30 mm. Prepare this and the next longer and shorter lengths of nail before the operation. After reduction, direct measurement is possible; subtract the exposed length of the reaming rod from its overall length of 950 mm or use the guide rod for comparison (Fig. 4.32).

Fig. 4.32 Measuring the length of nail for the femur.

a On the patient's uninjured leg, measure the distance L_+ from the tip of the greater trochanter to the intra-articular space of the knee. Subtract 20–30 mm to obtain the length L of the nail.

b Use the accurately positioned reaming rod to measure after reduction.
Subtract length A which remains exposed from the long reaming rod's total length of 950 mm.

c Comparative measurement. Hold the guide rod parallel to the accurately positioned reaming rod. Align the guide rod's tip with the point of insertion (i). The length from the free end of the reaming rod to the end of the guide rod is the nail length L.

Fig. 4.32

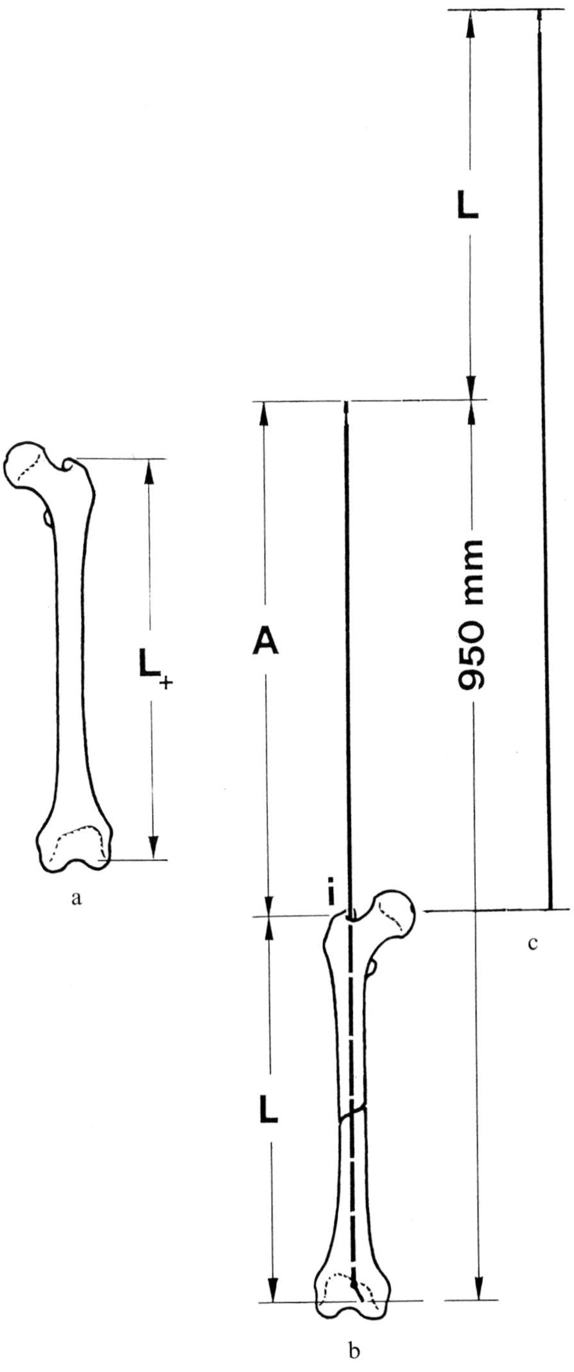

4.4.4 Opening the Medullary Canal

Starting from the greater trochanter, make a straight incision of about 8 cm directed proximally. Split the gluteal muscles to expose the piriform fossa.

Fit the centering pin in the universal chuck and position the assembly on the femur at the level of the piriform fossa. Turn and press simultaneously to introduce the centering pin at least 50 mm into the medullary canal, then remove the universal chuck (Fig. 4.33).

Pass the cannulated cutter over the centering pin and tighten the Allen screw to attach it to the centering pin. Rotate the cannulated cutter to open the medullary canal, then remove both instruments (Fig. 4.34). Under image intensification, introduce the 3.0-mm reaming rod with offset ball tip across the fracture site as far as the condylar mass. The reaming rod's angled tip facilitates threading up the fragments. Use the holding forceps to hold the reaming rod. Check correct position using the image intensifier in both planes (Fig. 4.35).

4.4.5 Reaming Technique

Before starting to ream, the correct position of the reaming rod must be checked fluoroscopically. Begin by using the flexible shaft with the 9.0-mm outer diameter fixed front-cutting reamer (Fig. 4.36).

Reaming then progresses with the 8.0 mm flexible shaft using interchangeable reamers in increments of 0.5 mm diameter to between 9.5 mm and 12.5 mm diameter.

If reaming exceeds 12.5 mm outer diameter exchange the 8-mm for the 10-mm flexible shaft and continue reaming in 0.5-mm increments.

When the required diameter is reached, pass the medullary tube over the reaming rod. Remove the reaming rod and replace it with the 4-mm guide rod (Fig. 4.37). The 4-mm guide rod cannot be used with the universal tibial nail but should be used in femoral nailing.

Fig. 4.33 Inserting the centering pin.

Fig. 4.34 Opening the medullary canal with the cannulated cutter.

Fig. 4.35 Inserting the reaming rod.

Fig. 4.36 Reaming with the front-cutting reamer over the reaming rod. Use the tissue protector on the medial side of the flexible shaft to protect the skin and soft tissue.

Fig. 4.37 Replacing the reaming rod. Use the medullary tube to exchange the reaming rod for the guide rod. During replacement, the medullary tube keeps the fragments in place.

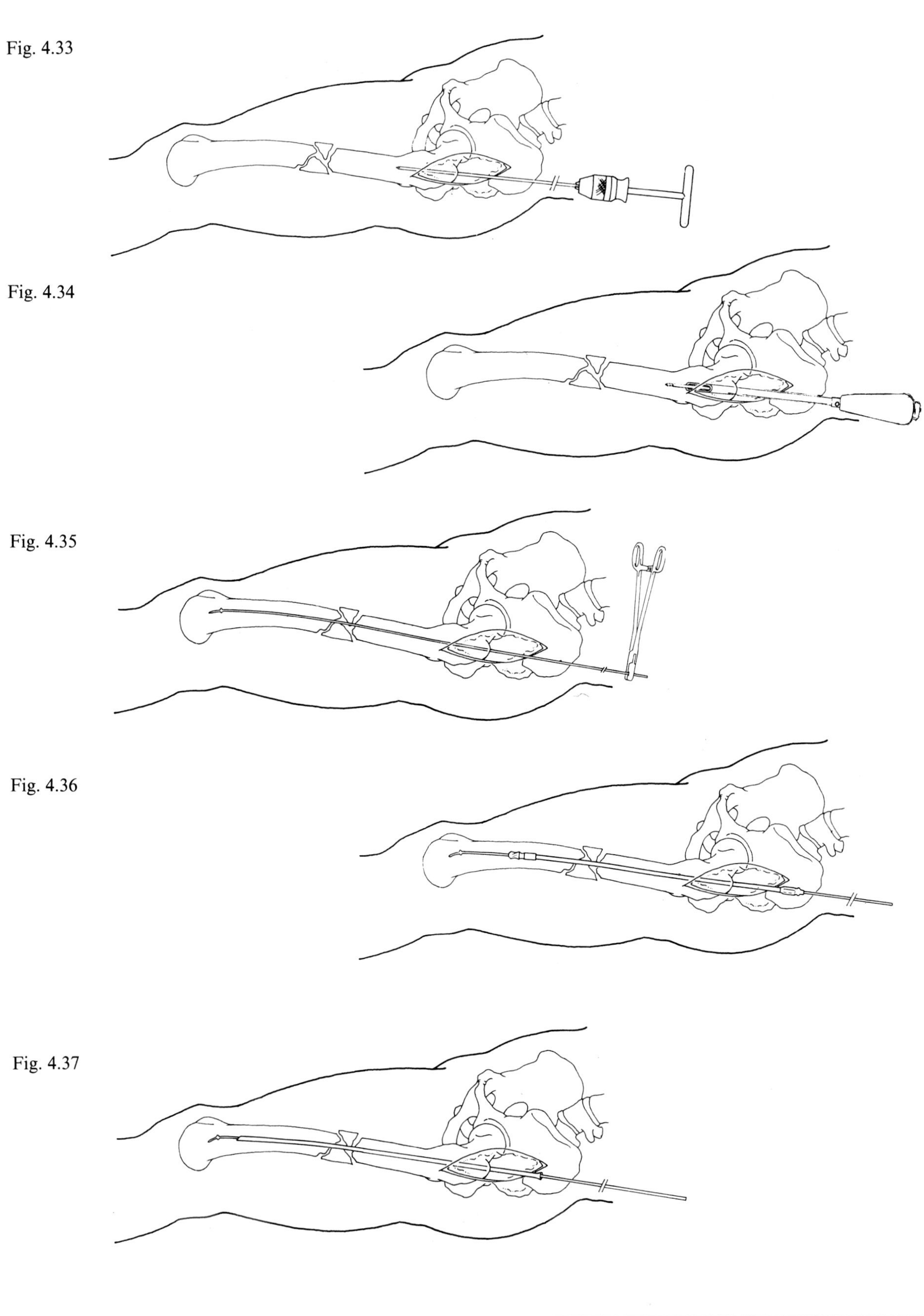
Fig. 4.33
Fig. 4.34
Fig. 4.35
Fig. 4.36
Fig. 4.37

4.4.6 Inserting the Nail

The outside diameter of the selected nail corresponds to the size of the last reamer used. Always double-check the nail diameter by using the special nail gauge.

Pass the nail over the guide rod and insert it as far as possible in the medullary canal. Fit the insertion handle and threaded conical bolt as described in Sect. 4.3. Screw the ram guide on the conical bolt. Check the orientation of the insertion handle relative to the nail (Fig. 4.38).

Use controlled blows with the ram to drive the nail into the medullary canal until its tip reaches the distal metaphysis and the proximal end is flush with the surface of the cortex at the point of insertion (Fig. 4.39). Hold the guide rod retainer on the guide rod to check and prevent the guide rod backing out of the nail due to inertia.

Each blow should advance the nail further into the medullary canal. Otherwise, remove the nail, and drill 0.5–1.0 mm more! (see Sect. 4.6).

If the tip of the trochanter roofs over the piriform fossa, it must be trimmed with a chisel to prevent the insertion handle from exerting a bursting force on the trochanter and/or the femoral neck.

4.4.7 Locking

The locking procedures for the universal intramedullary nails for femur and tibia differ only slightly. See the detailed description of the locking technique for universal femoral and tibial nails in Sect. 4.5.7.

Fig. 4.38 Assembly for inserting the universal femoral nail.

a Guide rod, 950 mm long, 3 mm outer diameter for tibia, 4 mm for femur.

b Insertion handle.

c Threaded conical bolt.

d Locking nut.

e Ram guide.

f Ram.

g Flexible grip.

h Guide rod retainer.

Fig. 4.39 Healing pattern of locked femoral nailing.

Fig. 4.38

Fig. 4.39

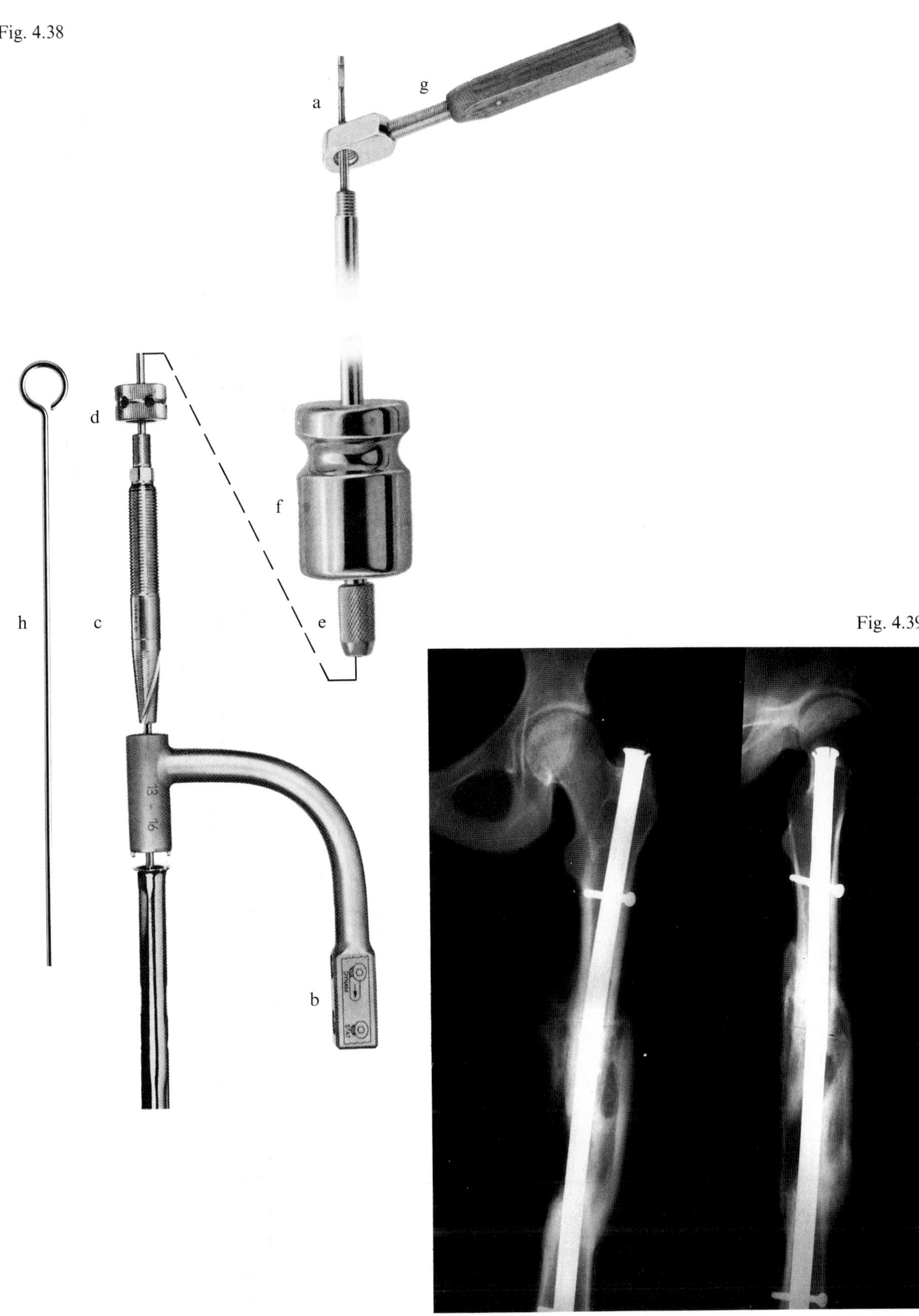

4.5 Intramedullary Nailing Technique for Closed Fractures of the Tibia

4.5.1 Anatomic Considerations

The implantation of a tibial nail differs from the method used for the femoral nail (see Höntzch and Weller 1986). The tibial nail – unlike the femoral nail – cannot be driven into the bone from the proximal side in prolongation of the axis of the tibial medullary canal, because this would necessitate penetrating the tibial intercondylar area and opening the knee. For this reason, the insertion point (i) is slightly offset medially, slightly proximal to the tibial tuberosity, and sufficiently below the tibial intercondylar area (Fig. 4.40) to avoid damage to the joint (see Heini 1987). The awl is used for opening the medullary canal (see Sect. 4.5.4).

On average, the insertion canal (ic) and the axis of the tibial medullary canal (a) form an angle of about 11° in the sagittal plane. During insertion, a straight nail would tend to penetrate the dorsal wall of the medullary canal. The tibial nail's specially tapered tip glides along the dorsal wall of the medullary canal (Fig. 4.41).

Fig. 4.40 Point of insertion and geometry of the tibial medullary canal.

Fig. 4.41 Reducing the insertion force using the specially tapered tip. This section in the sagittal plane shows the 11° angle between the insertion canal (*ic*) and the axis (*a*) of the tibial cavity; for greater clarity, the angle is drawn larger. During insertion, the straight distal part of the nail is aligned with the insertion canal (*ic*). Tip (*t*) of the nail is in close contact with the dorsal wall of the medullary canal. The special tapered tip guides the nail in the direction of the medullary canal (*a*). Its shape prevents it digging into the dorsal wall and jamming, and reduces the effect of the force necessary to insert the nail.

Fig. 4.40

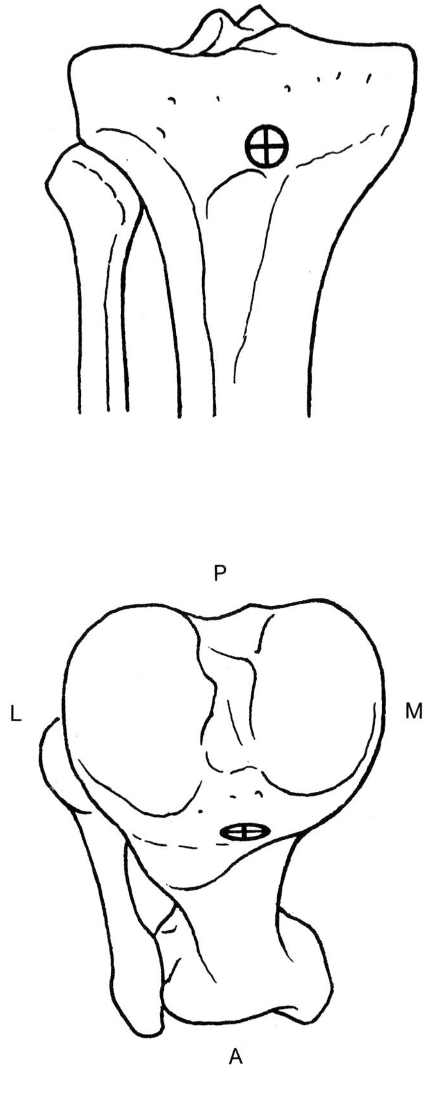

L

M

P

A

Fig. 4.41

11°

a

ic

t

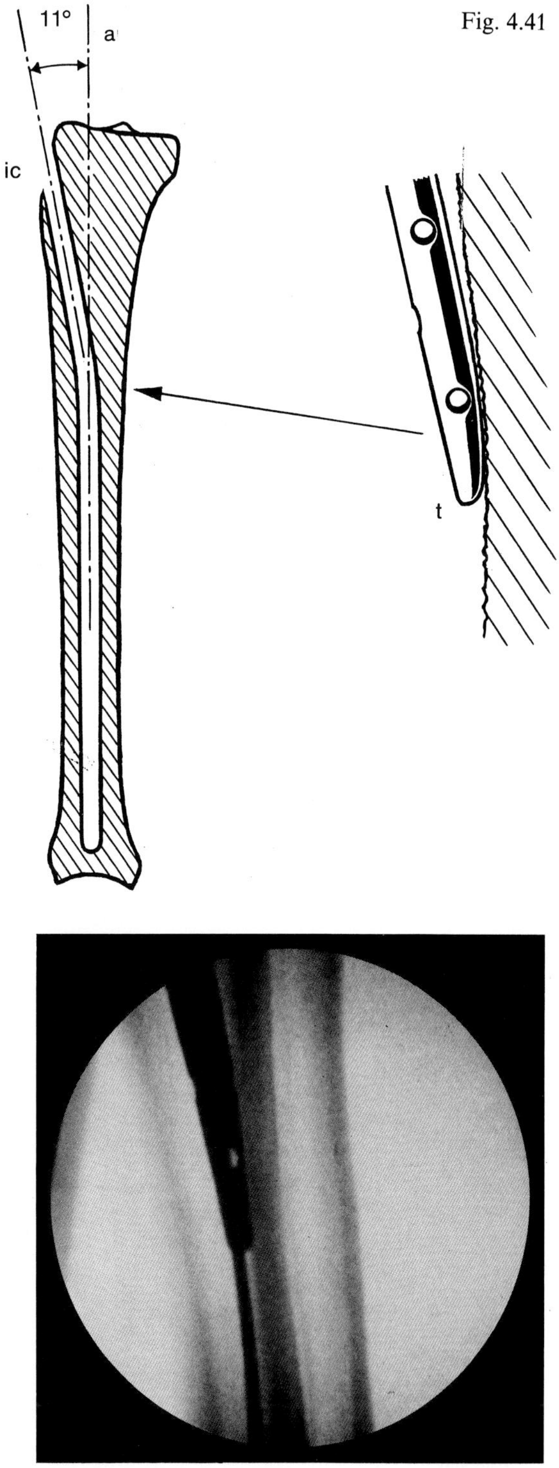

4.5.2 Preoperative Positioning of the Patient

As in the case of the femur, the fracture may be reduced by open or closed technique. An image intensifier is necessary for closed reduction (Figs. 4.42, 4.43). The large distractor is also useful in tibial nailing.

Fig. 4.42 Positioning on a fracture table for tibial nailing.

a In positioning on a fracture table, the patient is in the supine position, with the injured leg bent 90° at the knee and extended obliquely down. Extension is applied via a padded boot or a calcaneal traction pin. In distal locking, the calcaneal traction pin must be used, since the shoe extends too far proximally and obstructs the locking area. It is important to provide adequate padding to the popliteal fossa. The uninjured leg is also flexed.

The image intensifier must have free movement. The C arm in particular must be free to move in the anteroposterior and mediolateral directions. Reduction and the correction of rotation are difficult to achieve during the operation and must be carried out before sterile draping.

b Use a pad to support the distal femur at a sufficient distance from the popliteal artery and vein (*A*, *V*).

c If the pad is not properly posititioned, the force F used to insert the nail inhibits circulation in these vessels and may damage the vascular wall.

Fig. 4.43 Positioning on a standard table for tibial nailing. For positioning on a standard table, the table must be radiolucent. For reduction and temporary fixation the following alternatives may considered:

- Hanging leg.
- Stabilization by tight application of Ace bandages.
- Open reduction and temporary fixation of the fracture by a 4.5-mm DCP attached to the bone by Verbrugge clamps.
- Application of a distractor inserting the Schanz screws in a frontal plane as close to both tibial ends as possible.

Fig. 4.42

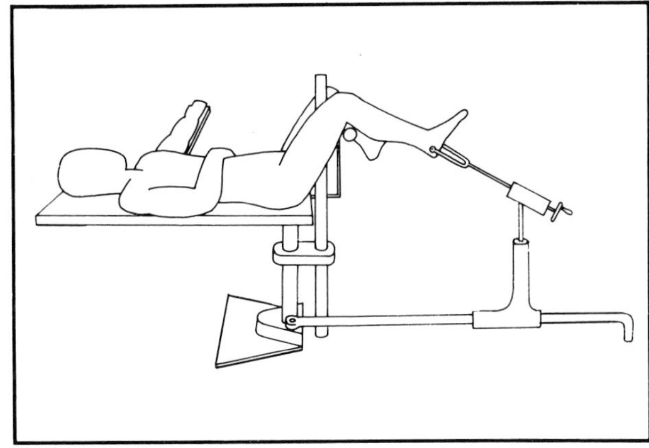

a

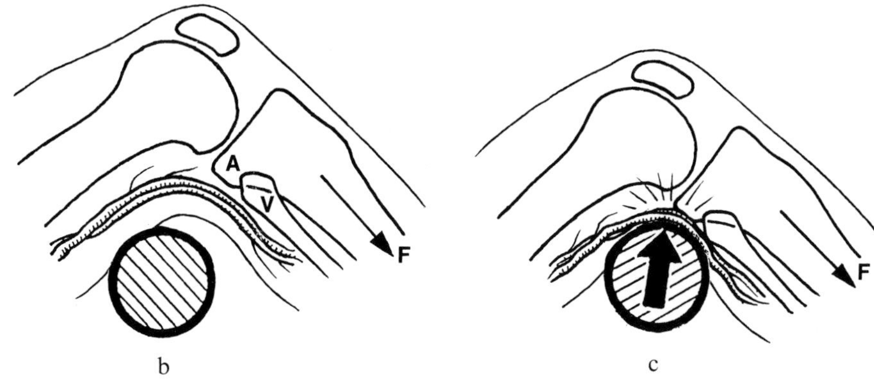

b c

Fig. 4.43

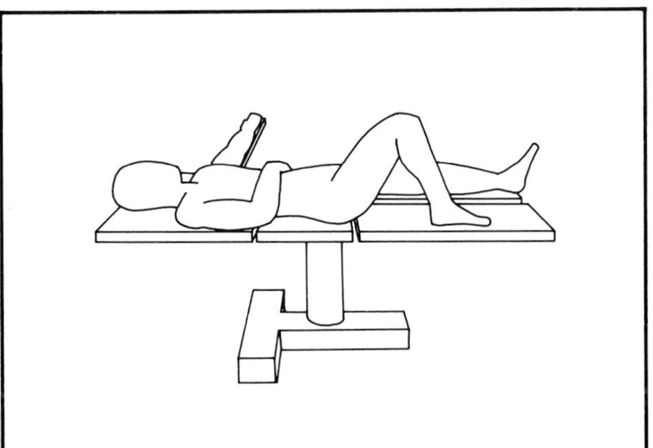

4.5.3 Choice of Nail Length

Measure the length from the intercondylar area of the tibial head to tibiotarsal joint of the uninjured leg and subtract 30–40 mm to obtain the required length of nail. Prepare this length of nail before the operation, together with 15 mm longer and shorter nails. The nail diameter depends on the bone's anatomy and the diameter of the reamed canal (Fig. 4.44; Sect. 4.5.5). To calculate the correct nail length, during operation measure the exposed length of the guide rod and subtract this from its total length of 950 mm.

Fig. 4.44 Measuring the length of nail for the tibia.

a On the patient's uninjured leg, measure the distance L_+ from the intercondylar area of the head of the tibia to the lower articular facet on the malleolar side. Subtract 30–40 mm to obtain the exact length L of the nail.

b Use the accurately positioned reaming rod to measure after reduction. Subtract length A which remains exposed from the reaming rod's total length of 950 mm.

c Comparative measurement. Hold the guide rod of the same length parallel to the accurately positioned reaming rod. Align the guide rod's tip with the point of insertion (i). The free length of the guide rod is then the nail length L.

Fig. 4.44

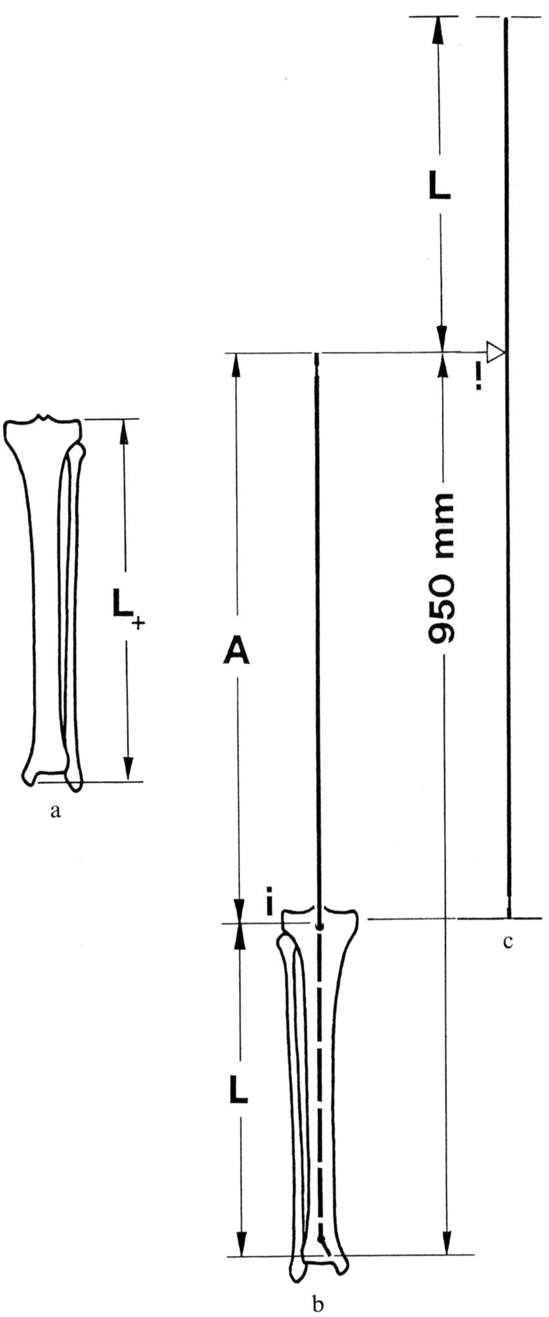

4.5.4 Opening the Medullary Canal

The classic technique which was recommended for years involves a longitudinal incision over the patellar ligament at the level of the joint, about 50–60 mm long (Fig. 4.45), splitting the tendon longitudinally, and insertion of an automatic wound spreader.

The current technique is to place the 60-mm incision medially to the patellar ligament and retract the tendon about 20 mm laterally (Fig. 4.46). Careful handling of the soft tissue is necessary to prevent damage to the lateral blood vessels and nerves. Use the awl to open the thin cortex at the point of insertion (i).

In order to obtain a circular hole, rotate the awl by more than 90° as you push it as far as possible into the medullary canal, until the handle is in line with the shaft axis. Remember that the insertion canal is at a slight angle to the axis of the bone. Tilt the awl into the axis of the tibia at an early stage to avoid penetrating the posterior cortex (Fig. 4.47).

Under image intensification, insert the 3-mm reaming rod with offset ball tip into the canal. Use brief exposures to check the position of the tip as it passes across the fracture site and into the malleolar region. The holding forceps controls the rotation of the reaming rod. The bent tip of the reaming rod facilitates reduction and picking up the fragments as it passes the fracture site (Fig. 4.48).

Use x-ray control to check that the reaming rod is in the correct axial and distal position (Fig. 4.49).

Fig. 4.45 Classic approach for nailing of the tibia. The ligamentum patellae is split longitudinally. We propose using the new core cutter instead of the awl, as the canal produced with the awl does not correspond to the bend of the new tibia universal nail. In short proximal fragments, this can lead to tilting of the fragment, or worse, splitting of the whole bone.

Fig. 4.46 As an alternative the ligamentum patellae is left untouched. It must, however, be pulled laterally in order to give access for the opening of the bone.

Fig. 4.47 In order to obtain the correct angle of introduction with the extra long Steinmann pin, which is held in the universal chuck, a tibia universal nail is placed against the crest of the bone (*left*). Once the Steinmann pin has been introduced a few centimeters (*right*), the cannulated core cutter is placed over it and a cylinder of bone is carefully cut out of the tibial head. As the instrument also sidecutts, care must be taken not to injure the ligamentum patellae, and for the same reason, a hammer should not be used.

Fig. 4.48 Inserting the 3-mm reaming rod.

Fig. 4.45

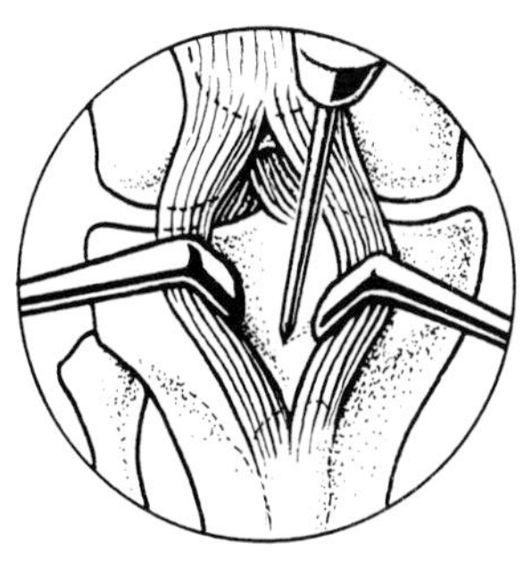

Fig. 4.46

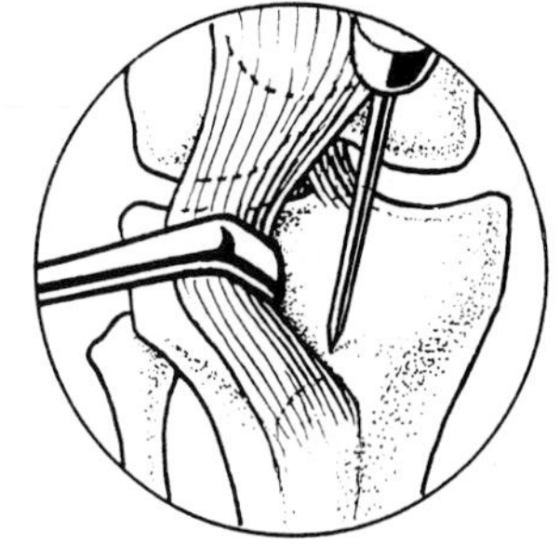

Fig. 4.47

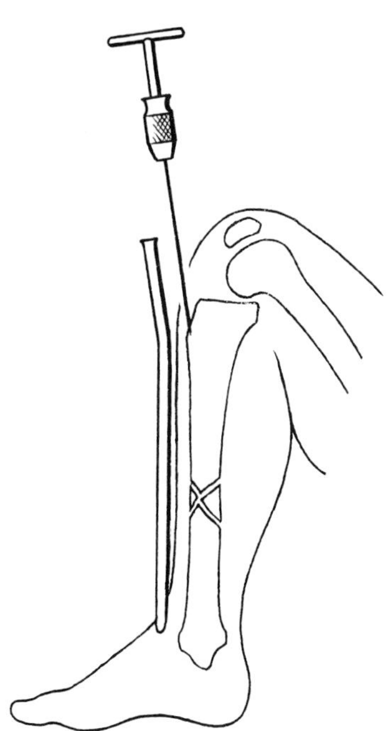

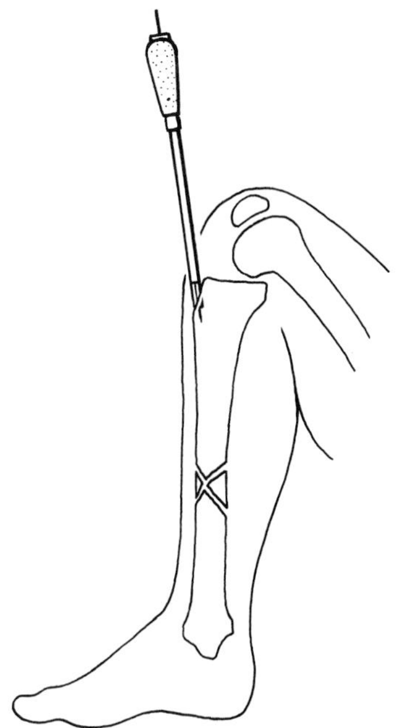

Fig. 4.48

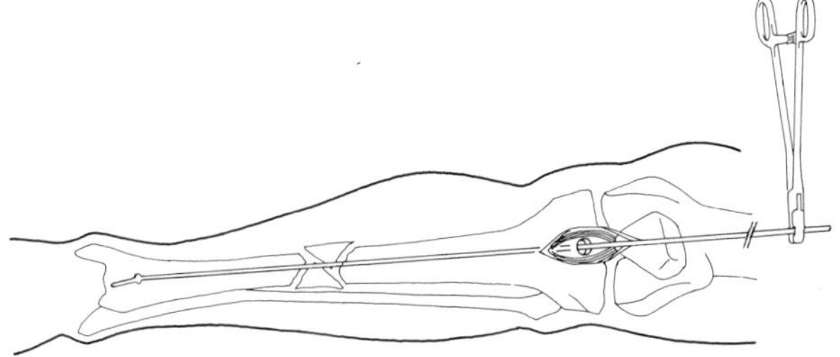

4.5.5 Reaming

Slide the flexible shaft with the 9-mm fixed front-cutting reamer over the reaming rod (Fig. 4.50) and open the medullary canal. Then replace the fixed front-cutting reamer by the 8-mm flexible shaft and interchangeable reamers.

Begin with the 9.5-mm outer diameter reamer and continue in 0.5-mm increments (Fig. 4.51). To protect the skin and the patellar ligament, slide the protection sleeve between the flexible shaft and the soft tissue. If reaming exceeds 12.5 mm, replace the 8-mm shaft with the 10-mm flexible shaft for the larger size of medullary reamers. Determine the length of nail by comparison with another reaming rod or by subtracting the exposed length of the reaming rod from its overall length. After reaming to the determined diameter, pass the medullary tube over the reaming rod and exchange the reaming rod for the 3-mm guide rod with flattened ends (Fig. 4.52).

Fig. 4.49 Exact final positioning of the reaming rod.

Fig. 4.50 Start of reaming with the 9 mm outer diameter front-cutting reamer.

Fig. 4.51 Change of reaming heads.

Fig. 4.52 Replacing the reaming rod by the medullary tube.

Fig. 4.49

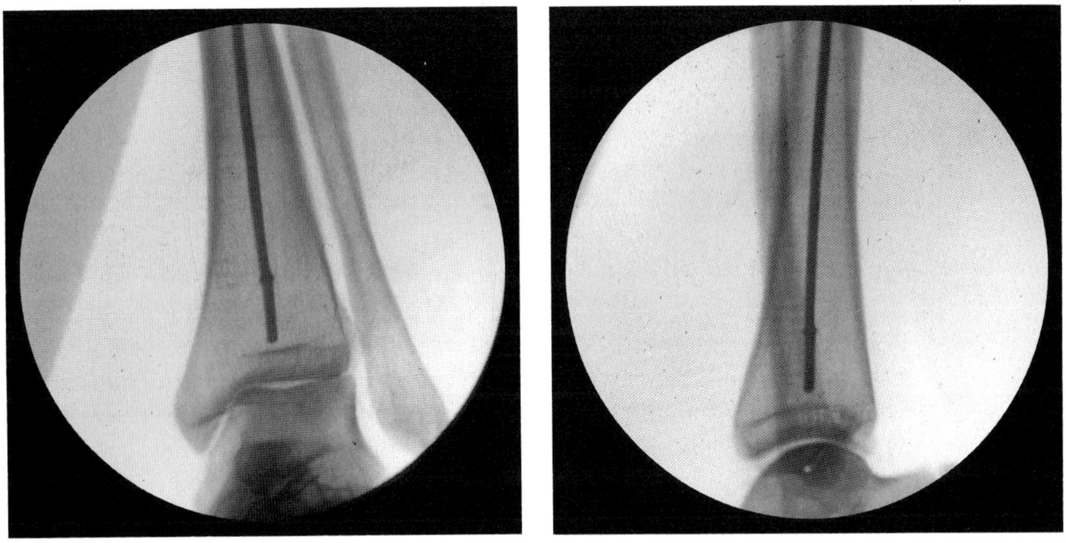

Fig. 4.50

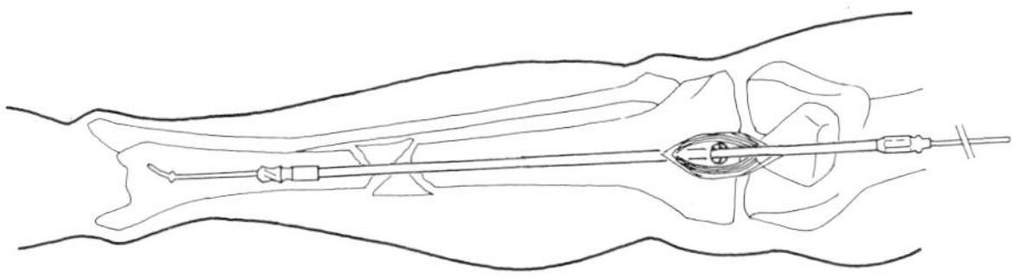

Fig. 4.51

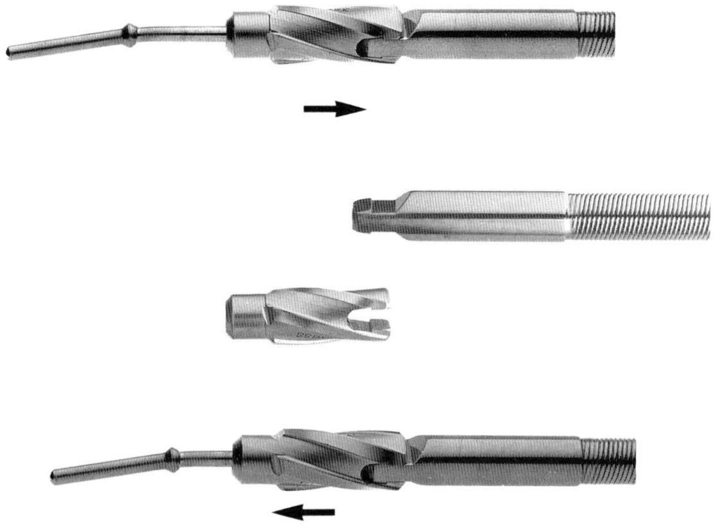

Fig. 4.52

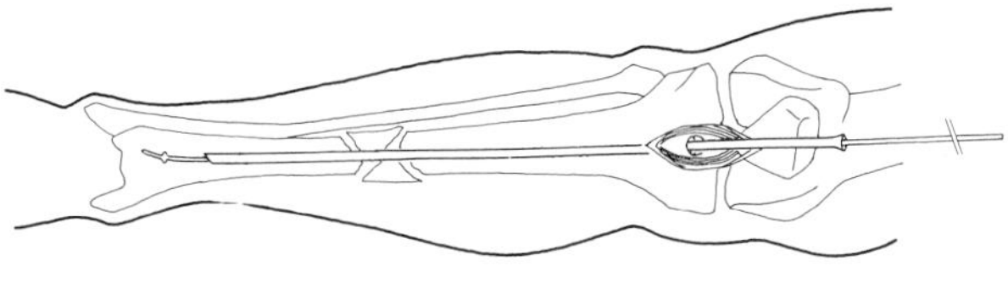

4.5.6 Inserting the Nail

The outside diameter of the nail should correspond to the diameter of the reamed canal, i.e. the diameter of the largest reamer used. Always double-check the nail diameter with the special nail gauge.

After choosing the appropriate intramedullary nail, insert the 3-mm guide rod in the medullary tube, then remove the medullary tube (Fig. 4.53).

Pass the nail over the guide rod and insert it as far as possible in the medullary canal. Fit the insertion handle, threaded conical bolt, and curved driving piece as described in Sect. 4.3.2 above. Screw the driving head on the curved driving piece.

Check the orientation of the insertion handle relative to the nail (Fig. 4.54). During insertion of the nail, the handle of the insertion handle must point in a medial direction.

Use the 700-g hammer to drive the nail into the medullary canal using controlled blows on the driving head, until the tip of the nail reaches the distal metaphysis and the proximal end is flush with the surface of the cortex at the point of insertion (Fig. 4.55). Each blow should advance the nail further into the medullary canal; otherwise, stop driving in the nail and ream 0.5–1 mm more (see Sect. 4.6).

The alternative method for inserting the nail is to use the ram. Instead of the driving head, screw the ram guide on the curved driving piece. This method is recommended when greater force is necessary and the direction of the blows must be controlled very accurately.[2]

The tendency of the nail to rotate is easily controlled with the insertion handle. If the nail rotates, release the locking nut, turn the handle 180° from its medial to the lateral position, and retighten the locking nut. This provides better guidance and control of the nail against twisting. Before starting the locking procedure, the locking handle is moved back to the medial position.

[2] An alternative method uses the ram guide screwed directly on the threaded conical bolt. The curved driving piece is not used. This changes the direction of the driving forces and cannot be recommended in the case of insufficient bone quality.

Fig. 4.53 Replacing the medullary tube by the 3 mm diameter guide rod.

Fig. 4.54 Correct assembly of the insertion instruments on the nail.

Fig. 4.53

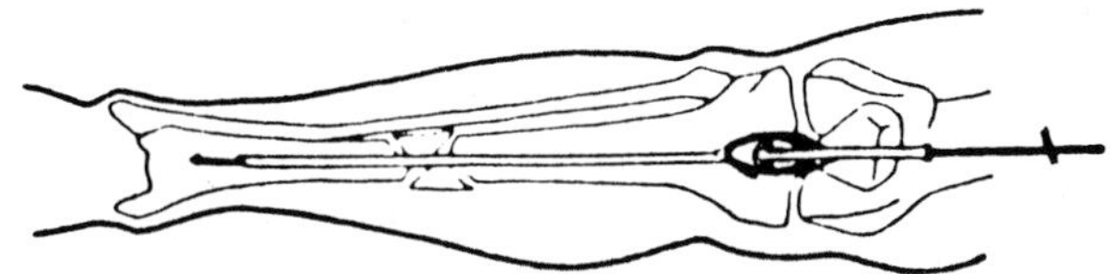

Fig. 4.54

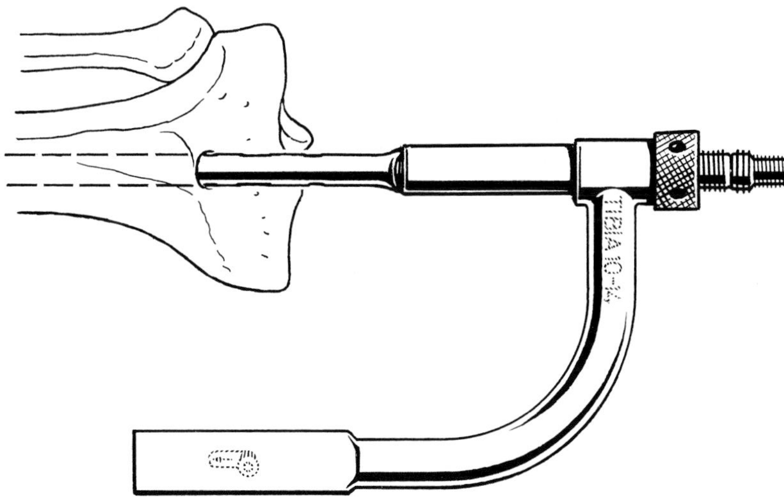

Fig. 4.55 Final position of the nail.

a Position of a nonlocked nail.

b Position of a locked nail.

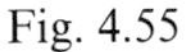

Fig. 4.55

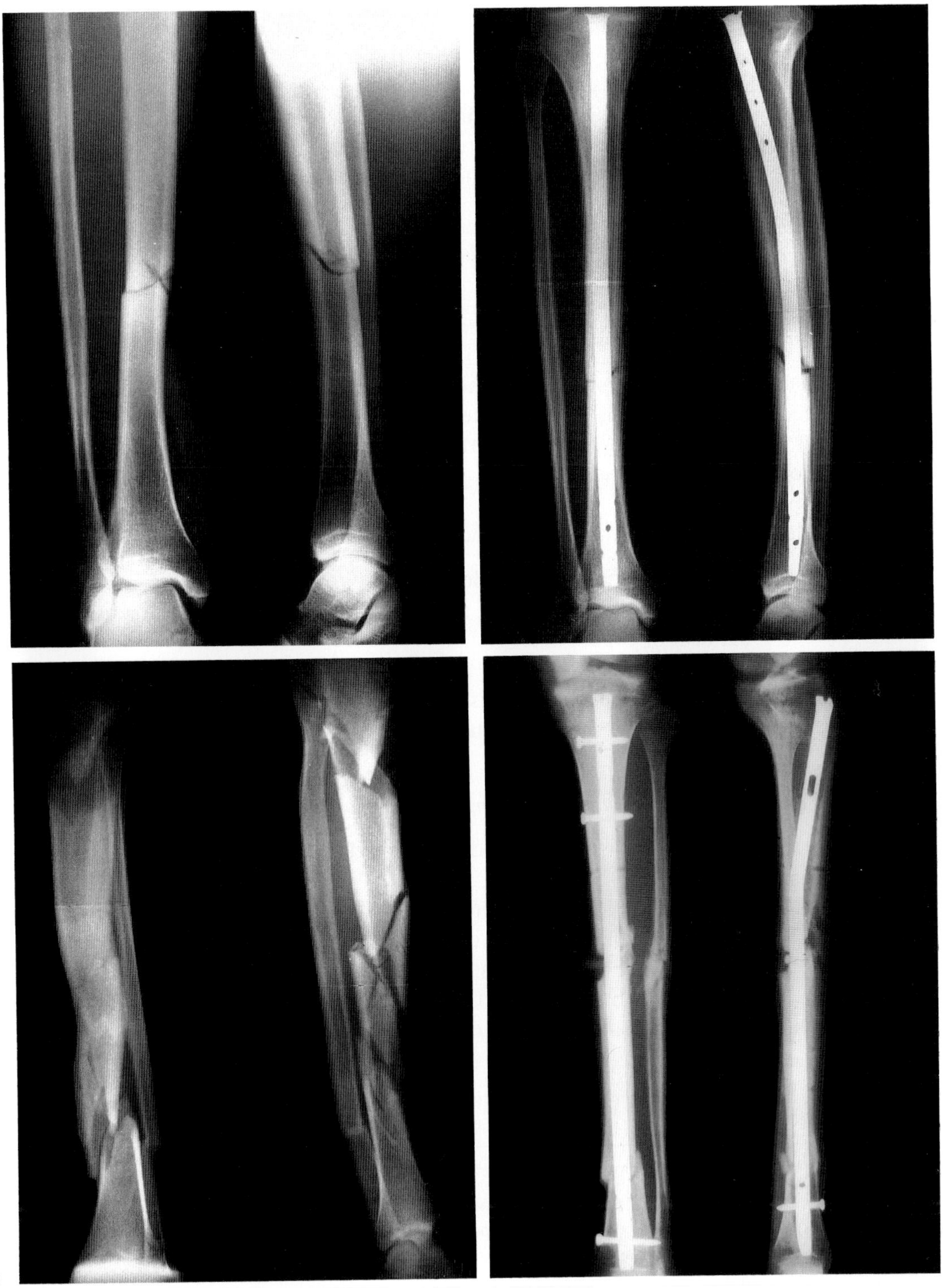

a

b

4.5.7 Locking of Universal Tibial and Femoral Nails

Locking is carried out in two stages, proximal and distal locking. Always perform the distal locking procedure first, for two reasons:

- After distal locking, you may have to manipulate the distal fragment. The best method for this is to use the insertion handle from the proximal end.
- Compression of the fracture area by proximal tension may be useful, either by distractor or manually by means of the insertion handle.

4.5.7.1 Distal Locking

Problems and Methods

Distal locking is impossible without an image intensifier (cf. Sects. 4.3.3 and 4.5.8). Mechanical aiming equipment fitted to the proximal side of the nail cannot compensate for nail deformation during insertion. In proximal locking, because the distance is so short, nail torsion is unimportant.

There are various techniques for positioning the distal locking bolt.

a) Use of a special distal aiming device. This is the recommended standard technique.
b) The so-called freehand aiming method. This is only suitable for use by surgeons with a great deal of experience.
c) Use of a radiolucent drilling attachment. This also permits the use of a freehand technique but under direct visual control on the x-ray image intensifier. This most likely will become the future standard.

Standard Technique with the Aiming Device

The patient's leg must be located between the source of the image intensifier and the aiming device.

First position the image intensifier so that the monitor shows the more proximal of the two transverse distal locking holes (Fig. 4.56). Move the image intensifier until the proximal locking hole appears as a perfect circle a little below mid-screen (Fig. 4.57a). Fix the C arm in this position. On no account move it again until you have finished drilling the 4-mm hole! *The x-ray on the monitor and the orientation of the leg should be identical.*

Fig. 4.56 Distal locking technique. Adjustment of the more proximal locking hole on the monitor, approximate positioning. The hole need not be a perfect circle at this point. Check whether the image intensifier shows the right diameter and whether zooming is necessary.

Fig. 4.57 Locking hole of left leg nailing in lower left quarter of monitor image.

a Rotation of the C arm to obtain a circular image of the more proximal hole. Incision above the locking hole.

b Alternative: Use of long scissors to protect surgeon's hand from radiation.

Fig. 4.58 Distal aiming device on the bone surface. The aiming trocar is inserted in the drill sleeve.

Fig. 4.56

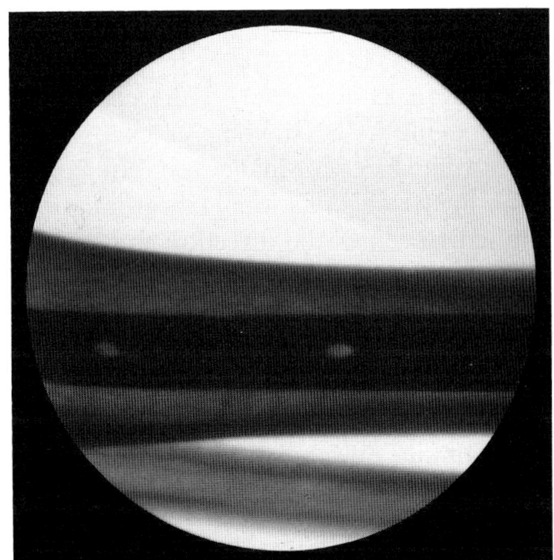

Fig. 4.57

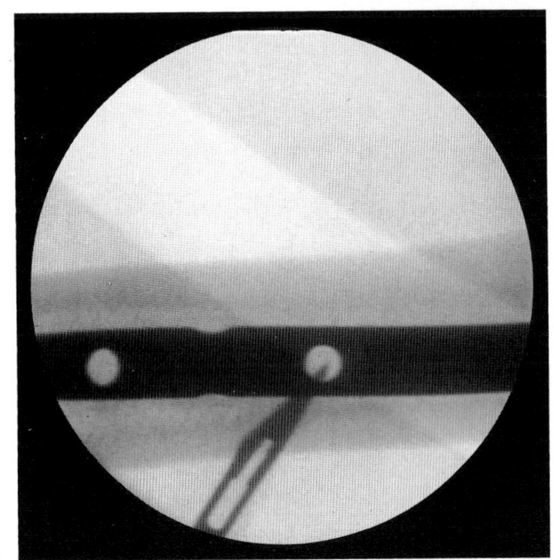

a

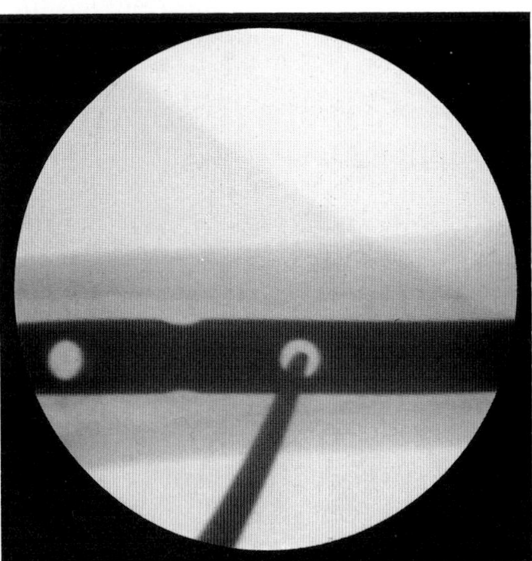

b

Fig. 4.58

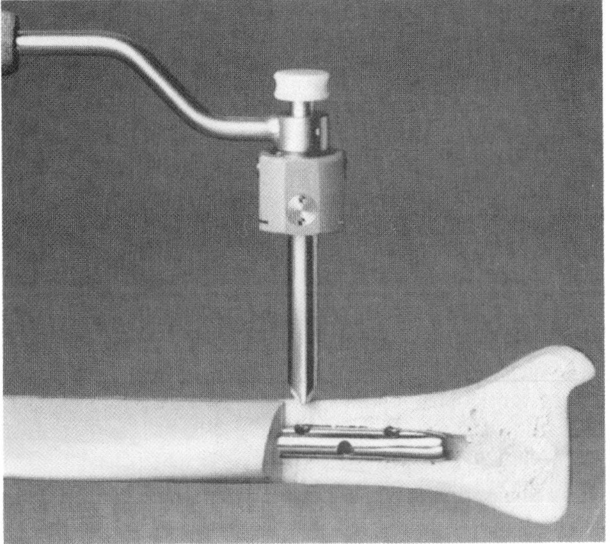

The part of the leg to be nailed should be covered with the sterile radiation shield. To prevent the radiation level being automatically raised, the shield should not extend into the central window. Mark the point by positioning the tip of the scalpel (Fig. 4.57a) or the tip of a scissors (Fig. 4.57b) in the center of the hole. The incision is located over the marked locking holes. In some cases a single incision (especially for the femur) is more convenient than are two smaller separate incisions.

The distal aiming device and aiming trocar are pressed on the nearby cortex (Fig. 4.58) and slightly rotated to center the direction finder's central dot in the circle. The aiming device is moved parallel along the axis of the bone until the central dot of the aiming trocar is centered in the locking hole (Fig. 4.59).

To prevent accidental lateral displacement, press the aiming device firmly against the surface of the bone and allow the tip to dig in slightly.

Remove the aiming trocar and replace it with the 4.5-mm drill sleeve (Fig. 4.60a). Recheck that the aiming device is correctly aligned. Its position is correct if the image of the locking hole in the nail is circular and concentric with the drill sleeve (Fig. 4.60b). Use the 4.0-mm outer diameter drill bit on the 4.5-mm shaft to drill through both cortices, passing through the locking hole in the nail. As you drill, keep checking the direction finder to keep the drill correctly aligned (Fig. 4.60b).

Fig. 4.59 Adjustment of distal aiming device. The centering dot of the aiming trocar is visibly centered in the locking hole, the correct position for drilling. The direction finder is also shown correctly centered.

Fig. 4.60 Distal locking technique.

a Protector sleeve in aiming device.

b Adjustment of the direction finder, dot centered. The locking hole is obscured by the trocar inserted in the drilling sleeve.

Fig. 4.59

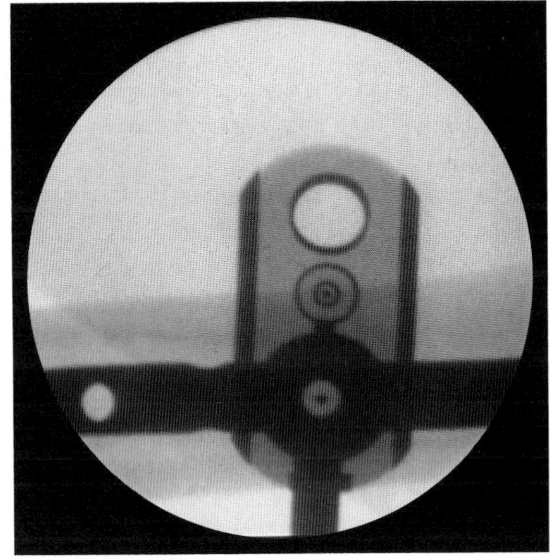

Fig. 4.60

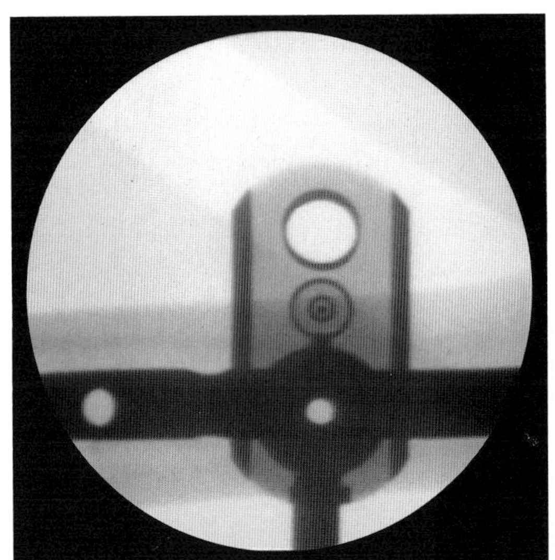

a

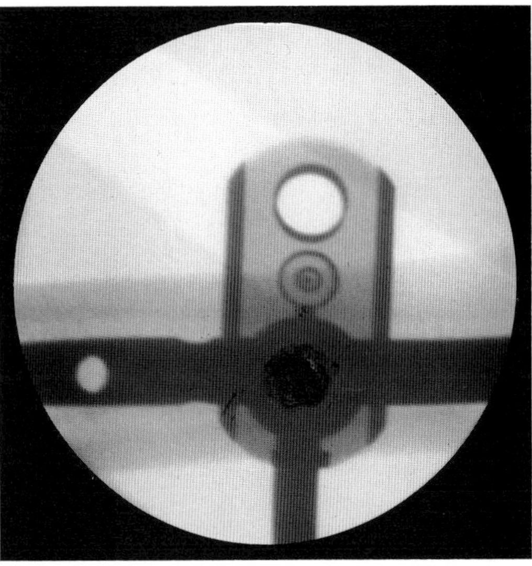

b

Remove the drill sleeve. Insert the depth gauge directly through the aiming device and measure the length of tibial locking bolt required (Fig. 4.61).

Insert the self-cutting tibial fixation bolt. This fixes the aiming device to the bone.

Insert the screwdriver in one of the Allen screws on the side of the direction finder (Fig. 4.62) and slacken the screw. Use the screwdriver to turn the direction finder until its guide markers on the monitor are parallel with the nail. Retighten the Allen screw. For insertion of the locking bolt the image intensifier is not needed.

Insert the 8-mm protection sleeve, with the metal trocar in place, through the distal hole of the aiming device, then replace the trocar with the 4.5-mm drill sleeve. Use the 4.0-mm/4.5-mm drill bit to drill the second hole like the first. Insert the depth gauge and determine the length of the locking bolt directly through the aiming device (see Sect. 4.6). Because of the specially shaped head of the locking bolt, add at least 2 mm to the measured length to maintain the locking bolt's nominal length. This is necessary to ensure that the tip of the bolt projects far enough out of the cortex to provide reliable support (Fig. 4.63).

Insert the distal locking bolt through the 8-mm protection sleeve. Then remove the fixation bolt in the proximal hole and replace it by the proximal locking bolt, then remove the aiming device.

If the anteroposterior locking hole is to be used, turn the C arm through 90° and use the same procedure as described above for the proximal locking hole. In this case the locking bolt can be inserted directly.

Fig. 4.61 Using the depth gauge to measure the length of the locking bolt.

Fig. 4.62 Using the screwdriver to turn the direction finder.

Fig. 4.63 Final position of the locking bolt in the opposite cortex.

Fig. 4.61

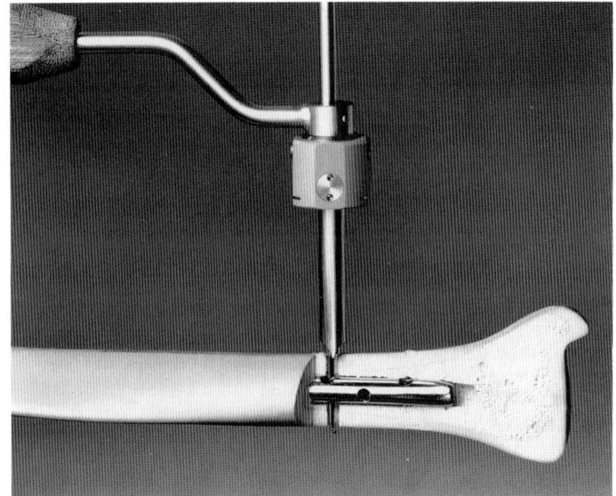

Fig. 4.62

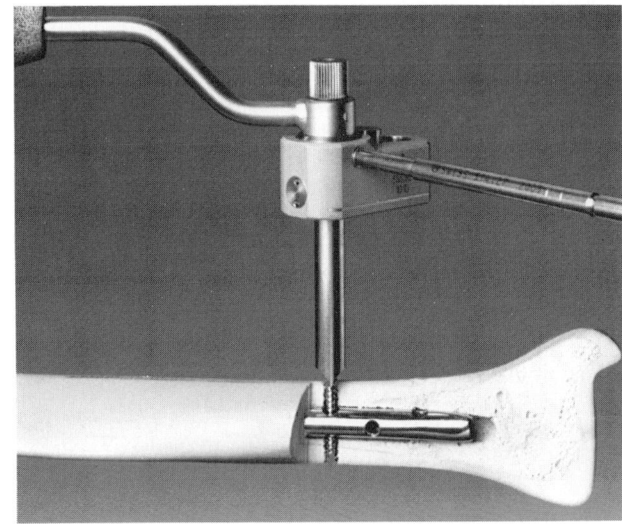

Fig. 4.63

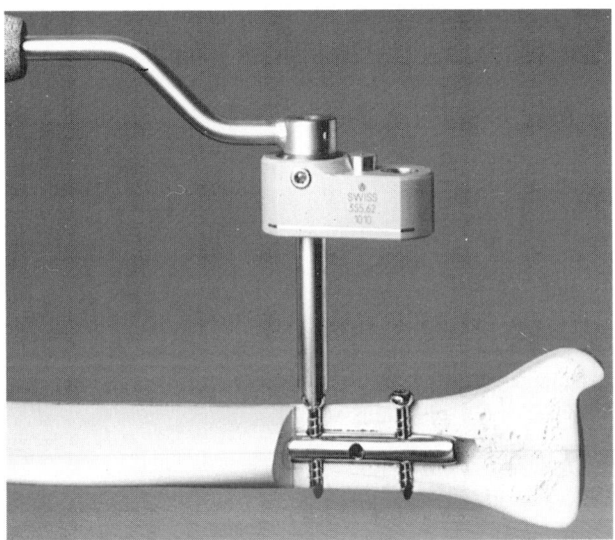

Freehand Aiming Method

Surgeons experienced in the locking technique use the drill bit itself as the aiming device. This greatly simplifies the aiming process. To prevent damage to the soft tissue, the oscillating attachment for the small air drill should be used.

Position the C arm as necessary to show the locking holes in the nail as perfect circles on the monitor. Insert the drill bit through the skin incision down to the bone near the locking holes. Tilt the drill and move it under visual control on the monitor until the tip of the drill bit is centered exactly over the locking hole (Fig. 4.64). Press the tip of the drill to the surface of the bone and raise it to a right-angled position with its axis exactly centered on the locking hole. Drill the hole in the bone directly through both cortices across the locking holes.

This method calls for a great deal of experience, exact alignment and perfect control of the drill during drilling. It permits no checking once drilling has started. The tip of the drill bit may slide out of position, particularly when the surface of the bone is not perpendicular to the drilling direction. This method cannot be recommended as standard procedure.

A safer variation of this method uses a drill guide instead of the aiming drill bit (Fig. 4.65a). The drill guide is set upright, its hole exactly centered on the locking holes (Fig. 4.65b), whereupon drilling through both cortices across the locking holes can be carried out. This method can also be recommended because it is very similar to the standard method.

When drilling is completed, the length of the first locking bolt is determined and the bolt is inserted. The same technique may be used for the second locking bolt. As an alternative, a tibial fixation bolt may be inserted in the first hole to fix the aiming device. This allows easy insertion of the second locking bolt through the aiming device as described in the standard procedure. Finally, after removal of the fixation bolt and screw the first locking bolt is inserted.

Fig. 4.64 Freehand drilling. Center the tip of the drill bit in the locking hole. Use the oscillating drill attachment to prevent damage to the soft tissue.

Fig. 4.65 Alternative freehand technique.

a Center the tip of the drill guide in the locking hole.

b Set the centered drill guide upright on the locking hole.

Fig. 4.66 Radiolucent drilling attachment. Correct alignment of the radiolucent drilling attachment. On the monitor, the drill bit completely fills the image of the locking hole.

Fig. 4.64

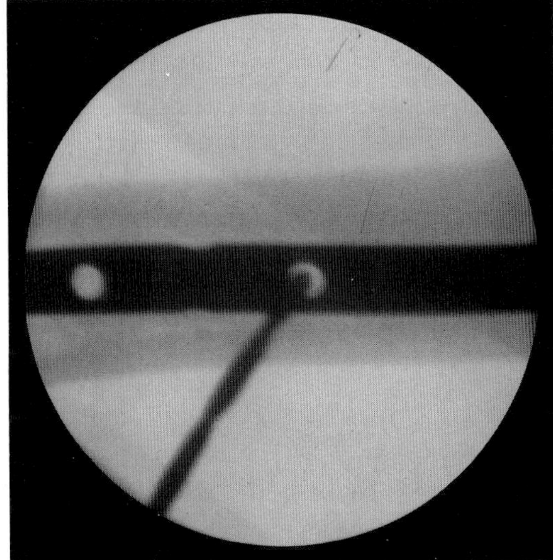

Fig. 4.65

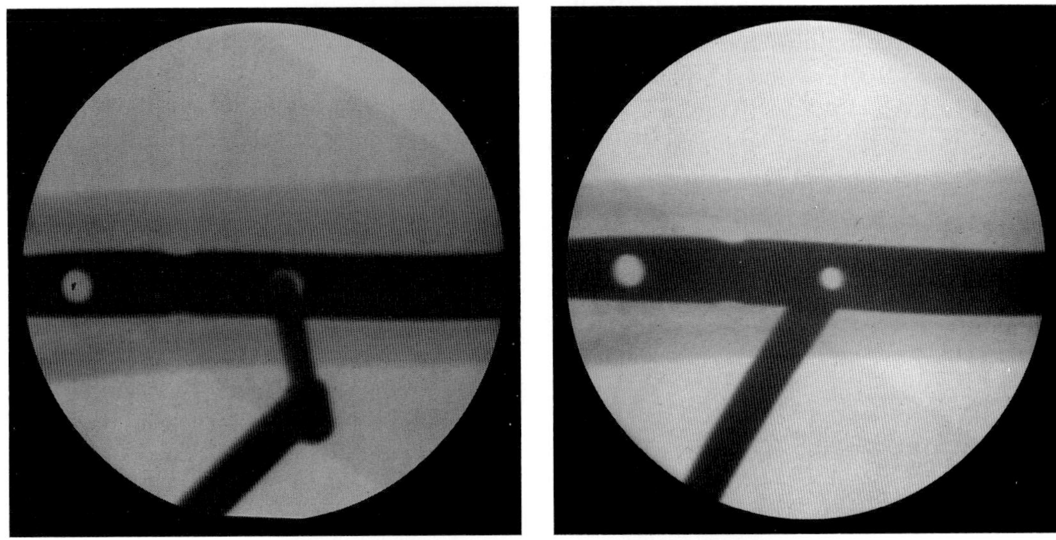

a b

Fig. 4.66

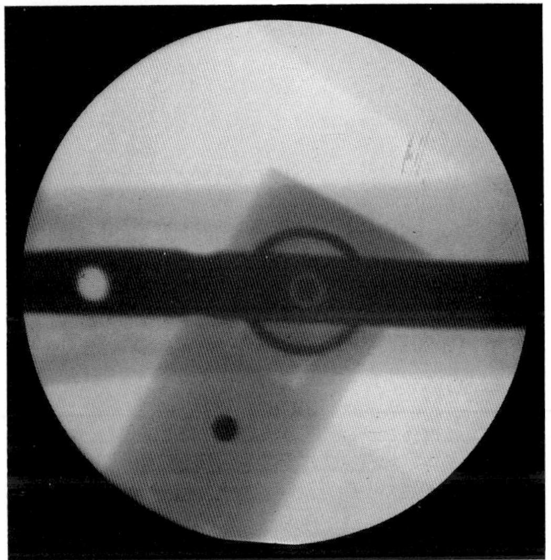

Freehand Aiming Method with Radiolucent Drill

A newly developed drilling attachment of synthetic material does not produce x-ray contrast. It allows accurate alignment of the drill bit within the hole. When the image of the drill bit completely obscures the locking hole (Fig. 4.66), the drill is correctly aligned to pass from cortex through the locking hole in the nail. The surgeon can follow the entire drilling process on the monitor. His hands should be protected by lead gloves or by an x-ray shield and remain outside the x-ray window (Fig. 4.67).

4.5.7.2 Proximal Locking

To insert the locking bolt in the proximal end of the nail, use the insertion handle. Proximal static and dynamic locking are both possible without x-ray control. The hole for dynamic locking is marked in capital letters on the insertion handle (Fig. 4.68). Make a stab incision over the appropriate locking hole. Introduce the 8-mm protection sleeve, with trocar inserted, through the appropriate hole in the insertion handle, until there is cortex contact (Fig. 4.69). Remove the metal trocar. Insert the 4.5 mm diameter drill sleeve and drill a 4 mm diameter hole with the 4.0-mm/4.5-mm drill bit (Fig. 4.70).

Remove the 4.5-mm drill sleeve. Use the depth gauge to determine the length of the locking bolt (Fig. 4.71). Add at least 2 mm (see Sect. 4.5.7.1) and insert the selected bolt through the 8-mm protection sleeve (Fig. 4.72). Repeat this procedure for a second locking bolt, if required.

Fig. 4.67 X-ray shield for use with the radiolucent drill. This shield may optionally be attached.

Fig. 4.68 Proximal locking. Guide hole in the insertion handle for dynamic locking.

Fig. 4.69 Inserting the protection sleeve with the trocar.

Fig. 4.67

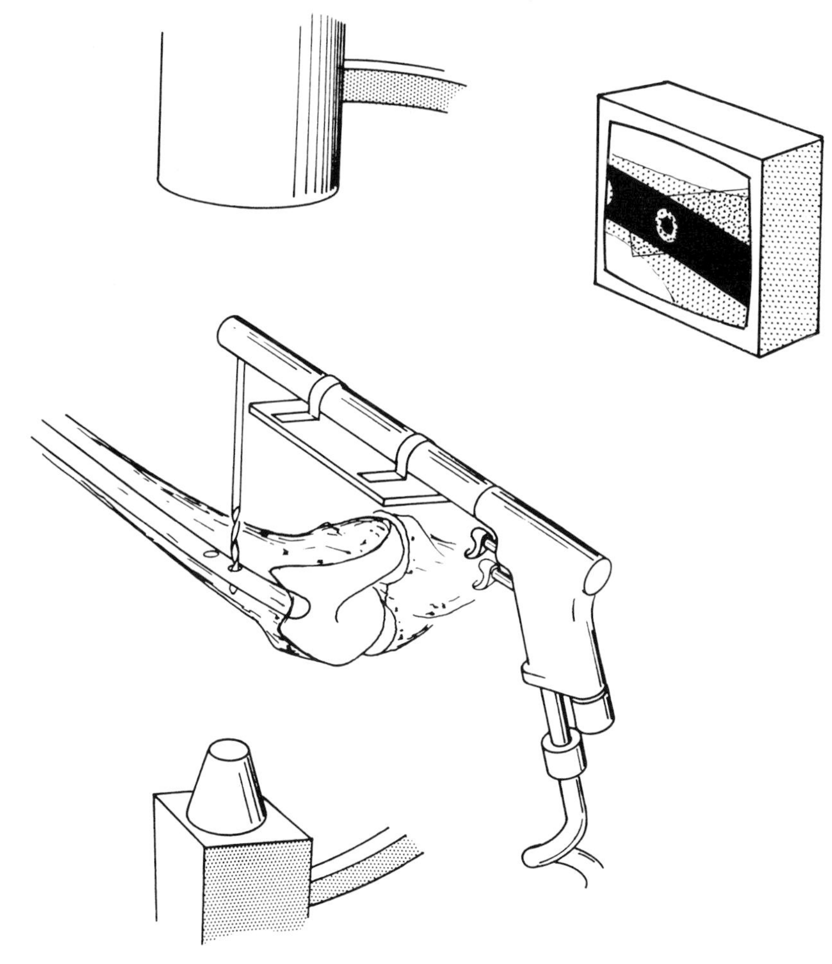

Fig. 4.68

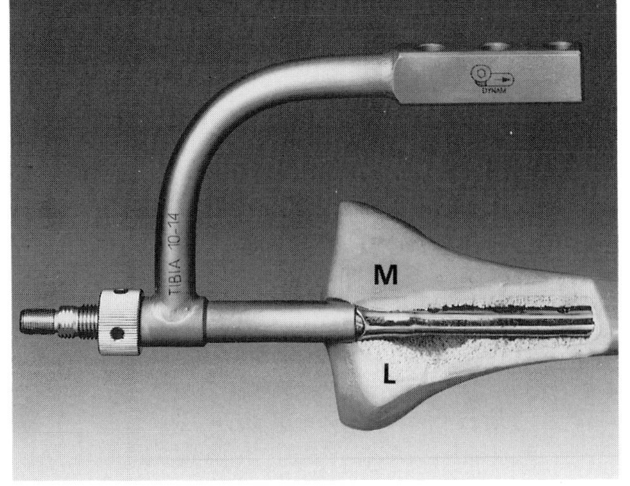

Fig. 4.69

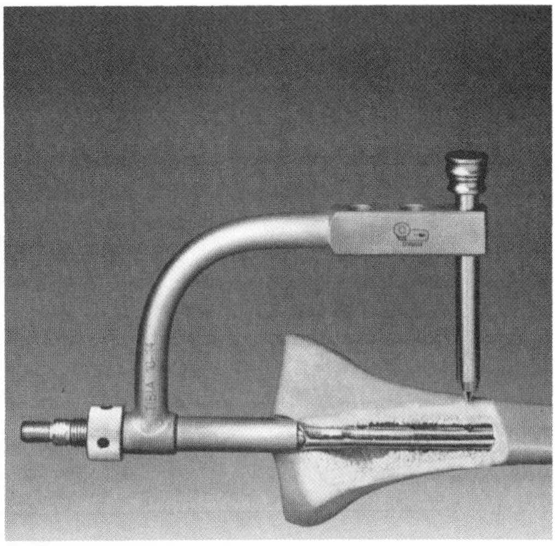

Fig. 4.70 Drilling with the 4.0-mm/4.5-mm drill bit.

Fig. 4.71 Measuring the length of the locking bolt.

Fig. 4.72 Inserting the locking bolt.

Fig. 4.70

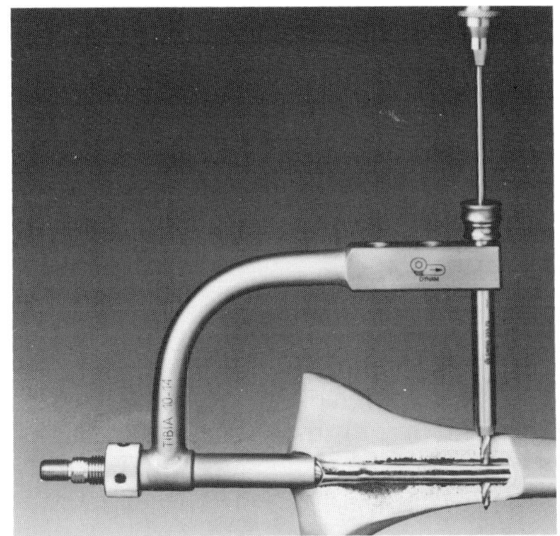

Fig. 4.71

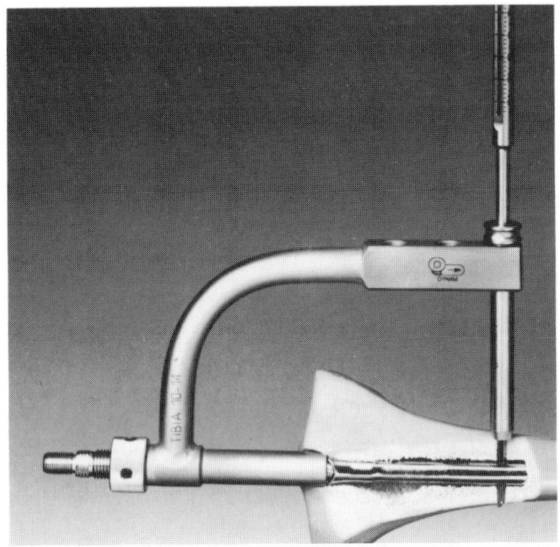

Fig. 4.72

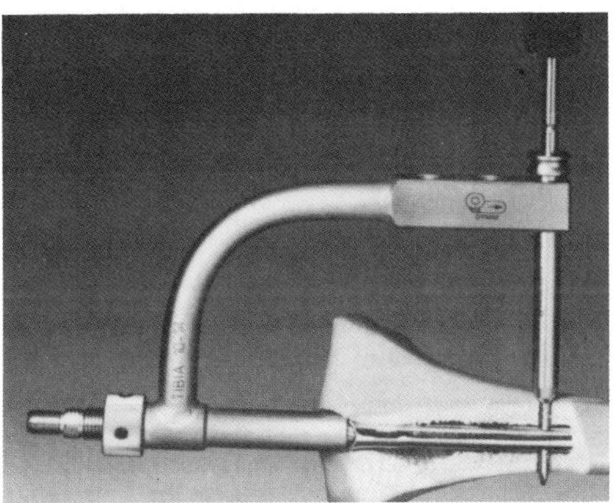

4.5.8 General Remarks on Using the Image Intensifier

For the locking procedure, position the image intensifier to leave adequate room for the operation on the side for surgical access. As shown in Figs. 4.73 and 4.74, leave space for aiming and drilling (a) on the medial side for the tibia, and (b) on the lateral side for the femur.

4.6 Complications

Turning the flexible reamer counterclockwise destroys the instrument. This has to be kept in mind when trying to disengage a jammed reamer by means of a handle. When introducing the nail one must be sure that the nail slides further into the medullary canal with each blow. If the nail jams, driving must be stopped at once. The nail has to be extracted, the guide rod exchanged for the reaming rod after insertion of the medullary tube and additional reaming of 0.5–1 mm performed.

To measure the length of the locking bolt with the depth gauge make sure that the opposite side of the nail is not erroneously taken for the opposite cortex!

4.7 Unreamed Nailing

4.7.1 Introduction

The treatment of fractures using the intramedullary nail is considered by many surgeons to be simple and effective. Nevertheless, it is still generally accepted that intramedullary nailing in combination with reaming should be avoided in treating severely open fractures (Kohlmann et al. 1988). The danger of intramedullary infection with the possible formation of a large cylindrical sequestrum has hitherto kept many surgeons from nailing

---

Fig. 4.73 Positioning the image intensifier. (Remember: Source close to the bone!)

a For the locking procedure on universal femoral nails, the image intensifier's source (*S*) or receiver (*R*) should be placed close to the medial side of the femur. This ensures adequate lateral distance (*d*) for drilling and locking.

b For the locking procedure of universal tibial nails, the image intensifier's source (*S*) should be placed close to the lateral (or posterior) side of the tibia. This ensures adequate distance (*d*) for drilling and locking from the medial side, or from the anterior aspect when the anteroposterior hole is used.

Fig. 4.74 Scale effect due to the position of the image intensifier.

a Normal window. Receiver (*R*) is positioned near the leg. Magnification is therefore similar to that of standard x-rays. This arrangement provides a good general view, but exact adjustment is difficult. This position does not work sufficiently well if the standard technique with the aiming device is used and should be avoided.

b Standard position (zoom effect). Source (*S*) is positioned near the object. This produces high magnification and permits exact positioning, but does not provide a general view. The distal aiming device is adapted to this position. Its tip must be directed to the source.

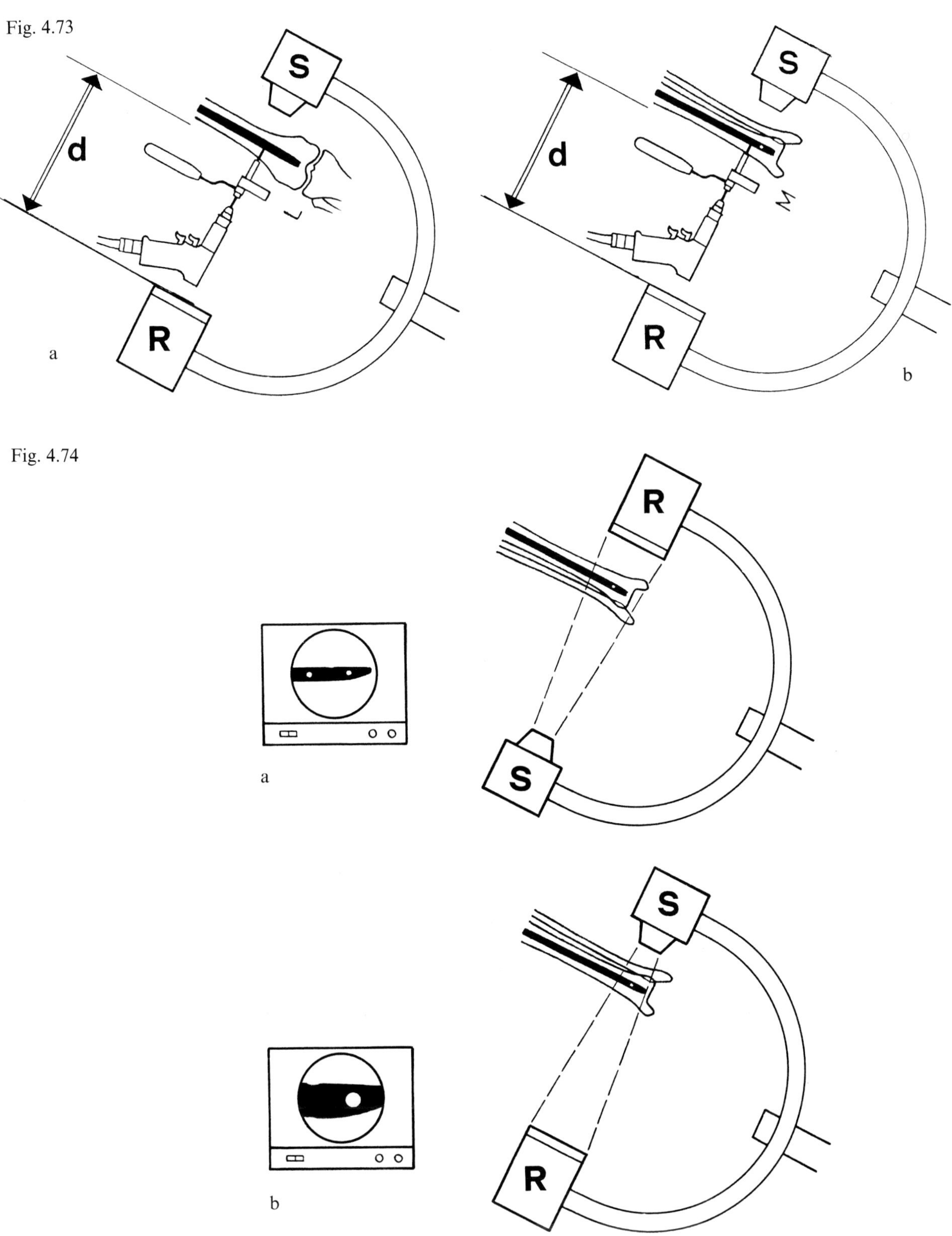
Fig. 4.73
S
d
L
R
a
S
d
M
R
b
Fig. 4.74
R
S
a
S
R
b

such fractures. Voigtlaender (1974), Harvey et al. (1975), Lhowe and Hansen (1988) and Brumback et al. (1989) reported the use of reamed nailing in treating open fractures which, when cautiously performed, may give good results.

4.7.2 History of Unreamed Nails

Velasco et al. (1983) used the Lottes nail, Chapman (1986), Wiss (1986) and Holbrook et al. (1989), the latter in a prospective study, used Ender-type unreamed nails. The problem with noninterlocked nails is that their use is precluded in the treatment of comminuted fractures. Helfet et al. (1990) obtained good results with interlocked unreamed nailing. Haas (personal communication 1990) used the solid AO unreamed and interlocked tibial rod with good success in severely open fractures. The obvious improvement in the results may be explained by the fact that no reaming was done prior to insertion of the nail. Extensive studies of the circulation following nailing procedures have been done by Rhinelander (1974). Recently Klein et al. (1989) demonstrated that the insertion of a nail without reaming results in better blood supply than with reaming. This is probably due to the avoidance of embolization in the intracortical blood vessels. This type of embolization might be induced by the pressure generated in front and at the side of the reamer (Danckwardt et al. 1970; Stuermer and Schuckardt 1980).

In earlier attempts to achieve stable fixation using a closely fitting nail in an unreamed medullary cavity, the nail frequently jammed. Also in this technique, the risk of an explosion fracture of the diaphysis was not to be neglected. Another problem using small, unlocked nails was a relatively high incidence of non-unions.

The smaller solid nail, combined with interlocking, may provide the same stability as a close fitting tubular nail but without the danger of jamming. Under these conditions, it makes sense to use a solid interlocking nail, as proposed by the AO.

In the treatment of open fractures, use of a solid nail avoids the large dead space present in a tubular nail, where bacteria can grow and defense is minimal. Current experience seems to indicate that certain open fractures can be treated using the unreamed nail without increasing the risk of a deleterious infection. Thus, the unreamed nail may be a good alternative to the external fixator in severely open fractures.

4.7.3 Design of the AO Unreamed Tibial Rod

The AO unreamed tibial rod consists of a solid rod with two main sections meeting at an obtuse angle (Fig. 4.75). The upper part is tapered, the circumscribed diameter of the lower part is constant. The proximal bend is based on the study of Heini (1987). The distal two-thirds are straight with a solid cross section corresponding to a triangle with a bowed baseline. The tip is beveled such that a posterior inclined surface is produced which guides the tip along the posterior wall (Fig. 4.76). The anterior surface of the

Fig. 4.75 The AO unreamed tibial rod.

Fig. 4.76 The beveled nail tip.

Fig. 4.77 The beveled anterior surface of the proximal end.

Fig. 4.75

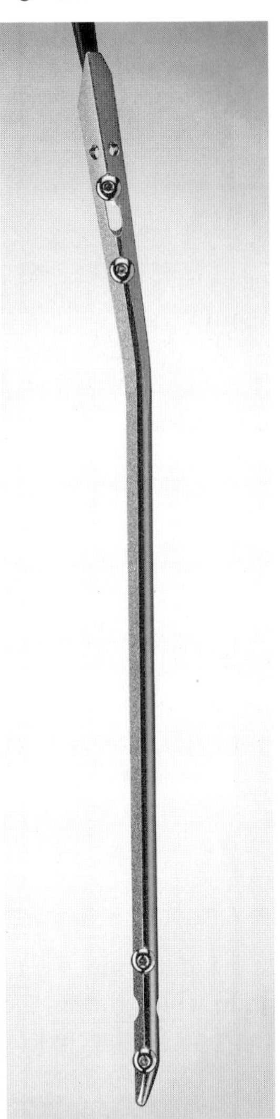

Fig. 4.76

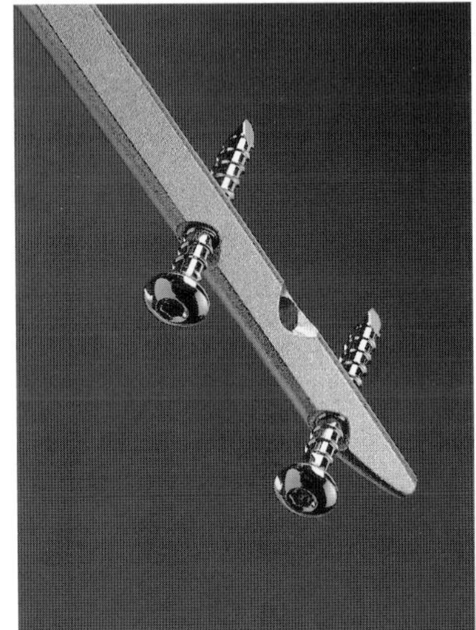

Fig. 4.77

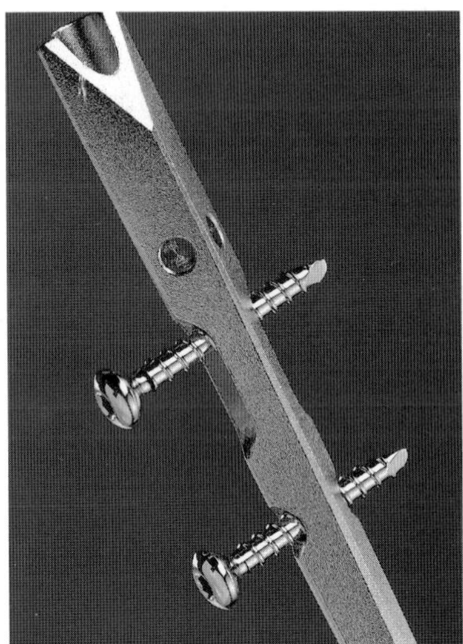

distal nail end is exactly straight so as to avoid angulation of the distal fragment, especially when the nail turns to adapt to the medullary cavity.

The proximal end flares to a somewhat larger diamond cross section to improve the guidance during insertion and the rotational stability within the proximal metaphysis and to allow for the connection of the insertion and extraction instruments. The anterior surface of the immediate proximal end is beveled thus preventing the edge from protruding over the anterior surface of the tibia (Fig. 4.77). Thus, trauma to the patellar ligament is minimized and rotational stability of the drive connection optimized.

Two distal and two proximal holes for interlocking are aligned in the frontal plane. They allow the use of a 3.9-mm locking bolt with shallow threads. This bolt has the same configuration as the 4.9-mm bolt and exerts radial preload. The nail is available in 8 and 9 mm circumscribed diameters.

4.7.4 Indications

The unreamed nail is advocated for temporary fixation in the treatment of fractures where maintaining the blood supply to bone has priority. This is especially the case in severe open fractures and fractures with blunt soft tissue trauma.

4.7.5 Contraindications

The unreamed nail is not recommended in metaphyseal fractures or in the case of acute or chronic infection.

4.7.6 Surgical Procedures

4.7.6.1 Preoperative Planning

Prior to surgery, the size of the medullary cavity must be determined radiologically. One should not use unreamed nails in the unlikely situation in which the smallest diameter of the cavity measures less than 8 mm. The length of the nail is selected according to the x-ray.

Fig. 4.78

Driving head.

Connecting screw.

Insertion handle.

Coupling block.

Unreamed tibial nail.

Fig. 4.79 Unreamed nail with insertion handle and proximal aiming device ready for insertion.

Fig. 4.78

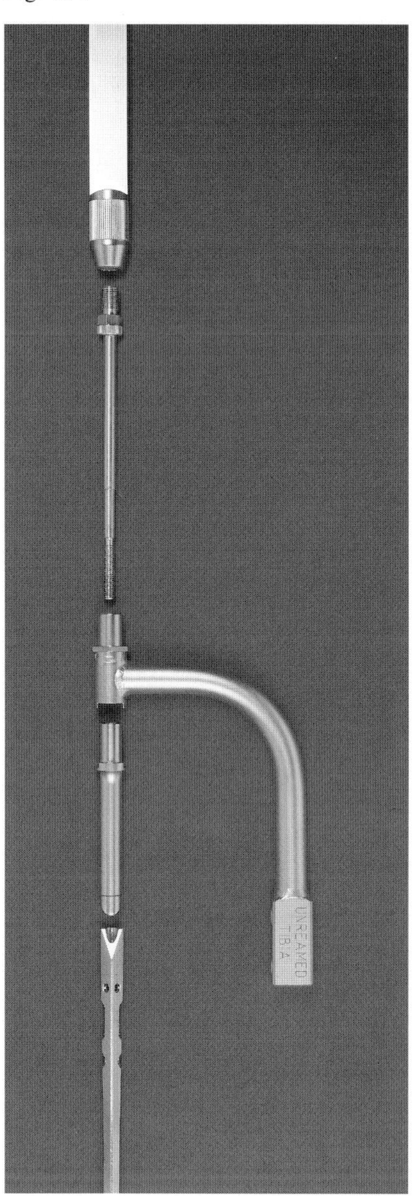

Fig. 4.79

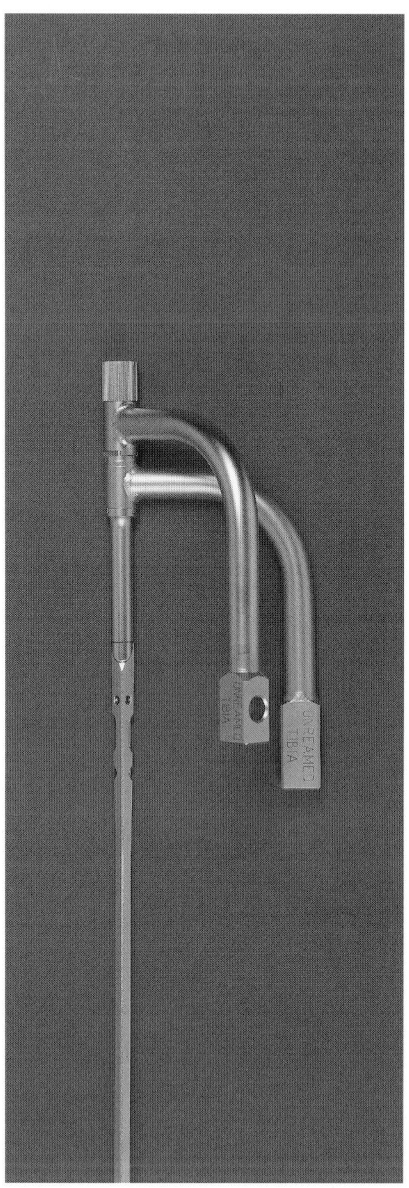

4.7.6.2 Implantation

The point of insertion is aligned with the long axis of the medullary cavity, i.e. slightly medial to the tibial tubercle. It should be located as proximally as possible without impinging on the anterior crest of the tibial plateau. The cortex is opened using the awl; care must be taken not to penetrate the posterior cortex. The nail is then inserted using the insertion handle and the driving head connected to the proximal end of the nail (Figs. 4.78, 4.79).

In most cases the nail can be inserted merely by hand. When necessary, the ram guide can be connected, and light blows with the ram serve to insert the nail. Under no condition should the nail be forced to advance against resistance. A smaller diameter should be selected instead. In the case of a narrow tibial cavity of less than 8 mm diameter, minimal reaming helps to avoid jamming. The nail should be inserted flush with the proximal anterior surface of the tibia.

4.7.6.3 Interlocking

The proximal 3.9-mm bolts are inserted using the insertion handle as an aiming device. The distal bolts are inserted after aiming using the x-ray technique as outlined for the universal tibial nail. The standard 3.2-mm drill bit is used. No tapping is necessary. The length of the bolt is determined using the depth gauge in the conventional manner. The locking bolts are normally inserted from medial to lateral.

4.7.6.4 Postoperative Care

A posterior splint may help to support the limb and prevent development of a drop foot. The rotational stability of the nail is sufficient. The nail was designed to be used temporarily and not for definitive treatment. The implant therefore is not strong enough to bear weight. Further procedures, e.g. secondary stabilization, depend on the circumstances.

References

Brumback RJ, Ellison PS Jr, Poka A, Lakatos R, Bathon GH, Burgess AR (1989) Intramedullary nailing of open fractures of the femoral shaft. J Bone Joint Surg [Am] 71:1324–1331

Chapman MW (1986) The role of intramedullary fixation in open fractures. Clin Orthop 212:26–34

Dagrenat D, Moncade N, Cordey J, Rahn BA, Kempf I, Perren SM (1988) Effect of the dynamization of an interlocking nail in sheep tibia. Internal report of the laboratory for experimental surgery. Davos, Switzerland

Dankwardt-Lilliestrom G, Lorenzi GL, Olerud S (1970) Intracortical circulation after intramedullary reaming with reduction of pressure in the medullary cavity. J Bone Joint Surg [Am] 52:1390–1394

Ender J, Simon-Weidner R (1970) Die Fixierung der Trochanterbrüche mit runden elastischen Condylennägeln. Acta Chir Austriaca 1:40–42

Faure C, Merloz P (1987) Transfixation. Atlas of anatomical sections for the external fixation of limbs. Springer, Berlin Heidelberg New York Tokyo

Hackethal KH (1961) Die Bündelnagelung. Springer, Vienna New York

Harvey FJ, Hodgkinson AH, Harvey PM (1975) Intramedullary nailing in the treatment of open fractures of the tibia and fibula. J Bone Joint Surg [Am] 57:909–915

Heini PF (1987) Untersuchungen der Tibia-Innenform im Zusammenhang mit der Marknagelung. Doctoral thesis, University of Berne, Switzerland

Heini PF, Schneider E, Perren SM (1987) Geometrical mismatch between tibia and intramedullary nail (in preparation)

Helfet DL, DiPasquale TG, Howey TD, Sanders R, Zinar D, Popman D, Brooker A (1990) The treatment of open and/or unstable tibial fractures with an unreamed double locked tibial nail. In: Proceedings of the American Association of Orthopedic Surgeons conference, New Orleans, Feb 1990

Herzog K (1953) Nagelung der Tibiaschaftbrüche mit einem starren Nagel. Dtsch Z Chir 276:227

Herzog K (1960) Die Technik der geschlossenen Narknagelung des Oberschenkels mit dem Rohrschlitznagel. Chirurg 31:465

Höntzsch D, Weller S (1986) Die Lagerung bei Ober- und Unterschenkelmarknagelung. OP-Journal 2:20–23

Höntzsch D, Weller S, Perren SM (1989) Der neue AO-Universal-Tibia-Marknagel. Klinische Entwicklung und Erfahrung. Aktuel Traumatol 6:225–237

Holbrook JL, Swiontkowski MF, Sanders R (1989) Treatment of open fractures of the tibial shaft: Ender nailing versus external fixation. A randomized, prospective comparison. J Bone Joint Surg [Am] 71:1231–1238

Klein M, Rahn BA, Frigg R, Kessler S, Perren SM (1989) Die Blutzirkulation nach Marknagelung ohne Aufbohren. Proceedings of the Osteosynthese International. Gerhard Kuentscher Kreis, Vienna, Austria, 16–18 Mar 1989

Klein MPM (1990) Aufbohren oder nicht Aufbohren? Zirkulationsstörung durch Marknagelung an der Hundetibia. Dissertation, University of Basel, Switzerland

Kohlmann H, Vecsei V, Rabitsch K, Haupl J (1988) Zur Indikation der Verriegelungsnagelung bei offenen Frakturen. Aktuel Traumatol 18:59–63

Küntscher G (1962) Praxis der Marknagelung. Schattauer, Stuttgart

Küntscher G (1970) Das Kallus-Problem. Enke, Stuttgart

Küntscher G, Maatz R (1945) Technik der Marknagelung. Thieme, Leipzig

Lhowe DW, Hansen ST (1988) Immediate nailing of open fractures of the femoral shaft. J Bone Joint Surg [Am] 70:812–820

Mueller JP, Moret O, Vasey H (1988) L'enclouage verouillé dans le traitement des fractures diaphysaires du fémur. Contrôle de la rotation et de la longueur. Med Hygiene 46:1714–1715

Müller ME, Allgöwer M, Schneider R, Willenegger H (1977) Manual der Osteosynthese, 2nd edn. Springer, Berlin Heidelberg New York

Perren SM (1987) Biomechanische Untersuchung zur proximalen Verriegelung des Verriegelungsnagels. Annual Meeting of the German Society for Traumatologic Surgery, Berlin, 1987

Pfister U (1983) Biomechanische und histologische Untersuchungen nach Marknagelung der Tibia. Fortschr Med 101(37):1652–1659

Pfister U, Frigg R (1969) Die Verklemmung des Marknagels in der Markhöhle der Tibia. Acta Orthop Scand [Suppl] 125:1–63

Pfister U, Harmel U (1987) Technik und Ergebnisse der Nagelung mit dem AO-Universal-Femur-Marknagel. OP-Journal 3:29–31

Rhinelander FW (1974) Tibial blood supply of human tibia. Clin Orthop 105:34–78

Sadakane T, Nagano K, Onoue Y, Sunam Y, Engelhardt P (1978) Anatomische und biomechanische Untersuchungen zur Femurmarknagelung. Arch Orthop Trauma Surg 91:31–37

Séquin F, Der AO-Femur-Universalnagel. OP-Journal 3:6–13

Stuermer KM, Schuckardt W (1980) Neue Aspekte der gedeckten Marknagelung und des Aufbohrens der Markhöhle im Tierexperiment. II. Der intramedulläre Druck beim Aufbohren der Markhöhle. Unfallheilkunde 83:346–352

Velasco A, Whiteside TE Jr, Fleming LL (1983) Open fractures of the tibia treated with the Lottes nail. J Bone Joint Surg [Am] 65:879–885

Voigtlaender H (1974) Marknagelung geschlossener und offener Unterschenkelbrüche. Ergebnisse in einem Kreiskrankenhaus. Monatsschr Unfallheilkd 77:20–28

Weller S (1972) Komplikationen bei der Marknagelung. Therapiewoche 22(47):4178

Weller S (1974) Die Marknagelung von Unterschenkelschaftbrüchen. 37th Annual conference of the Deutsche Gesellschaft für Unfallheilkunde, Berlin, 1973. Hefte Unfallheilkd 117:98–102

Weller S (1975) Die Marknagelung. Gute und relative Indikationen, Ergebnisse. Chirurg 46:152–154

Weller S (1987) Die Verriegelungsnagelung. OP-Journal 3

Winquist RA, Hansen ST (1980) Comminuted fractures of the femoral shaft treated by intramedullary nailing. Orthop Clin North Am II:633–648

Winquist RA, Hansen ST, Clawson DK (1984) Closed intramedullary nailing of femoral fractures. J Bone Joint Surg [Am] 66:529

Wiss DA (1986) Flexible medullary nailing of acute tibial shaft fractures. Clin Orthop 212:122–132

Zuber K, Schneider E, Eulenberger J, Perren SM (1988) Form und Dimension der Markhöhle menschlicher Femora im Hinblick auf die Passung von Marknagelimplantaten. Unfallchirurg 91:314–319

5 EXTERNAL FIXATION

5.1 Introduction

With improved components and a better understanding of the principles (Behrens and Searls 1986) that govern their safe and effective use, external fixators have become indispensable tools in the hands of the experienced trauma surgeon. The primary indications for external fixation are the stabilization of severe open fractures and infected non-unions, and the correction of both extremity malalignments and length discrepancies. Other indications include the initial stabilization of soft tissue and bony disruption in polytrauma patients, closed fractures with associated severe soft tissue injuries (crushing of the soft tissue sleeve, burns, dermatological conditions), severely comminuted diaphyseal and periarticular lesions, temporary transarticular stabilization of severe soft tissue and ligamentous injuries, certain pelvic ring disruptions, some children's fractures, arthrodeses and osteotomies.

External fixators have the unique capability to stabilize bone and soft tissues at a distance from the operative or injury focus. If correctly applied, they provide unobstructed access to the relevant skeletal and soft tissue structures for their initial assessment and also for those secondary interventions needed to restore bony continuity and a functional soft tissue sleeve. The additional vascular trauma to bone and soft tissue following the application of external fixation is minimal and, therefore, the risks of infection are much lower than with internal fixation devices.

5.1.1 History

The origins of external fixation go back to Malgaigne, who, in the nineteenth century, developed strapped-on metal points and "claws" to stabilize displaced fractures (Malgaigne and Connaissance 1853/54). Parkhill (1898) of Denver and Lambotte (1907) of Brussels built the first clinically useful external fixators around the turn of the century. Codivilla (1905) and Putti (1918) combined pins and plaster for leg lengthening. The introduction by the 1930s of transfixion pins, longitudinal distraction and compression mechanisms, and universal articulations led to the very sophisticated devices of Anderson (1936a, b), Stader (1937), and Hoffmann (1954). After World War II, Ilizarov (Ilizarov et al. 1972) developed highly complex, but versatile, ring fixators which appeared to be well suited to the correction of limb length discrepancies, malalignments and segmental transport after corticotomy. Simultaneously, surgeons and engineers in Western Europe and North America focused on the development of simple, mechanically sound devices which have become invaluable in the management of open and infected fractures. A recent study by Mears (1983) examined these devices.

5.1.2 AO External Fixators

The AO instrumentarium has successively included five external fixators: a small compression and distraction device for use in phalanges and metacarpals; the small external fixator for the wrist, hand and foot; the Wagner (1972) apparatus for bone lengthening; the fixator with threaded rods popularized by Weber (Weber and Magerl 1985); and the tubular external fixator. This chapter deals exclusively with the AO tubular fixator. This system is of a simple design, is easy to apply, and has proved to be highly versatile.

5.2 Components and Instrumentation of the Tubular External Fixator

The necessary instrumentation, implants and frame components are stored in an autoclavable stainless steel tray (Fig. 5.1).

5.2.1 Implants

The principal implant is a Schanz screw. Recent experimental evidence showed radial preload, using a Schanz screw with a shaft exceeding the diameter of the drill hole by 0.2 mm, to be superior to bending preload and hence more effective in preventing screw loosening. Therefore the two Schanz screws (Fig. 5.2e, f) were developed; a Schanz screw with conus exerting preload in the near cortex and anchoring with a deep thread in the far cortex, and Schanz screw with a shallow long thread exerting radial preload in both cortices. The latter needs one drill hole of 4.5 mm; the core diameter of the thread measures 4.7 mm.

5.2.2 Basic Frame Components (Fig. 5.2)

- Adjustable clamp: This is the basic articulation used to connect Schanz screws to the tubes or carbon fiber rods. The clamps allow screw insertion in any desired plane.
- Stainless steel tube and/or carbon fiber rods: These tubes have an outside diameter of 11 mm and vary in length from 100–600 mm.

Fig. 5.1 External fixator set in stainless steel sterilization tray.

Fig. 5.2 Basic frame components.

a Stainless steel tube, and/or

b Carbon fiber rod with outside diameter 11 mm, length 100–600 mm.

c Cap to hold loose clamps on rod or tube during mounting of the frame.

d Adjustable clamp.

e Schanz screw with conus: radial preload in near cortex, deep thread in far cortex.

f Schanz screw with shallow long thread: radial preload in both cortices.

g Steinmann pin, 5-mm diameter.

e has been discontinued in view of general applicability of *f*.

Fig. 5.1

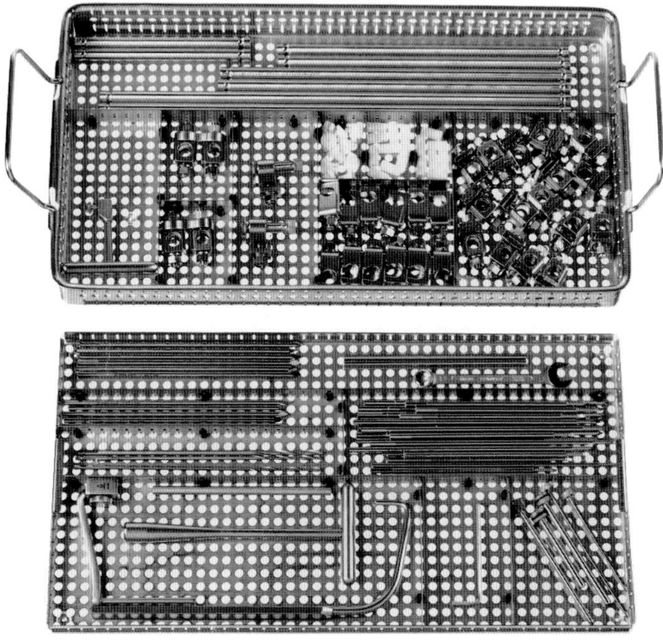

Fig. 5.2

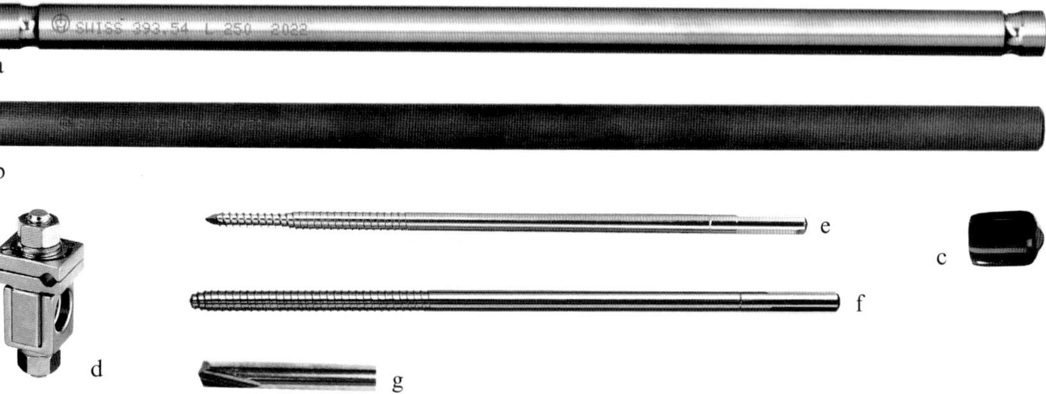

- Schanz screws with a core diameter of 4.7 mm.
- Steinmann pins with a diameter of 5 mm.

Schanz screws as the principal implant, the adjustable clamp, the stainless steel tube or carbon fiber rods as frame components, and the Steinmann pins are the four basic elements of the AO tubular external fixator.

5.2.3 Additional Components and Implants

For special situations, the following additional components and implants are available (Figs. 5.3A, 5.3B, 5.17A):

- Schanz screws with 5-mm diameter and a long thread.
- Schanz screws with 2.7/4.5-mm and 3.5/4.5-mm diameter for the wrist, hand, and foot (Fig. 5.17A).
- An open single clamp to facilitate the placement of additional Steinmann pins and Schanz screws after a frame has been applied.
- A pin-adjusting clamp (transverse clamp) for the stabilization of short fragments.
- A universal joint and a tube-tube clamp for the connection of two tubes and for a "modular" fixator.
- Carbon fiber rods. These are radiolucent and about 30% stiffer than the stainless steel rods.
- An open compressor/distractor.
- Threaded bars, short tubes of 7–10 cm length and transport nuts for fragment transport and lengthening.

Fig. 5.3A Additional components.

a Open single clamp.

b Universal joint.

c Tube-tube clamp.

d Schanz screw, 5.0-mm diameter with long thread.

e Cap for Steinmann pins.

Fig. 5.3B Components for segment transport and lengthening.

a Threaded rod, 8-mm diameter.

b Nuts for threaded rod.

c Short tubes (3 different lengths).

d Transport nut with distance markers.

e Pin-adjusting clamp (transverse clamp).

Fig. 5.3A

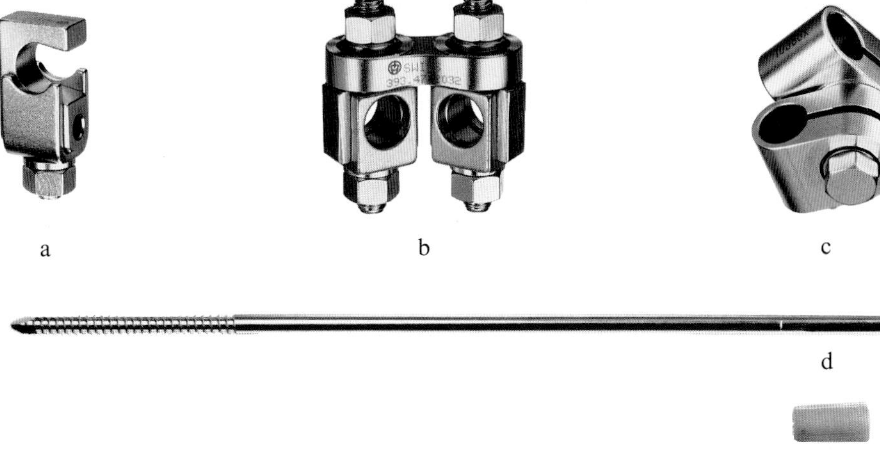

Fig. 5.3B

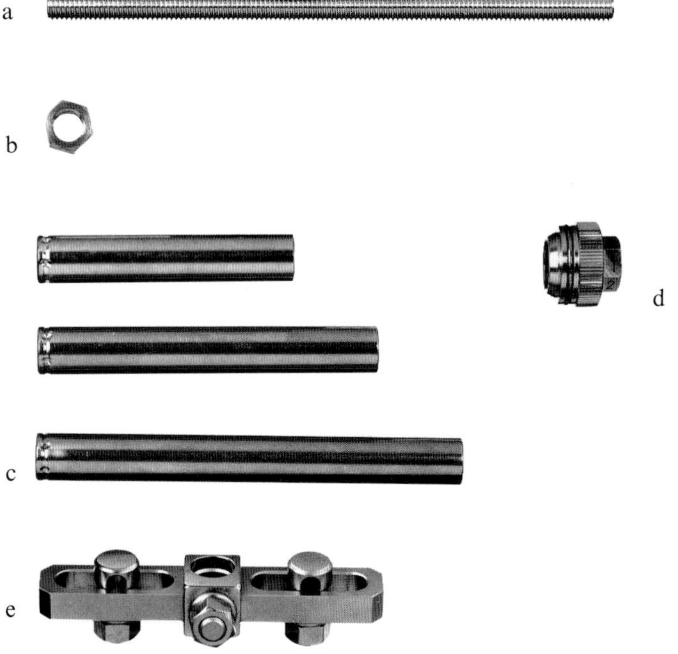

5.2.4 Instrumentation (Fig. 5.4A, B)

The triple trocar is a universal instrument for guiding insertion of the Schanz screw with conus. It consists of a 5-mm drill sleeve, a 3.5-mm drill sleeve, and a 3.5-mm trocar (Fig. 5.4). The screw holes are first predrilled with a 3.5-mm bit and then overdrilled in the near cortex with a long 4.5-mm drill bit. The universal chuck with a T handle holds the Schanz screws during insertion, while the wrenches are used to tighten the clamp nuts. The Schanz screw with a shallow long thread only needs a 4.5-mm drill sleeve with trocar and drilling through both cortices is performed using the 4.5-mm drill bit.

Fig. 5.4A Instruments.

- a Triple trocar: trocar 3.5 mm, drill sleeve 3.5 mm, drill sleeve 5.0 mm.
- b Drill bits, 3.5- and 4.5-mm diameter.
- c Open compressor/distractor.
- d Socket wrench.
- e Combination wrench.
- f Universal chuck with T handle.
- g Oscillating attachment to the small power drill.

Fig. 5.4B Bolt cutter comprising two handles (13- and 24-mm) and two cutting heads for 4.5- and 5.0-mm pins.

Fig. 5.4A

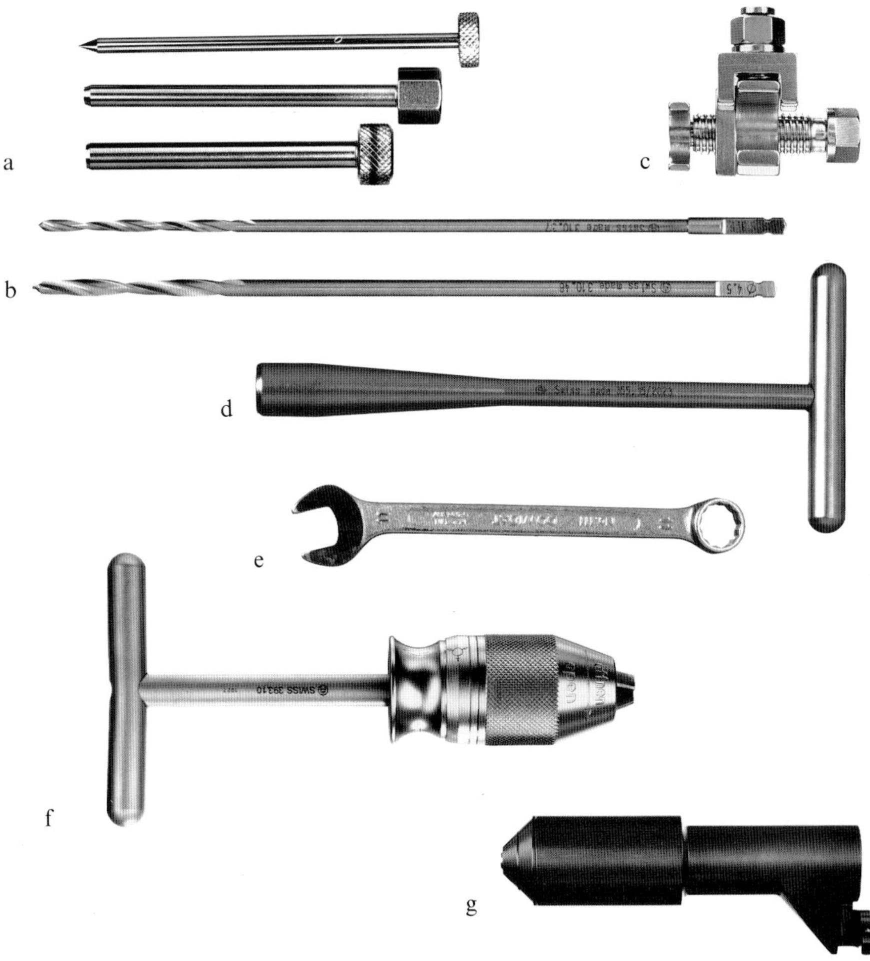

Fig. 5.4B

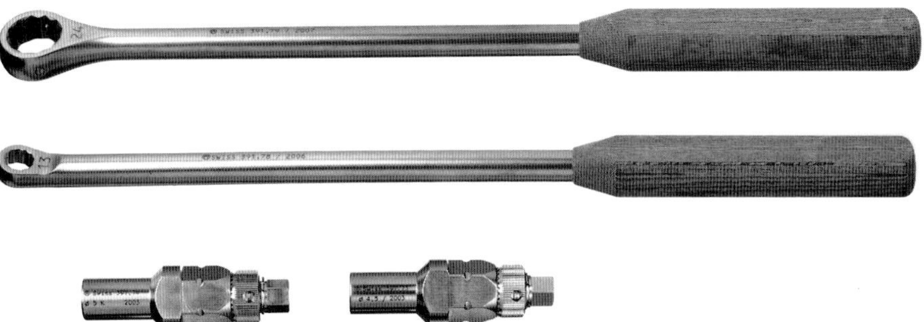

5.3 Basic Fixator Configurations

The fixator components are generally assembled into one of four basic frame types of configurations (Fig. 5.5), each of which has distinct clinical and mechanical properties (Behrens and Johnson 1985; Behrens et al. 1983; Behrens and Searls 1986; Evans et al. 1979; Hierholzer et al. 1978, 1985).

The two basic frame types, unilateral and bilateral, can be applied in both one- and two-plane configurations. The one-plane configurations are less obstructive and generally suffice for most injury situations. Two-plane frames are more effective in neutralizing multi-directional bending and torsional movements (Behrens and Johnson 1985; Behrens et al. 1983). However, they are only needed when dealing with severe comminuted fractures or with bone loss (Behrens and Searls 1986), and for arthrodesis as well as osteotomies.

5.4 Principles of External Fixation

To be safe and effective, an applied fixator should have a low rate of serious complications, be nonobstructive, be stiff enough to maintain alignment under adverse loading situations, facilitate full weight-bearing, and be adaptable to a wide variety of injury and patient conditions. Experience accumulated over the past decade has shown that these goals are best achieved by adhering to four basic principles (Behrens and Searls 1986) which demand that the applied frame optimally accommodates the vital limb anatomy, injury access for debridement and secondary procedures, mechanical demands of patient and injury, and patient comfort.

Fig. 5.5 The four basic configurations of external fixation.

a Unilateral frame, one plane.

b Unilateral frame, two planes (delta or V-frame).

c Bilateral frame, one plane.

d Bilateral frame, two planes.

In recent years, the two unilateral modalities have been almost universally applied except for arthrodeses and osteotomies where a parallel arrangement of compressive forces requires bilateral one- or two-plane external fixation.

Fig. 5.5

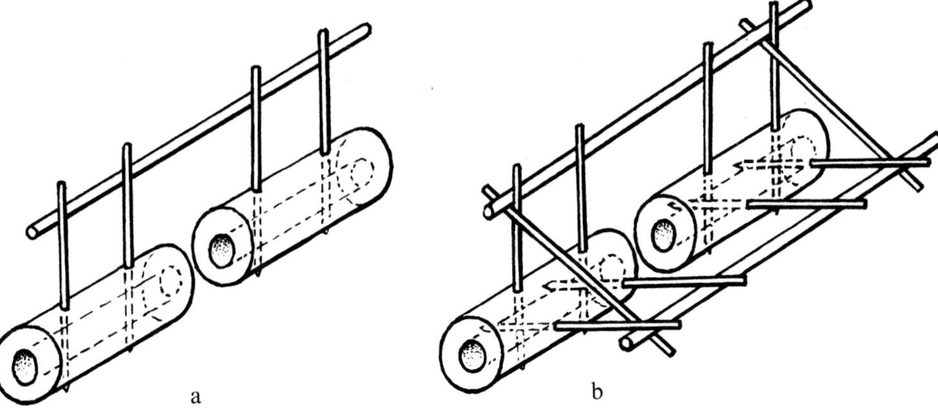

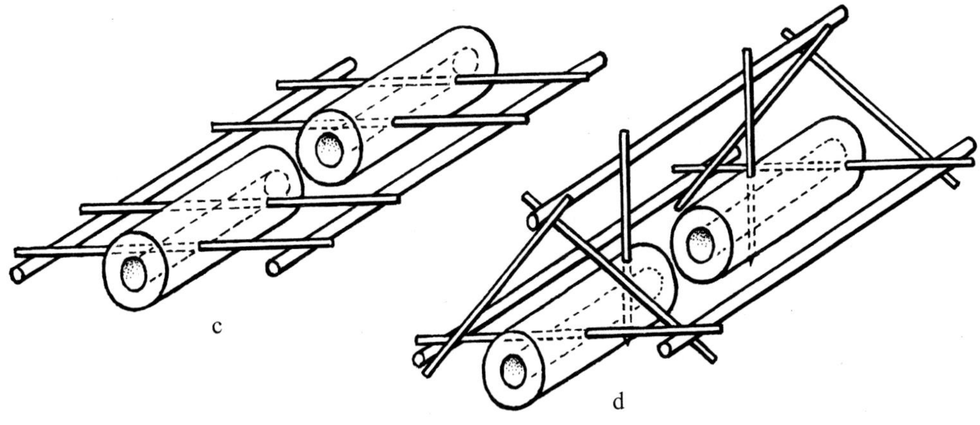

5.4.1 Limb Anatomy

Using the lower leg as an example (Fig. 5.6), it becomes evident that the safe soft tissue corridor, through which Schanz screws can be inserted without injuring the main vessels, nerves and musculotendinous units, lies anteromedially and varies in size from an arc of 220° close to the tibial plateau to one of 120° just above the ankle joint. To prevent injuries to the popliteal vessels in the proximal leg, the Schanz screw exit area should be limited to the medial part of the posterior tibia. Avoiding the distal two-fifths of the lateral tibial cortex will avoid injury to the anterior tibial vessels. The use, during drilling, of the oscillating attachment to the small power drill is strongly recommended to avoid damage to vessels and nerves.

The narrowness of the safe corridor in the lower leg and in most other body segments (Green 1981) limits the choice of safe frames to one- or two-plane unilateral configurations.

5.4.2 Injury Access

Within the safe corridor, the fixator frame is applied so as not to interfere with wound access either for the initial debridement or for secondary procedures, such as transfer of pedicled or free soft tissue flaps, sequestrectomies, or the placement of a bone graft.

5.4.3 Mechanical Demands

Clinical and experimental evidence (Behrens and Johnson 1985; Behrens et al. 1983; Behrens and Searls 1986) has shown that with the use of AO tubular components, one- or two-plane unilateral fixators can be made stiff enough to accommodate most injury conditions. The following seven frame characteristics have been shown to increase the stiffness of an applied frame and to diminish motion at the fracture site:

1. Placement of the principal frame in the sagittal plane.
2. Increasing the Schanz screw spread within each main bony fragment.
3. Preloading of Schanz screws – automatically done by slightly oversizing (+0.2 mm) the core.
4. Increasing the number of Schanz screws in each bony fragment.
5. Reducing the distance between the bone and the longitudinal tube.
6. Attaching a second longitudinal tube in the same Schanz screw plane with the clamps of each tube in close contact.
7. Creating a two-plane unilateral frame, i.e. constructing a second half frame within the safe corridor.

Fig. 5.6 The "safe corridor" for Schanz screw insertion in the lower leg.

At level A, proximal to the tibial tubercle, Schanz screws can be safely inserted within an arc of 220°. At level B, just below the tibial tubercle, the safe arc decreases to 140°. At C, in the distal third of the leg, the safe arc remains 140°, but anterior tibial vessels and deep peroneal nerves become vulnerable as they cross the lateral tibial cortex. At D, above the ankle joint, the safe arc is 120°. At levels E and F, Steinmann pins in the tarsal or metatarsal bones may be used to splint the ankle joint if neurological or soft tissue injuries prevent the application of an external support. The dotted area indicates where the tibia lies subcutaneously and Schanz screw insertion is safe particularly when using the oscillating attachment.

Fig. 5.6

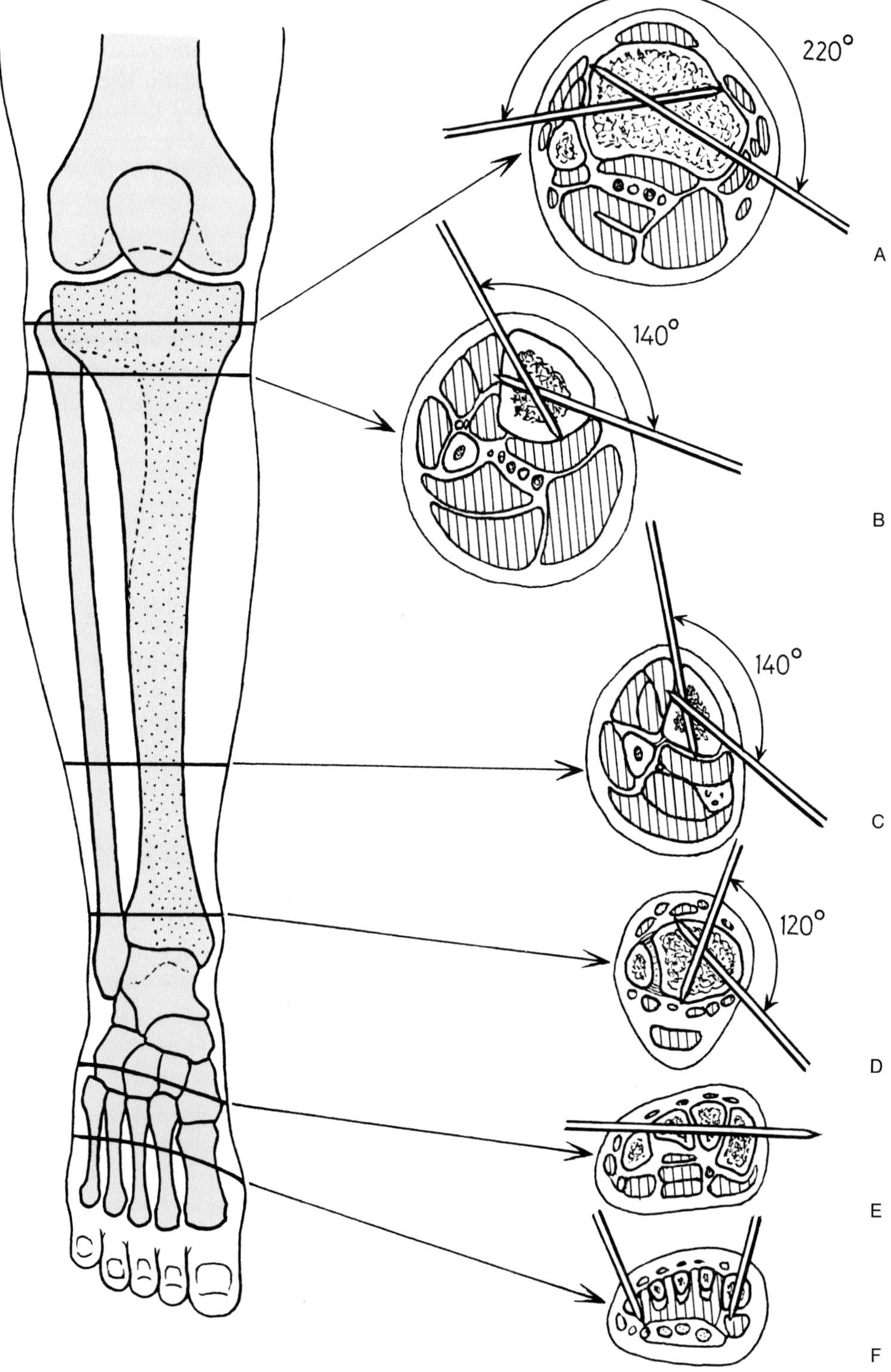

5.4.4 Patient Comfort

In the vast majority of cases, simple unilateral fixator configurations are sufficient, thus avoiding patient discomfort and the functional impairment characteristic of bilateral or circular assemblies. The Schanz screws can be shortened on the fixed clamps by means of the bolt cutter (Fig. 5.4B).

5.5 Application of a Fixator Frame

External fixators are usually applied under general or regional anesthesia with the limb draped free so as to leave all pertinent skeletal landmarks visible. An image intensifier facilitates screw placement, but skeletal alignment is assessed both clinically and with standard radiographs in two planes (Behrens et al. 1981).

5.5.1 Schanz Screw Insertion (Fig. 5.7A, B)

Insertion of Schanz screws with preload in near cortex and deep thread in far cortex (Fig. 5.7A): The triple trocar point is placed on the bony surface through a small stab incision. After the removal of the trocar, both cortices are pierced with a 3.5-mm drill bit. Following removal of the 3.5-mm sleeve, the near cortex is overdrilled through the 6.0/5.0-mm drill sleeve using a 4.5-mm drill bit. The depth gauge probe is inserted and the knurled disk advanced to the top of the drill sleeve, tightening the locking screw.

Fig. 5.7 Insertion of a Schanz screw.

A Application technique for the radial Schanz screw with preload in near cortex and deep thread in far cortex. (NB: This Schanz screw has been discontinued in favour of the screw illustrated in Fig. 5.7B.)

a Assemble the triple trocar and penetrate the soft tissue (through a stab incision) down to the bone surface.

b Remove the trocar and drill through both cortices using a long 3.5-mm drill bit.

c Remove the 3.5-mm drill sleeve. Through the remaining 6.0/5.0-mm drill sleeve, overdrill the near cortex using a long 4.5-mm drill bit. The use of the oscillating attachment combined with the three-fluted drill bit is strongly recommended.

d Insert the depth gauge probe through the drill sleeve hooking the far cortex.

e Loosen the locking screw, advance the knurled disk to the top of the drill sleeve and tighten the locking screw.

f Remove the probe. Place the threaded tip of the Schanz screw in to the Schanz screw recess of the knurled disk.

g Advance the universal chuck over the nonthreaded end of the Schanz screw until the tip of the probe touches the end of the universal chuck. Tighten the universal chuck onto the Schanz screw in this position.

h Insert the Schanz screw until the universal chuck nearly touches the top of the drill sleeve. The Schanz screw is now fully inserted into the far cortex.

i Remove the drill sleeve and attach the adjustable clamp.

Fig. 5.7A

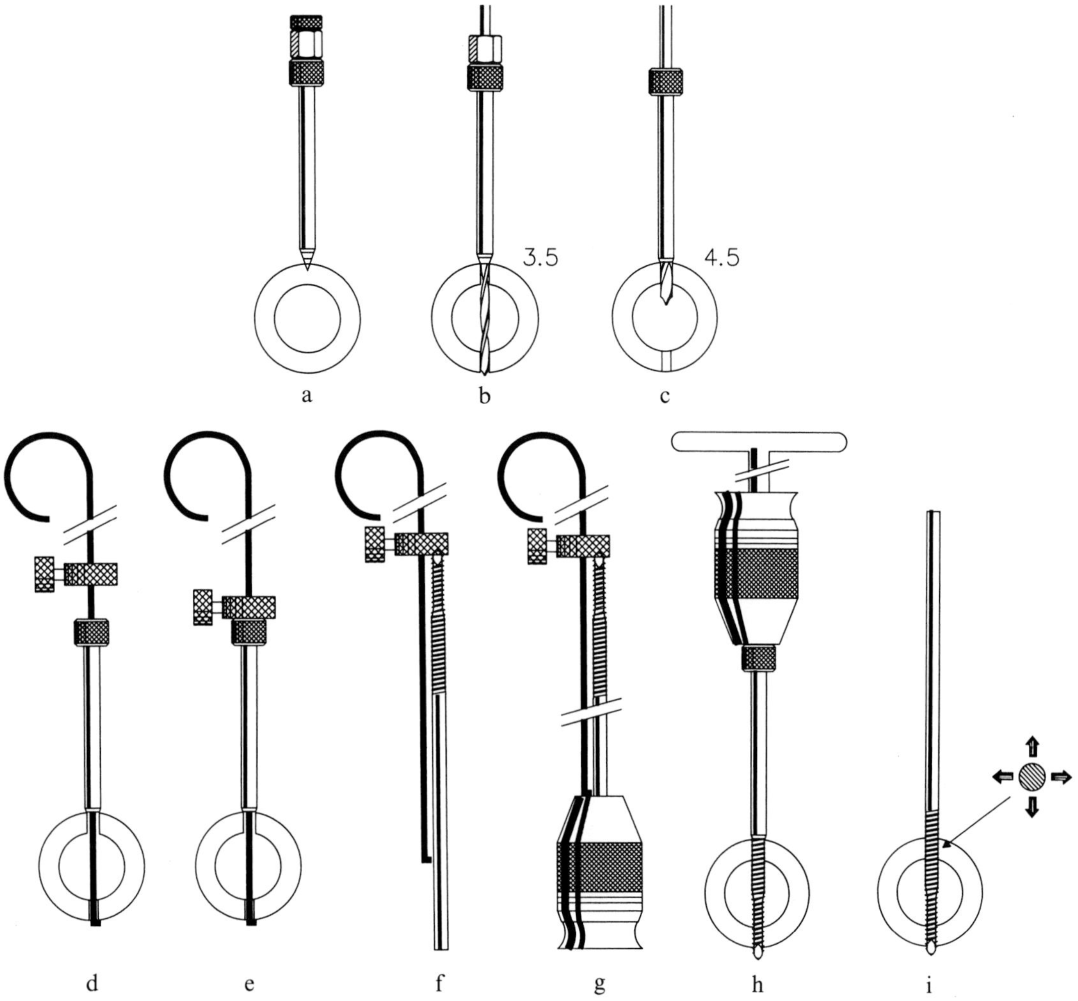

3.5
4.5

a b c

d e f g h i

Then the threaded tip of the Schanz screw is placed into the Schanz screw recess of the knurled disk and the universal chuck advanced over the nonthreaded end of the Schanz screw until the tip of the depth gauge touches the end of the universal chuck. After tightening of the chuck, the Schanz screw is inserted until the chuck touches the top of the drill sleeve. The Schanz screw is now fully inserted into the far cortex.

Insertion of Schanz screws with long shallow thread, exerting preload in both cortices (Fig. 5.7 B): The triple trocar point is placed on the bony surface, and the trocar, together with the 3.5-mm drill sleeve, removed. Both cortices are then pierced with a 4.5-mm drill bit. After measuring with the depth gauge, the Schanz screw can be fixed in the chuck and inserted across both cortices.

Fig. 5.7 Insertion of a Schanz screw (continued).

B Application of a Schanz screw with long shallow thread, exerting radial preload in both cortices.

a Assemble triple trocar and penetrate the soft tissue down to the bone through the stab incision.

b Remove trocar and 3.5-mm drill sleeve and drill both cortices with 4.5-mm drill bit. The use of the oscillating attachment (Fig. 5.4 Ag) is strongly recommended – as well as the three-fluted drill bit.

c–g Measure length and proceed to insert the long, shallow threaded screw (4.7 mm core diameter) by means of the universal chuck.

Fig. 5.7 B

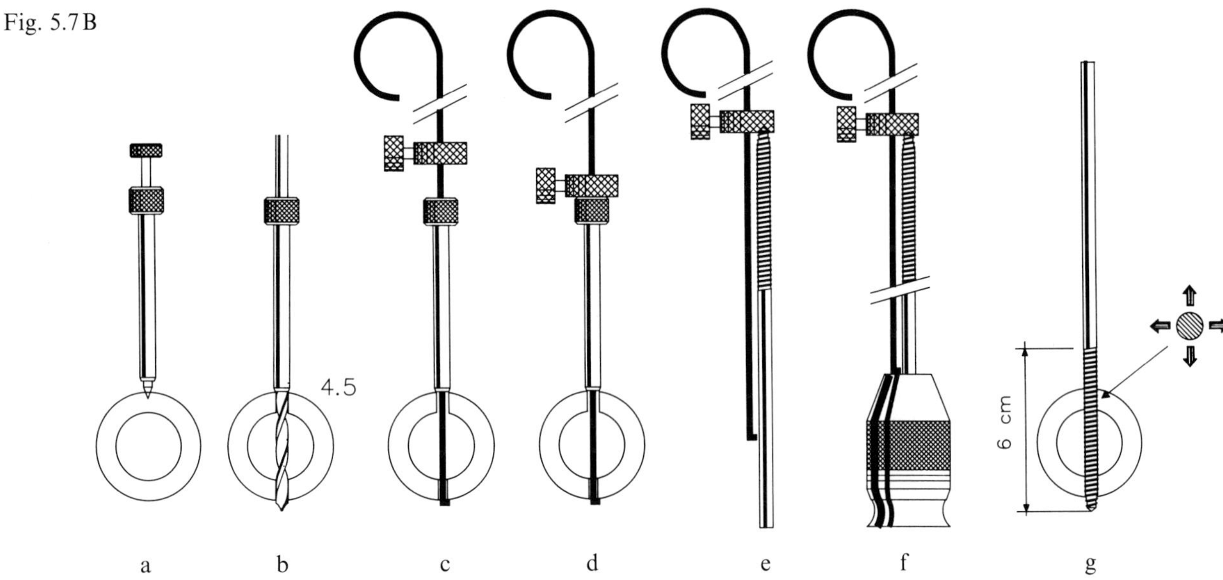

5.5.2 Mounting of Different Fixator Frames

5.5.2.1 Simple Unilateral Frame

Tubular fixator frames are applied in four steps (Fig. 5.8) (Behrens et al. 1981; Hierholzer et al. 1985).

Step 1. Gross alignment of the fracture and insertion of one Schanz screw in one main fragment. This initial screw is placed close to the joint. Application of the longitudinal tube fitted with the required number of clamps then follows:

Step 2. The fracture is reduced manually and the second Schanz screw is inserted into the other main fragment through the furthest opposite adjustable clamp. Reduction is secured by tightening the most proximal and distal clamps. At this stage, great care must be taken to secure proper length and rotational alignment before tightening the two clamps.

Step 3. Insertion of the remaining Schanz screws through the adjustable clamps, and tightening of the respective clamps.

Step 4. For angular adjustments in another plane, the longitudinal rod is replaced by two shorter tubes which are connected by a universal joint. To correct rotational malalignment, an intermediate tube has to be placed between two tubes, fixed to each of the proximal and distal main fragments, and connected to these two tubes by universal joints or tube-tube clamps (Fig. 5.9).

Warning: Insertion of conventional 4.5-mm Schanz screws into a 3.5-mm hole leads to potentially hazardous microcracks in the bone cortex.

When dealing with short fragments, two Schanz screws need to be inserted at the same level. The pin-adjusting clamp, however, is very versatile in its application – particularly in the area of the tibial head, where one should avoid interfering with the patellar ligament (Fig. 5.10).

Fig. 5.8 Application of the one-tube unilateral fixator.

This mode of external fixator application is the one most frequently used!

a Step 1: Application of the first Schanz screw close to the distal joint according to Fig. 5.7A or B.

b The tube with the planned number of adjustable clamps is fixed to the Schanz screw.

c Step 2: Application of the second Schanz screw across the most proximal adjustable clamp.

d At this time, three-dimensional reduction of fracture is easy, observing axis and rotation of the foot, by comparing it with the uninjured side.

e Step 3: The inner Schanz screws are inserted about 2 cm from the fracture area. The tubular fixator allows individualization of Schanz screw placement according to fracture configuration.

f Prevention of drop foot by connecting metatarsal I or II to tube by means of a Schanz screw.

Fig. 5.8

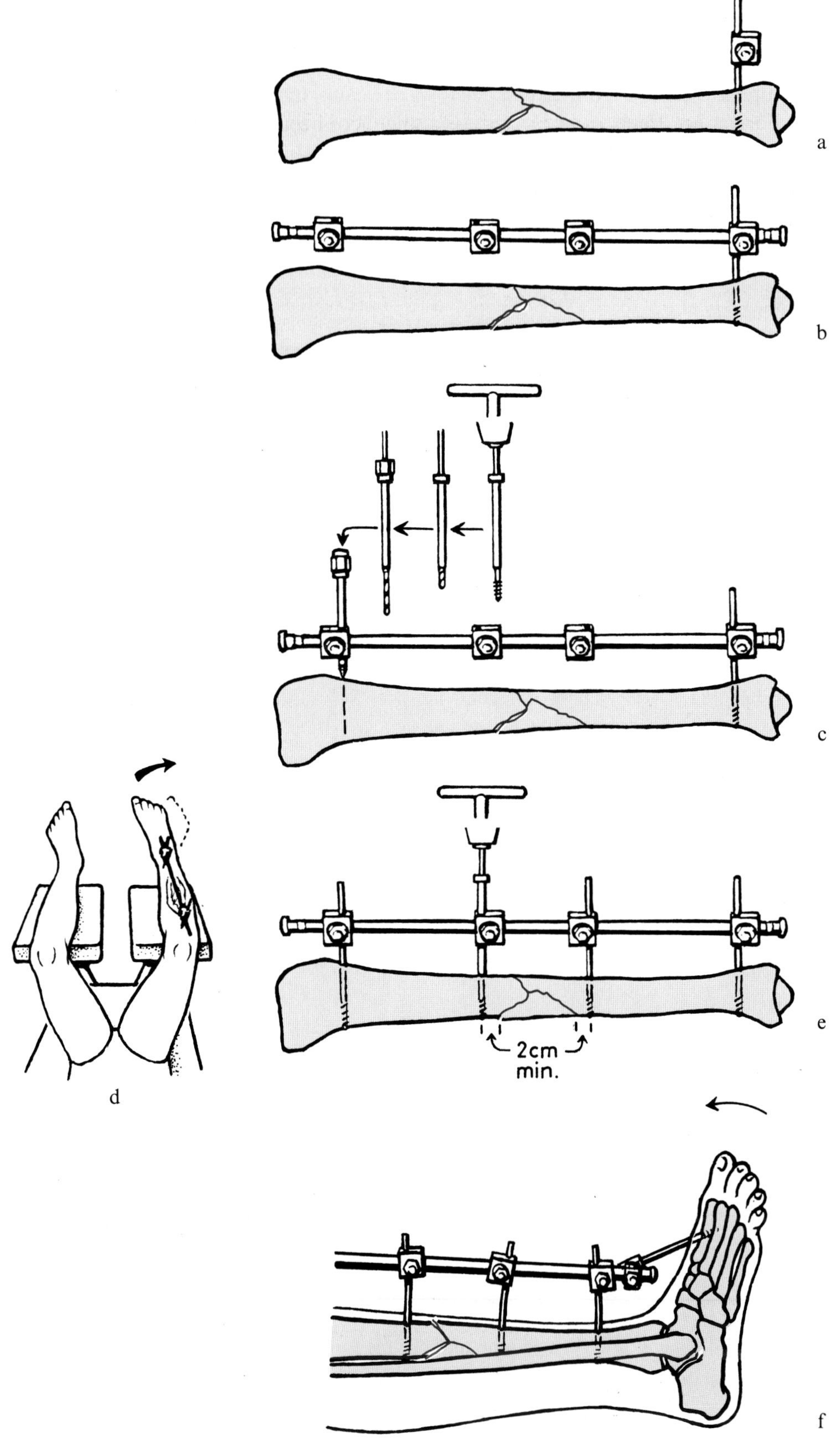

5.5.2.2 Modular Unilateral Frame – With Universal Joints or the Tube-Tube Clamp (Figs. 5.9, 5.11, 5.12)

For modular unilateral frames, manual reduction may be postponed until the whole frame is applied. Initially the Schanz screws in each main bony fragment are connected by a short tube. Each of these tubes is then connected by a universal joint or tube-tube clamp to an intermediate connecting tube. Alignment changes are easily made after loosening the two joints connecting the intermediate tube to the other two tubes.

Fig. 5.9 Modular application of the AO tubular fixator (preferably using metal tubes!). This permits three-dimensional secondary reduction.

a Each main fragment is provided with two Schanz screws and two relatively short tubes.

b Reduction and application of two tube-tube clamps and one connecting tube.

c Reduction stabilized by tightening tube-tube clamps on connecting tube.

Fig. 5.10 Fixation of a short metaphyseal fragment by the pin-adjusting clamp. An older alternative is the triple clamp/cardan double clamp with a fixed distance between parallel Schanz screws.

Fig. 5.9

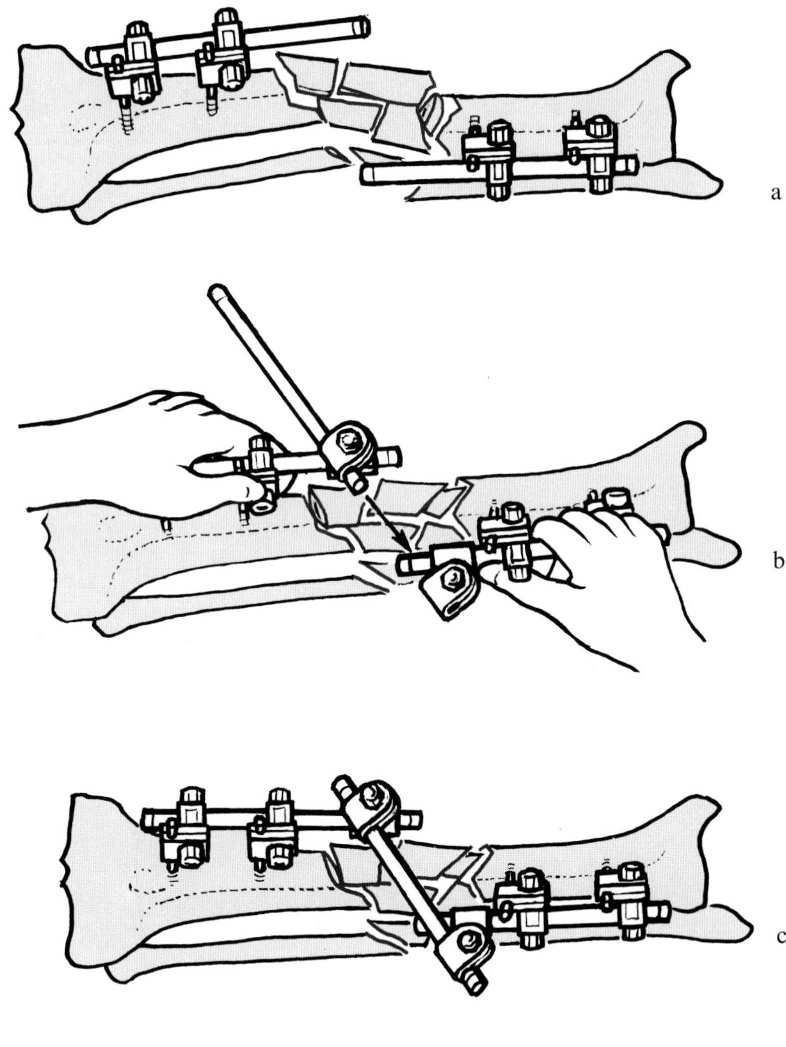

Fig. 5.10

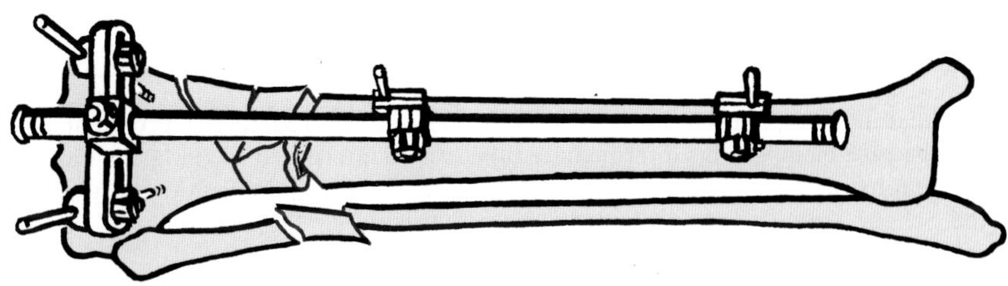

Fig. 5.11 Modular unilateral frame using an intermediate tube fixed to the proximal and distal tube by means of tube-tube clamps. This intermediate tube can be interposed secondarily and permits three-dimensional corrections of inadequate reduction. The figure illustrates application of this principle in the humerus, the Schanz screw being inserted at about 90° between the two pairs of screws to avoid interference with the radial nerve.

Fig. 5.12 Modular frame applied to the femur. For increased stability, two intermediate tubes have been used. If this fixation remains in place for more than a few days, a second set of tubes should be applied to the proximal as well as to the distal main fragment to increase stability. In contrast to tibial fractures, external fixation in compound femur fractures is very rarely used because, after soft tissue healing, internal fixation is carried out. If external fixation is chosen as the definitive treatment, the modular frame has to be replaced by a double-tube unilateral fixator with three pins in each main fragment. Cancellous autotransplants will have to be added.

Fig. 5.11

Fig. 5.12

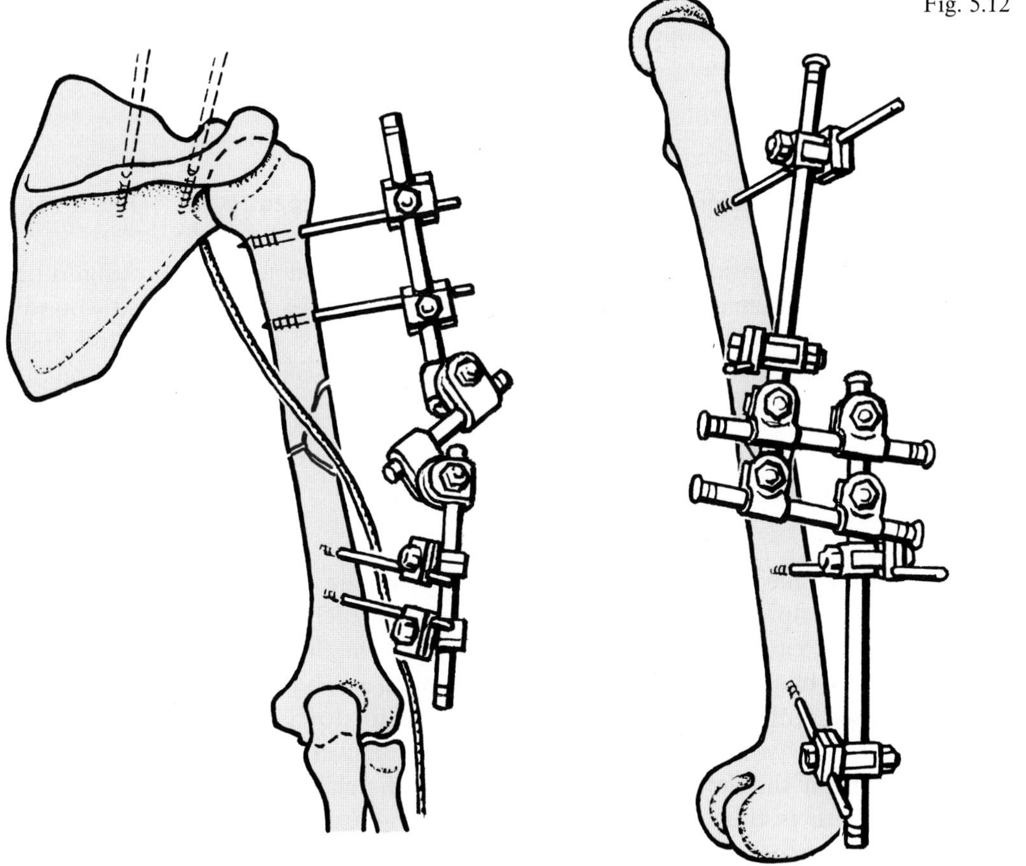

5.5.2.3 Double-Tube Unilateral Frame (Fig. 5.13)

For fractures with large areas of segmental comminution or bone loss, a stiffer frame such as the double-tube unilateral frame may be needed. We arrive at this configuration simply by stacking a second tube on top of the first after insertion of the first Schanz screw. There is, however, one prerequisite: all Schanz screws must be inserted in the same plane (Fig. 5.13) (Behrens and Johnson 1985; Behrens and Searls 1986). Therefore both tubes, provided with the necessary adjustable clamps, must be attached simultaneously. The remaining Schanz screws are then inserted through the two corresponding adjustable clamps.

5.5.2.4 Two-Plane Unilateral Frame – "Delta or V-Shaped Frame" (Fig. 5.14)

Another option for a stiffer frame is the two-plane unilateral configuration which consists of two interconnected simple unilateral frames. To allow optimal wound access, the plane for the second frame should lie at an angle of between 60° and 100° with the plane of the first frame (Fig. 5.14) (Behrens and Johnson 1985; Behrens and Searls 1986).

5.5.3 Additional Maneuvers

In simple transverse fractures, further stabilization at the fracture site can be achieved by compressing the main fragments against each other using the open compressor, taking care to avoid the tendency to angulate the fragments.

Oblique fractures in metaphyseal areas can be reduced anatomically and rigidly stabilized with interfragmentary screws. The fixator is then used as a neutralization frame. In diaphyseal fractures, however, this maneuver should only be considered when dealing with a simple two-fragment fracture with relatively long contact areas. In comminuted fractures this technique can lead to refracture when removing the external fixator and is therefore not recommended.

Fig. 5.13 One-plane double-tube unilateral fixator.

This allows for increased stability in a defect situation or with extensive comminution. The steps are identical to those of the one-tube fixator but both tubes provided with the adequate number of adjustable clamps have to be fixed simultaneously to the first (distal) Schanz screw.

Double-tube external fixation is the preferred mode in fractures of the femur, each of the two main fragments being provided with three Schanz screws.

a Insertion of distal Schanz screw.

b Addition of both tubes simultaneously – the clamps touching each other for better rotational stability and also for a less bulky arrangement.

c Control and correction of alignment after insertion of the proximal Schanz screw.

Fig. 5.14 Two-plane unilateral external fixator (delta or V-shaped frame).

First the ventral fixator is applied as illustrated in Fig. 5.9 in a nearly sagittal plane aiming somewhat toward the medial posterior tibial cortex. Next the medial fixator is applied at an angle between 60° and 100° and fixed with either two or four Schanz screws. The two tubes are then interconnected by two Steinmann pins, the pointed ends being covered by two protective caps.

Fig. 5.13

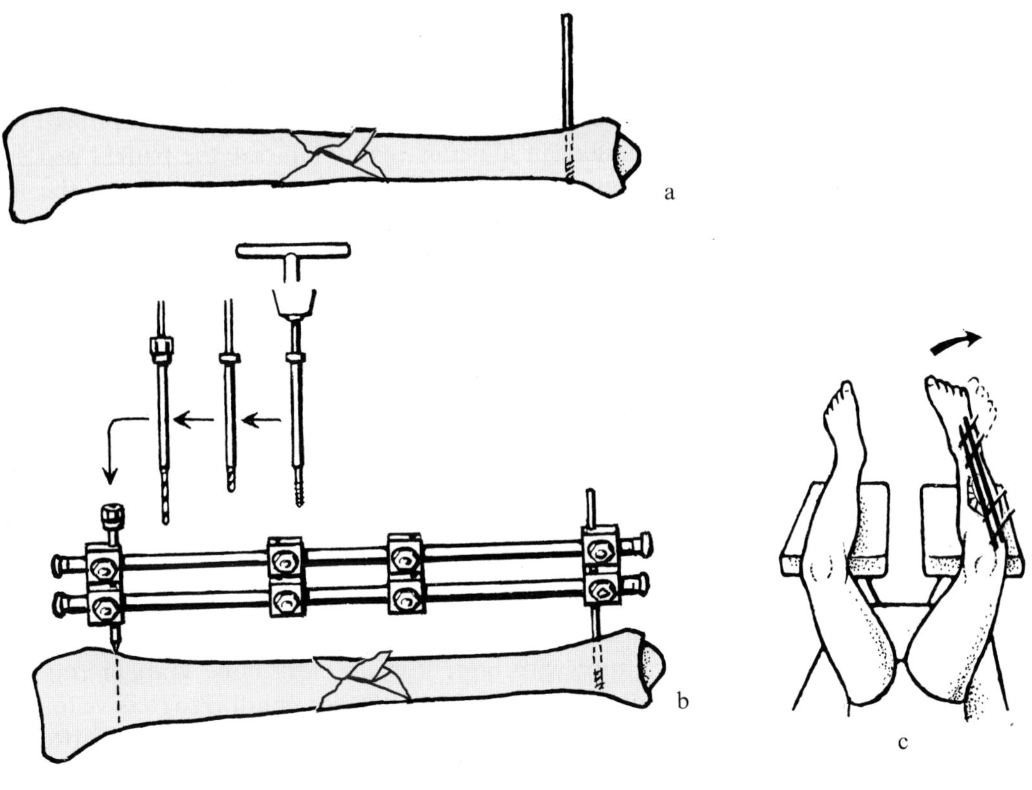

Fig. 5.14

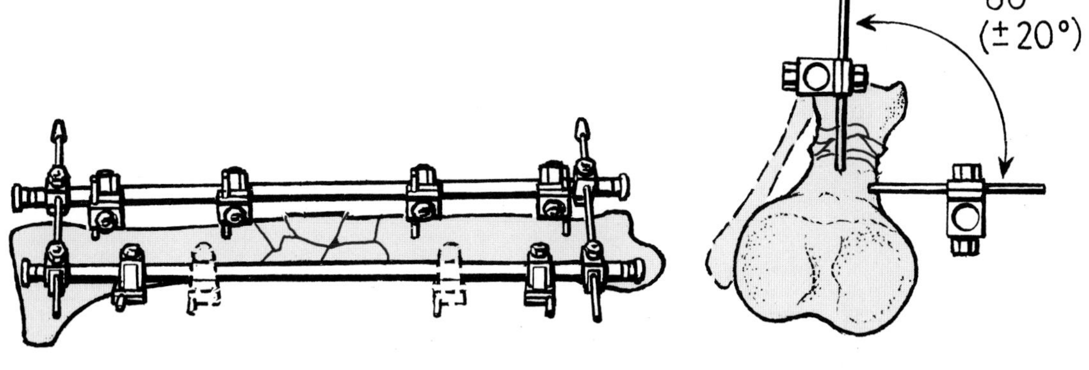

5.6 Postoperative Treatment

In the early postoperative period, the injured extremity segment is often supported by pillows or by balanced suspension. Adjacent joints are splinted in functional positions. As soon as the patient is reasonably comfortable, active joint motion and muscle strengthening exercises are initiated. In lower extremity injuries, the patient proceeds to partial weight-bearing with crutches, bearing increasingly more weight on the injured leg as the fracture consolidates (Behrens and Searls 1986).

Early during the stay in the hospital, the patient is taught Schanz screw and frame care (Searls et al. 1983). The Schanz screw entry sites are kept clean by taking a daily shower and cleansing the sites with a "Q-tip". After cleansing, the Schanz screw entry site can be covered with an antiseptic compound. The same cleansing policy applies in cases where Steinmann pins have been used to build a bilateral or triangular frame.

5.7 Fracture Healing and Frame Destabilization (Fig. 5.15)

Most fractures which have been stabilized with an external fixator consolidate by secondary bone union. In fractures with bone loss, an early bone graft or fragment transport may be necessary to assure bone healing and correct length. Progressive force transmission across the healing fracture site appears to stimulate bone formation. After consolidation of the soft tissues, patients are encouraged to walk with partial and then full weight-bearing. Once the patient has progressed to full, unsupported weight-bearing, a further increase in force transmission can be achieved through dynamization (Fig. 5.15) or gradual build-down of the fixator frame. Depending on the complexity of the initial frame, the build-down occurs sequentially:

1. Reducing a complex frame down to a one-tube configuration.
2. Moving the longitudinal tube away from the bone.
3. Sequential loosening of the clamps either to further decrease the stiffness of the frame or to allow for sliding of the clamps along the longitudinal tubes (Fig. 5.15a–d).

Fig. 5.15 Dynamization of the two types of unilateral fixator.

As explained in the text, gradual building down of the external fixator is one effective way of dynamization.

a If one intends to induce a rotationally and axially stable "telescoping" dynamization which preserves the longitudinal preload in a one-tube unilateral fixator, the addition of a short second tube connected to the long tube by means of a universal joint (b) permits a very elegant axial gliding mechanism.

b, c To this effect, the nut of the universal joint connecting to the short tube and the two nuts of the long tube have to be released (crosswise release!). It is best to remove the tube-nuts completely lest they get lost when the patient ambulates.

c Another possibility is dynamization, avoiding the need to use the universal joint.

d Dynamization of the unilateral one-plane double-tube fixator. Crosswise release of the tube-nuts permits longitudinal gliding provided that the Schanz screws are reasonably parallel.

Fig. 5.15

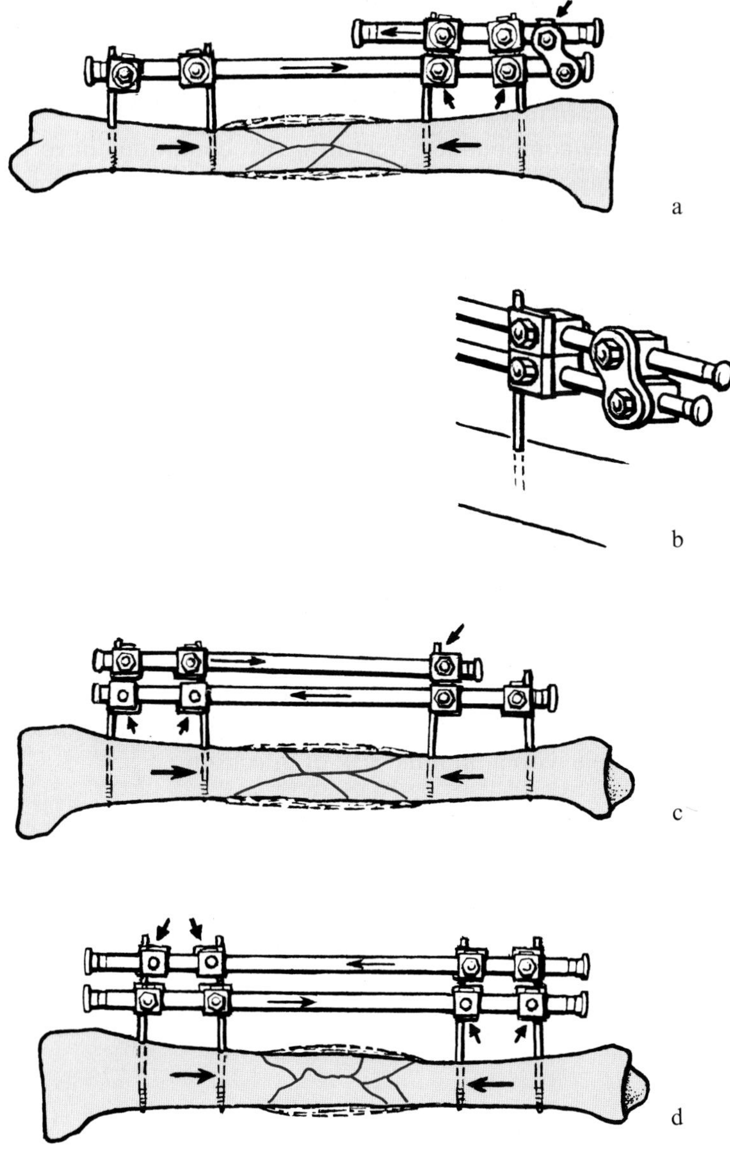

5.7.1 What Next After External Fixation?

Initially, the external fixator was used as a first procedure to allow healing of soft tissues, with an internal fixation performed as a secondary procedure after control of the soft tissue problem. Today, the number of secondary operations has strikingly diminished, as the external fixator is now being used successfully as both a primary and a definitive stabilization tool in a considerable number of cases.

In severely compounded fractures, two conditions have to be considered separately: simple, oblique or spiral fractures with severe soft tissue injuries, and complex fractures with severe soft tissue injury.

With simple fracture patterns, bone healing can occur within 3–4 months with an external fixator alone. One or two additional interfragmentary screws neutralized by a unilateral fixator may facilitate cortical healing. In severe complex fractures, a post-primary, autogenous, cancellous, onlay graft is recommended.

There remain, however, a number of cases where secondary stabilization appears necessary. If good callus formation is present, protection by a plaster cast and increasing weight-bearing will often suffice. In the face of delayed healing, internal fixation by plating or nailing is indicated after soft tissue healing. Secondary operative stabilization is still controversial. The question is whether it should be done directly or with a delay of 8–10 days after removal of the Schanz screws. The decision depends very much on the local tissue conditions.

If the fixator has been in place for less than 3 weeks and provided there are absolutely no inflammatory changes, removal of the device can be followed by immediate internal fixation. If the fixator has been in place longer, it should be removed and the limb temporarily stabilized in a cast for 8–10 days. Under antibiotic cover, plating or nailing is then possible with a minimal risk of infection.

5.8 Specific Locations and Indications

5.8.1 Lower Leg

With the use of AO tubular components, some 90% of all tibial fractures can be stabilized with a one-plane, unilateral frame (Behrens and Johnson 1985). Generally such a frame is applied within 30° to the lateral side of the sagittal plane. When a higher degree of stiffness is needed, as with extensive segmental comminution or bone loss, double-tube one-plane frames or two-plane unilateral configurations are more useful (Behrens and Searls 1986). Modified two-plane unilateral frames are most appropriate when dealing with short proximal or distal tibial fragments. If Schanz screws are placed within 2 cm of the tibial plateau, the knee must be moved through a full range of motion to ensure that they do not block the functions of the pes anserinus, the collateral ligaments, or the iliotibial band. Short proximal or distal fragments can also be held firm by the pin-adjusting clamp (Fig. 5.10) using a one-plane sagittal fixator (see also Sect. 5.8.6). Very distal tibial fractures or those involving the "pilon" can at least temporarily be stabilized with a frame that connects a calcaneal Steinmann pin to two anterior Schanz screws in the tibia. When the foot cannot be held with an external splint because of sensory deficits or a soft tissue injury, it is best stabilized by connecting a transtarsal or metatarsal Steinmann pin to the main frame. It is paramount that the ankle joint be splinted in about 5°–10° of dorsiflexion early in the treatment period to avoid a rapidly developing equinus contraction (Behrens and Johnson 1985; Behrens and Searls 1986).

5.8.2 Femur and Knee

Unlike the lower leg, the femur is covered circumferentially with a thick soft-tissue sleeve and, therefore, does not provide ideal corridors for Schanz screw insertion. To prevent screw track infections and knee stiffness, femoral fixators should only be applied for short periods and then replaced by other means of internal or external fixation. For most injury conditions, simple double-tube frames with six Schanz screws are satisfactory. The Schanz screws are generally inserted from a lateral direction, but any plane between the lateral intermuscular septum and the lateral border of the sartorius muscle can be chosen without risking major neurovascular injury. An exception, however, is the profunda femoris artery which has an inconsistent course. The application of a modular frame allowing secondary reduction of fragments is also possible (Fig. 5.12).

Occasionally, temporary transarticular fixation of the knee joint is indicated for a polytrauma patient, or when stabilizing osteoligamentous injury or a joint reconstruction. A simple anterior frame with a universal joint centered over the knee joint is generally most satisfactory and allows for immobilization in any desired position of knee flexion. To prevent undue knee stiffness, such fixators are usually removed within 2–4 weeks.

5.8.3 Pelvis (Fig. 5.16)

In the early management of a pelvic ring injury, an external frame may decrease blood loss, increase patient comfort, and facilitate nursing care. For most such urgently applied frames, the long-threaded 5-mm Schanz screws are inserted into the iliac crests. The first screw is placed 1–2 cm posterior to the anterior superior iliac spine and the second at the level of the iliac tubercle. Both Schanz screws are directed towards the sacroiliac joint and should pierce neither the inner nor the outer pelvic tables. It is generally possible to place these Schanz screws percutaneously, but in small and obese patients, open insertion after subperiosteal exposure of the anterior iliac crest is safer. The two corresponding Schanz screws in each crest are connected to one or more tubes. The tubes are placed so as to clear the abdominal wall of a sitting or standing patient by 2 cm. In a lean patient, a straight tube may achieve this goal, but in the obese a V-shaped connection is built with two short tubes connected by a universal joint (Fig. 5.16). Further stabilization of the frame is achieved by connecting the two tubes longitudinally with Steinmann pins or smaller tubes.

Simple frames are sufficient for emergency measures and for the stabilization of stable anterior and lateral compression injuries (Searls et al. 1983). More rigid configurations are needed to hold unstable compression injuries and vertical shear injuries (See Chap. 9).

Fig. 5.16 Pelvic frame.

5-mm Schanz screws with long thread are used and care has to be taken that the Schanz screws are obliquely inserted and that the tubes are fixed to the Schanz screws in such a way as to leave enough room for the abdomen in the sitting position. The modular frame using an intermediate tube fixed by tube-tube clamps to the lateral tubes greatly facilitates giving the abdomen its necessary freedom.

It must be noted that – contrary to the "open book injury", which is stable posteriorly – posterior instability of the pelvis cannot be fixed reliably by any kind of external frame. External fixation in such cases can only be considered as a temporary emergency procedure.

Fig. 5.16

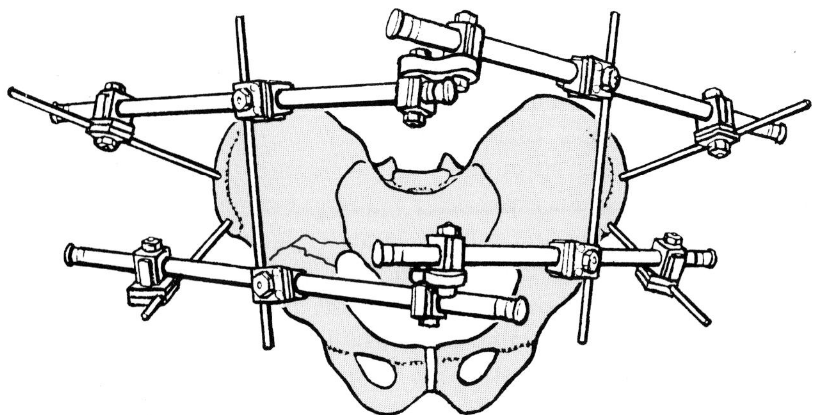

5.8.4 Upper Extremity

For the management of most *forearm and hand fractures*, internal fixation with screws and plates is preferable to the use of external fixation. However, the small external fixator is now popular among hand surgeons for lesions such as open fractures involving the distal forearm and the hand skeleton, as well as for certain wrist fractures. The tubular fixator (Fig. 5.17 A a–c) is a good alternative if employed using special Schanz screws (Fig. 5.17 B) with a 2.7-mm (Fig. 5.17 B a) or 3.5-mm (Fig. 5.17 B b) diameter thread and a 4.5-mm shaft which are held solid by the adjustable clamps. Due to its increased stiffness, it is well suited for complex fractures and fractures accompanied by bone loss.

When applying a fixator for a *wrist fracture*, the first Schanz screw (3.5/4.5 mm) is inserted into the radius close to the fracture and the second (2.7/4.5 mm) proximally into the second metacarpal after making 5-mm incisions and exposing the bone so as to avoid damage to the muscles and tendons. The Schanz screws are inserted at an angle of 30° to the radial direction. The reduction is checked with the image intensifier, corrected and preliminarily held with the tube and two single adjustable clamps. With two additional Schanz screws, one distally in the second metacarpal and one more proximally in the radius, a sufficiently stable assembly is achieved using only a single tube. If distraction alone does not result in a satisfactory reduction of the articular fragments, additional Kirschner wires must be used. Primary (or secondary) cancellous bone grafts are indicated in cases with marked cancellous defects or with severe metaphyseal comminution. When articular fragments are too displaced or impacted, secondary open reduction and internal fixation might be necessary.

When dealing with *extra-articular radial fractures* with distal fragments of at least 2-cm length, the distal fixator screws can be placed in this fragment, a variation which preserves some wrist motion during consolidation.

In the *forearm shaft*, external fixators are generally used as temporary devices until an open or infected lesion is covered with healthy soft tissues. The frames are then replaced by internal fixation.

In the *ulna*, the Schanz screws are placed through the dorsal subcutaneous border. The rare external fixation of a radial lesion should be preceded by a careful review of the relevant anatomy, followed by open Schanz screw insertion under direct vision through small incisions.

In the *humerus*, percutaneous Schanz screw placement is quite safe from a posterior direction in the distal third, and from laterally in the proximal third, but all other screw sites should be surgically exposed. The modular fixator, using three short tubes, is ideally suited to accommodate two pairs of Schanz screws inserted in two different planes (Fig. 5.11). To avoid the risks of screw-track infection and elbow stiffness, the external frames are replaced early either by braces or by internal fixation.

Fig. 5.17 A Use of the tubular external fixator for stabilization of the distal radius fracture.

Special 4.5-mm shaft Schanz screws either with a 3.5-mm thread for insertion into the radius or with a 2.7-mm thread for fixation to metacarpal II are available and provide a very simple as well as a very stable fixation. An alternative possibility with more flexibility: fix two short tubes to radius and metacarpal II and connect via an intermediate tube and two tube-tube clamps!

Fig. 5.17 B Special Schanz screws with 4.5-mm shaft and threads of (a) 2.7- and (b) 3.5-mm diameter with blunt trocar tip.

Fig. 5.17A

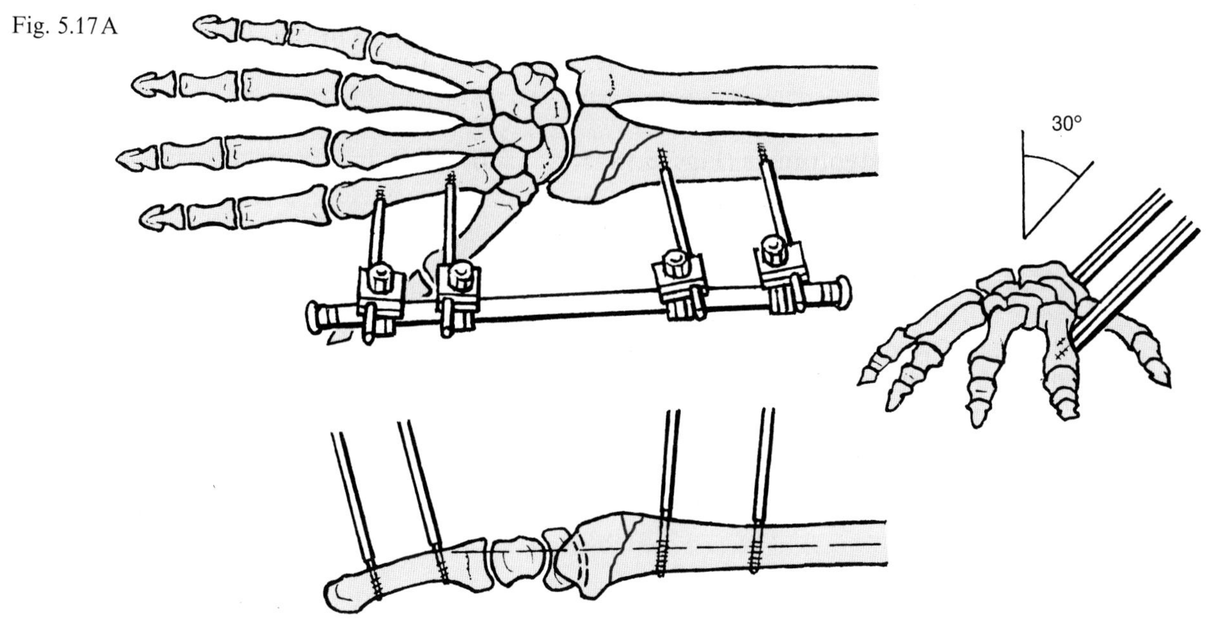

Fig. 5.17B

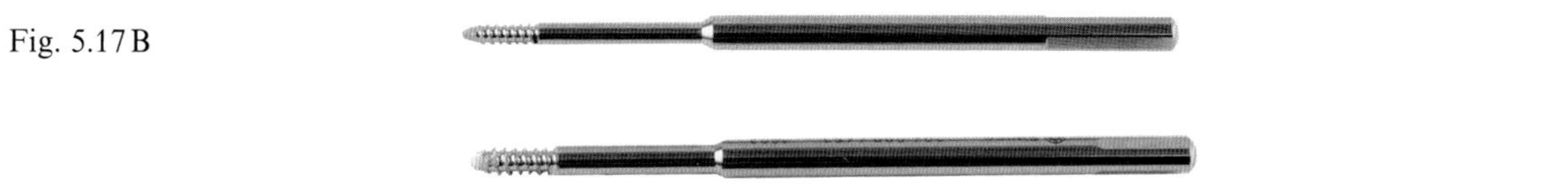

If the elbow is immobilized with an external fixator, the posterior Schanz screws are placed sagittally into the distal third of the humerus and the ulna.

For the exceptional situation demanding glenohumeral stabilization with an external fixator, the proximal Schanz screws are placed into the spine of the scapula (Fig. 5.11).

5.8.5 Fusions and Osteotomies (Figs. 5.18, 5.19, 5.20)

Fusions and osteotomies most often require symmetrical compression, which is best provided by a bilateral frame. Using the aiming device (Fig. 5.18), the bone is predrilled with a 3.5-mm drill bit. A 5-mm Steinmann pin is introduced *manually* through a 5-mm drill guide held by the adjustable clamp using a hand chuck. Longitudinal preload of the Steinmann pins provides compression fixation of the contact areas and prevents gliding of the Steinmann pins as well as pin-track infections. Figure 5.19 illustrates some of the procedures for joint fusions and Fig. 5.20 demonstrates how to fix correction osteotomies.

Fig. 5.18 A Aiming device for constructing a bilateral frame used for insertion of Steinmann pins.

a Bar with hook and sliding sleeve and with fixed 3.5-mm drill sleeve.

b 3.5-mm trocar.

c Long drill bits, 3.5- and 4.5-mm diameter. Use three-fluted drill bits!

d 5-mm drill sleeve for insertion over the fixed 3.5-mm drill sleeve of the aiming device. Once the 3.5-mm hole is drilled, the aiming device can be withdrawn and the 5-mm drill sleeve still remaining in the adjustable clamp will guide the Steinmann pin, which is driven in by the hand chuck.

Fig. 5.18 B Application of the aiming device.

A 5-mm drill sleeve is put on the fixed 3.5-mm drill sleeve of the aiming device and this assembly is inserted into the adjustable clamp on one side and the point of the aiming device into the adjustable clamp on the opposite side. The 3.5-mm trocar is placed on the bone surface across the aiming device through a stab incision. The trocar is replaced by a 3.5-mm drill bit which pierces both cortices. The aiming device is removed, the 5-mm drill sleeve remaining in place held by the adjustable clamp. Overdrilling the bone with a 4.5-mm drill bit and insertion of a 4.5- or 5-mm Steinmann pin by means of a universal chuck.

Fig. 5.18 A

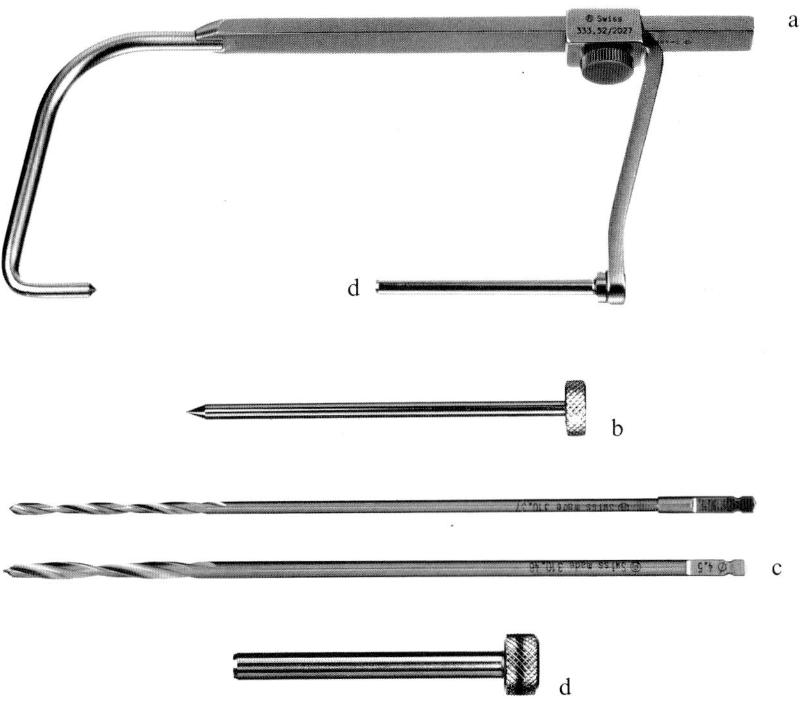

Fig. 5.18 B

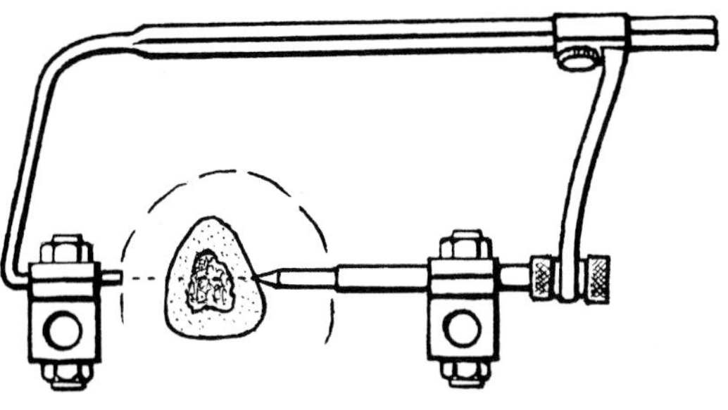

Fig. 5.19 Arthrodesis of various joints.

The external fixator allows very effective preload to be applied by bending the Steinmann pins against each other. For maximum stability, the Steinmann pins in the clamp should be kept at 90° to the tube so that they describe a double bend. To this effect, open the tube nuts only, use the compressor with the Steinmann nut tightly closed and then retighten the tube nut.

a, b Arthrodesis of the elbow. This is one of the most difficult arthrodeses to perform. The position of the nerves and vessels make a tension band fixation impossible. Most often we combine axial compression, obtained by means of external compression clamps, with a cancellous lag screw inserted in the axis of the humerus. The surfaces of the trochlea of the humerus and of the olecranon fossa are resected to fit. The osteotomy is reduced and a thick Kirschner wire is driven through the olecranon into the medullary canal of the humerus. The head and neck of the radius are then resected as far as the insertion of the biceps tendon. A Steinmann pin is then inserted transversely through the olecranon in line with the anterior cortex of the humerus. The Kirschner wire is removed and is replaced with a long cancellous bone screw. This cancellous bone screw should be as long as possible and should be supported with a washer to prevent its head from sinking into the olecranon. A second Steinmann pin should be inserted and the compression of the arthrodesis increased by means of the external fixators.

c–g Arthrodesis of the knee.

c, d Make a straight longitudinal incision directly over the middle of the patella. With a broad chisel, resect from the patella as large a cube of bone as possible. Open the joint widely so that you can flex the knee to 90°. Keeping the knee flexed at 90°, resect the distal articular surface of the femur in line with the long axis of the tibia. This means that the cut is at 90° to the long axis of the femur. Next the proximal surface of the tibia is cut, sloping the cut slightly to the back, so that the arthrodesis, when reduced, will be in 10° of flexion.

e The position of the arthrodesis once reduced is checked with a long string which, when stretched from the anterior superior spine to the web space between the first and second toe, should cross the middle of the knee joint. The flexion and the valgus should be about 10° each.

f Once the surfaces have been suitably trimmed to obtain correct alignment of the leg, four Steinmann pins are inserted. The two posterior pins are inserted as close to the arthrodesis as possible. The two anterior ones are inserted about 4 cm away from the arthrodesis. The external fixator is installed and axial compression is applied.

f′ Check once again the alignment of the arthrodesis. Finally, slot in the cube of bone which you removed from the patella as a bridge across the arthrodesis.

g Alternative fixation possibility (Hierholzer) using a bilateral frame in two planes, the anterior tube acting as a very effective tension band. Access and resection are identical with the procedure described above.

Fig. 5.19

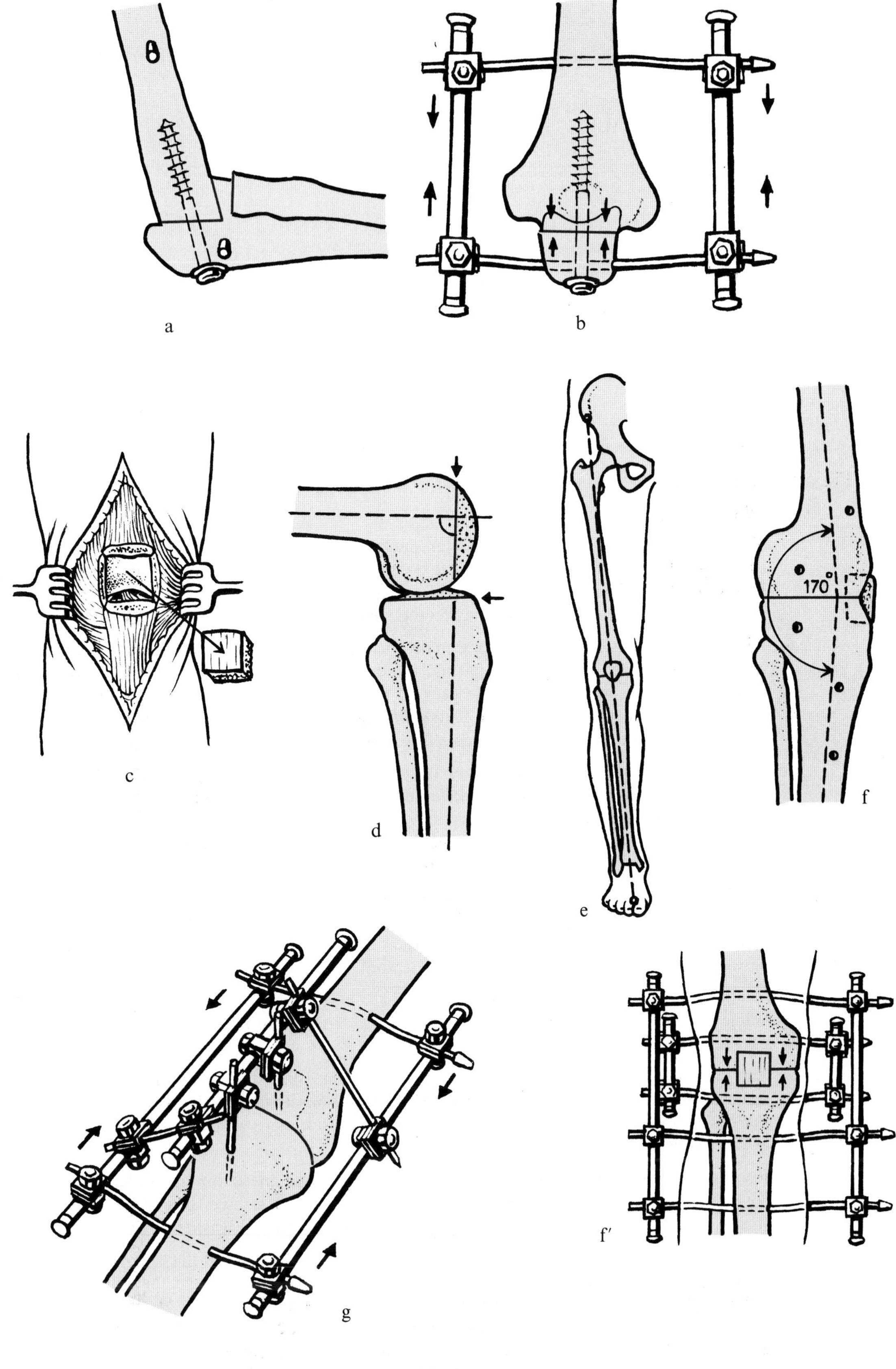

Fig. 5.19 Arthrodesis of various joints (continued).

h–o Tibiotarsal arthrodesis.

h–i The procedure is carried out under pneumatic tourniquet control. The whole limb is prepared and draped to expose the knee and ankle. The first Steinmann pin is then inserted 6–7 cm above the ankle joint. It is inserted in a lateral to medial direction and in 20° of external rotation with respect to the knee joint axis. To ease the insertion of the Steinmann pin, predrill the bone with a 4.5-mm drill bit.

h Make an 8-cm incision over the lateral malleolus and a 5-cm-long medial incision over the medial malleolus. If no great deformity exists, particularly as far as rotation is concerned, it is best to insert two 2.5-mm Kirschner wires through the neck of the talus and the tibia, at the point where the Steinmann pins will subsequently be inserted. The point of the second Steinmann pin lies directly in the neck of the talus, in line with the anterior edge of the tibia.

i The Steinmann pin and Kirschner wire are now removed so that they are not in the way of the surgeon during the procedure. The lateral malleolus is osteotomized obliquely about 3 cm from its tip. The distal articular surface of the tibia is now resected either with a chisel or an oscillating saw. Great care must be taken to resect the posterior lip of the tibia. The resection is completed through the medial incision: the medial malleolus is resected; the distal medial flare of the tibia is flattened.

j The knee is flexed to 90° and the foot externally rotated so that its external rotation corresponds to the external rotation of the uninvolved leg. Two Kirschner wires are now inserted into the previous drill holes through the tibia and neck of the talus respectively. In a woman we aim for a right angle between the long axis of the tibia and the foot. In a man with a mobile midtarsal joint we prefer 10° of dorsiflexion.

k While the foot is held in the desired position, the articular surface of the dome of the talus is resected parallel to the distal osteotomy through the tibia.

l The proximal Steinmann pin is now inserted into the tibia. The position of the foot is checked once again and if all is well the second Steinmann pin is inserted into the hole previously drilled through the neck of the talus. The foot is now displaced posteriorly, which improves the posterior lever arm as well as the forwards roll of the foot from heel to toe.

m Fix the external fixators to the two Steinmann pins and place the arthrodesis under maximal axial compression. The lateral malleolus is now shaped to fit and is used as a bridge across the arthrodesis. It is fixed with a malleolar or a small cancellous bone screw and a washer.

n, o Pantalar arthrodesis. Resect the whole talus. Resect the articular surface of the navicular, the cuboid and the articular surfaces of the os calcis. Reduce the foot and shape the talus as a free bone graft in such a way that it fits accurately between all the resected surfaces. At the end, one Steinmann pin is inserted into the tibia, another into the os calcis and a third across the cuboid and navicular, taking great care not to damage the neurovascular bundle. Axial compression is then obtained between the different segments by using four or six external compression units.

Fig. 5.19

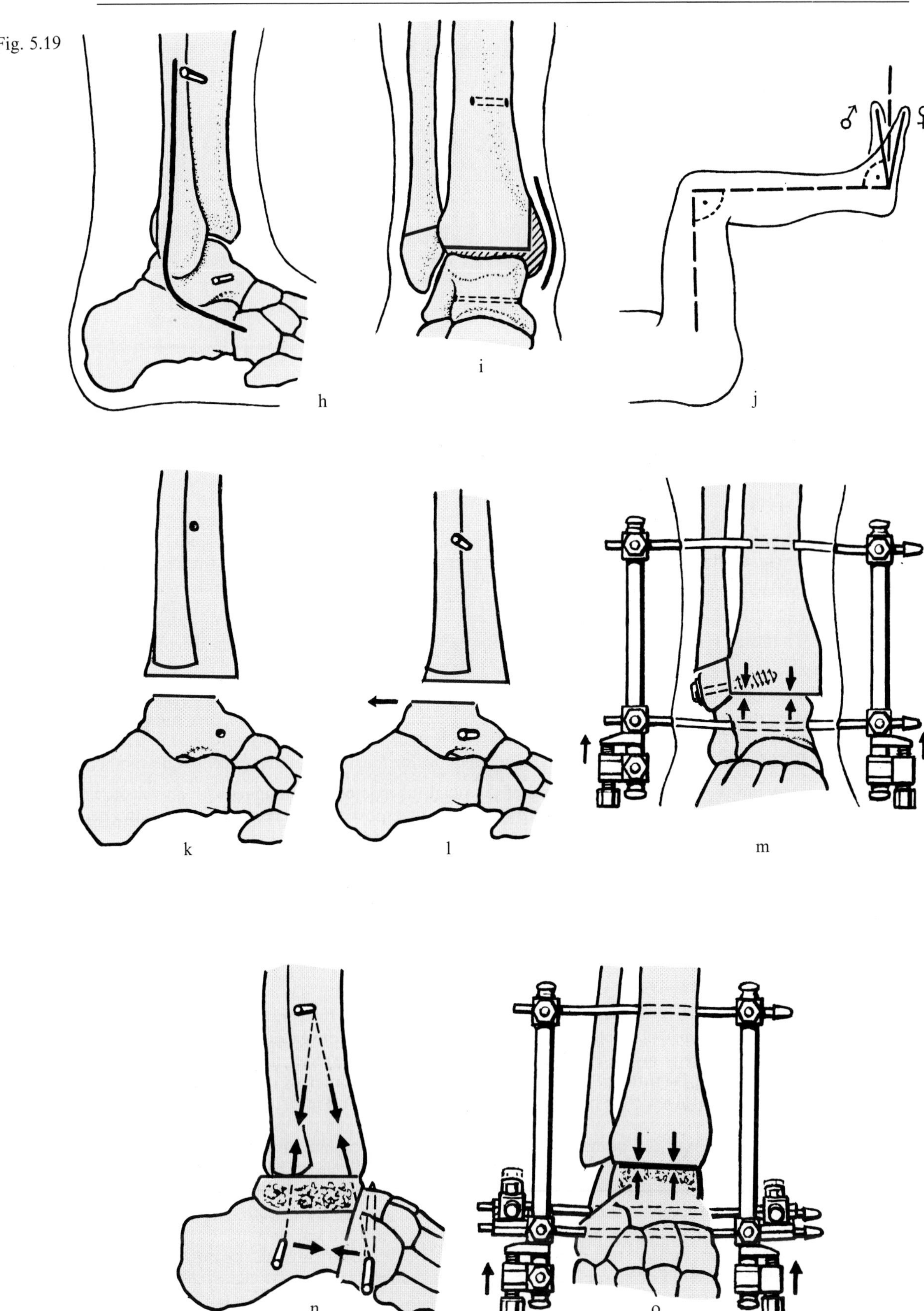

Fig. 5.20 Proximal and distal tibial osteotomies.

If no soft tissue problems exist, internal fixation is usually preferred. Compression fixation by means of a bilateral one-plane external fixator also leads to a rapid bony union in the osteotomized metaphysis.

a Proximal tibia (Müller et al. 1979). First osteotomize the fibula. Then make your anterior incision and insert the first Steinmann pin about 1–2 cm distal to the knee joint and parallel to it. A Kirschner wire introduced distally subtends with the Steinmann pin an angle which corresponds to the angle of correction. To maintain rotational control, two further Kirschner wires are inserted in a sagittal direction on each side of the osteotomy at right angles to the Steinmann pin and parallel to one another.

b Carry out the osteotomy at the level of the tibial tubercle by undermining with an osteotome the distal insertion of the infrapatellar tendon. The wedge is removed either medially or laterally, depending on whether you are carrying out a valgus or a varus osteotomy.

c Displace the tibia until the Steinmann pin and the Kirschner wire come to lie parallel to one another. Remove the Kirschner wire and replace it with a 4.5-mm Steinmann pin, the two AP Kirschner wires remaining parallel!

d Compress the osteotomy with two external fixators. This will impact the osteotomy surface. The distance between the osteotomy and the Steinmann pin should be about 1–1.5 cm. Inadequate fixation of the fragments will result if the distance is greater.

e Distal tibia. The choice is between an opening osteotomy on the concave side (with varus malalignment medially, and valgus laterally) or a wedge resection on the convex side. If there is length to be gained, the opening osteotomy is to be preferred. This procedure requires the insertion of a corticocancellous wedge removed from the pelvis which needs to be fixed by internal fixation and is not illustrated here. The partial wedge resection on the convex side is illustrated in Fig. 5.20e–h according to M.E. Müller.

Resect a small segment of the fibula and insert a Steinmann pin parallel to the distal articular surface of the tibia. From the medial side and proximal to the planned osteotomy insert a 3.2-mm drill bit into the tibia. This drill bit should subtend the desired angle of correction with the Steinmann pin. Into the anterior crest insert two Kirschner wires, one on each side of the osteotomy. They will serve to control the rotational alignment as well as the angulation of the osteotomy.

f Carry out the osteotomy between the Kirschner wires.

g Correct the deformity.

h Remove the drill bit and replace it with a Steinmann pin. Reduce the osteotomy and compress it with two external fixators.

Fig. 5.20

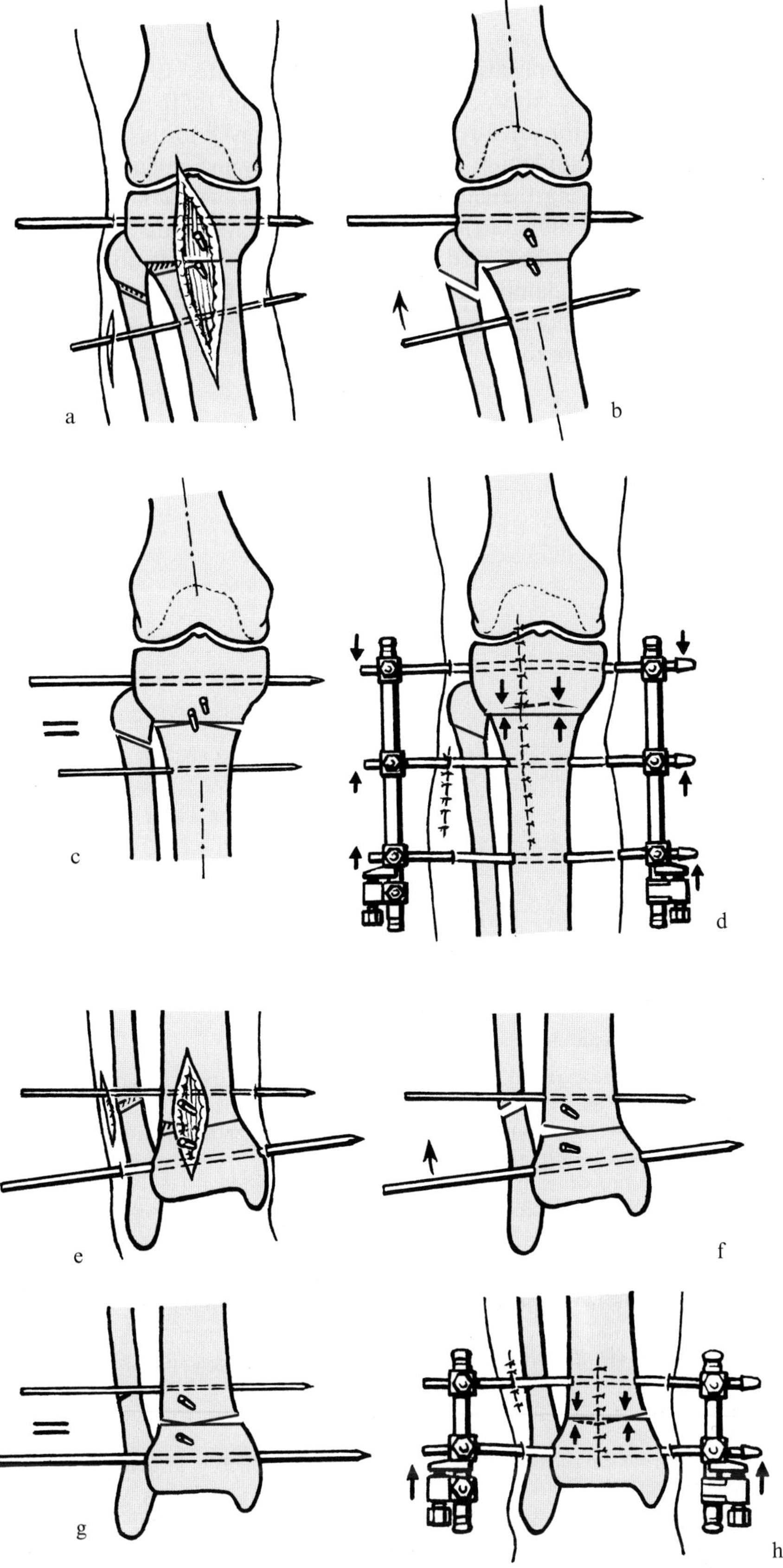

5.8.6 Segment Transport and Bone Lengthening

The most recent application of the external fixator is its use for bone lengthening or fragment transport after corticotomy according to Ilizarov. The tubular fixator, with the addition of a threaded rod, lends itself very well to this procedure (Fig. 5.21).

The gradual elongation in four to five daily increments, totalling about 1.0 mm/day, is achieved by fixing the gliding fragment using two Schanz screws connected to a short tube which glides along a threaded rod driven by a transport nut. In the tibia, the metaphyseal fragment is best held by two Schanz screws introduced through a pin-adjusting clamp (transverse clamp) or a double clamp. Figure 5.21d demonstrates that fragment transport can be achieved by means of a simple double-tube arrangement, using the compressor to move the fragment.

Fig. 5.21 Segment transport and lengthening of diaphyseal bones.

a The fully assembled external fixator used for segment transport. Basically, the arrangement corresponds to a double-tube unilateral fixator: the inner tube is replaced by a threaded bar on which a mobile short tube, driven by a transport nut, glides. At both ends of the threaded bar, two short tubes are locked in position by two ordinary nuts.

The actual procedure is such that after a lag period of 4–6 days, transport starts. The transport nut has indentations which, when turned in increments, cause a segment displacement of 0.2 mm with each indentation. Four to five daily partial turns will result in a transport totalling 0.8–1.0 mm per day.

b For segment transport, the tubulator fixator needs a few additional elements, which are illustrated in this figure.

A pin-adjusting clamp (transverse clamp)
B threaded rod
C ordinary nut
D transport nut
E short tube which glides on the threaded bar and which is also used to fit the threaded bar to the Schanz screws.

When proceeding with the application of the external fixator for segment transport or lengthening, it is best to fully prepare the threaded bar as well as the tube with the necessary adjuncts as depicted in this figure.

Fig. 5.21

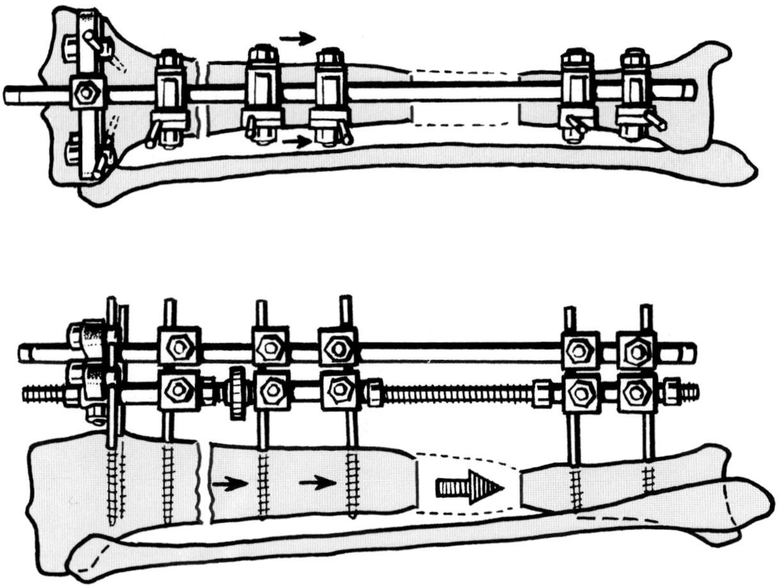

a

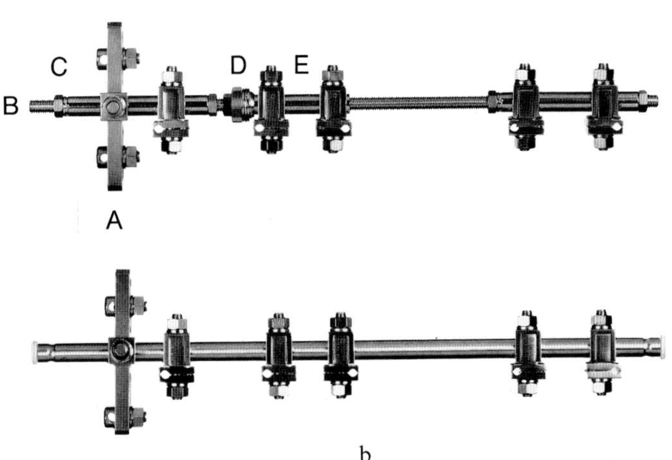

b

5.9 Complications

With rigorous adherence to the basic principles of external fixation referred to earlier, such major complications as injuries to neurovascular structures and iatrogenic joint stiffness have virtually disappeared (Green 1981). It is estimated that 10%–30% of all patients will have increased drainage at the Steinmann pin/Schanz screw track while the fixator remains in place. About 10% of patients show reddening of the pin/screw entry sites with or without positive cultures. This condition is best handled with increased attention to pin/screw care, wrapping of the entry/exit areas, enlargement of the pin/screw sites with a knife under local anesthesia, or a short course of systemic antibiotics. Out of a hundred patients, two may develop a ring sequestrum, which is reliably treated by overdrilling the infected hole. Occasionally pins/screws may loosen, particularly in metaphyseal areas. They should be promptly removed and, if needed, replaced in a different site (Searls et al. 1983).

Fig. 5.21 Segment transport and lengthening of diaphyseal boner (continued).

c Schematic representation of the individual steps when proceeding to diaphyseal lengthening (*right*) or to segment transport (*left*).

Step 1: Insert Schanz screws distally and proximally close to the joints.

Step 2: Prepare rod and tube with all necessary adjuncts needed for stabilization and transport.

Step 3: Fix rod and tube to the two Schanz screws across the adjustable clamps. If pin-adjusting clamps (transverse clamps) are being used for a metaphyseal fragment, they are provided with Schanz screws secondarily.

Step 4: Carry out corticotomy in the metaphyseal area by means of a sharp osteotome through a small skin incision.

Step 5: After 4–6 days, transport is begun in four to five daily increments totalling 0.8–1.0 mm. During transport, partial weight-bearing is encouraged.

Step 6: This applies to segment transport only. As soon as there is contact between the transport segment and the distal fragment, a cancellous onlay graft is applied over the contact area. After lengthening, internal fixation may be considered to protect the lengthened segment.

d The double-tube external fixator lends itself very well for segment transport, the fragment being pushed in five daily increments of about 0.2 mm by means of the compressor – one full turn corresponds to 1.5 mm. A motor-driven device providing very slow continuous elongation (developed by Korsinek and Tepich) seems to induce neocortex formation more rapidly!

Fig. 5.21

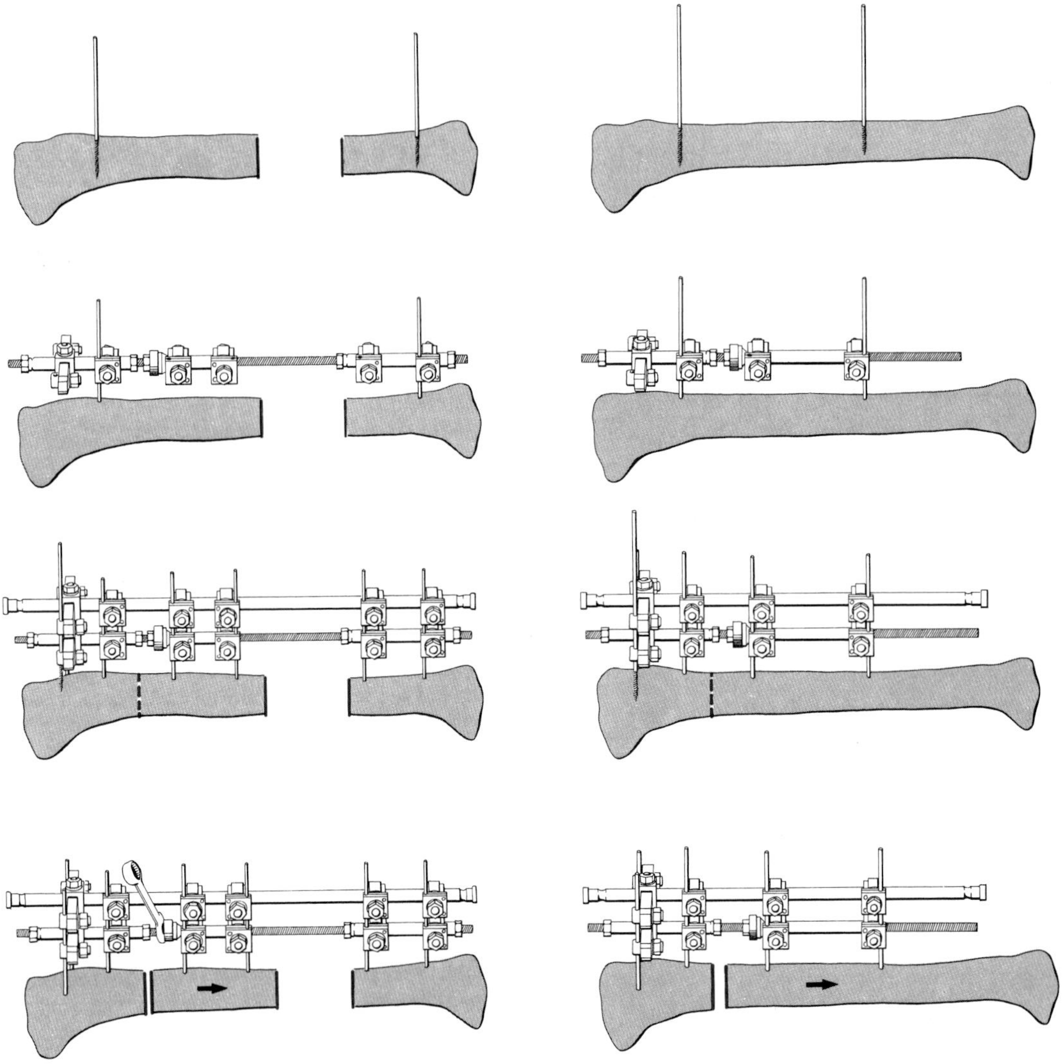

c

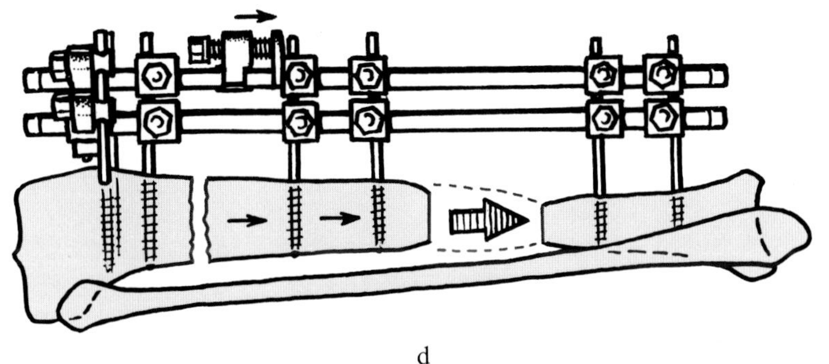

d

References

Anderson R (1936a) Femoral bone lengthening. Am J Surg 31:479–483

Anderson R (1936b) An ambulatory method of treating fractures of the shaft of the femur. Surg Gynecol Obstet 62:865–873

Behrens F, Johnson WD (1985) Variables altering the mechanical characteristics of fixator frames. In: Perren SM, Schneider E (eds) Biomechanics: current interdisciplinary research. Martinus-Nijhoff, Dordrecht, pp 525–530

Behrens F, Searls K (1986) External fixation of the tibia. Basic concepts and prospective evaluation. J Bone Joint Surg 68 [Br]:246–254

Behrens F, Fischer D, Jones R (1981) External fixator application. Mosby, St Louis, pp 125–143 (AAOS instructional course lectures, vol XXX)

Behrens F, Johnson WD, Koch TW, Kovacevic N (1983) Bending stiffness of unilateral and bilateral fixator frames. Clin Orthop 178:103–110

Codivilla A (1905) On the means of lengthening in the lower limbs. Am J Orthop Surg 3:353–369

Evans M, Kenwright J, Tanner KE (1979) Analysis of single sided external fracture fixation. Eng Med 8:133–137

Green SA (1981) Complications of external skeletal fixation. Thomas, Springfield, Ill

Hierholzer G, Kleining R, Hoerster G, Zemenides P (1978) External fixation. Classification and indications. Arch Orthop Trauma Surg 92:175

Hierholzer G, Ruedi T, Allgöwer M, Schatzker J (1985) Manual on the AO/ASIF tubular external fixator. Springer, Berlin Heidelberg New York Tokyo

Hoffmann R (1954) Ostéotaxis, ostéosynthèse externe par fiches et rotules. Acta Chir Scand 107:72

Ilizarov GA, Kaplunov AG, Degtarev VE, Ledaiev VI (1972) Treatment of pseudarthroses and ununited fractures, complicated by purulent infection, by the method of compression-distraction osteosynthesis. Ortop Travmatol Protez 33:10–14

Lambotte A (1907) Le Traitement des fractures. Masson, Paris

Malgaigne JF, Connaissance J (1853/54) Med Pratique 16:9

Mears DC (1983) External skeletal fixation. Williams and Wilkins, Baltimore

Müller ME, Allgöwer M, Willenegger H, Schneider R (1979) Manual of internal fixation, 2nd edn. Springer, Berlin Heidelberg New York

Parkhill C (1898) Ann Surg 27:553

Putti V (1918) La trazione per doppia infissione e l'allungamento operativo dell'acto inferiore. Chir Organi Mov 2:421

Searls K, Heichel S, Neimuth P, Behrens F (1983) External fixation. General principles of patient management. Crit Care Q 6:45–54

Stader O (1937) A preliminary announcement of a new method of treating fractures. North Am Vet 18:37

Wagner H (1972) Technik und Indikation der operativen Verkürzung und Verlängerung von Ober- und Unterschenkel. Orthopädie 1:59–74

Weber BG, Magerl F (1985) Fixateur externe. Springer, Berlin Heidelberg New York Tokyo

6 PRE-, INTRA- AND POSTOPERATIVE GUIDELINES

6.1 The Timing of Surgery

In 1958, the AO started an endeavour to improve the then surprisingly poor results of fracture treatment: one-third of all tibia fractures, two-thirds of femur fractures and almost all severe fractures involving major joints ended with a relatively high degree of permanent impairment. At this time, the four basic treatment principles which aimed to improve these results were formulated: early operative anatomic reduction; stable internal fixation; atraumatic surgical technique; and very early active mobilization. To judge from the experience of the Swiss Accident Insurance (SUVA), increasing application of these principles has indeed reduced both the proportion of cases in which compensation is paid after long bone fractures (Table 6.1) and the subsequent degree of permanent impairment.

Table 6.1. The decrease between 1945 and 1975 in the proportion of patients (according to SUVA) receiving temporary or permanent compensation after fractures.

Bone(s) fractured	Decrease
Humerus	49%
Radius/ulna	28%
Femur	34%
Patella	20%
Tibia/fibula	45%
Malleoli	31%
Metatarsus	17%

Source: Morscher (1985)

It soon became obvious that this aggressive approach to trauma surgery not only caused no harm to the patient as a whole by increasing trauma sequelae like so-called fat embolism, pulmonary insufficiency and multiple organ failure, but in fact decreased the frequency and severity of these complications. These observations were published as early as 1963 (Allgöwer) and again in 1975 (Rüedi and Wolff) and 1978 (Wolff et al.). The data published by Rüedi and Wolff had previously been submitted to the *Journal of Trauma* but refused on the basis that no prospective comparisons were available. The results were so obvious, however, that we no longer felt able to deny this kind of trauma treatment to a group of "control patients".

Since then, ample evidence with hard data has been published: the most careful study compares pathophysiological consequences of conservative versus early operative treatment in the multiply injured patient with particular emphasis on early fixation of femur fractures and was carried out by Border's group in Buffalo, NY (Seibel et al. 1985). They analyzed polytraumatized fracture patients of whom half were treated conservatively and the other half had immediate operative reduction with internal fixation. Both groups of patients had similar operations for lesions of the body cavities and they had the same intensive care policy. The number of days on the respirator, days in intensive care, febrile days and the number of metabolic disturbances were all significantly smaller in the patients receiving immediate total care, including fixation of fractures, particularly of the femur. Of special interest was the comparison of the alveolar arterial oxygen difference in these two groups of patients. Normalization of the gradient took only two to three days in patients receiving immediate total care including internal fixation but more than 10 days in the group of patients treated conservatively or by delayed internal fixation. Similar observations have been published by Riska (1976, 1982) Goris et al. (1982), Johnson et al. (1984), Border (1987) and Bone et al. (1989).

From these data, it is quite obvious that many complications seen in multiply injured patients are not due to the initial trauma but rather to the treatment modalities such as the so-called "crucifix position" with the femur in traction. The planning of emergency treatment in multiply injured patients must, therefore, include stabilization of fractures of the long bones, despite the priority given to lesions of the body cavities.

Summarizing the experiences of the last two decades, it may be said that the so-called "aggressive trauma treatment" which includes internal fixation of the long bones and pelvic fractures not only has many advantages in terms of rapid and complete restoration of the localized injury but is also significant in preventing morbidity and mortality for the patient as a whole.

With regard to treatment of the local lesions, fractures are best operated on immediately and before the primary swelling occurs. Hematoma can be evacuated and the fracture fragments are freely mobile, so that minimal fragment devitalization is likely to occur. Debridement of devitalized tissue and precise evacuation of hematomas is more difficult in late operations, resulting in the danger of leaving more bacterial nutrients behind.

In acute tibial fracture surgery, the pretibial skin must be treated with "loving care". Its normal vasculature is rather poor and the trauma leading to the fracture may have further compromised its viability. If there is any question about the viability of the pretibial skin as a consequence of contusion, the surgery should be delayed until microcirculation of the contused skin is fully restored, which usually takes 6 to 10 days. If internal fixation is contraindicated by the state of the soft tissues, early fracture fixation can still be accomplished by application of an external fixator either as a temporary or as a definitive solution to the problem (see Chap. 5).

6.2 Organizational Prerequisites

The asepsis of the operating room must be guaranteed. A high degree of professional expertise and discipline from all members of the surgical team – surgeons and nurses – is as important as the technical refinements of the equipment. The best index of asepsis is the infection rate, which should not exceed 2% for elective cases and closed fractures. Statistics of postoperative infections, subdivided into anatomic regions, are mandatory. The individual figures for one institution must be comparable to established standards.

6.3 Preventing Wound Infection

Avoidance of infection is primarily achieved by reducing additional bacterial contamination before operation. Dressings put on at the roadside should be left in place until the operating team is ready and the delay before surgery should be kept to a minimum so as to prevent the spread of the bacteria. Exact reduction and operative stabilization of the fracture and prevention and postoperative hematomas, fluid collection and edema formation are important elements of infection prophylaxis. See Chap. 20 for infection prophylaxis by antibiotics.

The wound infection rate in open fractures is a function of the whole emergency care system and not just of the surgery performed. In a third degree open fracture with much soft tissue devitalization, routine re-exploring of the wound and re-excising at 48 h is recommended and often reveals a surprising extent of devitalization. If extensive postoperative swelling and inflammatory reaction develop, the wound should be re-explored, cleaned and left open. An initially closed fracture will have to be left open for the same reason as in open fractures. Removal of bacterial nutrients, dead tissue and hematoma is the key to preventing and treating wound infection.

Wounds are left open to drain and not to dehydrate. This means loose approximation of viable tissues but does not imply leaving the wound massively open. Skin may be approximated where not under tension but has to be left open where closure causes tension. The resulting skin defect may then be partially closed to prevent dehydration with Ringer solution-soaked compresses or with some "artificial skin" such as Biobrane or Epigard used in a way that allows gravity drainage.

In all of these measures are accomplished properly, then the administration of antibiotics started in the emergency room or preferably at the roadside and continued for up to 24 h will further reduce the rate of wound infection and osteitis (Rittmann and Perren 1974). However, the benefits of antibiotics are small relative to those of good wound management.

6.4 General Guidelines for Operative Procedures

6.4.1 Preoperative Planning

See Chap. 2.

6.4.2 Preparation of the Operative Field

To avoid further trauma, detailed instructions based on adequate preoperative planning are needed for the immobilizing of the fracture during the positioning of the patient on the operating table as well as during skin disinfection.

Extensive shaving of the operative field is unnecessary and can even be dangerous if it is done some hours before surgery. It is sufficient to shave one hand's breadth at the location of the planned incision just prior to surgery.

Surgery on extremities is commonly performed under pneumatic tourniquet. The tourniquet may be left inflated for up to 2 h. The pressure has to be clearly defined and controlled with a gauge. Contraindications for the use of the tourniquet are acute or chronic circulatory problems and, in certain instances, open fractures.

A tourniquet reduces bleeding and, therefore, sponging and shortens operative time due to a clean and "dry" operative field. The hazard lies in increased, at times irreversible, ischemic damage.

Stick-on transparent plastic sheets are controversial and their use is not mandatory. They are of benefit only if they firmly stick to the skin throughout the procedure. Otherwise, they may be counterproductive and even increase bacterial contamination in the wound area.

6.4.3 Preoperative Instructions and Preparation of Instruments and Implants

Since internal fixation is best carried out in the acute phase immediately after admission of the patient, a sufficient supply of all the necessary instruments and especially the commonly needed implants is of utmost importance.

The operating room team needs precise instructions about the surgeon's intentions for the planned internal fixation. This includes instructions for standard sets, special instruments, as well as for the possibly needed implants. A perfectly prepared lay-out on the instrument table is essential so that the the operation can be performed without any delay. All surgical equipment should be under constant quality control. Proper maintenance of instruments is essential.

6.4.4 The Operation

For cosmetic reasons, incisions are preferably made parallel to Langer's lines, especially in diaphyseal regions of bones. As a rule, straight incisions are made along lines which have fixed anatomical references and which may be extended to adjacent regions during either the same procedure or future operations. Around joints, particularly the knee, the pattern of blood supply, the need to gain adequate exposure, and the possibility of later insertion of an artificial joint all necessitate longitudinal incisions at 90° to the Langer's lines. Soft tissue must be handled with utmost care and delicate instruments are required. We try to minimize further devitalization and avoid creation of necrotic tissue resulting from extensive use of either ligatures or diathermy. All these factors are essential to prevent infection.

Throughout the procedure, and specifically during drilling, we irrigate the operative field regularly with Ringer solution. We do this for two reasons: one is that the irrigation physically removes bacterial contamination deposited both from the air and by the operating team; the second is that it prevents the drying out of tissues. The addition of locally active antibiotics may be of some benefit but there are no data to prove this point. If used, they should differ from the systemic antibiotics applied. We use suction rather than sponging to remove blood and tissue fluids. A special suction device overcomes the annoyance of frequent plugging.

Once the soft tissue dissection is completed, the exposure of the fracture itself is carried out with the aid of bone levers. Because they are levers, one must remember that they multiply the force applied to them! Therefore, they have to be handled with care and should have their position changed often to prevent tissue necrosis from pressure. Extensive periosteal stripping is to be avoided. Sufficient exposure of the fracture can usually be gained by periosteal stripping 2 to 3 mm along the fracture edge. Next, the whole fracture is exposed and the fracture surfaces carefully cleaned of clots and tissues. Reduction must be carried out as atraumatically as possible.

See Chap. 2 for reduction principles.

6.4.5 Cancellous Bone Grafts

In fresh fractures where cortical defects remain after reduction, autologous cancellous bone grafting is recommended. In principle, and on the basis of preoperative planning, the site for harvesting of cancellous bone has to be prepared together with the main operative field. If a bone graft is required, it should be removed before exposing the fracture.

The greater trochanter is an excellent source for pure cancellous bone. Cortico-cancellous grafts are best taken from the wings of the ilium leaving the crest intact. The most abundant source of cancellous as well as cortico-cancellous autotransplants is the parasacral region of the iliac bone (see Fig. 19.2).

Bone grafts should be kept in a sponge moistened with Ringer solution or blood until used. Immersion in Ringer solution should be avoided.

6.4.6 Wound Closure

Success or failure of internal fixation depends to a large degree on the handling of the soft tissue during exposure and wound closure. The fascia is closed loosely with resorbable sutures. Wherever there is the slightest danger of a compartment syndrome, such as in the anterior tibial compartment, the fascia should be left open. Compartments with elevated pressures may have to be released by fasciotomy.

Once the deep fascia is loosely reapproximated, no further sutures are inserted, particularly not into the subcutaneous tissue. We use suction drainage for 24 to 48 h to prevent formation of hematomas or seromas.

For good cosmetic results, perfect adaptation of the dermis is paramount. The skin is closed with vertical mattress sutures, either interrupted or with the same stitch as a running suture (Fig. 6.1). Perfect adaptation of the dermis by staplers is difficult. 4.0- or 3.0-mm nonresorbable sutures are used.

Wound closure under tension has to be avoided. In these cases, only approximation of the skin without tension is performed. If there is any doubt, the wound should be left open. Temporary coverage may be provided by synthetic skin (Epigard). Flaps as a primarily procedure are not recommended. Special tissue transfers may, at a later date, be considered in open fractures (see Chap. 17).

For *positioning of the patient* after the operation, see Fig. 6.3.

Fig. 6.1 Wound closure: the most important aspect for a good cosmetic result is precise adaptation of the dermal layer!

a The classical Donati mattress stitch, which gives very good cosmetic results provided both wound lips have unimpaired microcirculation.

b The Allgöwer modification of the Donati stitch where the wound lip with the more precarious microcirculation (particularly if there is a flap) is grasped only intradermally.

c The same modified Donati stitch used as a running suture.

Fig. 6.2 The double U splint. This splint is particularly useful after pilon fractures and malleolar fractures to prevent equinus position of the foot.

a Two plaster slabs are applied with the knee and ankle at 90°.

b The double U splint protects the heel and allows early active dorsiflexion of the ankle.

Fig. 6.1

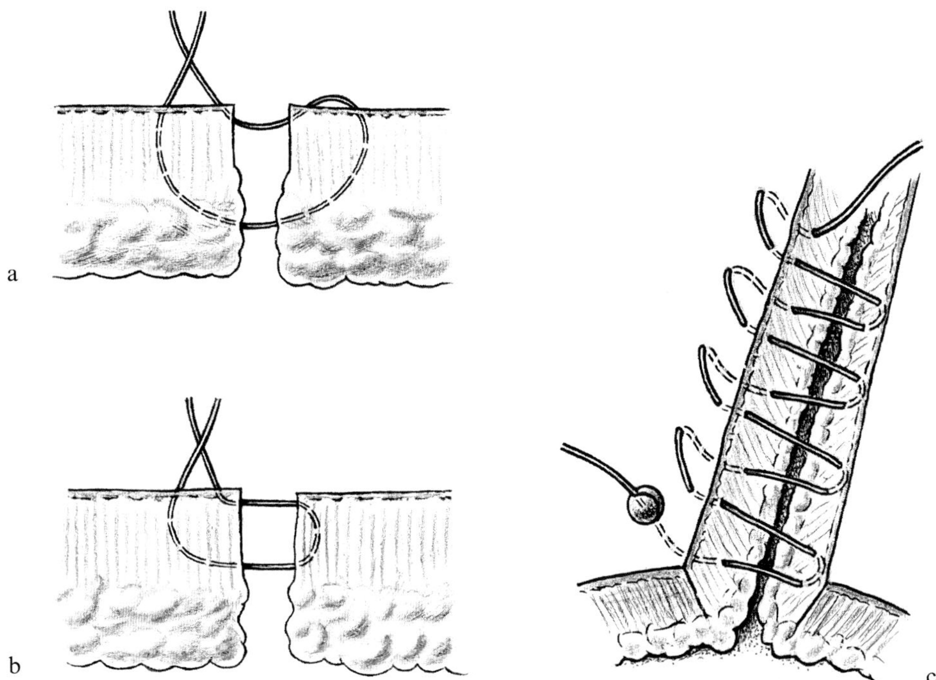

Fig. 6.2

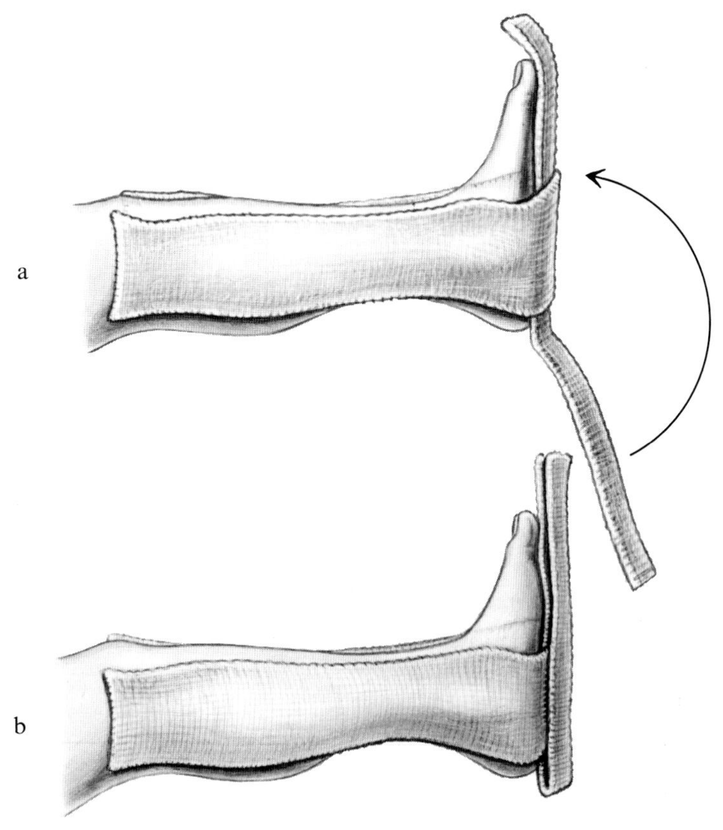

Fig. 6.3 The three standard postoperative positions of the patient.

a Fractures of the tibia are elevated on a special frame which is padded with plastic sponge. The knee is flexed to 45° and the ankle kept at 90°. The splint is so arranged that the foot is higher than the knee and the sole rests firmly against the foot rest.

b Fractures of the middle and distal femur are positioned in this way (the 90/90/90 position) for the first 4–6 days. This position prevents wrong adhesions of the quadriceps and immediate postoperative mobilization is easily possible. The patient can get out of bed after 4–6 days but remains in this position when lying down until he has a range of motion of the knee from 0° to 120°.

c Positioning of the limb after fracture of the forearm and hand. The elbow is bent to between 80° and 90° and the limb is suspended from an intravenous pole by means of a sling. The hand is kept in supination.

Fig. 6.3

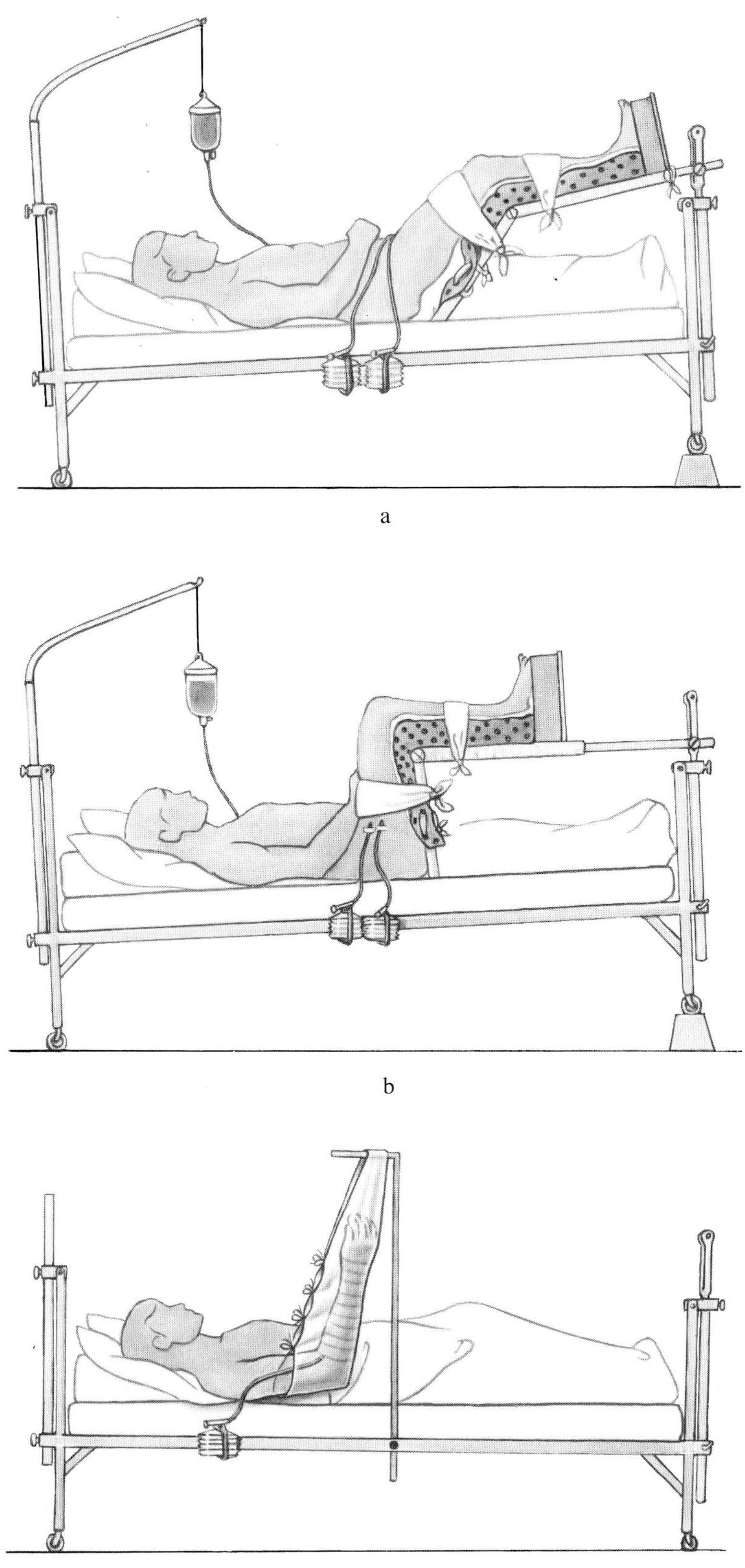

6.5 Antibiotics

The risk of infection must be evaluated: it depends on the type of fracture, its anatomic site, its precise localization on the extremity and its complexity (open fracture, injury mechanism, time elapsed since injury). Relative to these factors, antibiotics play a secondary role.

Provided the infection rate in a given institution for closed fracture treatment with open reduction and internal fixation (ORIF) remains consistently below 2%, antibiotics are not mandatory in fresh, simple closed fractures of the upper and lower extremities in patients without additional risk factors. Patients with complex fractures involving articulations and any fractures of the hip and pelvis, as well as those with open fractures, should receive prophylactic antibiotics. The drug has to be applied intravenously at induction of anesthesia or on admission to the emergency ward. Prophylactic antibiotics do not in any way replace meticulous wound debridement and a thorough wound lavage with copious amounts of isotonic Ringer solution during and at the end of a procedure (see Chap. 20 on infection). It is the mechanical element of the lavage that is effective. Locally added antibiotics have not been shown convincingly to lower infection rates. The use of a pressure spray may be helpful in performing wound cleaning.

6.6 Prevention of Thromboembolism

Active, early, painless mobilization would appear to best normalize local blood flow – this is one reason for early ORIF with subsequent active mobilization under the guidance of a physiotherapist.

Four possibilities are available for the prevention of thromboembolism – Dextran, Heparin, Dicoumarin and mechanical devices. In the trauma patient, the last-named are rarely applicable.

The most straightforward prophylaxis during short-term immobilization (up to 1 week) is achieved by the infusion of dextran, with a mean molecular weight of 70000. At induction of anesthesia, 500 ml of dextran is infused. An identical second dose is given after 8 h and a third dose after 24 h so long as no contraindication prevents the application of 1500 ml of dextran within 24 h (e.g. elderly patients with cardiac disease). Anaphylactic reaction should be prevented by injection of hapten before the infusion of Dextran. In addition to the extreme simplicity of this prophylactic treatment, dextran may be part of an early blood volume restoration.

In the case of prolonged bed rest, the use of heparin, with two daily doses of 2500–5000 units injected subcutaneously, is recommended. The dose depends on body weight. Bleeding is rarely a problem.

A valid alternative to heparin is long-term anticoagulation by means of the dicoumarins. These are particularly useful when the start of mobilization cannot be predetermined and for any pelvic and hip fractures. In the elderly patient, the risks of long-term anticoagulation have to be weighed against the probability of pulmonary embolism.

6.7 Radiological Follow-Up of Bone Healing

6.7.1 General Remarks

The radiological aspect of bone healing is closely related to the treatment modalities. We have to keep in mind that nature's response to the loss of bony continuity is a gradual stabilization by periosseous granulation tissue which occupies a large area surrounding the fracture area (endosteal granulation tissue forms as well, but has little bearing on eventual solid bone formation due to the large lever arms of the fragments relative to the small medullary cavity).

This sleeve-like three-dimensional periosseous tissue accumulation – called callus – considerably reduces the lever arms between bone fragments and regenerating area. Calcification starts at the periphery and moves slowly towards the fracture center where the initially formed woven bone is gradually transformed into mature haversian systems.

It was Cave (1958) of Boston who remarked that nature has the potential to use a short cut in cortical healing. He stated that relatively stable cortical fractures treated conservatively only need a minimum of visible callus formation to become solidly united. Danis (1947) had clearly demonstrated that stable internal fixation of vascular bone brings this potential fully into play. Haversian remodeling in the vascular cortex adjacent to the fracture is stimulated and leads to "welding" of the adapted and stably fixed fragments. Based on the radiological aspect of this callus-free direct bone healing, Danis called this healing modality "*soudure autogène*".

Schenk and Willenegger (1964), in their remarkable histological analysis of the osteotomized and stably fixed radius of dogs, fully confirmed the purely empirical claims of Danis and demonstrated the "callus free healing" by haversian osteon remodeling with a minimal amount (not radiologically visible) of callus formation. In analogy to the familiar terms used to characterize wound healing as primary or secondary, the term of primary (or direct) bone healing was coined.

The AO has unfortunately gone on record with the plated transverse osteotomy of the dog radius showing beautiful primary contact and gap healing. It has not been sufficiently appreciated that in this particular case, illustrating exclusive use of a plate fixation to bridge a transverse defect, the defect was well protected by the intact ulna.

Over the last two decades, two things have become very obvious:

First, internal fixation of transverse or short oblique fractures in weight-bearing bone using only a plate does not provide adequate stability and therefore requires additional measures to ascertain stabilization of the opposite cortex. In large bones such as the femur and tibia, this is best achieved by interfragmentary lag screws. It is advantageous to apply such screws through the plate. At times, the nature of the fracture demands a plate-independent interfragmentary lag screw. In smaller bones like the radius and the humerus, overbending of the plate exerts adequate compression on the opposite cortex to allow cortical healing provided there is no bone defect or severe comminution present. It is quite obvious that the principles of overbending and of additional interfragmentary screws can be combined to good advantage.

A corollary of these findings is the necessity to compensate for any defect in the cortex opposite to a plate by an onlay graft of autologous concellous bone.

The second fact that has to be stressed is that the AO has been misunderstood to advocate primary bone healing as a general principle to be aimed at in all forms of operative fracture treatment. Nothing could be farther from the truth. Primary direct bone healing is important for one treatment modality only: compression fixation by lag screws, most of the time protected by neutralization plates. Treatment by medullary nailing as well as by external fixation as a rule requires radiologically visible callus formation, thus depending very much on nature's response to less rigid fracture stabilization.

6.7.2 X-Ray Assessment of Fractures Stabilized by Lag Screws and Plates

Ideally, fractures treated by stable compression fixation unite without radiologically visible periosseous callus formation: this is "primary" or "direct" bone healing. At the beginning of the era of stable osteosynthesis, 30% primary bone healing was present in fractures of the shaft of the tibia (mainly simple screw fixations; Corrodi 1962), whereas a later series (mainly plate osteosynthesis) showed 70% primary healing (Müller et al. 1963). Any deviation from primary bone healing (especially the appearance of callus) must be considered a warning sign and its cause must be investigated.

Routine clinical and X-ray follow-up is usually indicated at 6, 10 and 16 weeks after osteosynthesis. The follow-up after 16 weeks is especially important, as by that time most fractures are clinically healed and any disturbed bone healing can be clearly recognized and dealt with by secondary cancellous bone grafts, reosteosynthesis, etc.

The radiological aspects of the fracture lines in postoperative X-rays are interesting. Ideally, the lines are hardly visible immediately after operation, but in the further course of healing they may develop in two directions. Normally, they become less distinct and disappear within 8 to 12 weeks as the fracture area becomes ready to accept increasing loads. In contrast, however, these fracture lines may become more visible, indicating osteolysis, which must be interpreted as a sign of mechanical movement in the fracture area. After compression osteosynthesis, this phenomenon represents a warning sign. In this case, the patient must reduce or even stop weight-bearing but can continue with active mobilization of adjacent joints. Osteolysis should regress within about 4 weeks without significant development of a periosteal or endosteal callus. (Apart from mechanical causes, osteolysis zones localized around screw threads are encountered mainly in advanced infections.)

The appearance of periosseous callus always indicates an instability of the fracture fixed by lag screws and plates. We essentially distinguish two callus types: "irritation callus" and "fixation callus". We speak of an irritation callus when cloudy, poorly delimited callus develops which does not yet bridge the fracture zone. Irritation callus requires complete abstention from weight-bearing. Within a few weeks, this abstention generally causes the irritation callus to change into the sharply delimited fixation callus of homogeneous structure, indicating that the fracture will tolerate weight-bearing.

If the osteolysis or irritation callus formation, i.e., the delay in healing, is not correctly diagnosed and treated between 15 and 20 weeks after the operation, the plate will soon undergo fatigue failure and break. Plate fractures are hardly ever due to faulty material but are rather the result of "biomechanical mistakes" in the operative techniques or the postoperative treatment and/or of a noncompliant patient!

6.8 Special Guidelines for Postoperative Treatment and Patient Guidance in the Most Common Fractures

6.8.1 General Recommendations

Postoperative treatment and patient guidance have to keep a somewhat precarious balance between avoiding fracture disease, in particular patchy demineralization of the bone, instituting early functional challenge by movement and partial weight-bearing and jeopardizing the internal fixation by over-enthusiastic activity. In principle, the surgeon who carried out the operation is best placed to evaluate the result and thus to make suggestions with regard to the postoperative treatment plan, concerning weight-bearing, X-ray controls, etc.

As a general rule, partial weight-bearing of some 10 to 15 kg and – with regard to the upper extremity – active mobilization will prevent the fracture disease discussed in Chap. 1. This amount of physiological challenge should be possible in a majority of all fractures treated by internal fixation.

It must be stressed that the indications for postoperative treatment given here are related to "state of the art internal fixation" and that the time after operation takes the operation date as day zero.

The treating physician/surgeon will relate his recommendations for the patient to the *individual* healing process, as evaluated by clinical signs and radiological criteria. Every patient on increasing weight-bearing and mobilization should be made aware of the classical alarm signs of *pain, edema and inflammatory reddening* of the injured limb. These alarm signs dictate complete rest until re-evaluated by the treating physician/surgeon.

Elevation of the injured limb above the level of the heart is a very general recommendation during the first postoperative days, but this does not preclude patients with lesions to the upper extremity getting out of bed very early. Even for patients with fractures of the lower extremity, temporary interruption of the elevation is recommended, combined with sitting up (upright chest position!) and early training for the upright positioning of the body as a whole. In polytraumatized patients, early upright chest position, sitting position and training of upright out-of-bed position are the most efficient means to prevent cardiopulmonary complications.

6.8.1.1 Plan for Weight-Bearing and X-Ray Controls of the Fractures of the Lower Extremity

X-rays are essential at 6 and 12 weeks, the latter being the moment where normal bone healing has occurred and which as a rule is compatible with full weight-bearing and function of the extremity, except for contact sports or other strenuous activities. At 12 weeks, impending complications are usually visible clinically as well as radiologically and can normally be corrected by appropriate changes in the treatment plan.

6.8.2 Scheme of Gradually Increasing Functional and Weight-Bearing Challenge to Typical Fractures of the Lower Extremity

6.8.2.1 Schedule Following "State of the Art ORIF"

Lower Extremity (Table 6.2)

Active Movements: 24 h after operation.

Continuous Passive Movement (CPM): immediately after operation for fractures around the knee.

Partial Weight-Bearing: of about 10 kg, usually after 3–4 days but in certain joint fractures with small fragments only after 8–10 days.

Upper Extremity

There are practically no stably fixed fractures of the upper extremity which cannot be actively mobilized. For better patient comfort, fractures of the distal forearm should have removable splints for 3–4 weeks with daily exercises out of the splint. Fractures around the elbow should be treated by CPM from the beginning.

6.9 Metal Removal

6.9.1 Upper Limb

In the upper limb, as a rule, metal implants can be left in place. Metal removal should only be considered if inflammatory reactions are present or if the implant bothers the patient mechanically. Plate removal from the humerus or the proximal radius may jeopardize the radial nerve and should only be undertaken if significant clinical symptoms or complications are present.

6.9.2 Lower Limb

In the lower limb, indications for metal removal depend on the type of implant and its metallurgic composition. Isolated screws made of 316L steel as well as plates and screws made of pure titanium can as a rule be left in place. Titanium implants therefore have a distinct advantage over stainless steel implants by obviating the necessity of a second operation. Stainless steel implants in the weight-bearing bones are usually removed at the times indicated in Table 6.3.

Table 6.2. Timetable of recommended X-ray and clinical follow-ups and expected full weight-bearing.

Fracture type		X-ray and clinical controls (weeks)	Full normal activity without strenuous or contact sports (weeks)
44	A1, 2, 3	4/8	8/12
	B1, 2		
	B3	4/8/12	12
43	A1, 2	8/12	12–16
	A3	8/12/16	16
	B1	8/12	12
	B2, 3	8/12/16	16
	C1	8/12	12
	C2, 3	8/12/16	16
42	A1, 2 lag screw + neutralization plate	8/12	12–16
	A1, 2, 3 MN	8/12	4–8
	B1, 2 lag screw + neutralization plate	8/12	12
	B3 lag screw + neutralization plate	8/12/16	16
	C1 bridging plate	8/12/16	16–20
	C2 lag screw + neutralization plate	8/12/16	16–20
	C2 MN	8/12/16	8–12
	C3 bridging plate	8/12/16	16–20
	C3 MN interlocking	8/12/16	12–20
41	A1, 2	CPM! 8	8
	A3	CPM! 8/12/16	16
	B1	CPM! 4/8	8
	B2, 3	CPM! 4/8/12[a]	12–16
	C1	CPM! 4/8/12	8
	C2	CPM! 4/8/12	12
	C3	CPM! 4/8/12[a]	12–16
33	A1, 2	4/8/12	12–16
	A3	4/8/12/16	16–20
	B1, 2	4/8/12	8–12
	B3	4/8/12/16	12–16
	C1	4/8/12	12
	C2	4/8/12/16	16–20
	C3	4/8/12/16	16–24
32	A1, 2 plate	4/8/12/16/20	16–20
	A1 MN conventional	8/16	12–16
	A2, 3 MN conventional	8/16	6–10
	B1, 2, 3 plate	4/8/12/16/20	16–24
	B1, 2, 3 MN interlocking	8/16/20	16–20
	C1, 3 bridging plate	4/8/12/16/20	16–24
	C1, 2, 3 MN interlocking	4/8/12/16	12–20
31	A1	8/12	8–12
	A2, 3	4/8/12	12–16
	B1	4/8	1–2
	B2	8/12	12–16
	B3	4/8/12	12–30
	C1, 2, 3	4/8/12	10–?

MN, medullary nail.

[a] Tomography at 12 weeks.

Table 6.3. Timing of metal removal.

Bone/fracture	Time after implantation
Malleolar fractures	8–12 months
Tibial pilon	12–18 months
Tibia shaft:	
Plate	12–18 months
Medullary nail	18–24 months
Tibial head	12–18 months
Patella, tension band	8–12 months
Femoral condyles	12–24 months
Shaft of the femur:	
Single plate	24–36 months
Double plates	From month 18, in 2 steps (interval 6 months)
Medullary nail	24–36 months
Pertrochanteric and femoral neck fractures	12–18 months
Pelvis (only in case of complaints)	From month 10
Upper extremity (optional)	12–18 months

These data essentially relate to recent fractures with uncomplicated healing processes and do not apply to osteosyntheses in pseudarthroses, major fragments or after infections, which must be considered on an individual basis.

References

Allgöwer M (1963) Shock treatment and immediate operative stabilisation of fractures. In: Müller ME, Allgöwer M, Willenegger H (eds) Technik der operativen Frakturbehandlung. Springer, Berlin Göttingen Heidelberg, pp 324, 325

Bone L, Johnston K, Weigelt G, Scheinberg R (1989) Early versus delayed stabilisation of femoral fractures, a prospective randomised study. J Bone Joint Surg [Am] 71:336–340

Border JR, Hassett J, LaDuca J, Seibel R, Steinbert S, Mills B, Losi I, Border D (1987) The gut origin septic states in blunt multiple trauma (ISS=40) in the ICU. Ann Surg 206:427–448

Cave EF (1958) Fractures and other injuries. Year Book, Chicago

Corrodi E (1962) Nachkontrolle einer konsekutiven Serie von 113 verschraubten Frakturen (Nov. 1957–59). Inaugural dissertation, Basel

Danis R (1947) Théorie et pratique de l'ostéosynthèse. Masson, Paris

Goris JA, Gimbrère JSF, van Niekerk JLM, Schoots FJ, Booy LHD (1982) Early osteosynthesis and prophylactic mechanical ventilation in the multitrauma patient. J Trauma 22:895–903

Johnson K, Johnston G, Parker B (1984) Comminuted femoral shaft fractures: treatment by roller traction, cerclage wires and intramedullary nail, or an interlocking intermedullary nail. J Bone Joint Surg [Am] 66:1222–1235

Morscher E (1985) Ist unser Gesundheitswesen wirklich so schlecht. Schweiz Ärztezeitung 66:1708–1714

Müller ME, Allgöwer M, Willenegger H (1963) Technik der operativen Frakturbehandlung. Springer, Berlin Göttingen Heidelberg

Riska E, Myllynen P (1982) Fat embolism in patients with multiple injuries. J Trauma 22:891–894

Riska E, von Bonsdortt H, Hakkinen S (1976) Prevention of fat embolism by early internal fixation of fractures in patients with multiple injuries. Injury 8:110–116

Rittmann W, Perren SM (1974) Cortical bone healing after internal fixation and infection. Springer, New York Berlin Heidelberg

Rüedi T, Wolff G (1975) Vermeidung posttraumatischer Komplikationen durch frühe definitive Versorgung von Polytraumatisierten mit Frakturen des Bewegungsapparates. Helv Chir Acta 42:507–512

Schenk R, Willenegger H (1964) Histologie der primären Knochenheilung. Langenbecks Arch Klin Chir 308:440–452

Seibel R, LaDurca J, Hassett J, Babikian G, Mills B, Border D, Border JR (1985) Blunt multiple trauma (ISS=36), femur traction and the pulmonary failure septic state. Ann Surg 202:283–295

Wolff G, Dittmann M, Buchmann B, Allgöwer M (1978) Koordination von Chirurgie und Intensivmedizin zur Vermeidung respiratorischer Insuffizienz. Unfallheilkunde 81:425–442

7 SCAPULA, CLAVICLE, HUMERUS

7.1 Fractures of the Scapula

Fractures of the scapula are rare injuries and mainly result from a severe direct force to the shoulder and thorax. They are, therefore, often found in the multiply injured patient. As the major parts of the scapula are enveloped by muscles which act as a splint, most fractures of this bone are minimally displaced and may be treated nonoperatively.

7.1.1 Classification of Scapula Fractures

We can distinguish between stable extra-articular, unstable extra-articular and intra-articular fractures of the scapula depending on their location in relation to the glenoid and on the stability of the whole shoulder.

Stable extra-articular fractures (Fig. 7.2a) comprise the injuries of the body and processes of the scapula, which can be simple or combined. Fractures of the neck of the scapula, in spite of some displacements, usually appear to be quite stable fractures and also fall into this category.

The unstable extra-articular fractures of the neck (Fig. 7.3a) are usually associated with a fracture of the coracoid process or acromion and most typically with a fracture of the clavicle. This latter combination – fracture of the neck and clavicle – renders the entire shoulder joint quite mobile with a tendency to caudad rotation due to the weight of the arm. The severe force necessary to cause such a complex injury – similar to a pelvic ring fracture – often also results in fractures of the upper three to four ribs and may damage the brachial nerve plexus and major vessels as well.

Intra-articular fractures (Fig. 7.1a) are much rarer and as a rule present with a transverse fracture through the glenoid. Large lip fractures of the glenoid are usually associated with a luxation or partial dislocation of the head of the humerus.

7.1.2 Indications for Surgery

Stable extra-articular fractures (Fig. 7.2a) should be treated non-operatively in most instances, with a sling or Desault bandage, as bony union practically always occurs and functional deficits are rare. Only severely displaced and unstable fractures of the neck, acromion, or coracoid process are indications for surgery (Fig. 7.2b).

In unstable fractures of the neck and clavicle (Fig. 7.3a), the clavicle should be approached first and fixed with a 3.5-mm dynamic compression plate (DCP) (Fig. 7.3b) or reconstruction plate (Fig. 7.6b). This maneuver usually partially reduces the neck fracture and renders the whole shoulder stable so that no fixation of the neck fracture is necessary. Grossly displaced neck and body fractures (Fig. 7.2a) may however also require open reduction and internal fixation with either single screws, a short 3.5-mm DCP or a one-third tubular plate (Fig. 7.2b). Internal fixation for transverse fractures of the glenoid (Fig. 7.1a) and for lip fractures is best performed with small cancellous bone screws (Fig. 7.1b).

Fig. 7.1

a Displaced intra-articular fracture of the glenoid.

b After open reduction and fixation with two 3.5-mm cortex screws in lag fashion.

Fig. 7.2

a Extra-articular fracture of the glenoid.

b Open reduction and internal fixation with a short 3.5-mm DCP or one-third tubular plate is only indicated in cases of gross displacement of the glenoid in regard to the rest of the scapula. Minor dislocations – treated nonoperatively – hardly interfere with functional aftertreatment or with a good result.

Fig. 7.3 Combination injury with fractures of the glenoid, spine, and clavicle due to a heavy blow to the shoulder.

a This results in an unstable joint with a tendency of secondary caudad displacement of the whole shoulder. Associated injuries of the thorax and neural plexus are quite common.

b If approached early, the plating (3.5-mm DCP or reconstruction plate) of the clavicle is usually sufficient to approximate the other fractures as well, thus permitting functional aftercare. Only exceptionally is there a need to stabilize the scapular fractures per se.

Fig. 7.1

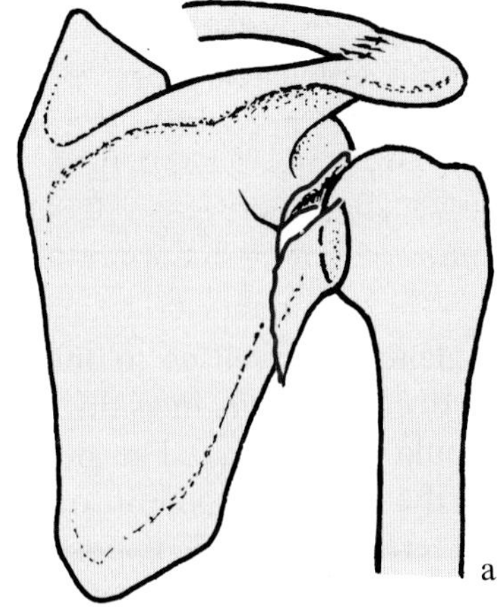

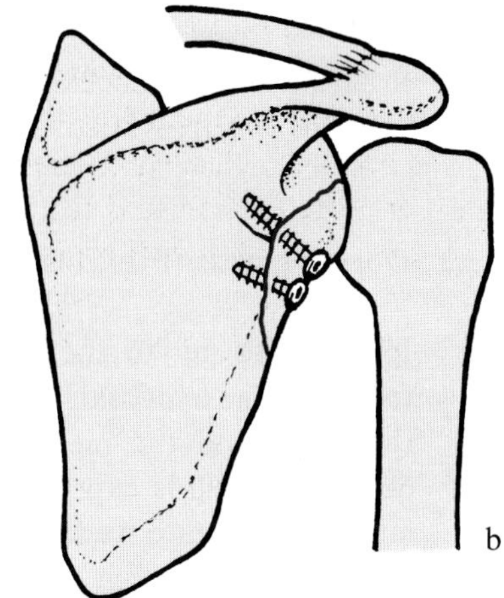

Fig. 7.2

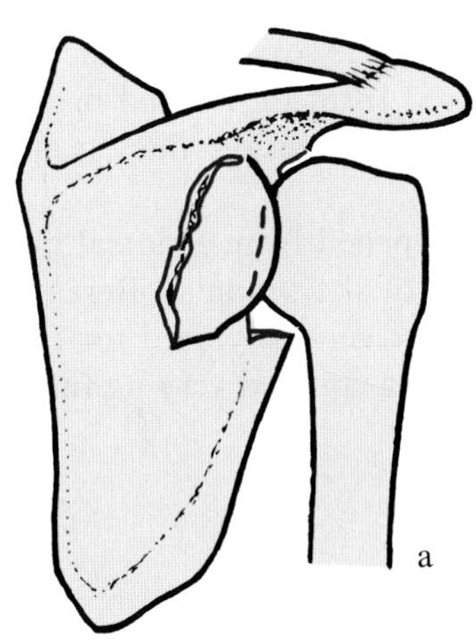

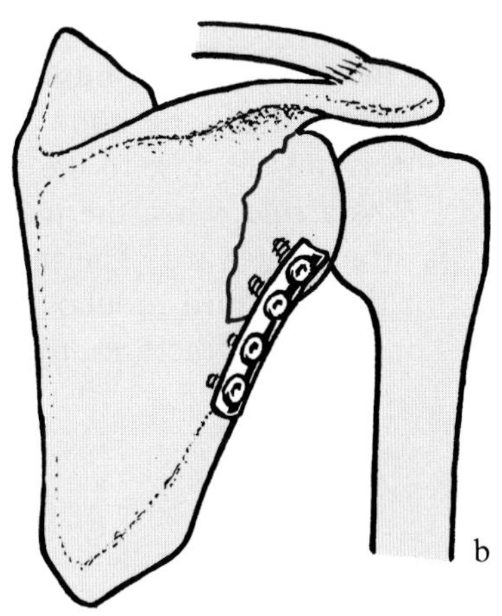

Fig. 7.3

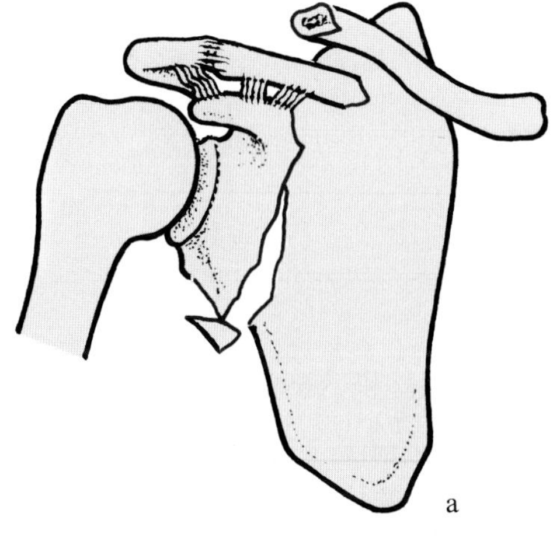

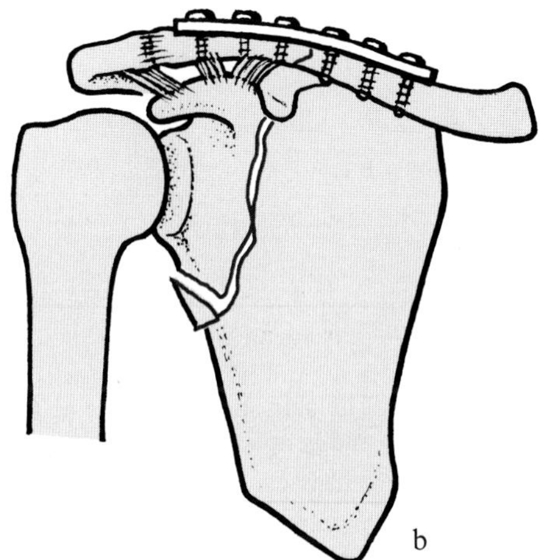

7.1.3 Approach to the Shoulder Joint

Fractures of the neck and body of the scapula are usually best approached through a dorsal access, while fractures of the glenoid are best approached ventrally.

7.1.3.1 Dorsal Access (Fig. 7.4)

In order to get to the dorsal aspect of the glenoid as well as to the lateral margin of the scapula, a dorsal approach is used with a curved skin incision running parallel to the spine and the medial border of the scapula (Fig. 7.4a). The posterior part of the deltoid muscle is exposed and detached from the scapular spine in order to be retracted laterally. Beneath we find the infraspinous and teres muscles. To expose the lateral margin, the interspace is split between infraspinous and teres minor (Fig.7.4b). Two neurovascular structures have to be carefully respected: the suprascapular nerve which curves through the suprascapular notch and innervates the supra- and infraspinous muscles and the axillary nerve and vessels which swing around the neck of the humerus and may be injured close to the glenoid. To expose the body of the scapula – which is rarely necessary – the infraspinous muscle can also be removed from the medial margin of the scapula and peeled off the bone, which is probably less dangerous than transecting the origin of this muscle close to the tubercula.

As a rule, when the joint capsule has been opened from a dorsal direction, reduction is straightforward. The massive lateral margin of the scapula offers a solid attachment for the one-third tubular plate or DCP which are generally used for fixation (Fig. 7.2b). For extensive fractures, the reconstruction plate has proved very useful.

Fig. 7.4

a The skin incision starts at the palpable posterior border of the acromion, running parallel to the spine and gently curving towards the inferior angle of the scapula.

1 Clavicle; *2* Acromion; *3* Suprascapular nerve; *4* Axillary nerve.

b The deltoid muscle has been detached from its origin at the scapular spine and swung laterally. The posterior aspect of the shoulder joint and the lateral margin of the scapula are exposed between the infraspinous and teres minor muscles. This interspace is devoid of neurovascular structures; however, care has to be taken not to injure the axillary nerve and the posterior circumflex vessels of the humerus.

1 Articular capsule; *2* Deltoid muscle; *3* Circumflex scapular vessels; *4* Axillary nerve, posterior circumflex vessels of humerus; *5* Infraspinous muscle; *6* Teres minor muscle.

Fig. 7.4

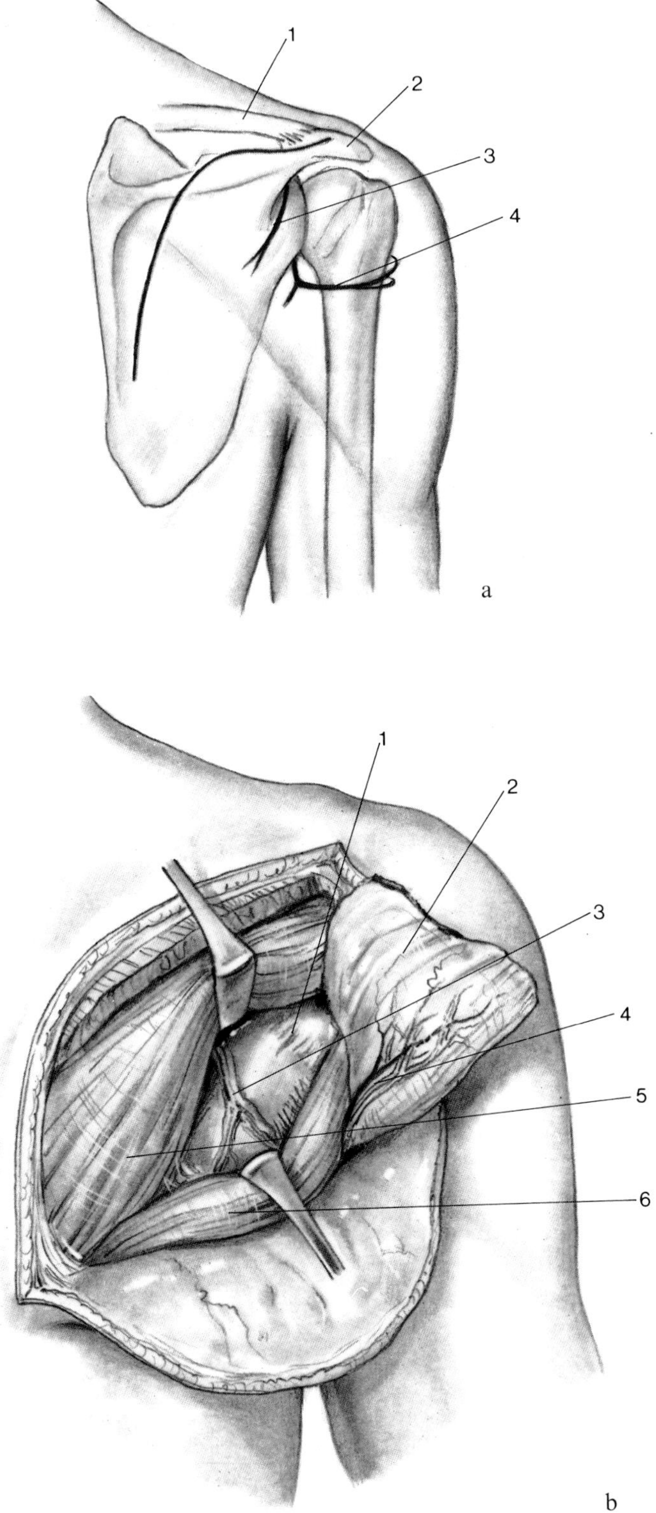

7.1.3.2 Ventral Access (Fig. 7.5)

The anterior and inferior margins of the glenoid are approached via the classical route of the deltopectoral groove. Depending on the fracture situation, it may not be necessary to incise the tendon of the subscapular muscle. Reducing the fragments of the inferior glenoid (origin of the triceps muscle) can be rather difficult. For improved visualization, it may be necessary to perform an osteotomy of the tip of the coracoid or to use an axillary or even a dorsal approach.

7.1.4 Postoperative Treatment

Temporary immobilization in a Gilchrist or Desault bandage of 3–4 days and thereafter careful passive and active mobilization.

Fig. 7.5

a The skin incision starts at the coracoid process and runs in a gentle curve along the anterior border of the deltoid muscle to the lateral bicipital sulcus.

1 Axillary nerve; *2* Coracoid process; *3* Acromion; *4* Clavicle.

b After identification of the cephalic vein, which runs between the deltoid and the pectoralis major muscles, the two are separated, thus exposing the proximal end of the humerus. For a more extensive exposure (e.g. to the greater tubercle) the deltoid muscle may be detached from the clavicle and the acromion may even be osteotomized.

1 Cephalic vein; *2* Long head of biceps muscle; *3* Deltoid muscle; *4* Pectoralis major muscle; *5* Short head of biceps muscle, coracobrachial muscle; *6* Subscapular muscle.

Fig. 7.5

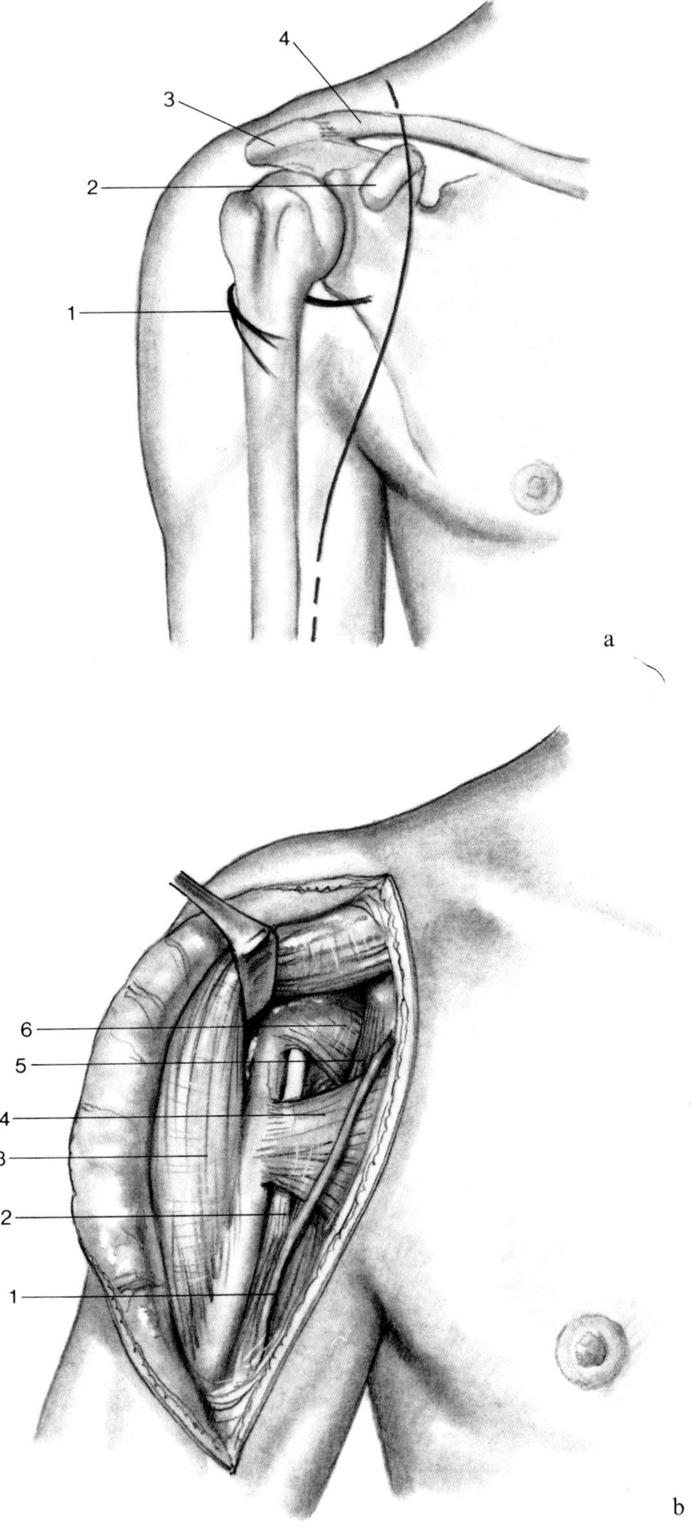

7.2 Clavicular Fractures (Including Luxation of Adjacent Joints)

Clavicular shaft fractures usually heal even without immobilization and are therefore treated conservatively in the majority of cases. Surgery often leads to ugly, painful scars and not infrequently to non-unions, which are rather rare after conservative treatment.

7.2.1 Indications for Surgery

The following types of injuries are considered indications for surgery: open fractures; fractures associated with neurovascular lesions; and fractures combined with scapula neck fractures. Exceptions when surgery may be advocated are: if a fragment threatens to perforate the skin; grossly displaced lateral fractures; and painful non-unions.

7.2.2 Approach to the Clavicle

The saber cut incision running parallel to Langer's lines usually gives adequate access to the bone and is cosmetically preferable to the incision parallel to the clavicle.

7.2.3 Choice of Implant

The most appropriate implants are the 3.5-mm DCP and the 3.5-mm reconstruction plate. Due to the forces acting on the clavicle, the plates chosen should have a minimum of six to seven holes. The reconstruction plate is best placed on top of the clavicle (Fig. 7.6a). If it is placed on the anterior margin, more dissection is required but much longer screws can be anchored in the bone and the plate is better protected underneath the skin (Fig. 7.6b).

Unstable displaced lateral fractures of the clavicle may need a tension band fixation through the acromioclavicular joint or a small fragment T plate (Fig. 7.6c).

If non-unions of the clavicle are painful or disabling, they should be treated by ORIF. A hypertrophic callus may be trimmed to better accept the 3.5-mm DCP or reconstruction plate. In poorly vascularized bone, a cancellous autograft may be required.

Fig. 7.6 Depending on the fracture pattern of grossly displaced mid-shaft fractures of the clavicle, a 3.5-mm DCP or 3.5-mm reconstruction plate is chosen.

a The reconstruction plate may be contoured to fit precisely on top of the S-shaped clavicle.

b The 3.5-mm DCP may be placed onto the anterior or ventral aspect of the clavicle, whereby much longer screws will find excellent purchase in the bone.

c The lateral fracture of the clavicle appears to be rather unstable and difficult to reduce by nonoperative means. To fix this fracture, we may use a small T plate.

Fig. 7.6

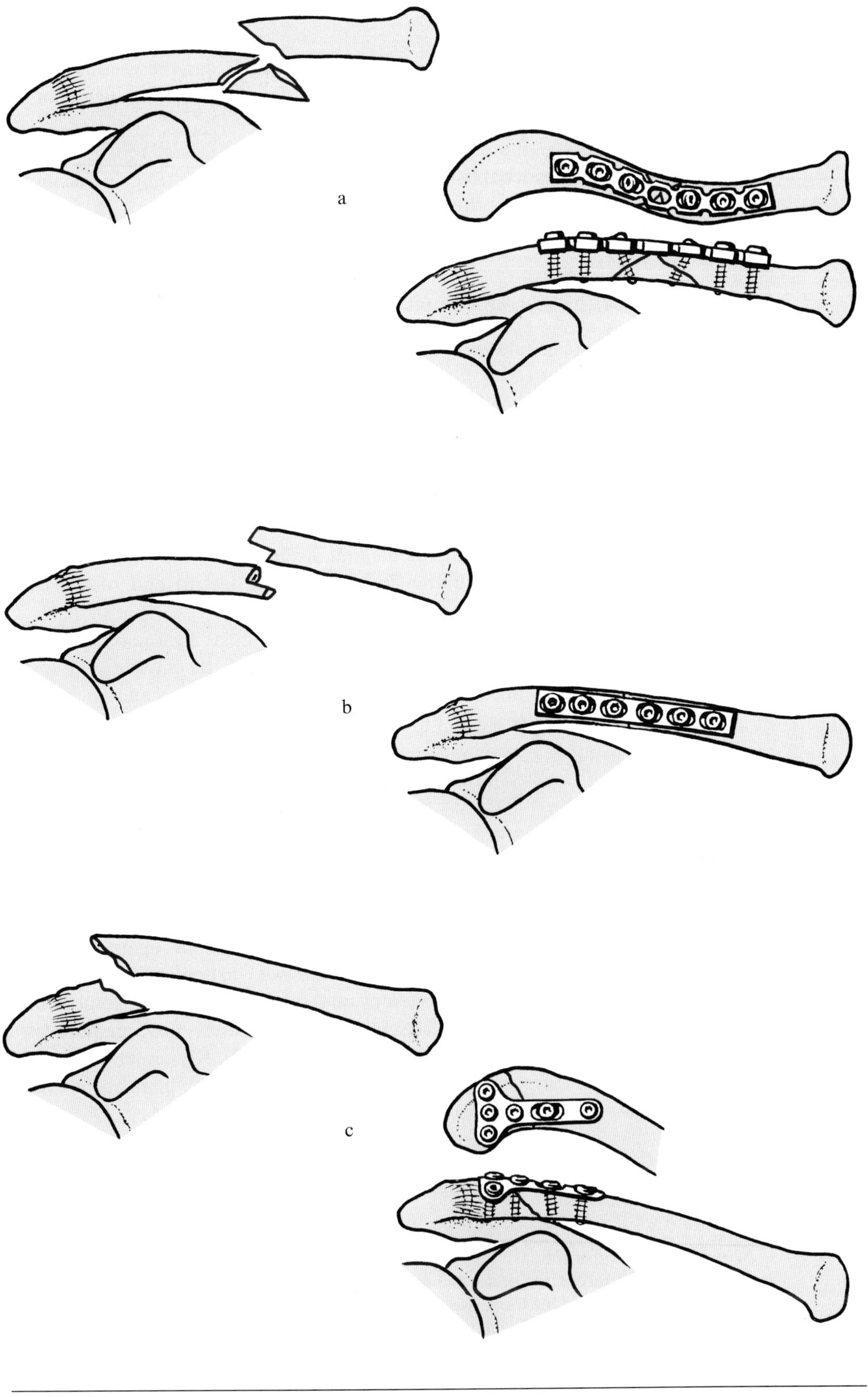

7.2.4 Dislocation of the Sternoclavicular Joint

Two forms, an anterior and a posterior dislocation, can be distinguished. Depending on the extent of the injury to the capsular and costoclavicular ligaments, we speak of complete or incomplete ruptures.

Although unstable, there is rarely an indication for primary repair. If surgery is decided upon, transosseous resorbable sutures with Maxon or PDS slings is recommended. Metal wires should not be used as they tend to migrate.

7.2.5 Dislocation of the Acromioclavicular Joint

The acromioclavicular (AC) joint plays an important part in the architecture and function of the shoulder. Total dislocation or a partial rupture of the ligaments may cause pain and loss of shoulder function. Tossi (Tossi et al. 1963) describes three types of AC joint injuries:

Type I: Tear and partial rupture of the AC ligaments. The stress X-rays show only a slight displacement of the clavicle.

Type II: Rupture of the AC ligaments and stretching of the coracoclavicular ligaments. On stress films, half the diameter of the lateral end of the clavicle projects by half its diameter beyond the acromion.

Type III: Total rupture of both AC and coracoclavicular ligaments; piano key phenomenon? The X-ray shows total displacement of the clavicle. The distance between the coracoid process and the clavicle is clearly greater in comparison to the opposite side (Fig. 7.7a).

7.2.6 Indications for Surgery

Tossi type III injuries are indications for surgery in the young adult or athlete. Surgery consists of a primary suture of the AC ligaments and temporary fixation of the joint. The conoid and trapezoid sections of the coracoclavicular ligament are only repaired if some ligamentous tissue is present. A destroyed articular disk should be removed. There are various methods for the temporary fixation of the AC joint which range from cerclage wires with one or two Kirschner wires to screw fixation between clavicle and coracoid process (Fig. 7.7b) to a special hook plate. As Kirschner wires tend to migrate, we recommend the temporary screw fixation combined with ligamentous repair or, exceptionally, the use of the hook plate.

Fig. 7.7

a Acromioclavicular disruptions, Tossi type III, may be an indication for surgery. Of the many possibilities offered by the literature, we prefer the direct repair of the cuff-like avulsed acromioclavicular ligament and capsule with resorbable transosseous sutures in combination with a 4.5-mm cortex or 6.5-mm cancellous bone screw reducing the clavicle to the coracoid process. To prevent loosening or fatiguing of the screw, the hole in the clavicle is slightly overdrilled.

b The screw is usually removed after 6–8 weeks.

Fig. 7.7

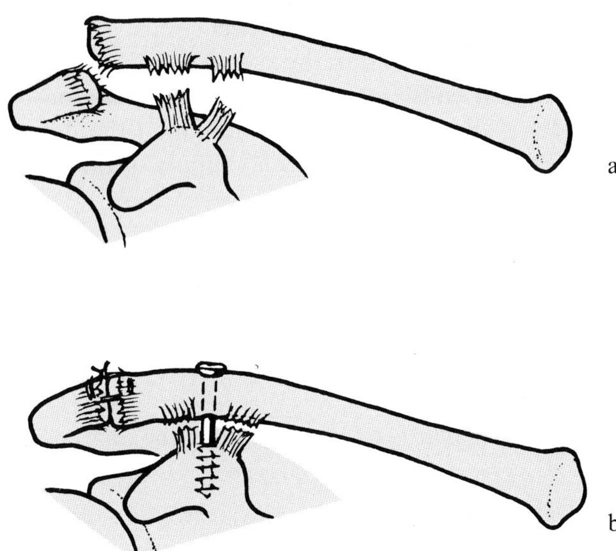

7.3 Fractures of the Humerus

As in the other long bones, fractures of the humerus and their treatment differ considerably depending on the site – proximal, diaphyseal, or distal. The following sections must therefore be considered independently.

7.3.1 Fractures of the Proximal Humerus

Fractures of the proximal humerus occur most typically in the older patient after a fall against the shoulder or arm. In the younger patient, more severe injuries (type C fractures) are observed as a consequence of high-energy traffic or sports accidents, for instance, skiing accidents. The prognosis depends upon the degree of fragment displacement and on the damage to the delicate vascular supply of the humeral head.

7.3.1.1 Classification (see also Chap. 1)

Type A: Extra-articular fractures with one fragment (tubercle or metaphyseal).
Type B: Extra-articular fractures with two to three fragments (both tubercle(s) and metaphysis).
Type C: Intra-articular fractures involving the anatomic neck.

7.3.1.2 Indications for Surgery

The majority of fractures of the proximal humerus are type A fractures, which, with rare exceptions, are treated nonoperatively. Surgery may be indicated for luxation fractures, grossly displaced unstable fractures, and polytrauma patients. In some instances, the biceps tendon is caught between the shaft and the head fragments which then prevents closed reduction.

If the fracture situation appears unstable after closed reduction, percutaneous Kirschner wires may be used. However, stable fixation allowing functional aftertreatment can only be achieved by ORIF with a three- or four-hole T plate placed so as not to interfere with the biceps tendon (Fig. 7.8 b). Fully threaded 6.5-mm cancellous bone screws

---

Fig. 7.8

a Avulsion fractures of the greater tubercle (A1) are usually treated nonoperatively. In the case of major displacement, however, reduction is essential.

b Refixation may be performed with one or two cancellous bone screws,

c or a tension band wire.

Fig. 7.9

a Displaced extra-articular fractures (collum chirurgicum) of the head of the humerus (A3). If closed reduction fails, open reduction and internal fixation may be the only way to treat this fracture.

b With a large head fragment, a short T plate is the best way to stabilize the fracture. Care must be taken not to interfere with the biceps tendon.

Fig. 7.8

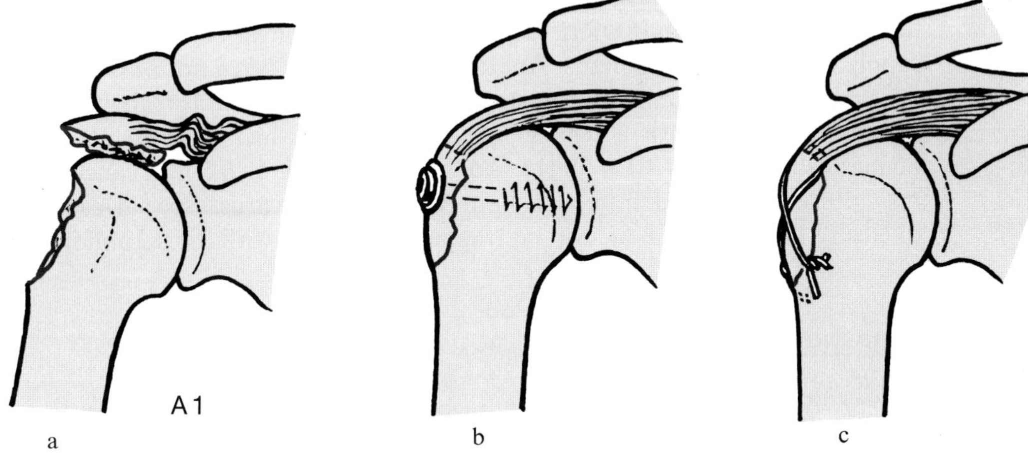

a b c

Fig. 7.9

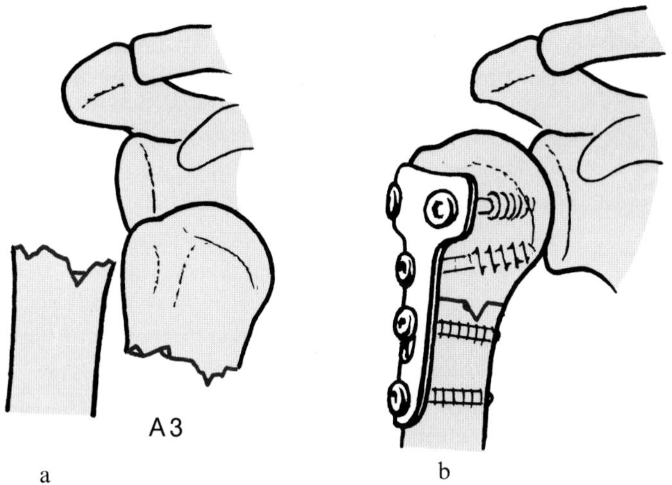

a b

usually have a good purchase in the head fragment, while standard 4.5-mm cortex screws are used for the shaft. Displaced avulsion fragments of the tubercle must be reduced and fixed with screws (Fig. 7.9 b) or tension band wire (Fig. 7.9 c).

In type B and C fractures (Fig. 7.10 and 7.11), the indication for surgery depends upon the degree of fragment displacement and the patient's age. In the elderly patient, most fractures are treated nonoperatively, while in the younger age group, displaced fractures are treated operatively. Again, threaded Kirschner wires may be applied percutaneously (Fig. 7.11 a). If ORIF is chosen, much care must be taken to ensure the vascular supply to the head of humerus. Anatomic reduction is often not possible and functionally not necessary. The main aim is restitution of the rotator cuff (greater and lesser tubercle). This is best done with a tension band wire loop which anchors the tubercles to the humeral shaft (Figs. 7.10 b, 7.11 c). Additional 4.0-mm or 6.5-mm cancellous bone screws may prevent the head fragment from slipping into varus. Special care must be taken to ensure that during abduction no fragment interferes with the acromion.

7.3.1.3 Approach (see Fig. 7.5)

The proximal humerus is best approached through an incision along the deltopectoral groove which may be extended by detaching the deltoid muscle from the clavicle and acromion. In subcapital fractures, the shaft almost always lies subcutaneously and can be eased back under the head by using a small bone retractor.

7.3.1.4 Postoperative Treatment

Postoperatively, the arm should be placed in an abducted position and all physiotherapy started from that position. Lengthy immobilization of the shoulder joint should be avoided.

Fig. 7.10

a Extra-articular fractures involving three fragments (tubercle and surgical neck) with derotation of the head fragment (B2). Open reduction is the only way to anatomically reduce the fragments.

b Fracture fixation may be carried out with a T plate (Fig. 7.9 b) but it appears quite adequate to combine the tension band principles (wire) for the tubercle with one or two lag screws for the fixation of the head fragment.

Fig. 7.11

a Intra-articular three- and four-part fractures with impaction of the small head fragment onto the humerus shaft (*C*).

b Closed reduction and percutaneous Kirschner wire placement may be attempted. If open reduction is chosen to disengage the fragment of the tubercles, care must be taken not to strive for anatomic reduction of the head fragment and not to interfere with vascular supply to the head fragment.

c By pulling the greater and lesser tubercles with one, two or even three wire loops (tension bands) in a caudal direction, it is usually possible to partly reduce the impacted fragments in a gentle way.

c′, c″ Depending on the individual situation, additional lag screws or Kirschner wires may be added.

Fig. 7.10

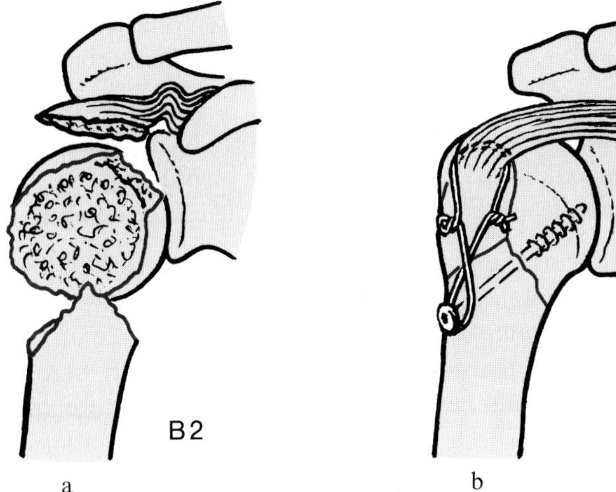

a b

Fig. 7.11

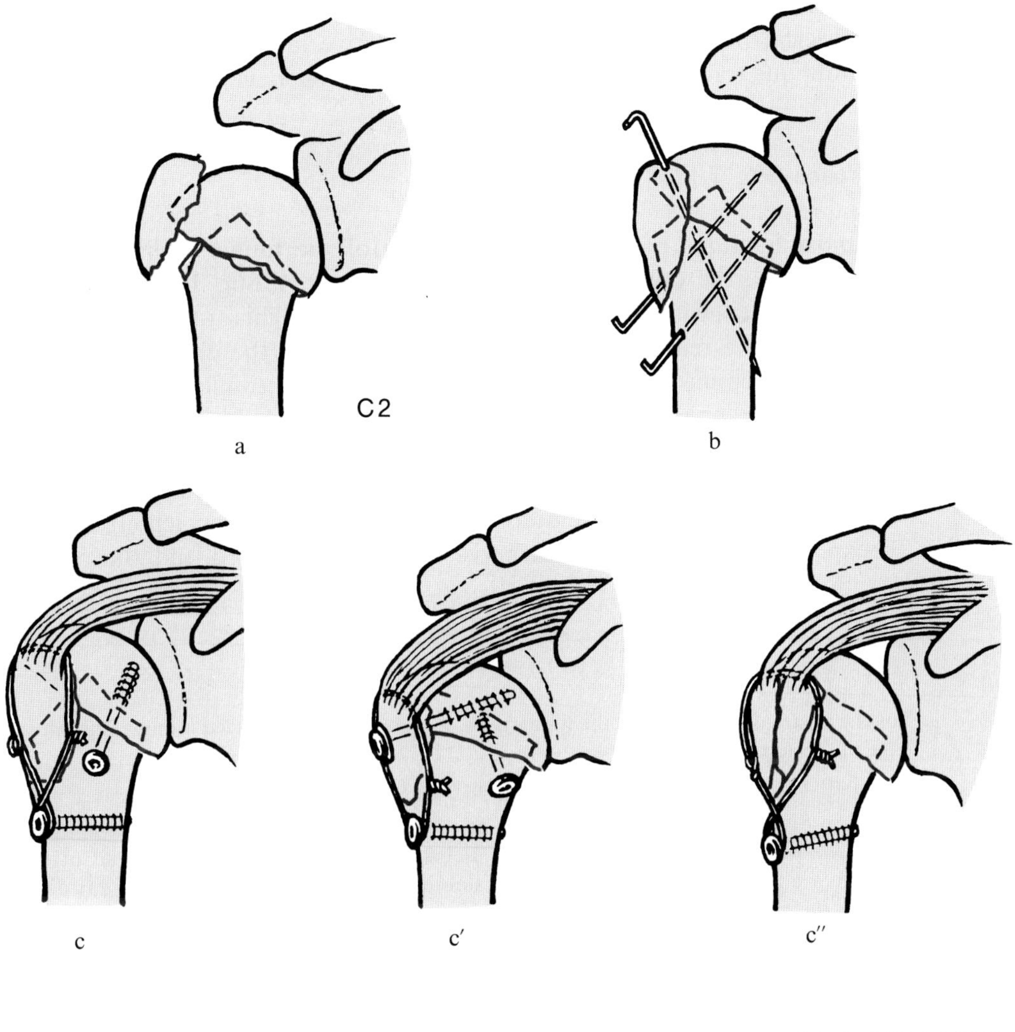

C2

a b

c c′ c″

7.3.2 Fractures of the Humeral Shaft

7.3.2.1 Classification (see also Chap. 1)

Type A: Simple fractures: transverse, spiral, or oblique.
Type B: One additional fragment: wedge or butterfly.
Type C: Complex fractures: spiroid, two levels, or comminuted.

Most fractures of the humeral shaft can be successfully treated conservatively by means of primary immobilization for 1–2 weeks in a Desault or Gilchrist bandage. As soon as the pain and swelling have subsided, a custom-made brace is applied following Sarmiento's technique. Evidence of clinical union can usually be observed after 3–6 weeks. However, the brace should be kept in place until the fracture appears solidly healed, normally at about 8–10 weeks.

7.3.2.2 Indications for Surgery

Indications may be divided into absolute and relative. Absolute indications are: open fractures; fractures with primary or secondary radial nerve palsy or vascular injury; patients with multiple injuries; bilateral shaft fractures; serial fractures on the same arm; pathological fractures; and non-unions. Relative indications are unstable transverse or short oblique fractures as well as a general illness such as Parkinson's disease.

7.3.2.3 Approach (Fig. 7.12)

For most fractures of the distal two-thirds of the humeral shaft, the safest approach appears to be the dorsal one described by Henry (1966). The patient is best placed in a prone position, with the elbow resting on a support. This automatically gives the humerus an approximate reduction. The skin incision lies on the dorsal surface of the humerus along a line connecting the dorsal margin of the acromion with the olecranon. After separating the superficial fascia, the forefinger is inserted in the V-shaped sulcus between the two superficial heads of the proximal triceps (long and lateral heads). The two are split in a distal direction as far as is needed by blunt or sharp dissection. Deep to the V lie the radial nerve and the accompanying radial vessels which cross the humeral shaft. To expose the bone, the radial nerve is gently mobilized and the medial head of the

---

Fig. 7.12

a For the posterior approach of the humerus, a straight incision is placed along a line between the posterior edge of the acromion and the olecranon.

1 Axillary nerve; *2* Radial nerve; *3* Ulnar nerve; *4* Olecranon.

b The deep dissection is started proximally at the posterior border of the deltoid muscle. With the index finger, we identify the "V"-shaped interval between the long and lateral head of the triceps muscle. The two are then separated bluntly in a distal direction. After separation of the two portions, we safely identify the radial nerve and the deep brachial vessels as they transverse the medial head of the triceps and the humeral shaft in an oblique direction. The aponeurosis of the triceps muscle is then split in a distal direction as far as is needed.

1 Deep brachial artery; *2* Radial nerve; *3* Posterior cutaneous nerve; *4* External intermuscular septum; *5* Articular capsule.

Fig. 7.12

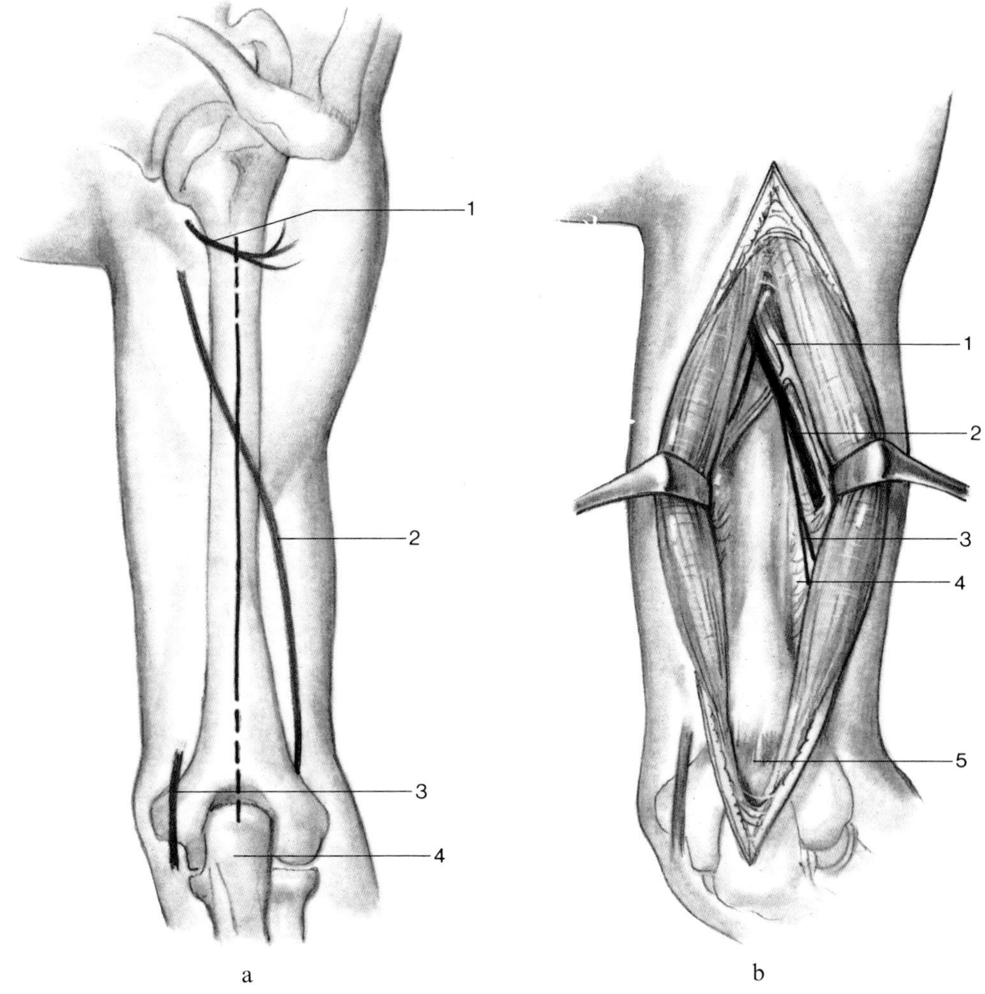

triceps is split. To prevent entrapment of the radial nerve, the lateral intermuscular septum should be cut.

For fractures extending into the proximal third, an anterolateral approach is recommended. As the bone in that area is covered by the brachial muscle, the muscle should be split longitudinally so that the bone can be reached.

7.3.2.4 Choice of Implant

Lag screws by themselves (Fig. 7.13a), even in long spiroid fractures, and the narrow 4.5-mm DCP (Fig. 7.13b) do not provide adequate fixation in fractures of the humerus shaft. They are best stabilized by a broad 4.5-mm DCP placed on the dorsal surface of the bone to act as a tension band (Fig. 7.14a, b). The plate may be slipped underneath the radial nerve and vessels and, because of this position, implant removal is not advocated. The proximal and distal main fragments must be held by at least three screws each which means that long plates must be used. For transverse and short oblique fractures an interfragmentary screw should be used wherever possible (Fig. 7.14a), and in multifragment fractures an autologous cancellous bone graft is advocated (Fig. 7.14b).

7.3.2.5 Postoperative Treatment

Immediate active physiotherapy is suggested.

Fig. 7.13

a For fractures of the shaft of the humerus, lag screw fixation is always inappropriate.

b The narrow 4.5-mm DCP is not our primary choice for fixation. We generally prefer the broad 4.5-mm placed on the dorsal surface.

Fig. 7.14 For plating the humeral shaft, a long broad 4.5-mm DCP is the only suitable implant.

a In case of a short transverse fracture, a lag screw should be placed across the fracture, and to obtain a good reduction and compression of the opposite cortex, the plate may be slightly prebent.

b If there is an area of comminution, an autologous cancellous bone graft is advocated.

In cases where the broad 4.5-mm DCP appears too large for a small humerus, the narrow 4.5-mm DCP or, preferrably, the narrow 4.5-mm LC-DCP may be used.

Caution: Care must be taken that the screws are inclined against each other sideways as much as the plate holes allow, in order to avoid longitudinal cracks in the far cortex.

Fig. 7.13

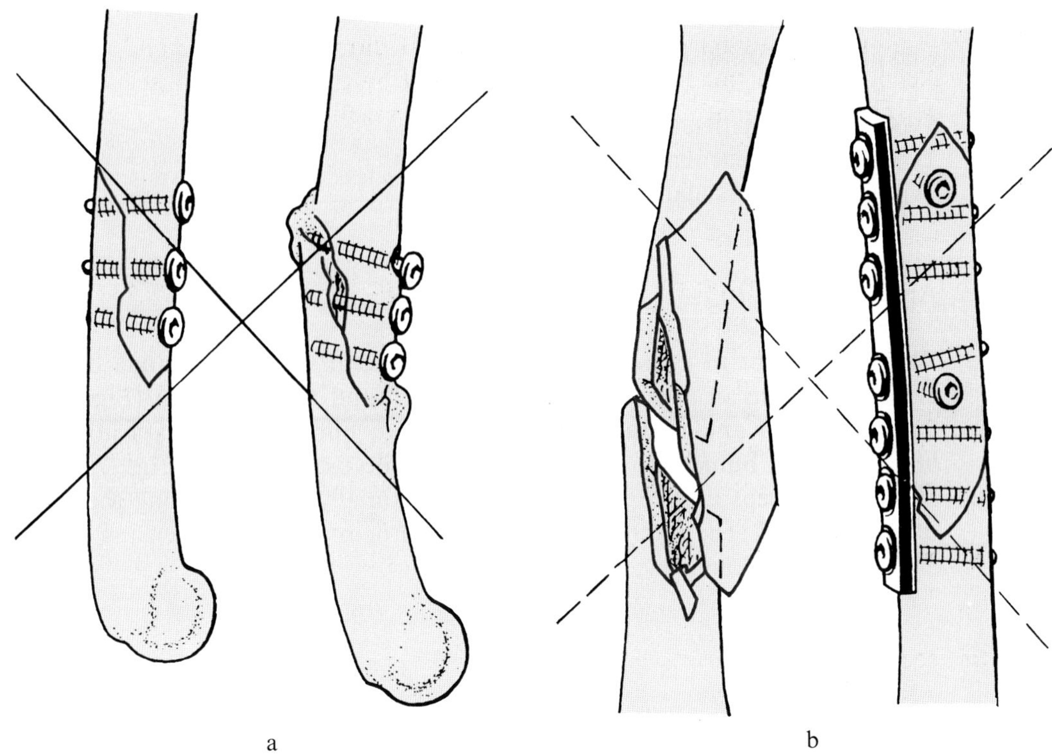

a b

Fig. 7.14

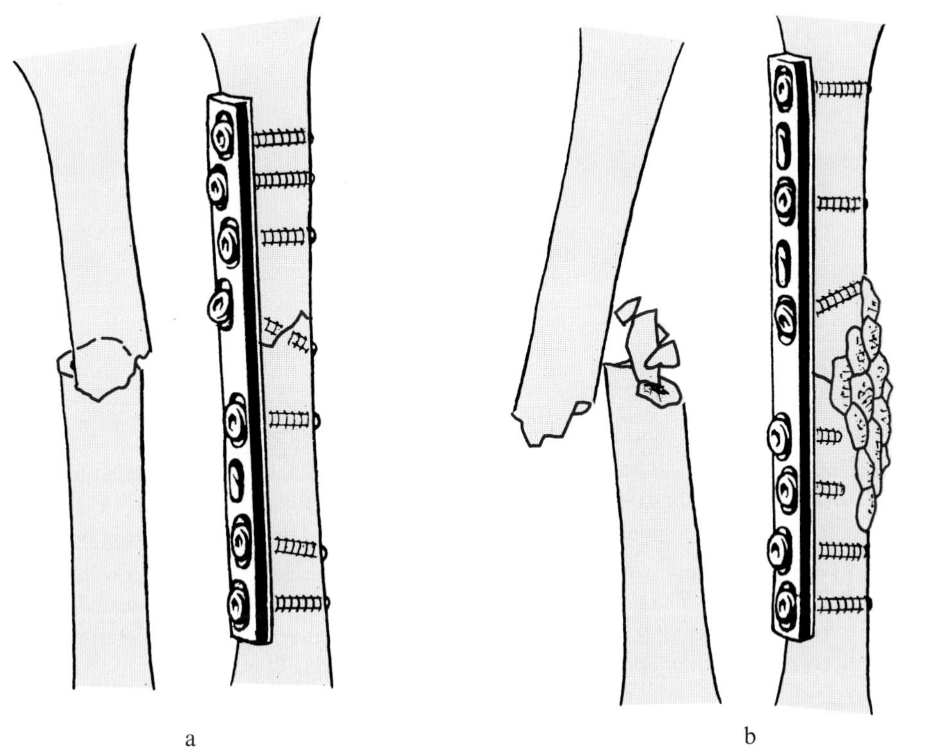

a b

7.3.3 Fractures of the Distal Humerus

7.3.3.1 Classification (see also Chap. 1)

Type A: Extra-articular fractures.
Type B: Intra-articular, unicondylar fractures.
Type C: Intra-articular, bicondylar fractures.

7.3.3.2 Approach (Fig. 7.15)

With the patient in a prone position (see humeral shaft) the standard approach to the elbow joint runs in a gentle curve radially around the olecranon (Fig. 7.15a). The skin flap is elevated and the ulnar nerve identified. For improved exposure of the trochlea and capitulum humeri, the olecranon should be osteotomized (Figs. 7.15b, 7.16a). This allows the triceps muscle to be reflected proximally, thus exposing the entire distal end of the humerus. The olecranon is later reapproximated with a tension band wire and/or a 6.5-mm cancellous bone screw (Fig. 7.16b, c).

Fig. 7.15

a The skin incision starts over the posterior middle of the distal humerus and curves radially past the tip of the olecranon to the posterior crest of the ulna.

1 Radial nerve; *2* Superficial branch of radial nerve; *3* Ulnar nerve; *4* Deep branch of radial nerve.

b In order to achieve a broad exposure of the joint, the olecranon is osteotomized and displaced medially and proximally. The ulnar nerve must be identified in the sulcus of the medial epicondyle.

1 Triceps muscle; *2* Radial nerve, external intermuscular septum; *3* Posterior cutaneous nerve; *4* Ulnar nerve; *5* Olecranon (osteotomized); *6* Anconeus muscle.

Fig. 7.16

a The osteotomy of the olecranon should be made with a small wedge to prevent rotational instability.

b For refixation of the olecranon, we like to combine a tension band either with a 6.5-mm cancellous bone screw as an internal splint,

c or with two Kirschner wires.

Fig. 7.15

Fig. 7.16

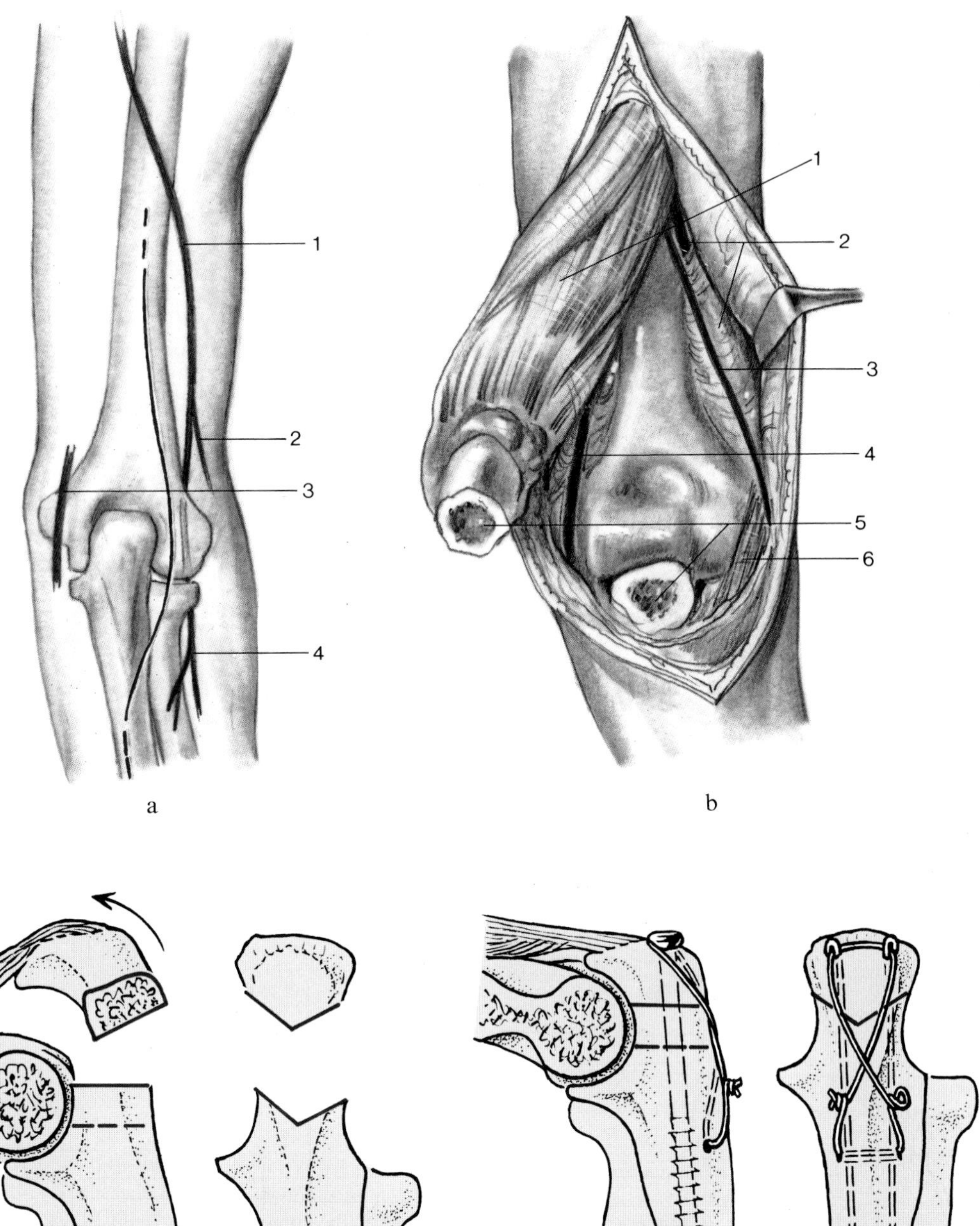

7.3.3.3 Fractures of the Distal Extra-articular Humerus (Type A)

Fracture type A is rare in adults but rather frequent in children, who are treated nonoperatively or by Kirschner wire pinning. As there is a tendency to delayed union in adults, internal fixation is indicated.

In the case of epicondyle avulsions (Fig. 7.17), fixation by lag screws, using 4.0-mm cancellous bone or 3.5-mm cortex screws, is advocated. If possible, these screws should be anchored in the opposite cortex. Splitting of the fragments may be avoided by predrilling with a 2.5-mm drill bit.

In the case of transverse or oblique metaphyseal fractures, a contoured 3.5-mm DCP is normally used. A rarely used alternative would be one- and two-third tubular plates. The position of the plate depends on the fracture configuration (Fig. 7.18).

7.3.3.4 Fractures of the Distal Intra-articular Humerus (Types B and C)

Unicondylar fractures (type B) must be reduced anatomically and are best fixed with 4.0-mm cancellous bone or 3.5-mm cortex lag screws (Fig. 7.19). Larger fragments may necessitate additional stabilization with a small plate.

In the more complex fractures involving trochlea and capitulum (type C), the reconstruction of the trochlea and capitulum humeri are the most important steps in internal fixation. Although the fragments are often severely displaced or rotated, they must be fitted back together accurately, and if this is done, permanent defects will be rare. If there is a defect after reconstruction, it must be filled with autologous cancellous bone.

Fig. 7.17 Extra-articular unicondylar avulsion fracture of the ulnar condyle fixed by (a′) one, or better (a″) two 4-mm cancellous bone screws.

Fig. 7.18 Supracondylar extra-articular fractures of the humerus, typical in children, are quite rare in adults.

a They usually require internal fixation by 3.5-mm DCP or even two one-third tubular plates.

b Depending on the fracture configuration, the plate is placed on the dorsal aspect of the bone or on either side. Additional lag screws are often required.

Fig. 7.19

a Intra-articular unicondylar fractures (type B) are stabilized by lag screws (4.0-mm cancellous bone or 3.5-mm cortex screws).

b Fracture of the radial condyle, fixed by two 4-mm cancellous bone screws.

At the time of injury, the elbow has usually been subluxated, resulting in considerable joint instability. It is therefore advisable to fix the condylar fragments back operatively with either one or two lag screws (4.0- or 6.5-mm cancellous bone screws) or exceptionally with a tension band wire.

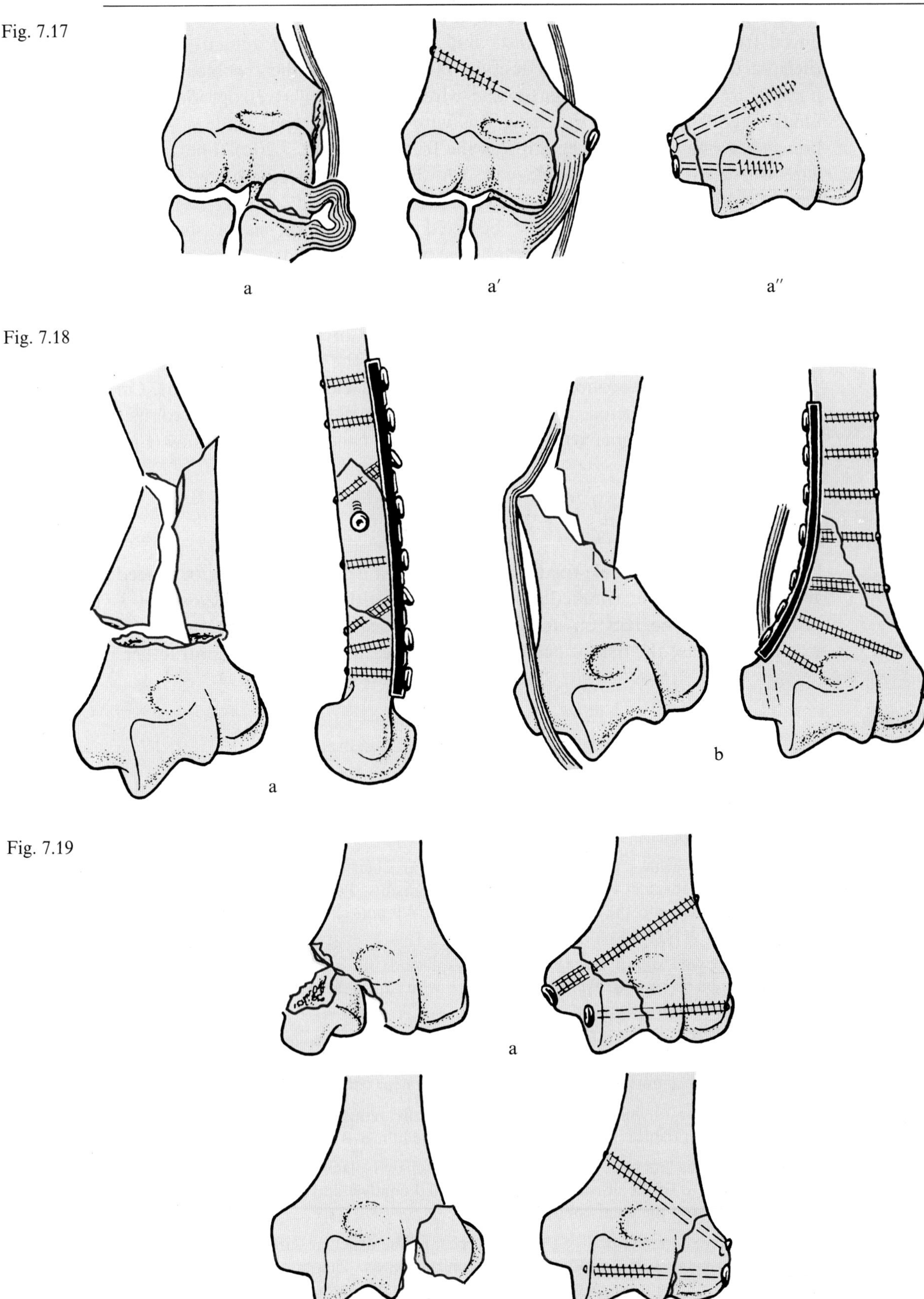
Fig. 7.17
a
a′
a″
Fig. 7.18
a
b
Fig. 7.19
a
b

Kirschner wires are used for reduction and temporary fixation. The first wire is introduced from the fracture plane into and across the radial fragment (Fig. 7.20a). It may then be used as a lever for reduction purposes. Once the trochlea and the capitulum humeri are anatomically aligned, the wire is drilled in a retrograde direction into the ulnar fragment (Fig. 7.20b). Using this wire as a directional guide, a 4.0-mm cancellous bone screw may be used to compress the fragments (Fig. 7.20c). The 1.25-mm Kirschner wire will then serve as a guide wire for the additional cannulated screw (Fig. 7.20d). Once the articular fragments are accurately reduced and securely fixed with one or two screws, this articular block must be fixed to the metaphysis or shaft of the humerus (Fig. 7.20c). One-third tubular plates (five to seven holes) or 3.5-mm reconstruction plates are the most suitable implants for this purpose. Considerable contouring of the plates is necessary. On the radial side of the metaphysis, the plate – preferably a reconstruction plate – is best placed on the dorsal flat surface of the bone. The best choice for the ulnar side is a one-third tubular plate, which fits the crest of the bone well (Fig. 7.20f). The olecranon and coronoid fossae must be kept clear of any implant. Once the distal humerus is reconstructed, the osteotomy of the olecranon is secured using a tension band wire with Kirschner wires or with a 6.5-mm cancellous bone screw (Fig. 7.16).

7.3.3.5 Postoperative Treatment

Postoperatively, if a stable fixation has been obtained, the arm may be placed in a removable splint. However, immediate active mobilization without any splint is preferable. Emphasis must be laid on active exercises in elbow injuries as passive physiotherapy seems to increase the risk of periarticular calcification and elbow contracture.

Fig. 7.20

a A Kirschner wire, 1.25 mm in diameter and sharpened at both ends, is driven from the fracture plane into the radial fragment.

b Having served as a lever to help reduction of the articular fragments, this guide wire is drilled in the reverse direction through the reduced trochlea fragments. Parallel to this first wire, a 2.5-mm hole is drilled from radial into the ulnar fragment and a 4.0-mm cancellous bone screw with a short thread is introduced after tapping.

c The Kirschner wire still in place now serves as a guide for a second, cannulated screw. A cannulated 3.5-mm drill bit is slipped over the Kirschner wire and a hole is drilled which does not go all the way across the trochlea fragment.

d A 3.5-mm cannulated fully threaded cancellous bone screw may be introduced to give additional support to the articular fragments. Depending on the fracture situation, it may be used as a lag screw (overdrilling) or just as a spacer screw (for a spacer screw, only the near cortex will be drilled).

e Once the articular fragments have been anatomically reduced to form an articular block, Kirschner wires may serve to reduce this block to the rest of the humerus.

f To firmly join the humerus to the articular block, two plates are applied: a 3.5-mm reconstruction plate contoured to fit the dorsal aspect of the radial condyle and a one-third tubular plate which nicely fits onto the crest of the ulnar condyle.

g In case of severe comminution of the middle part of the articular surface, a cancellous bone graft must be introduced between the capitulum and trochlea humeri. This bone graft should not be compressed: a fully threaded 3.5-mm cortex or a 4.0-mm cancellous bone screw is used.

h In case of good quality bone and simple fracture lines, the capitulum humeri may be fixed with only two lag screws. It is however always necessary that at least one plate be applied as a buttress.

Fig. 7.20

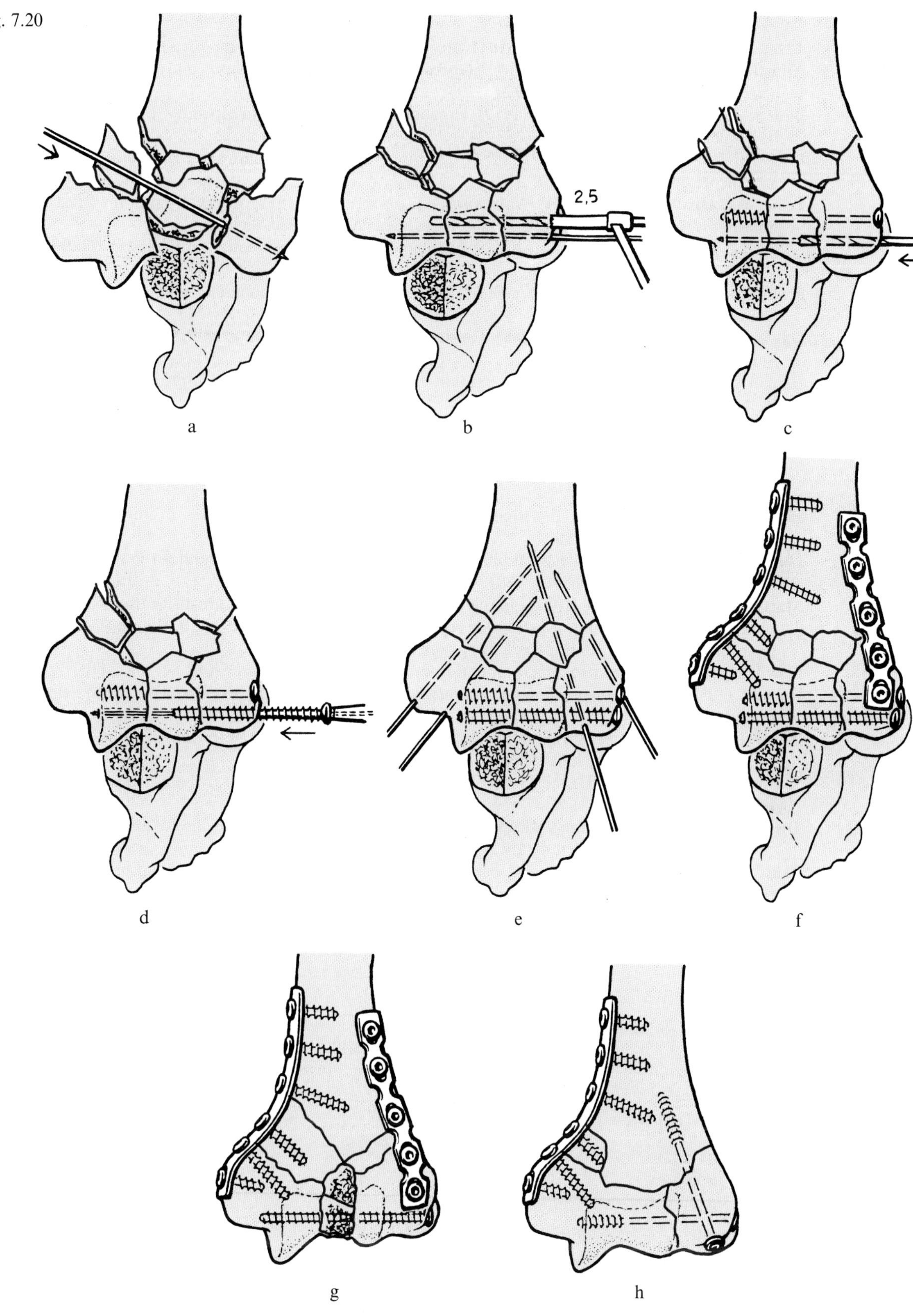

References

Armstrong CP, Van der Spuy J (1984) The fractured scapula: importance and management based on a series of 62 patients. Injury 15:324–329

Blömer J, Muhr G, Tscherne H (1977) Ergebnisse konservativ und operativ behandelter Schlüsselbeinbrüche. Unfallheilkunde 80:237–242

Bone LB (1988) Fractures of the shaft of the humerus. In: Chapman M (ed) Operative orthopedics. Lippincott, Philadelphia

Foster RJ, Dixon GL, Bach AW, Appleyard RW, Green TM (1985) Internal fixation of fractures and non-unions of the humeral shaft. J Bone Joint Surg [Am] 67:857–864

Giebel G, Tscherne H, Reissmann K (1986) Die gestörte Frakturheilung am Oberarm. Unfallchirurgie 89:353–360

Hardegger FH, Simpson LA, Weber BG (1984) The operative treatment of scapular fractures. J Bone Joint Surg [Br] 66:725–731

Hawkins RJ, Bell RH, Gurr K (1986) The three-part fracture of the proximal humerus. J Bone Joint Surg [Am] 68:1410–1414

Heim U, Pfeiffer KM (1988) Internal fixation of small fractures, 3rd edn. Springer, Berlin Heidelberg New York

Henry AK (1966) Extensile exposure. Livingstone, Edinburgh

Jakob RP, Kristiansen T, Mayo K, Ganz R, Müller ME (1984) Classification and aspects of treatment of fractures of the proximal humerus. In: Bateman JE, Welsh RP (1984) Surgery of the shoulder. Mosby, St Louis

Jupiter JB, Neff U, Holzach P, Allgöwer M (1985) Intercondylar fractures of the humerus. J Bone Joint Surg [Am] 67:226–239

Lee CK, Hansen HR (1981) Post-traumatic avascular necrosis of the humeral head in displaced proximal humeral fractures. J Trauma 21:788–791

Marti R, Lim TE, Jolles CW (1987) On the treatment of comminuted fracture dislocations of the proximal humerus: internal fixation or prosthetic replacement. In: Kölbel R, Helbig B, Blauth W (eds) Shoulder replacement. Springer, Berlin Heidelberg New York

Neer CS (1970) Displaced proximal humeral fractures. J Bone Joint Surg [Am] 52:1077–1103

Rüedi T (1989) The treatment of displaced metaphyseal fractures with screw and wiring systems. Orthopedics 12:55–59

Rüedi T, Chapman M (1988) Fractures of the scapula and clavicle. In: Chapman M (ed) Operative orthopedics. Lippincott, Philadelphia

Schweiberer L, Poeplau P, Gräber S (1977) Plattenosteosynthese bei Oberarmschaftfrakturen. Unfallheilkunde 80:231–235

Tossi JD, Newton CM, Sigmond HD (1963) Acromic-clavicular separations: useful and practical clarification for treatment. Clin Orthop 28:111–119

Van der Griend R, Tomasin J, Ward EF (1986) Open reduction and internal fixation of humeral shaft fractures. J Bone Joint Surg [Am] 68:430–433

Weber BG (1988) Fractures of the distal humerus. In: Chapman M (ed) Operative orthopedics. Lippincott, Philadelphia

8 FOREARM AND HAND/MINI-IMPLANTS

8.1 Introduction

The forearm is an exceptionally mobile unit of two bones and five articulations for the positioning of the hand and the transmission of forces.

For internal fixations in this area, small fragment implants are recommended as they are the most atraumatic, need little space and afford good stability. The 3.5-mm cortex screw, used with the 3.5-mm dynamic compression plate (DCP) to stabilize diaphyseal fractures, fulfills all these demands. Tension band wiring with Kirschner wires is the fundamental technique for simple fractures of the olecranon.

T plates are used on the distal radius. Only the radial head – an extremely fine structure with a double articulation – needs smaller screws of 2.0 or 1.5-mm diameter.

For anatomic and biomechanical reasons, osseoligamentous injuries of the forearm should be divided into proximal, diaphyseal and distal lesions.

8.2 Proximal Lesions

8.2.1 Proximal Ulna (Olecranon)

Fractures of the olecranon are usually caused by direct trauma or hyperextension. Open fractures are rare, but skin contusions and abrasions frequent.

A fracture of the olecranon causes a discontinuity of the extensor mechanism. It is a classical indication for internal fixation to permit functional restoration. The subcutaneous position of the fragments makes the reduction and stabilization comparatively easy. We must distinguish between transverse, oblique and complex fractures, which sometimes may extend into the diaphyeal area.

8.2.1.1 Positioning and Approach (Figs. 8.1–8.3)

Position: Supine, with the forearm lying across the chest or on an armboard.

Approach: The midline posterior incision is curved radially to avoid the point of the olecranon. It can be enlarged in either direction depending upon the fracture itself. The ulnar nerve should be identified, and isolated and protected with a rubber band if it is vulnerable.

Fig. 8.1 Dorsal and lateral incisions and approaches to the forearm.

a (*1*) The extensile exposure of Boyd and Thompson: proximal curved incision for fractures of the olecranon. Extension distally for shaft fractures by directing the incision towards the styloid process of the radius.
(*2*) The approach to the shaft of the ulna is between flexor carpi ulnaris and extensor carpi ulnaris.
(*3*) The approach to the middle and distal third of the radius is between extensor digitorum communis and extensor carpi radialis brevis.

b Cross section through the proximal third of the forearm to illustrate the proximal dorsal approach to the radius from the ulnar aspect as well as the position of the plates on the radius and ulna. The arrow (*4*) shows the volar approach of Henry between brachioradialis and pronator teres, the radial artery being retracted to the ulnar side.

c Cross section through the middle third of the forearm illustrating the surgical approaches to the radius and ulna by separate incisions (*2, 3*) or by the volar approach of Henry (*4*).

d The extensile approach of Boyd and Thompson, illustrating the approach to the proximal radius after partial detachment and reflection of the *supinator* muscle together with the posterior interosseous nerve. More distally the approach is developed between extensor digitorum communis and extensor carpi radialis brevis.

Fig. 8.1

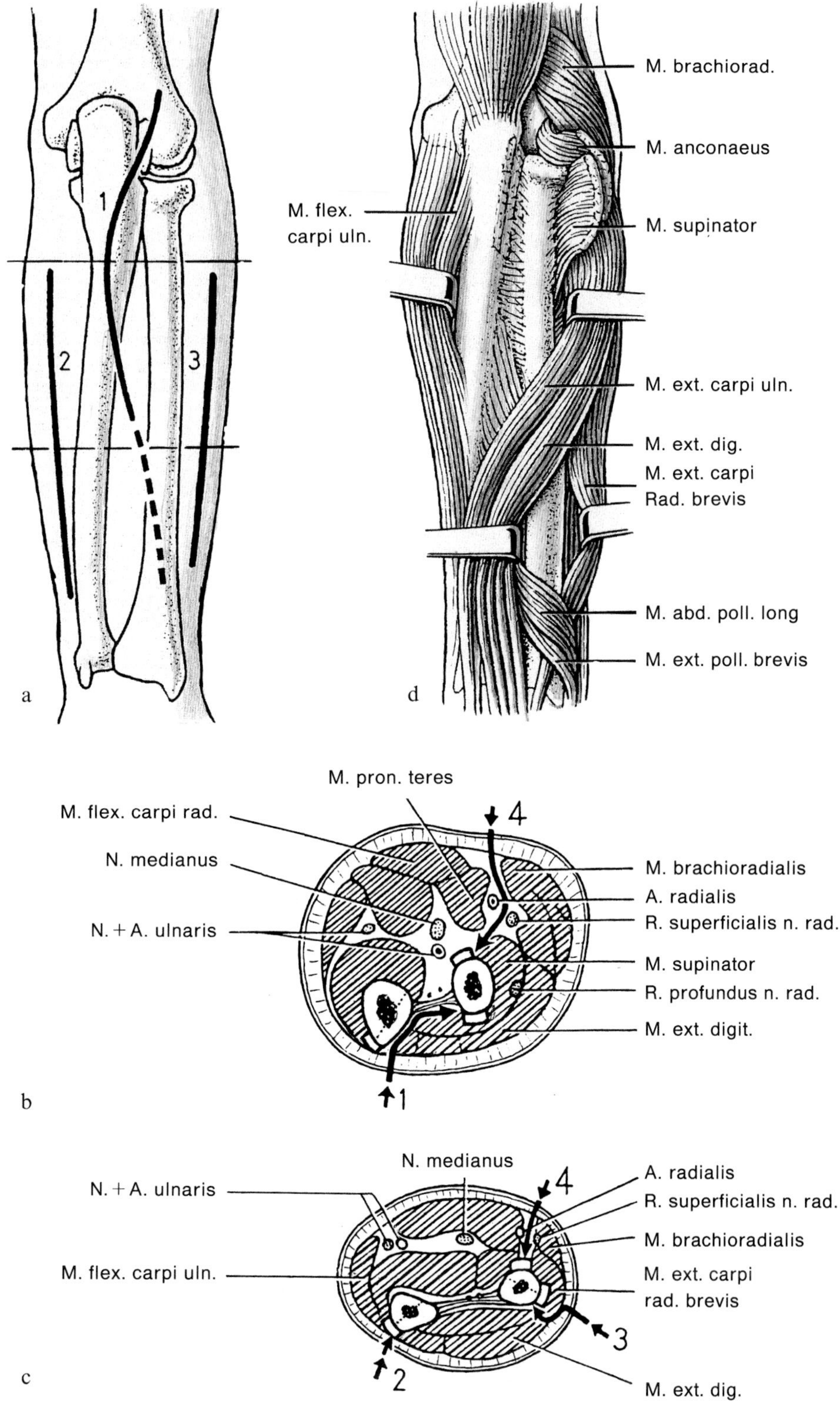
1
2
3
a
M. flex.
carpi uln.
M. brachiorad.
M. anconaeus
M. supinator
M. ext. carpi uln.
M. ext. dig.
M. ext. carpi
Rad. brevis
M. abd. poll. long
M. ext. poll. brevis
d
M. pron. teres
M. flex. carpi rad.
N. medianus
N. + A. ulnaris
4
M. brachioradialis
A. radialis
R. superficialis n. rad.
M. supinator
R. profundus n. rad.
M. ext. digit.
1
b
N. medianus
N. + A. ulnaris
M. flex. carpi uln.
4
A. radialis
R. superficialis n. rad.
M. brachioradialis
M. ext. carpi
rad. brevis
3
2
M. ext. dig.
c

Fig. 8.2 The volar approach of Henry (see Fig. 8.1 b, c for cross sections).

a Skin incision. The incurvation over the elbow joint prevents contractures.

b The brachioradialis muscle and the superficial branch of the radial nerve are retracted radially exposing the radial artery and its branches, which should be carefully ligated.

c Under the retracted artery, the radius is visualized, the supinator muscle partially detached after identification of the deep radial nerve (see d). The attachment of the pronator teres muscle is preserved.

d Detail of the anatomy: the deep branch of the radial nerve entering the supinator muscle through the arcade of Frohse.

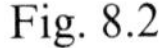
Fig. 8.2

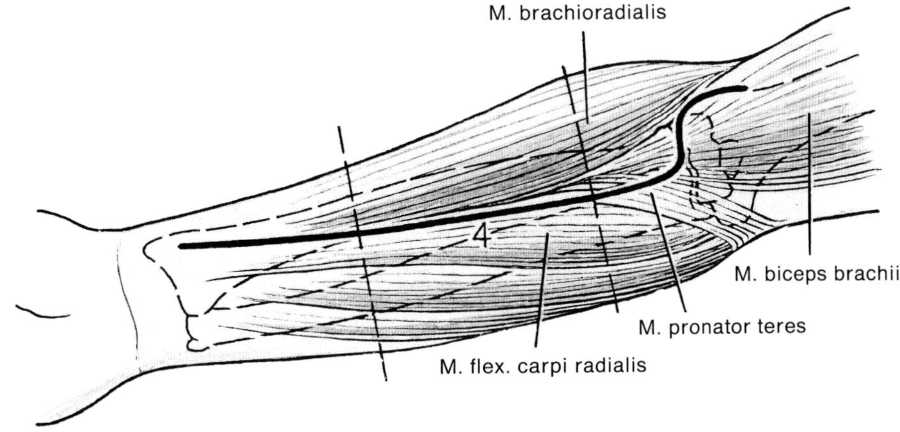

M. brachioradialis
4
M. biceps brachii
M. pronator teres
M. flex. carpi radialis

a

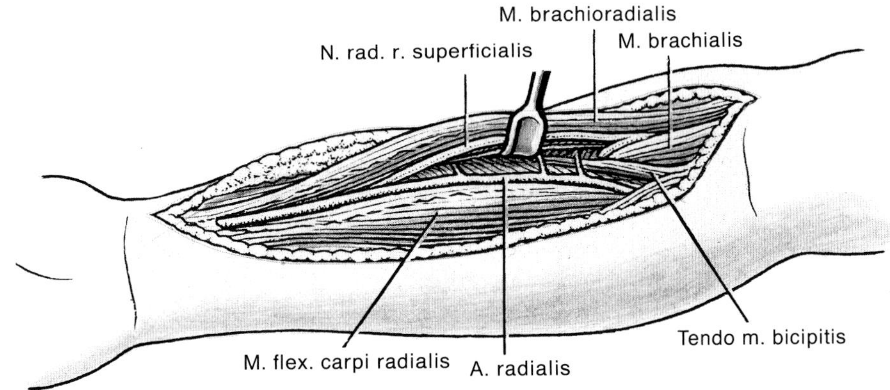

M. brachioradialis
M. brachialis
N. rad. r. superficialis
Tendo m. bicipitis
M. flex. carpi radialis
A. radialis

b

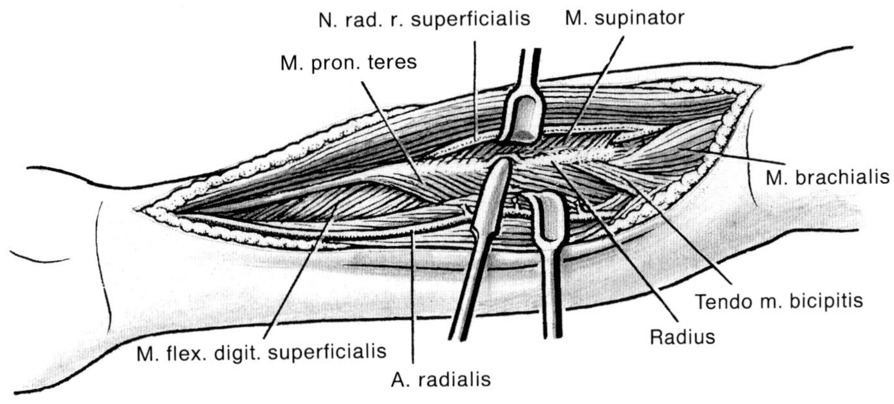

N. rad. r. superficialis
M. supinator
M. pron. teres
M. brachialis
Tendo m. bicipitis
Radius
M. flex. digit. superficialis
A. radialis

c

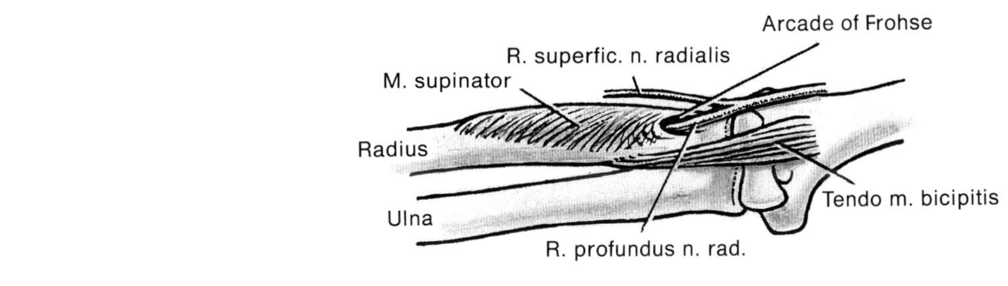

Arcade of Frohse
R. superfic. n. radialis
M. supinator
Radius
Ulna
Tendo m. bicipitis
R. profundus n. rad.

d

Fig. 8.3 Prone and lateral positions of the patient for the treatment of complex fractures or fracture dislocations in the elbow area. The hanging forearm can be flexed over 90°.

Fig. 8.4 Approach to the radial head.

a The longitudinal radiodorsal incision, dorsally extended. Incision of the muscle fibers and joint capsule along with the annular ligament. The proximity of the deep branch of the radial nerve has to be kept in mind!

b Extended approach into the articulation with osteotomy of the epicondyle. The collateral ligament remains attached to the bone. The reconstruction with a small cancellous screw and plastic washer with points is prepared. Cancellous bone is harvested from the osteotomy side. The Hohmann retractor is placed against the condyle to avoid compression of the deep radial nerve branch.

Fig. 8.3

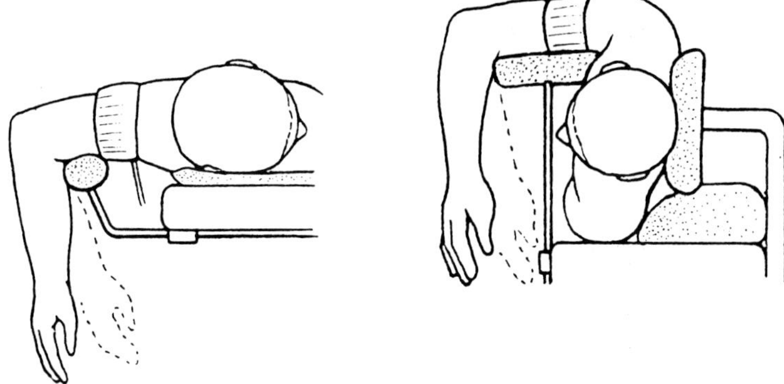

Fig. 8.4

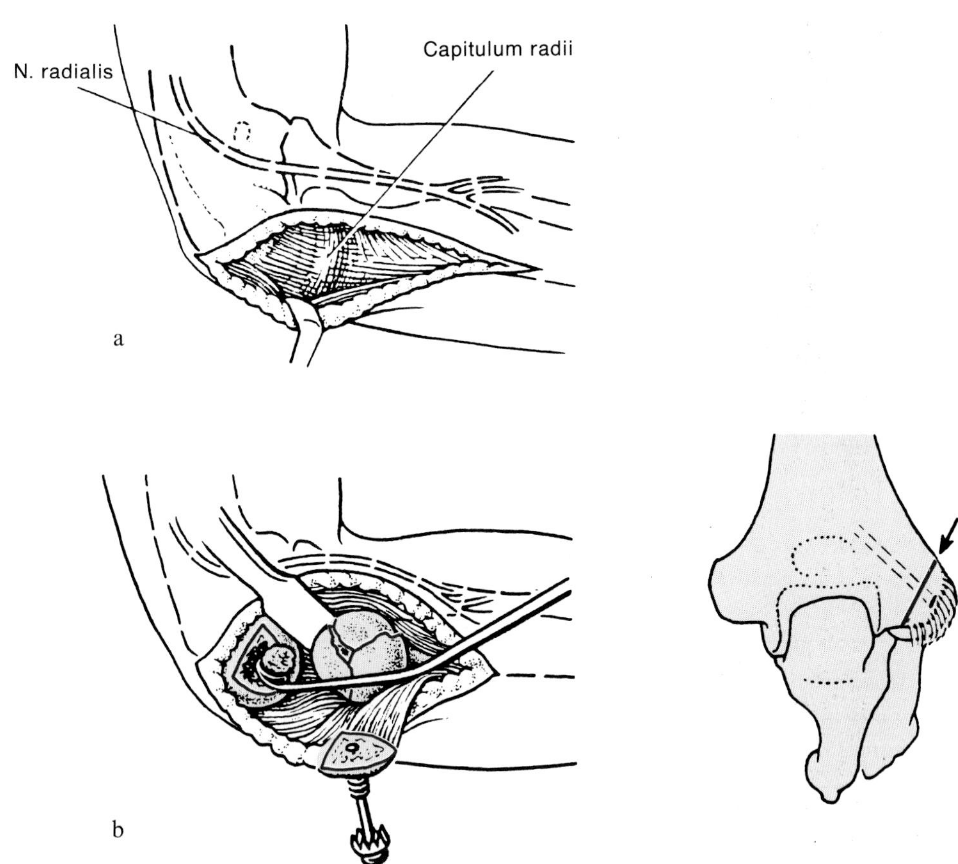

8.2.1.2 Tension Band Technique in Transverse Olecranon Fractures (Fig. 8.5)

The classical technique uses two Kirschner wires and a figure-of-eight wire loop.

Begin by drilling a superficial hole in the distal fragment to allow the introduction of the tip of the pointed reduction forceps. The other tip of the forceps catches the proximal fragment and reduces the fracture. Inspect the precision of the reduction on both sides of the bone.

Introduce two parallel Kirschner wires (1.6 mm diameter) from the center of the proximal fragment in a slightly oblique anterior direction until you feel the resistance diminishing after the perforation of the anterior cortex.

Drill a transverse 2.5-mm hole in the distal fragment through both cortices. Push a wire of 1.0 or 1.2 mm through this hole after having made a loop near one end, cross the two ends of the wire and pass one end under the triceps and the Kirschner wires. Instead of one long wire loop, two separate loops may be used (Fig. 8.5f).

Both sides of the wire must be separately tightened to produce a symmetrical tension. The tightening advances in several stages. The base of each twist is gripped with a parallel or special twisting forceps which pulls on the wire perpendicular to the axis of the bone. The wire is then twisted whilst slightly diminishing the tension. This procedure is repeated until the wire lies flat on the surface of the bone. Examine for correct stability and tension. The Kirschner wires are then slightly pulled back, cut short obliquely to leave a sharp point and bent over at the protruding ends to form little hooks. Drive these back into the bone over the tension wire. After the examination of the tension, the twists are shortened and bent over to lie flat on the bone.

Fig. 8.5 Tension band wire and Kirschner wires for a transverse fracture of the olecranon.

a Reduction of the fracture with pointed forceps. The distal branch is introduced in a previously drilled cortical hole.

b Drilling of two parallel Kirschner wires of 1.6-mm diameter obliquely from proximal to distal until they perforate the volar cortex. Drilling of a transverse 2.5-mm hole in the distal fragment.

c Insertion of a cerclage wire with a prefabricated loop, creating a figure of eight through the transverse hole and under the triceps tendon and the Kirschner wires. The wire end is introduced in a curved large injection needle used as a guide.

d The free ends of the cerclage wire are crossed and bent. Alternatively, tightening of the loops by pulling and rotating creates interfragmentary compression. The free ends of the cerclage wire are cut and the loops bent to the bone.

e The ends of the Kirschner wire are cut obliquely for sharpening, then bent 180° and hammered into the bone.

f Alternative: the same technique using two separate cerclage wires.

Fig. 8.5

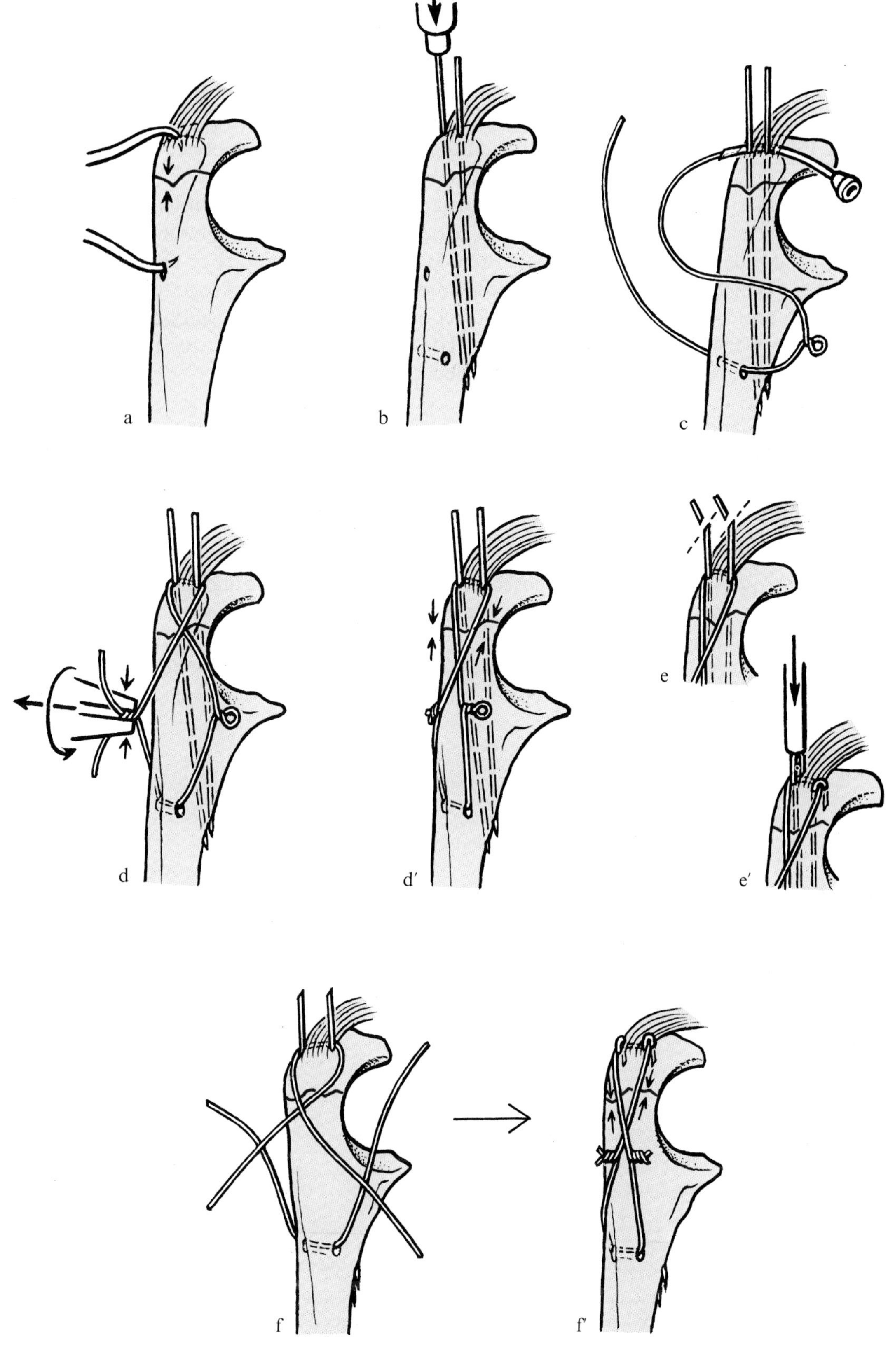

8.2.1.3 Internal Fixation in Oblique Fractures (Fig. 8.6b)

After reduction, first introduce an interfragmentary lag screw and then apply Kirschner wires and tension wire as indicated in Sect. 8.2.1.2.

8.2.1.4 Stable Internal Fixation in Comminuted Fractures (Fig. 8.6a)

In situations where proximal olecranon fractures extend into the diaphysis, priority is given to the reduction of the articular fragments using pointed forceps or Kirschner wires for the provisional fixation. Butterfly fragments are re-united to the main fragment by lag screws. Finally, the main fragments are connected together using either a one-third tubular plate, a 3.5-mm reconstruction plate or a 3.5-mm DCP, the choice being dependent on the type of fracture. These plates must be bent to fit the anatomic situation exactly and tightened using the tension device.

8.2.1.5 Screw Fixation of the Coronoid Process of the Ulna (Fig. 8.6c)

Internal fixation of large coronoid fragments is indicated to restore the stability in the hinge joint of the trochlea.

Approach from the ulnar side, identifying and securing the ulnar nerve. Osteotomize the ulnar epicondyle with a fine chisel. The epicondyle with its muscles and the nerve are retracted anteriorly. The coronoid process is now visualized and can be fixed under direct vision with a screw introduced dorsally. The epicondyle is then reduced and fixed with a previously prepared screw, and finally the nerve is replaced in its bed.

8.2.1.6 Fracture Dislocations of the Elbow

See Sect. 8.2.3.

Fig. 8.6 Fixation of olecranon fractures with lag screws and the one-third tubular plate.

a, a′, a″ A three-part fracture of the olecranon is fixed with a long one-third tubular plate applied as a tension band. The tension device is used to obtain fine reduction and optimum compression.

b, b′ For an oblique fracture, a lag screw is combined with a tension band wire.

c Fixation of the coronoid process with a 4.0-mm cancellous bone screw.

Fig. 8.6

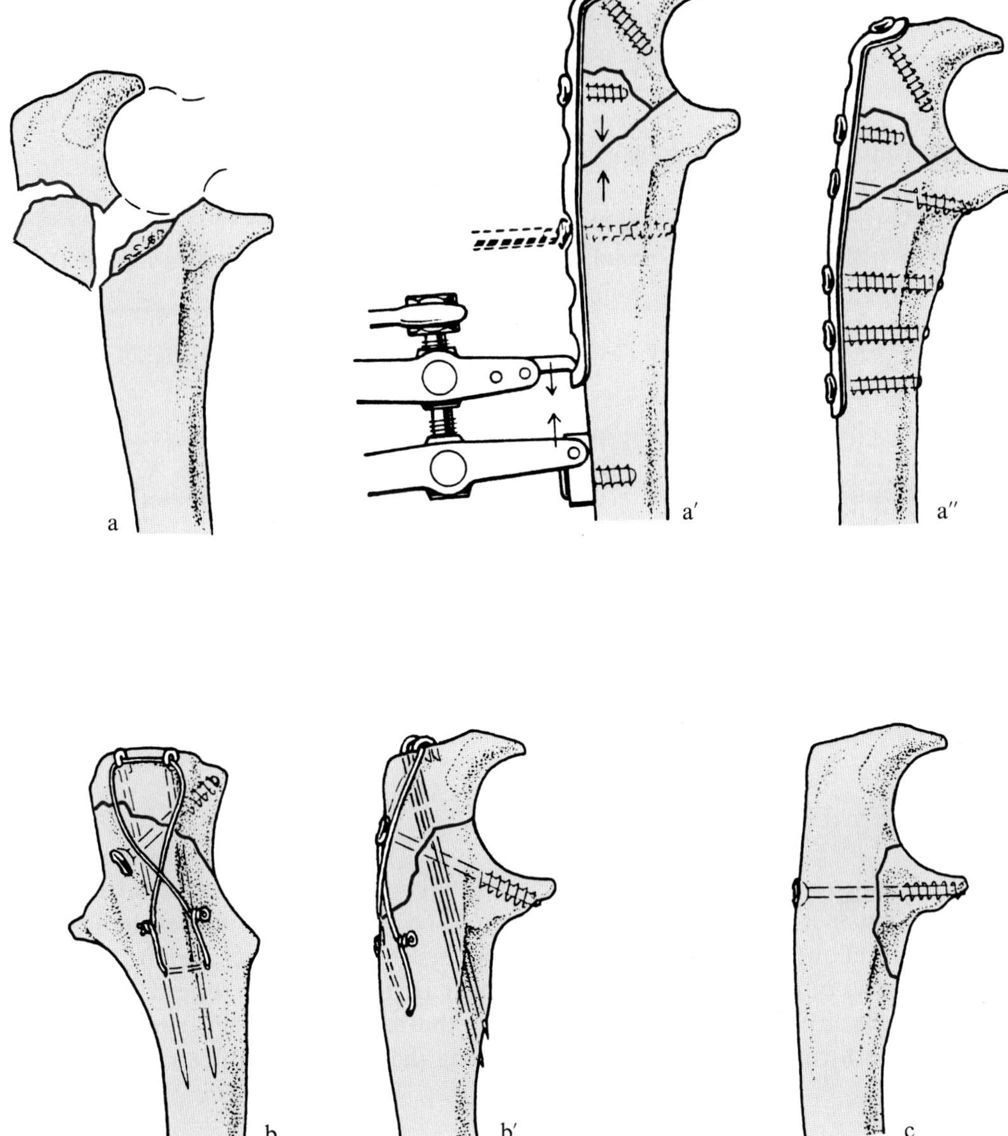

8.2.2 Fractures of the Radial Head

The radial head transmits axial forces and is an important stabilizer of the elbow joint. So-called isolated fractures are often combined with ligamentous ruptures and avulsions of capsular ligamentous structures, especially on the medial side. Avulsions of humeral articular cartilage and its interposition between the radial fragments should be sought.

8.2.2.1 Classification (Fig. 8.7a–c)

Vertical separation fractures, central depressed fractures, or neck fractures which produce a tilt of the head (especially common in children). Devitalization of fragments is rare, even in the presence of comminution. Periosteal connections between the fragments should be preserved.

8.2.2.2 Positioning and Approach (Fig. 8.3, 8.4)

Position: Place the elbow on an armboard in medium flexion with the forearm in pronation.

Approach the radial head through a dorsolateral longitudinal incision. The incision can be enlarged proximally by an osteotomy of the lateral epicondyle with the collateral ligament attached. This allows a nearly circumferential view of the fracture area. Special care has to be taken as the deep branch of the radial nerve runs near the bone in the supinator muscle with particular danger of paralysis from pressure of retractors.

8.2.2.3 Internal Fixation (Fig. 8.7a–c)

Reduction is obtained with a special narrow forceps used in hand surgery, or with fine Kirschner wires. Depressed areas must be reduced and the resultant defects filled with cancellous bone graft taken from the nearby epicondyle. Stabilization is achieved with screws of 1.5- or 2.0-mm diameter which are introduced in different planes and at different levels. Their heads must be sunk in the cartilage of the articulation. Wound closure is performed in one layer after inspecting the stability and free rotation.

Fig. 8.7 Screw fixation of radial head fractures.

a Screw fixation of a wedge fracture. *Top left:* The displacement seen from above and from the side. *Bottom left:* There may be entrapment of cartilage between the fragments and distraction of the ulnar collateral ligaments. *Right:* After removal of the entrapped cartilage and reduction by pushing (oblique arrow), the lag screw technique is used in both simple and multifragmentary fractures.

b Screw fixation and cancellous graft of a depressed fracture. *Left:* The centrally depressed area with a partially intact wall of the radial head. *Right:* Reduction and central grafting of the defect and lag screw fixation.

c Depressed fracture of the neck of the radius. *Left:* The depressed area under the intact articular surface. AP view with valgus angulation after rupture of the collateral ulnar ligament. *Right:* Obliquely introduced screw in buttress position and small cancellous bone graft.

Fig. 8.7

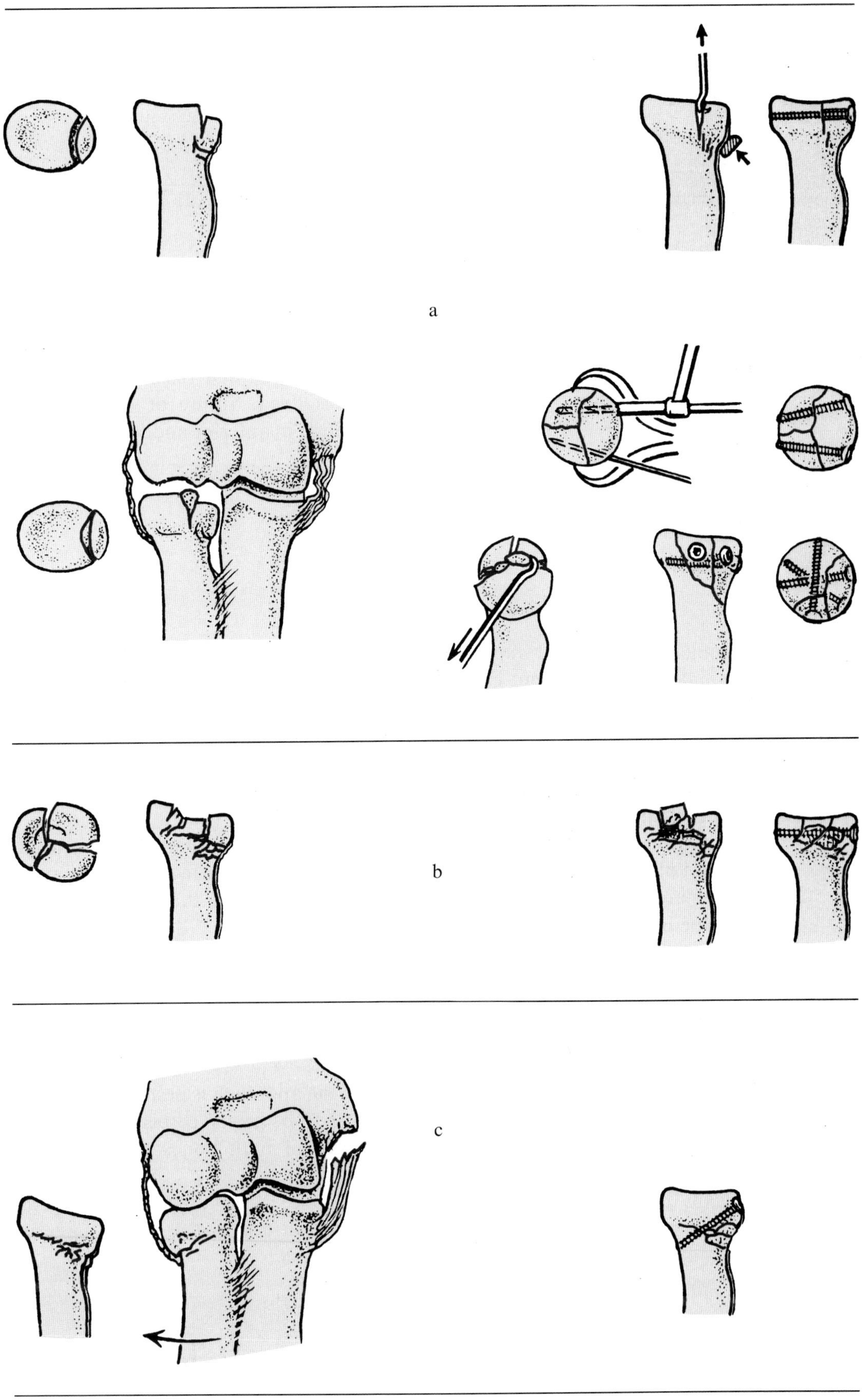

a

b

c

8.2.2.4 Postoperative Treatment

This is functional, with movements beginning from a dorsal splint applied in medium flexion. It is not necessary to remove the screws.

8.2.3 Posterior Fracture Dislocations of the Elbow (Posterior Monteggia Injury)

Fracture dislocations where the radial head is displaced dorsally are comparatively rare. The fracture of the ulna can be of various configurations, situated from the olecranon to the diaphysis. Comminution is frequent. The radial head is nearly always fractured and lies on the dorsal side, easily accessible in the prone position with a hanging forearm Fig. 8.3. The fracture of the radial head is reduced and fixed by the above-mentioned technique as a first step, before the ulna is fixed. Suture of the annular ligament is rarely necessary. The indications are the same as in anterior and lateral Monteggia injuries (see Sect. 8.3.6.1).

8.3 Forearm Shaft

During pronation and supination, the radius describes an important rotation around the ulna. For this reason, isolated fractures of the radius are unstable and an indication for internal fixation. This is also the case when both bones are broken. Isolated non-displaced fractures of the distal third of the ulna may sometimes be treated by nonoperative methods.

Radiological examination for shaft fractures should always include the distal and the proximal joints.

Immediate surgery leads to better functional results than delayed internal fixation. The use of a tourniquet is recommended. As for any major internal fixation, it is advisable to prepare the iliac crest preoperatively for a removal of the cancellous graft, especially for type B and C fractures.

8.3.1 Approaches to Forearm Bones (Figs. 8.1, 8.2)

For fractures of the middle and distal thirds, the approach is best achieved by two separate incisions. A sufficiently broad skin bridge has to be preserved between the incisions.

Complex fractures of the proximal thirds of both bones can be approached by a single incision according to Boyd (1963) (Fig. 8.1).

For the radial shaft, there is a choice between the dorsolateral approach and the anterior approach of Henry (1966) (Fig. 8.2).

8.3.1.1 Shaft of the Ulna

The entire length of the bone can easily be exposed by virtue of its subcutaneous situation.

Position: The arm is placed on an upholstered armboard with medium elbow flexion and full forearm pronation.

Landmarks: The subcutaneous border of the ulna between the olecranon and the ulnar styloid process.

Interneural Approach: This is between the extensor carpi ulnaris muscle (posterior interosseous nerve) and the flexor carpi ulnaris muscle (ulnar nerve).

Dangers: The ulnar nerve lies proximally under the flexor carpi ulnaris and on the flexor digitorum profundus. It should be carefully preserved in the event of proximal dissection. The ulnar artery is endangered in cases of damage to the flexor carpi ulnaris.

8.3.1.2 Shaft of the Radius

Access to the radius is difficult because of its deep position. The full length can only be exposed by the volar approach of Henry, which should be preferred for aesthetic reasons. For fractures of the proximal third of both bones, Boyd's dorsal approach may be easier; the dorsolateral approach is often used for the distal two-thirds of the radius.

Anterior Approach (Henry)

Position: The arm is placed on an armboard with straight elbow and full forearm supination.

Landmarks: The biceps tendon and the styloid process of the radius.

Interneural Approach: This is between the brachioradialis muscle (radial nerve) and the flexor carpi radialis muscle (median nerve).

Surgical Dissection: The fascia is incised between the brachioradialis and flexor carpi radialis muscles. Preserve the antebrachii lateralis nerve which lies subcutaneously and the superficial branch of the radial nerve lying along the brachioradialis muscle, which is retracted radially. The brachioradialis muscle is supplied by several branches of the radial artery which must be ligated. The radial artery and accompanying veins are retracted medially. In the middle third, the insertion of the pronator teres muscle should be preserved if possible. Proximally, the supinator muscle must be incised at its insertion on the radius and retracted laterally together with the deep branch of the radial nerve within its substance.

Dangers: The radial artery is vulnerable during the mobilization of the brachioradialis, especially when using a tourniquet, as it appears surprisingly small. The deep branch of the radial nerve (posterior interosseous) runs within the mass of the supinator muscle. The supinator insertion should be exposed in full supination and detached from the radius as close as possible to the bone.

Dorsolateral Approach (Thompson) for Distal Two-Thirds of Radius (Fig. 8.1)

Position: The arm is placed on an armboard, with a flexed elbow, and midpronation of the forearm.

Landmarks: The lateral epicondyle of the humerus and Lister's tubercle.

Interneural Approach: This is between extensor carpi radialis brevis (radial nerve) and extensor digitorum communis (posterior interosseous nerve).

Surgical Dissection: The fascia between the extensor carpi radialis brevis and the extensor digitorum communis is incised. In the distal third, abductor pollicis longus and extensor pollicis brevis emerge obliquely. By gentle dissection, separate both muscles from the shaft of the radius, just sufficiently for a plate to be slipped beneath. Proximally, identify the radial nerve before it enters the supinator and then emerges distally from the muscle. Spreading the muscle fibers of the supinator enables identification and preservation of all muscular branches.

Danger: Damage to the radial nerve, which should be identified and protected within the supinator.

8.3.1.3 Proximal Shaft of Both Forearm Bones (Boyd) (Fig. 8.1)

Position: The patient may be placed either prone or in the lateral decubitus position, with the forearm hanging, the elbow at 90° and the upper arm supported on a rest (Fig. 8.3). Alternatively, with the patient supine, the arm may be placed on an armboard with the elbow in flexion, and midpronation of the forearm.

Landmarks: The lateral epicondyle of the humerus and styloid process of the ulna.

Wound Extension (Boyd and Thompson): The skin incision may be extended distally for further access to the radius between the extensor digitorum communis and the extensor carpi radialis brevis, as in the dorsoradial approach.

Surgical Dissection: Detach anconeus, extensor carpi ulnaris and supinator muscles from their periosteal insertions into the ulna until you arrive on the interosseous membrane. Avoid damage, by the pressure of retractors, to the posterior interosseous artery and to the radial nerve within the supinator.

8.3.2 Reduction

8.3.2.1 General Considerations

The reduction must be atraumatic and is achieved using small forceps. Periosteal bridges should be preserved. Wedge fragments should be connected with a main fragment by preliminary lag screws, even if devitalized. To avoid rotational deformities and shortening, it is necessary to preserve small devitalized fragments as guides to the precision of the reduction. If they have to be removed later, they should be replaced by autologous cancellous iliac bone graft.

In fractures with a defect, the plate is provisionally fixed to one of the main fragments by a screw, and to the second main fragment with forceps. The final fixation of the plate has to wait until it is adapted to the shape of the bone, pronation and supination are free and the correct length of the bone has been confirmed radiologically. Defects are filled with grafts of iliac cancellous bone.

8.3.2.2 Reduction Tactics in Fractures of Both Bones

We begin with the fracture which is easiest to approach and to reduce – usually that of the ulna. After reduction, a plate is provisionally fixed to one main fragment with a screw and to the other with a reduction forceps (or a screw).

The second bone is then approached and its fracture exposed. If reduction is impossible, loosen the plate on the first bone. After reduction and provisional fixation of both bones, examine the pronation and supination, which should be free before other screws are introduced into the plates.

8.3.3 Internal Fixation (Figs. 8.8–8.10)

8.3.3.1 Implants

A diaphyseal fracture of the forearm is best fixed with a plate. Each main fragment should have at least seven cortex holes. The 3.5-mm DCP has proved to be the ideal implant, requiring an eight-hole plate in a transverse or short oblique fracture and a nine- or ten-hole plate when there is a third fragment. Very short fragments of the proximal radius do not always accept these long plates (Fig. 8.11).

Wedge fragments should first be fixed to the main fragment by lag screws placed so as to avoid collision of the screw heads with the later position of the plate. The plate should be contoured perfectly to the shape of the bone. To achieve this, malleable, colored templates may be useful as guides.

The position of the plate holes over an oblique fracture should be planned to permit the introduction of an interfragmentary lag screw through one of the central holes of the plate and across the fracture after the axial compression has been applied. This technique has been shown to significantly increase the stability of the fixation.

These details are very important because there will be strong rotational forces acting against our internal fixation during the postoperative functional treatment.

8.3.3.2 Bone Graft

Experience shows that the surgeon usually overestimates the quality of his reduction and stabilization. In case of doubt about the quality of the reduction or suspicion of devitalization, the osteosynthesis is improved biologically with an additional autologous cancellous bone graft. The graft should be placed away from the interosseous border to avoid formation of radio-ulnar bridging callus.

8.3.3.3 Wound Closure

The tourniquet is released after the stabilization so that the local and distal circulation can be examined and to secure hemostasis. Suction drainage is inserted in the depth of the wound. The fascial layers are not sutured. Skin suture is performed only when there is neither tension nor danger of postoperative swelling. Alternatively, the wound is left open and is covered with a nonadhesive gauze dressing. The closure of the skin is performed in steps after swelling has subsided (local anesthesia). There is rarely an indication for a secondary skin graft in closed fractures.

A padded dressing is applied and the arm elevated. This helps to reduce pain and swelling and can be removed for functional treatment.

Fig. 8.8 A simple transverse fracture of the distal ulnar shaft (22-A1). Fixation with a six-hole 3.5-mm DCP inducing axial compression.

Fig. 8.9 Fractures of both bones of the forearm (22-B3). The oblique fracture of the ulna is fixed with a seven-hole 3.5-mm DCP and an interfragmentary lag screw. The butterfly fragment on the radius needs preliminary fixation to a main fragment with a separate 2.7-mm lag screw. The 3.5-mm DCP must be longer than the ulna plate.

Fig. 8.10 Complex fracture of radius with simple fracture of ulna (22-C2). In case of devitalization or defect, the plate – which is bridging – should then be longer. Packed cancellous bone graft avoiding the interosseous membrane.

Fig. 8.8

Fig. 8.9

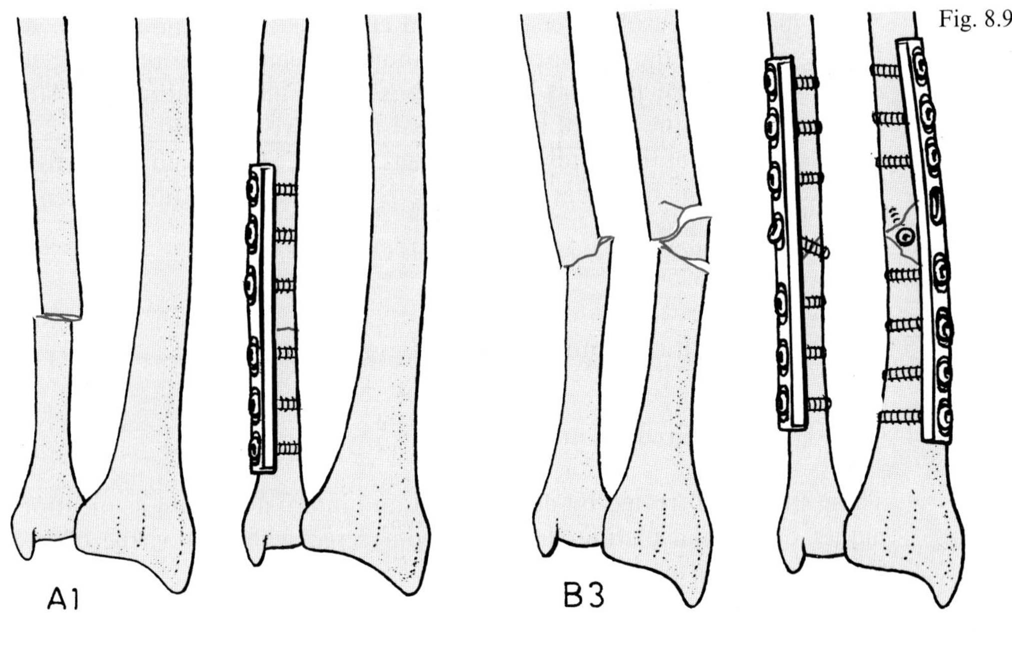

Fig. 8.10

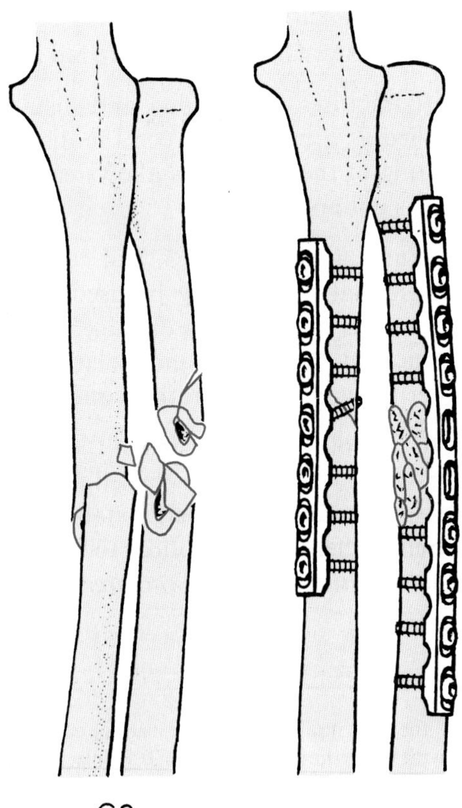

8.3.4 Postoperative Treatment

Active mobilization of fingers, wrist and elbow should begin as early as the pain allows. During exercises, the exterior splints should be temporarily removed; their definitive removal should take place as early as possible. Full pronation and supination is often gained only with the help of passively assisted active physiotherapy.

The removal of the plates in diaphyseal fractures should not be performed until 2 years after the fixation. It appears that these is no strict indication for removal of proximal plates on the radius.

8.3.5 Particular Situations and Special Osteosyntheses

8.3.5.1 Open Fractures Grades 2 and 3

These should be treated by debridement and internal fixation as mentioned above. Techniques other than plating should be considered when, by virtue of loss of soft tissue, there is a danger of exposing the plates.

8.3.5.2 Application of the External Fixator

The primary use of the external fixator has proved helpful in two situations:

(a) Combined shaft fractures of the ulna and distal comminuted radius fractures. The fixator is then applied as a bridge between the distal radius and the second metacarpal, combined with plating of the ulna. This allows early mobilization in cases where plating on the distal radius is not appropriate.

(b) Compound fractures, grades 2 and 3, and complex fractures, especially with defects. In such cases the external fixator may be used as a primary stabilization, if a plating is not possible for reasons of soft tissue damage. In such cases, it is important to perform extensive fasciotomies on the dorsal and volar sides, including the flexor retinaculum at the wrist, in order to avoid postoperative compartment syndromes.

To avoid damage to the soft tissue, the tips of the Schanz screws should not be introduced too deeply. When the soft tissues are healed, it is usually better to change from the fixator to a plate fixation which gives better stability.

In smaller patients, there is the option to use the small external fixator system as described in *Internal Fixation of Small Fractures* (Heim and Pfeiffer 1987).

Fig. 8.11 Complex fracture of the proximal third of the radius combined with a simple ulnar fracture (22-C2): the radius is fixed with a six-hole 3.5-mm DCP. Only two screws are fixing the proximal fragment (four cortices).

Fig. 8.12 Combined fracture of the ulnar diaphysis (22-B1) and the distal radius (23-C2). Articular fracture of the distal radius reduced and fixed with provisional Kirschner wires after classical synthesis of the ulnar fracture. The stability is then secured by a small external fixator with pins introduced in the radius and the second metacarpal bone. (External fixation can be accomplished in this case by means of the tubular fixator and the special Schanz screws described in Chap. 5.)

Fig. 8.11

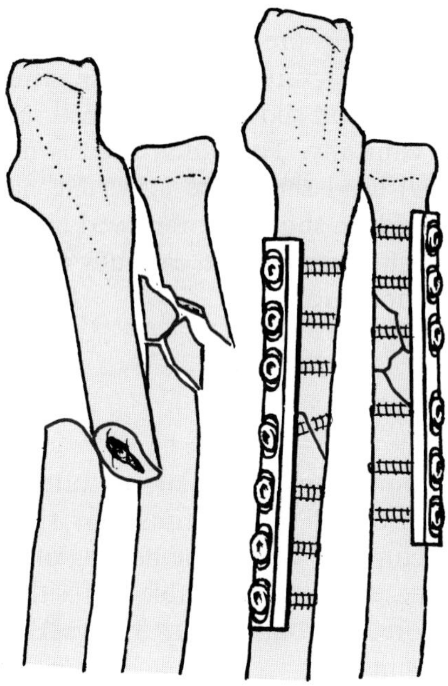

C 2

Fig. 8.12

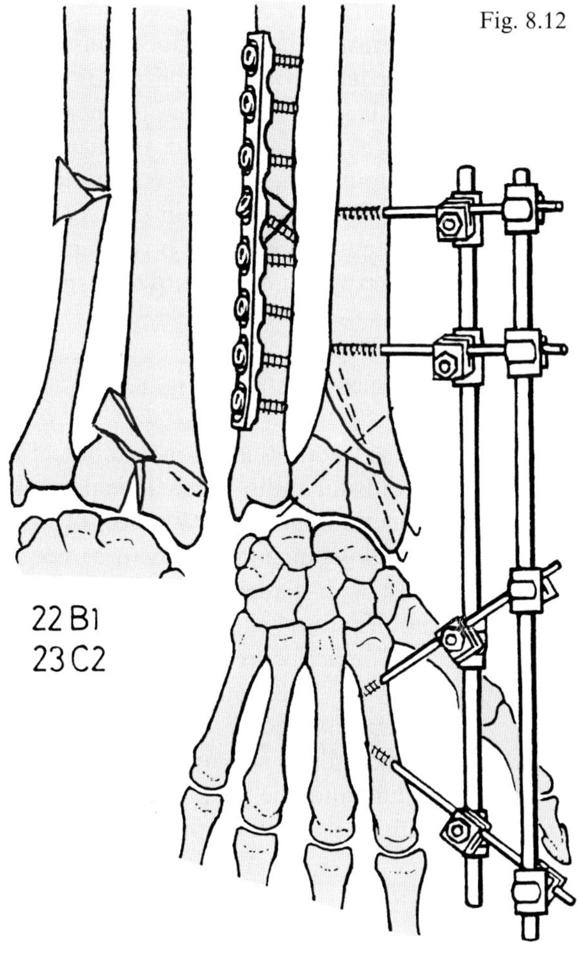

22 B1
23 C2

8.3.6 Fracture Dislocation of the Forearm Bones

All these fractures are indications for stable internal fixation. It has been shown that the functional result is better after immediate surgery.

8.3.6.1 Monteggia Fractures (Fig. 8.13b)

Anterior or lateral dislocations of the proximal radius are usually spontaneously reduced by reduction and stabilization of the ulna shaft fracture. Nevertheless, after reduction and fixation of the ulna, the position of the radial head should be examined radiologically, and the pronation and supination examined clinically. The radial head is usually stable in supination. If there is any doubt, the radial head should be inspected via a separate approach. Interposition or avulsions of the cartilage should be removed and the annular ligament sutured. The postoperative treatment should consist in carefully controlled physiotherapy out of a removable splint put on in supination.

8.3.6.2 Galeazzi Fractures (Fig. 8.13a)

These fractures are not rare but, if the dislocation is unspectacular, are often overlooked. The distal radio-ulnar articulation is mostly reduced spontaneously by the anatomical reduction and stable fixation of the radial fracture. However, the healing of the ruptured capsuloligamentous structures needs more time, and it is advisable to fix the elbow and wrist with a removable splint in a medium forearm rotation for 3–4 weeks. Full active mobilization begins after the removal of the splint.

The perfect reduction in the distal radio-ulnar joint should be radiologically examined after the stabilization of the radius. If a subluxation remains, the articulation should be approached through a dorsal incision which will allow a suture of the triangular fibrocartilage and/or of the ruptured dorsal capsule and ligaments. Transfixation of the radius and the ulna in medium rotation for a short period is recommended by some authors if such an open reduction and capsular suture has proved necessary.

Fig. 8.13 Fracture dislocations of the forearm bones.

a Galeazzi fracture (22-A2) reduced and fixed with a seven-hole 3.5-mm DCP and an interfragmentary lag screw.

b Monteggia fracture (22-A1): fixation of the transverse ulna fracture with an eight-hole 3.5-mm DCP and interfragmentary compression.

Fig. 8.13

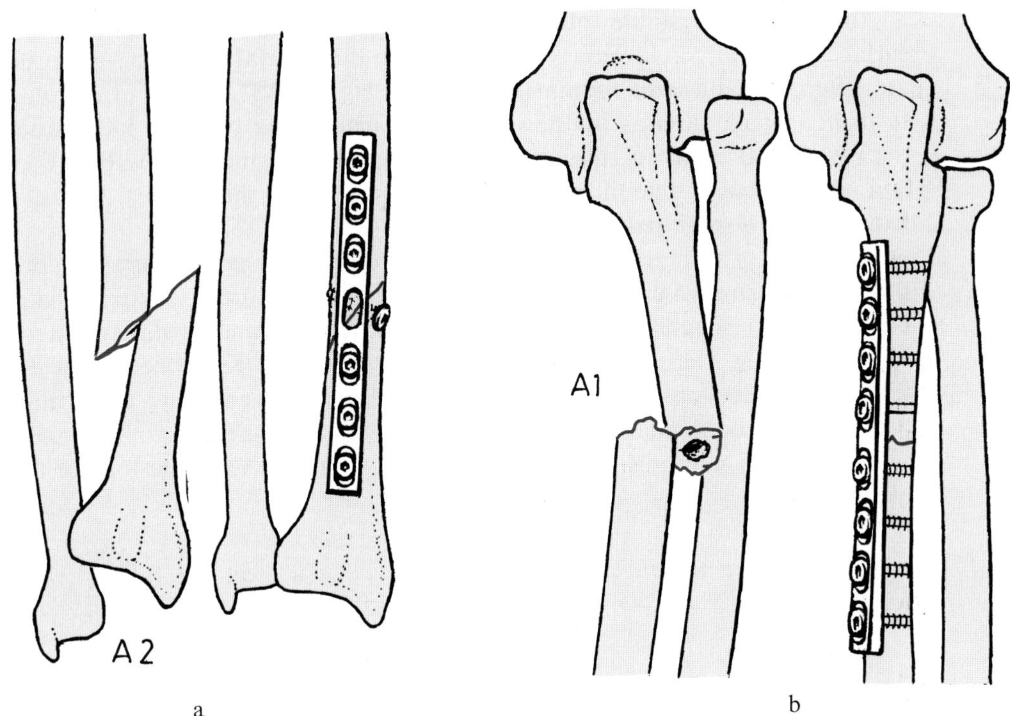

8.4 Distal Forearm

8.4.1 Fractures of the Distal Radius

Fresh extra-articular fractures (e.g. Colles fractures) very rarely require internal fixation. If reduction cannot be maintained, they are commonly fixed with percutaneous Kirschner wires (Fig. 8.14a). In cases of secondary displacement of extension-type fractures, internal fixation with a dorsally applied small T plate has proved successful (Fig. 8.16). Reduction is still possible many weeks after the accident.

Indications for stable internal fixation are frequent in fractures where the articular surface is partially involved (type B). Gaps in the sagittal plane (styloid process of radius) are often unstable and require fixation by lag screws. Special attention must be paid to osteoarticular lesions in the adjoining carpus. The classical indication for ORIF is the reversed Barton fracture with a small palmar fragment (type B3). Closed reduction and, in particular, retention are rarely possible. For these cases, we advocate internal fixation with a small palmar T plate (Fig. 8.15).

In complex fractures of type C, open reduction is mandatory if depressed areas in the articular surface cannot be reduced by traction (ligamentotaxis!). Plates should only be considered if screws can be anchored safely in intact distal fragments. When this is not possible, the reduction may be maintained by Kirschner wires and the defects filled with cancellous bone. The fixation is then achieved by an external fixator applied between the second metacarpal and the radial shaft (Fig. 8.12).

In all these fractures, attention should also be paid to the lesions of the distal radio-ulnar joint.

Fig. 8.14 Internal fixation of fractures of the distal radius with Kirschner wires and screws.

a Three Kirschner wires are necessary in the case of an intra-articular dorsal ulnar fragment.

b Screw fixation of a radial styloid fracture.

Fig. 8.15 Internal fixation of a type B volar fracture. Right angle or oblique T plate on the palmar side.

Fig. 8.16 Internal fixation of a dorsally angulated type A fracture with an oblique T plate applied to the dorsal radius. After preliminary reduction, the plate is temporarily attached to the proximal fragment with a screw in the proximal oval plate hole. Final reduction is carried out and the remaining plate screws are inserted.

Fig. 8.14

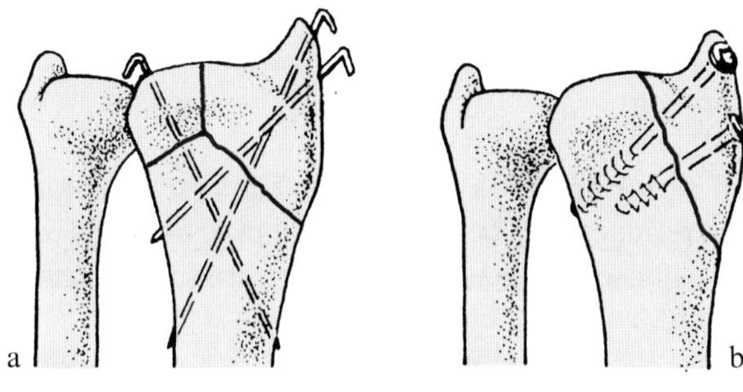

Fig. 8.15

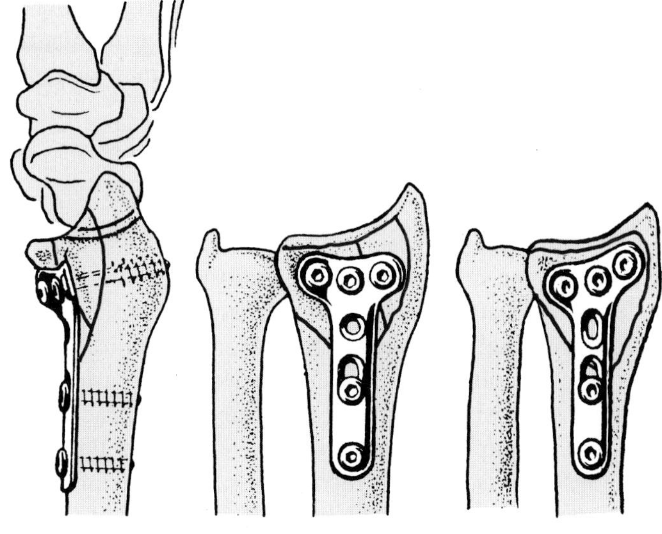

Fig. 8.16

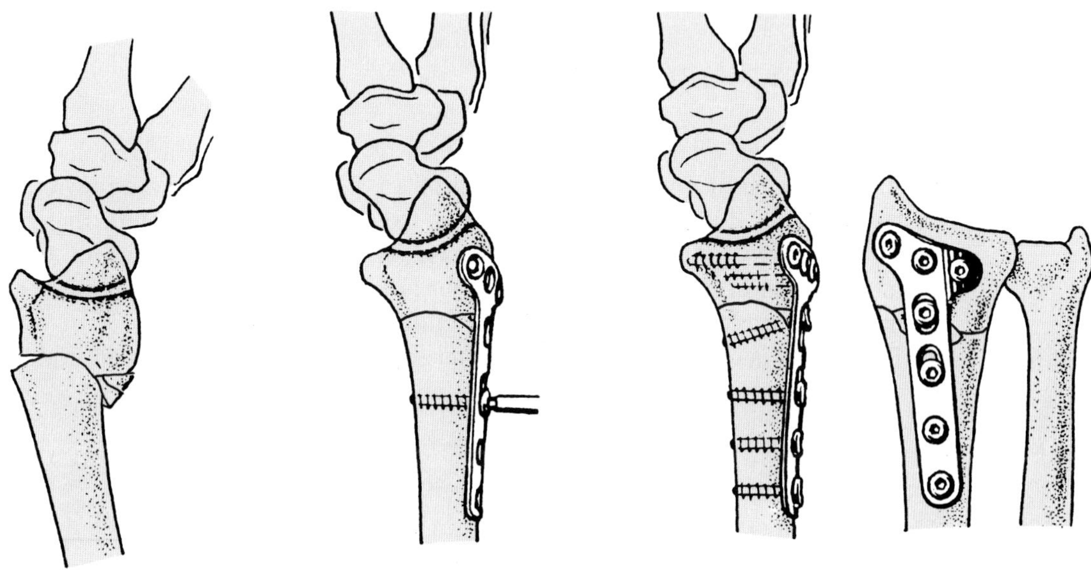

8.4.2 Approaches to the Distal Radius

8.4.2.1 Dorsal Approach

A Z-shaped skin incision is employed. The distal radius can be approached by dividing the extensor retinaculum between the compartment of extensor carpi radialis brevis and longus, and extensor pollicis longus. This broadly exposes the compartment of the extensores digitorum.

The access to the styloid process of the radius is more distal and radial between the tendons of extensor pollicis longus and the compartment of the extensores pollicis brevis and abductor pollicis longus.

In cases of complex fractures where palmar fragments have also to be reduced, one may select an incision of the first extensor compartment just palmar to abductor pollicis longus. This incision provides access to the palmar side of the radius for reduction by digital or instrumental pressure.

8.4.2.2 Volar Approach (Fig. 8.17)

A long angular incision begins proximally over the radius shaft and proceeds to the ulnar side of the distal crease of the wrist, then follows the longitudinal thenar crease near to the proximal transverse creases of the hand. We advocate a complete section of the flexor retinaculum on its ulnar border. Access to the radius is between the palmaris longus tendon and the median nerve. The nerve is retracted radially to protect the sensitive branch of the thenar together with the tendon of flexor carpi radialis and the radial artery. The fracture is exposed through a radial incision of pronator quadratus. Its fibers are raised from the surface of the bone. If reduction of the articular surface needs control by direct vision, the articulation can be opened by a transverse incision. The strong ligament should afterwards be resutured.

8.4.2.3 Implants

Dorsal or palmar internal fixation of the distal radius is best accomplished using the small right angled or oblique T plates (Figs. 8.15, 8.16). The plates are previously adapted to the anatomic situation and then loosely fixed to the bone through the oval hole by means of a screw. Then follows the precise reduction and placement of the plate and the introduction of the screws into the other holes. Defects and comminuted areas should be filled with autologous cancellous bone grafts.

The wound is closed by skin suture after introduction of deep suction drainage. Suturing of the palmar retinaculum or fascias is not recommended.

Fig. 8.17 Volar approaches to the distal radius.

a Long, slightly angled skin incision.

b Cross section at the level of the distal radius showing the approach to the radial attachment of the pronator quadratus muscle. The median nerve is retracted radially.

c The fracture and the pronator quadratus muscle are exposed. The muscle is incised at its radial attachment.

d Exposure of the fracture after partial detachment of the pronator quadratus muscle.

Fig. 8.17

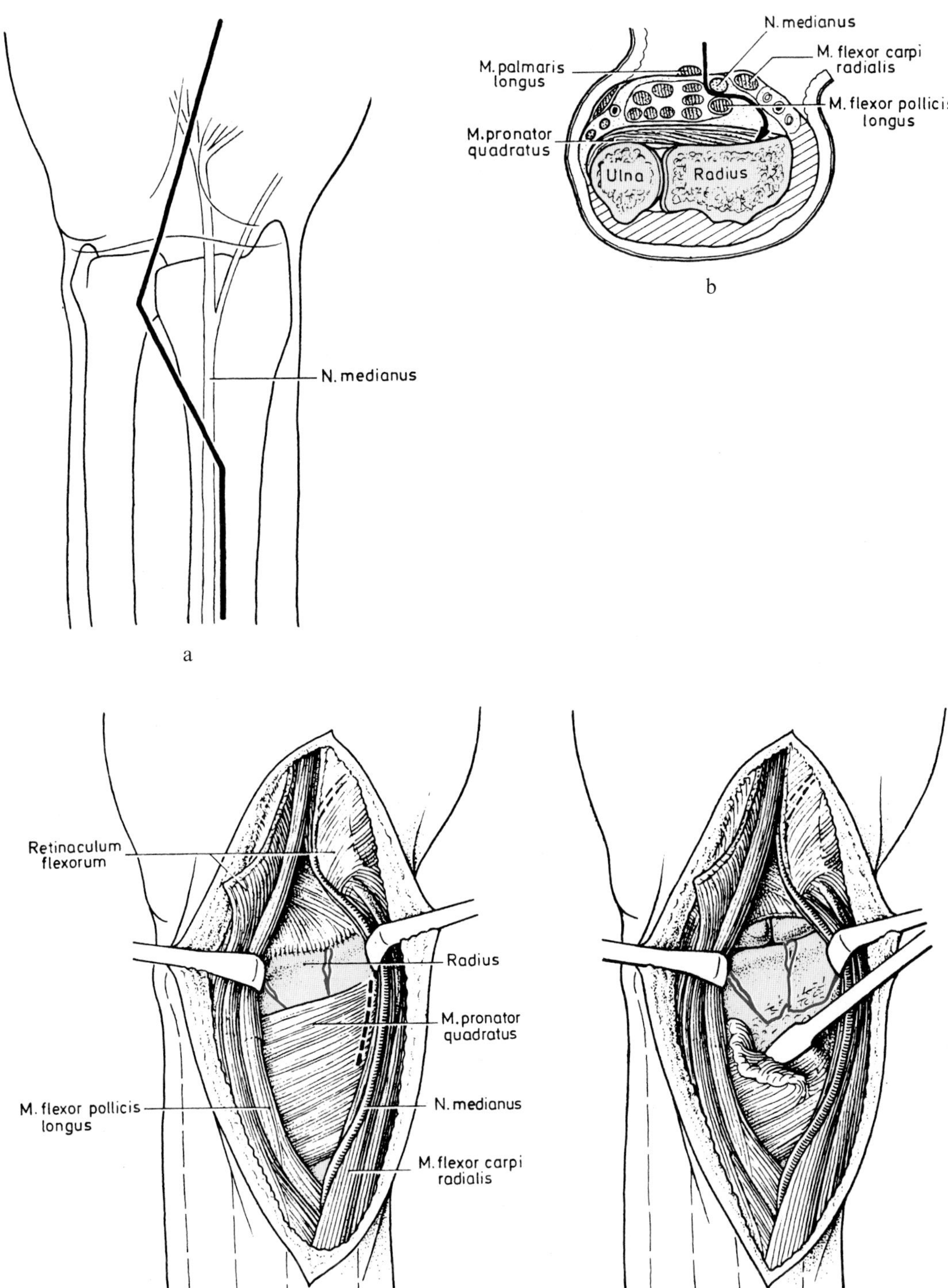
N. medianus
a
N. medianus
M. flexor carpi radialis
M. palmaris longus
M. flexor pollicis longus
M. pronator quadratus
Ulna
Radius
b
Retinaculum flexorum
Radius
M. pronator quadratus
M. flexor pollicis longus
N. medianus
M. flexor carpi radialis
c
d

8.4.2.4 Distal Ulna

The rotation of the radius also involves the distal ulna and therefore may jeopardize previously undislocated fractures of the ulna. Stable internal fixation is recommended. According to the type of fracture, application of a 3.5- or 2.7-mm DCP is indicated. The one-third tubular plate rarely provides adequate stability.

Attention has to be paid to the protection of the sensitive branch of the ulnar nerve which crosses to the dorsal side over the distal ulna.

8.5 Internal Fixation in the Hand Skeleton

8.5.1 Fractures of the Hand Skeleton

The majority of the fractures of the hand skeleton are treated conservatively. If maintenance of reduction is impossible, internal fixation is indicated. This applies particularly to multiple fractures. Stable internal fixation has proved superior when nerves and tendons are damaged. The postoperative treatment can then be conducted according to the requirements of the repaired soft tissues. Internal fixation is also often used to good advantage in microsurgery (e.g. replantations).

8.5.2 Approaches (Figs. 8.18, 8.19)

It is important for functional and aesthetic reasons to choose the correct type of skin incision. For the approach to metacarpal bones, we advocate longitudinal incisions between two bones. They may be enlarged (Y- or L-shaped). One incision can give access to two, exceptionally to three, metacarpals. If an articulation has to be opened, we prefer slightly curved dorsolateral incisions which can also be enlarged (Y-shaped). In phalanges we prefer the classical dorsolateral skin incision which allows access to the fracture and fully respects the extensor apparatus. Atraumatic surgery is crucial, particularly with regard to the delicate gliding layers, the veins and the nerves.

Fig. 8.18 Skin incisions over the hand skeleton.

a Dorsoradial approach to the thumb with extensions, avoiding the branches of the radial nerve.

b Angled incision for fractures of the scaphoid.

c Approaches to the metacarpus between the bones, with angled or Y-shaped extensions.

d Dorsoradial incision at the middle finger with a small angulation at the PIP joint.

Fig. 8.19 Approach to the base of the first phalanx and to the PIP joint.

a Longitudinal incision of the extensor apparatus and the articular capsule. Screw fixation of an oblique fracture.

b Approach to the palmar side of the PIP joint in flexion of the finger.

Fig. 8.18

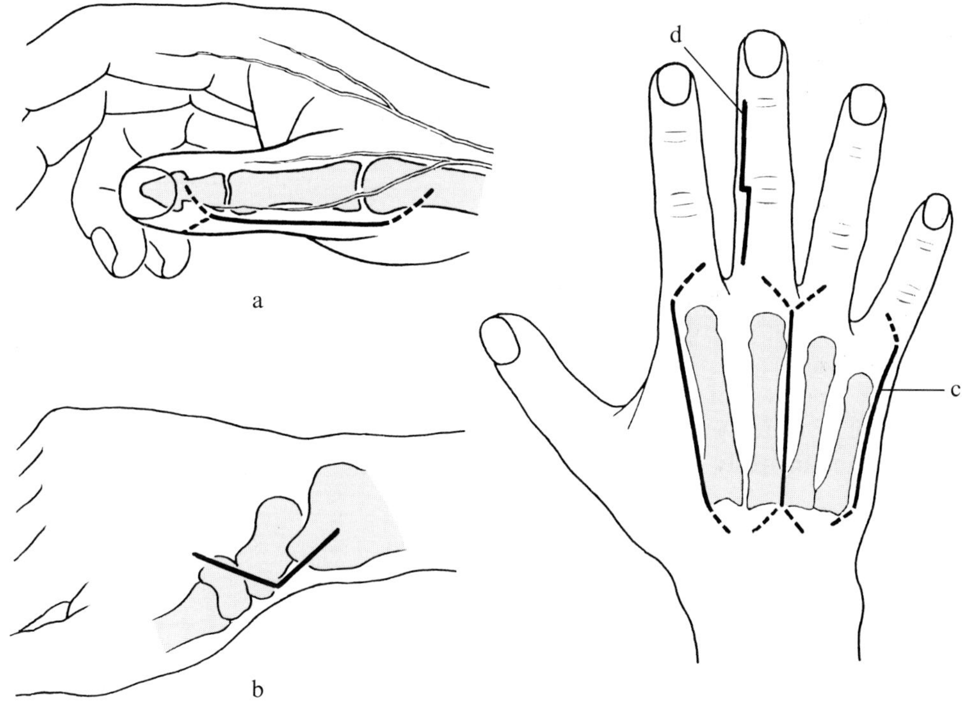

Fig. 8.19

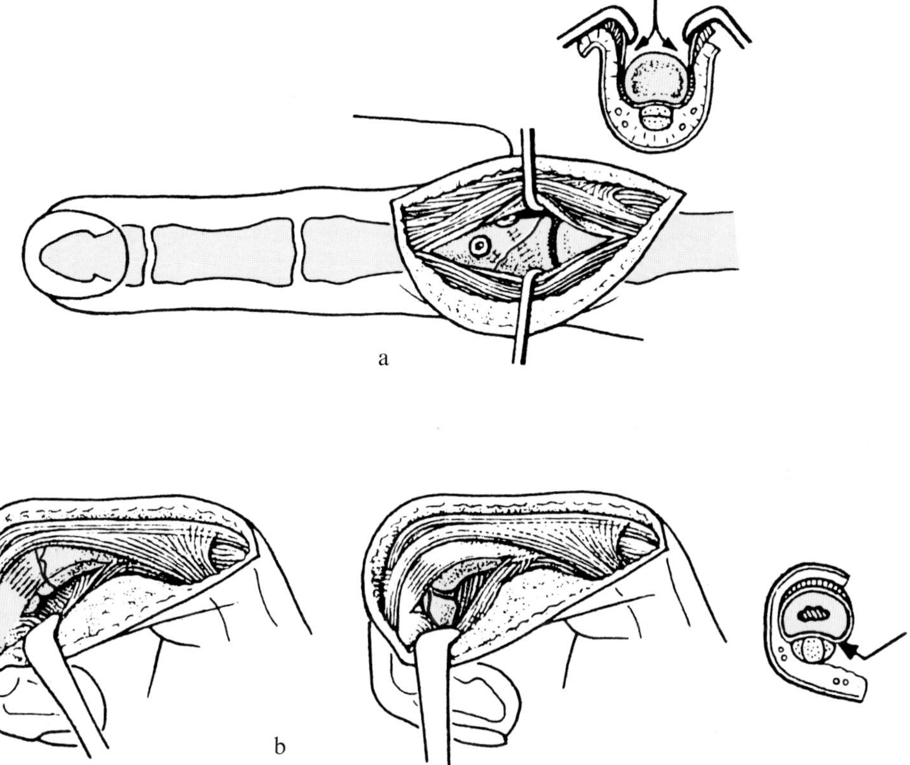

Fragments are often small and not easily accessible. Reduction and preliminary fixation can prove to be difficult. Bending and shearing forces will come to bear fully during functional postoperative treatment. For this reason, the choice of fine implants of adequate stability, applied if possible on the tension side, is very important.

8.5.3 Postoperative Treatment

Elevation of the injured limb and active mobilization are of utmost importance. In special situations and for noncompliant patients, removable splints may be necessary for some weeks.

Removal of the implants – if advisable at all – is performed after fracture healing, usually after 4 months. If there are adhesions at this time, tenolysis can be carried out simultaneously.

Fig. 8.20 Screw fixation of a scaphoid fracture using the dorsoradial approach.

a Combination of 2.7-mm lag screw and a Kirschner wire left in place for rotational stability.

b Fixation with two small lag screws (2.7 or 2.0 mm).

Fig. 8.21 Internal fixation of typical fractures of the base of the first metacarpal.

a Extra-articular fracture with palmar angulation.

b Bennett fracture: shortening and adduction of the distal fragment by traction of the abductor pollicis longus muscle.

c Internal fixation of a Bennett fracture with a dorsally introduced lag screw and a Kirschner wire (for rotational stability).

d Rolando fractures stabilized with a simple T plate or a combination of plate and lag screw.

Fig. 8.22 Typical internal fixation of fractures of the hand skeleton.

Shaft fractures of the first and second metacarpals are fixed with 2.7-mm plates. The metaphyseal fracture of the fifth metacarpal is stabilized by an L plate. Fractures of the first phalanx of the thumb and of the middle finger are fixed with mini-plates in lateral position. A subcapital phalangeal fracture is fixed with a shortened mini-condylar plate. Torque fractures of the central metacarpals and the phalanges and articular fractures are fixed with 2.7-mm or mini lag screws.

Fig. 8.20

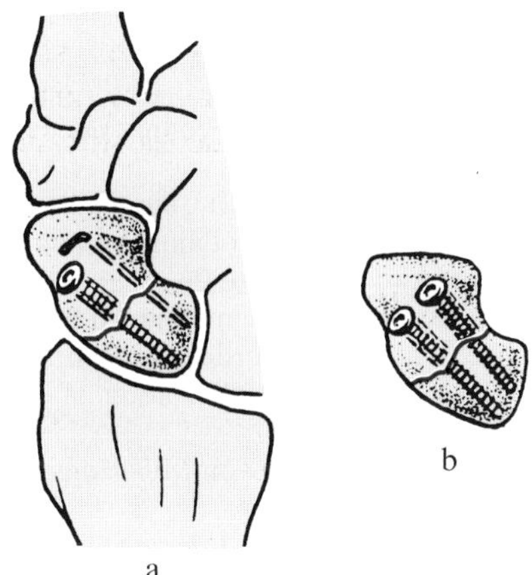

Fig. 8.21

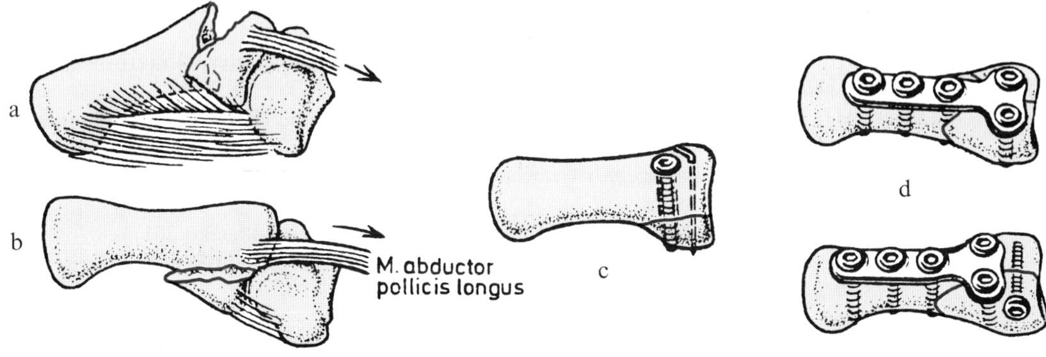

Fig. 8.22

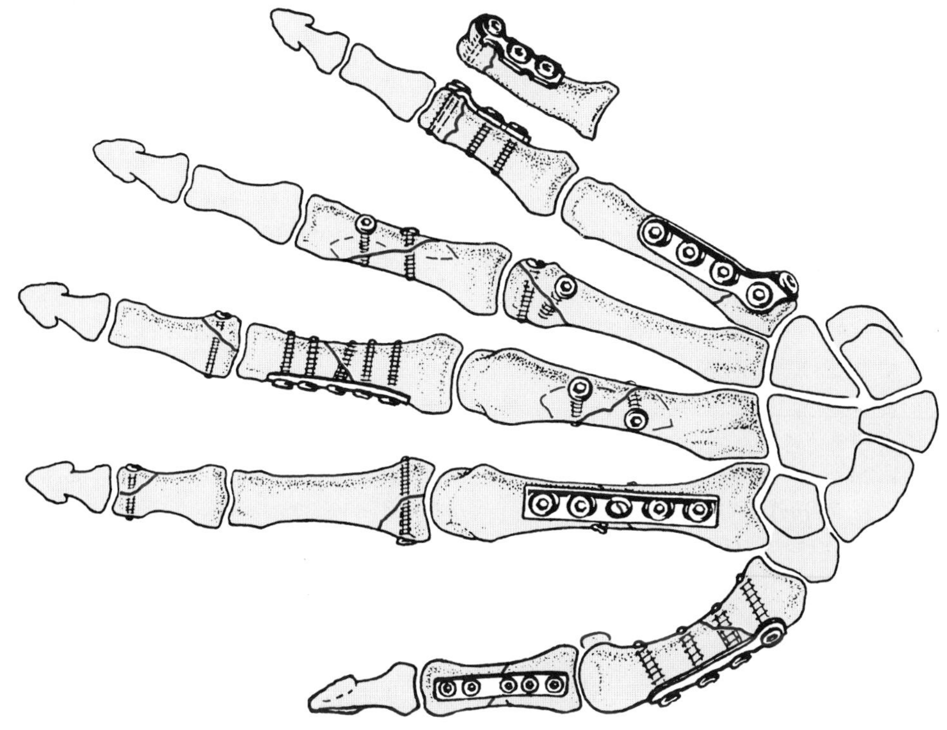

References

Beaufils P et al. (1983) Traumatismes complexes de l'extrémité supérieure des deux os de l'avant-bras. Rev Chir Orthop 69:303–316

Boyd HB (1963) see Crenshaw AH (ed) Campbell's orthopaedics. Mosby, St Louis

Deluca PA et al. (1988) Refracture of bones of the forearm after the removal of compression plates. J Bone Joint Surg [Am] 70:1372–1376

Eitel F (1983) Olekranonfrakturen. Unfallheilkd 86:143–151

Gross E (1979) Osteosynthese bei Vorderarmschaftfrakturen. AO Bulletin

Heim U, Pfeiffer KM (1987) Internal fixation of small fractures, 3rd edn. Springer, Berlin Heidelberg New York

Heim U, Zehnder R (1989) Analyse von Mißerfolgen nach Osteosynthesen von Unterarmschaftfrakturen. Hefte Unfallheilkd 201:243–258

Henry AK (1966) Extensile exposure. Livingstone, Edinburgh

Josten C et al. (1989) Verfahrenswechsel bei offener distaler Unterarmfraktur. Hefte Unfallheilkd 201:116–119

Moed BR et al. (1986) Immediate internal fixation of open fractures of the diaphysis of the forearm. J Bone Joint Surg [Am] 68:1008–1017

Müller ME, Allgöwer M, Willenegger H (1963) Technik der operativen Frakturbehandlung. Springer, Berlin Heidelberg New York

Oestern HJ, Tscherne H (1983) Ergebnisse der AO-Sammelstudie über Unterarmschaftfrakturen. Unfallheilkunde 86:136–142

Szyszkowitz R (1978) Spätergebnisse nach Plattenosteosynthese am Unterarmschaft. Hefte Unfallheilkd 132:415–418

Tscherne H (1989) Chirurgische Zugänge am Unterarm. Hefte Unfallheilkd 201:1–8

Vince KG, Miller JE (1987) Cross union complicating fracture of the forearm. J Bone Joint Surg [Am] 69:640–653

9 PELVIS

9.1 Introduction

Since the second edition of this book was published a decade ago, traumatic disruption of the pelvic ring has become a major focus of interest. Previously, conventional orthopedic wisdom held that surviving patients with disruption of the pelvic ring had few long-term problems following a musculoskeletal injury. However, more recent evidence indicates that patients with an unstable pelvic ring disruption may benefit from operative fixation. Stabilization may also be important for the survival of the patient, as has been proven for fractures of the femur, and it can also improve the long-term functional results of these pelvic injuries. These are serious injuries with an associated mortality rate of more than 10%, with 4% of this total due to pelvic hemorrhage. Retroperitoneal hemorrhage associated with pelvic trauma remains a difficult management problem. Hence the inclusion in this third edition of a chapter on fractures of the pelvis.

Vertically stable injuries to the bony pelvis, approximately 65% of the total, do not usually require stabilization; with some exceptions the unstable pelvic injury is, however, best treated by some form of stabilization, which can be internal or external.

9.2 Pelvic Stability (Fig. 9.1)

The stability of the pelvic ring depends upon the integrity of the posterior weight-bearing sacroiliac complex, which includes the sacroiliac joint and the major sacroiliac, sacrotuberous and sacrospinous ligaments as well as the muscles and fascia of the pelvic floor. The extremely strong posterior sacroiliac ligaments maintain the normal position of the sacrum in the pelvic ring. The sacrospinous ligaments resist external rotation of the hemipelvis, whereas the sacrotuberous ligaments resist rotational forces in the sagittal plane.

The major forces acting upon the pelvis are external rotation, internal rotation and vertical shear, each producing a different type of pelvic fracture (Fig. 9.2).

Fig. 9.1

a, b Osseo-ligamentous structures essential for pelvic stability. (From Tile 1984.)

c Analogy of a suspension bridge.

Fig. 9.2 Forces acting on the pelvic floor, particularly on the ligamenta sacrospinosa and sacrotuberosa.

Fig. 9.1

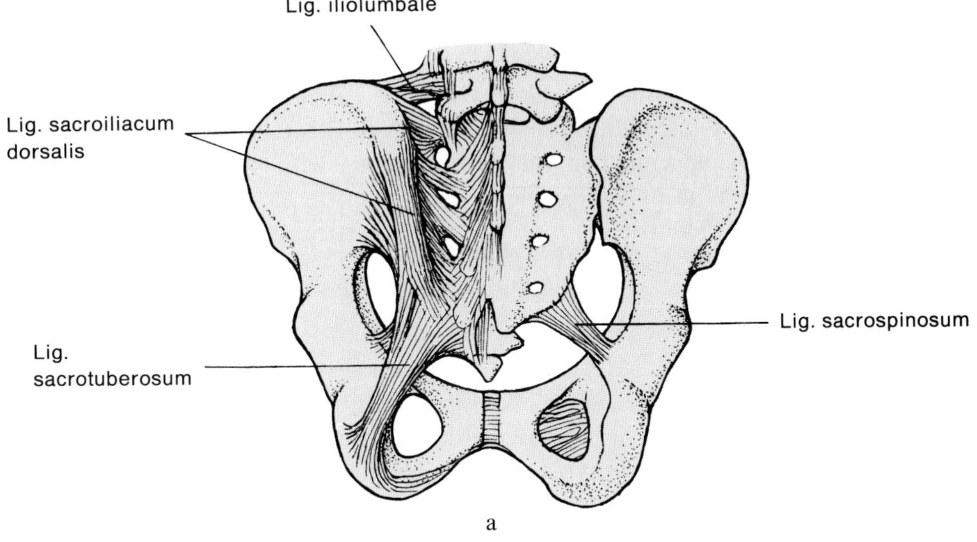
Lig. iliolumbale
Lig. sacroiliacum dorsalis
Lig. sacrospinosum
Lig. sacrotuberosum

a

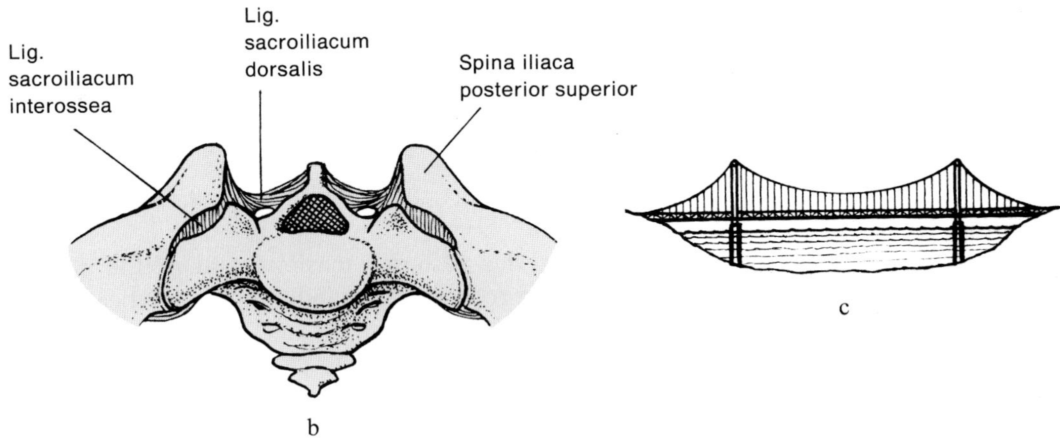
Lig. sacroiliacum interossea
Lig. sacroiliacum dorsalis
Spina iliaca posterior superior

b

c

Fig. 9.2

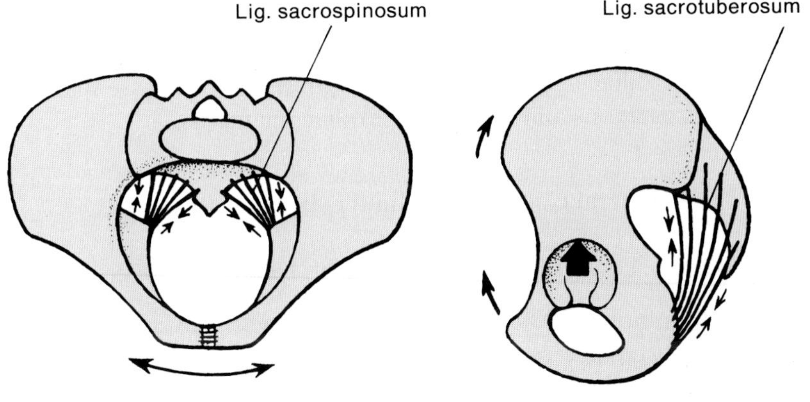
Lig. sacrospinosum
Lig. sacrotuberosum

9.3 Classification (According to Tile 1988)

Fractures of the pelvis are divided into three types. The type A fracture is stable, minimally displaced and does not usually involve the pelvic ring. The clinically relevant disruptions show rotatory instability, either alone (type B) or in association with vertical instability (type C). Displacement in the vertical plane with posterior and cephalad migration of the hemipelvis is only possible if the posterior sacroiliac complex and the pelvic floor is disrupted; therefore, an injury which is vertically stable (type A or B) cannot by definition be vertically displaced.

9.3.1 Type A – Stable, Minimally Displaced (Fig. 9.3)

In this type, the pelvic ring is stable and the displacement is insignificant. In type A1, the pelvic ring is not involved. This includes avulsions of the anterior superior spine, anterior inferior spine and/or ischial tuberosities. In type A2, the pelvic wing may be fractured without involvement of the pelvic ring or the pelvic ring may be fractured without displacement. The rami may be fractured unilaterally or bilaterally (straddle fracture). An associated posterior lesion may be identified, often only on scanning techniques, but no displacement is present and the pelvic ring is stable.

The type A3 fractures are transverse fractures of the sacrum and coccyx not involving the pelvic ring. There may be an undisplaced transverse fracture through the sacrum; displaced transverse fracture through the sacrum; or a coccygeal fracture.

9.3.2 Type B – Rotationally Unstable, Vertically Stable (Figs. 9.3, 9.5)

In this particular type of injury, the posterior tension band of the pelvis and of the pelvic floor remains intact, allowing rotational instability but no vertical instability.

9.3.2.1 Type B1 – Open Book Injury, External Rotation

This injury is caused by an external rotatory force which disrupts the symphysis pubis and causes the pelvis to open like a book. The hemipelvis is unstable in external rotation; the end point is reached when the posterior superior iliac spine abuts against the sacrum. In this particular injury, the posterior ligamentous structures remain intact so no vertical instability is possible. The lesion may be unilateral or bilateral. If the symphysis pubis is open less than 2.5 cm, only the symphysis is disrupted but not the sacrospinous or anterior sacroiliac ligaments. If the symphysis is open more than 2.5 cm there is disruption of the sacrospinous and anterior sacroiliac ligaments.

9.3.2.2 Type B2 – Lateral Compression Injury, Internal Rotation

Type B2.1 – Lateral Compression Injury, Ipsilateral Type

A lateral compressive force applied to the hemipelvis, usually through the greater trochanter, crushes the sacroiliac complex and causes an anterior injury on the same side. The anterior injury may be a fracture of both the superior and inferior pubic rami,

---

Fig. 9.3 Classification of pelvic fractures (overview).

Fig. 9.3

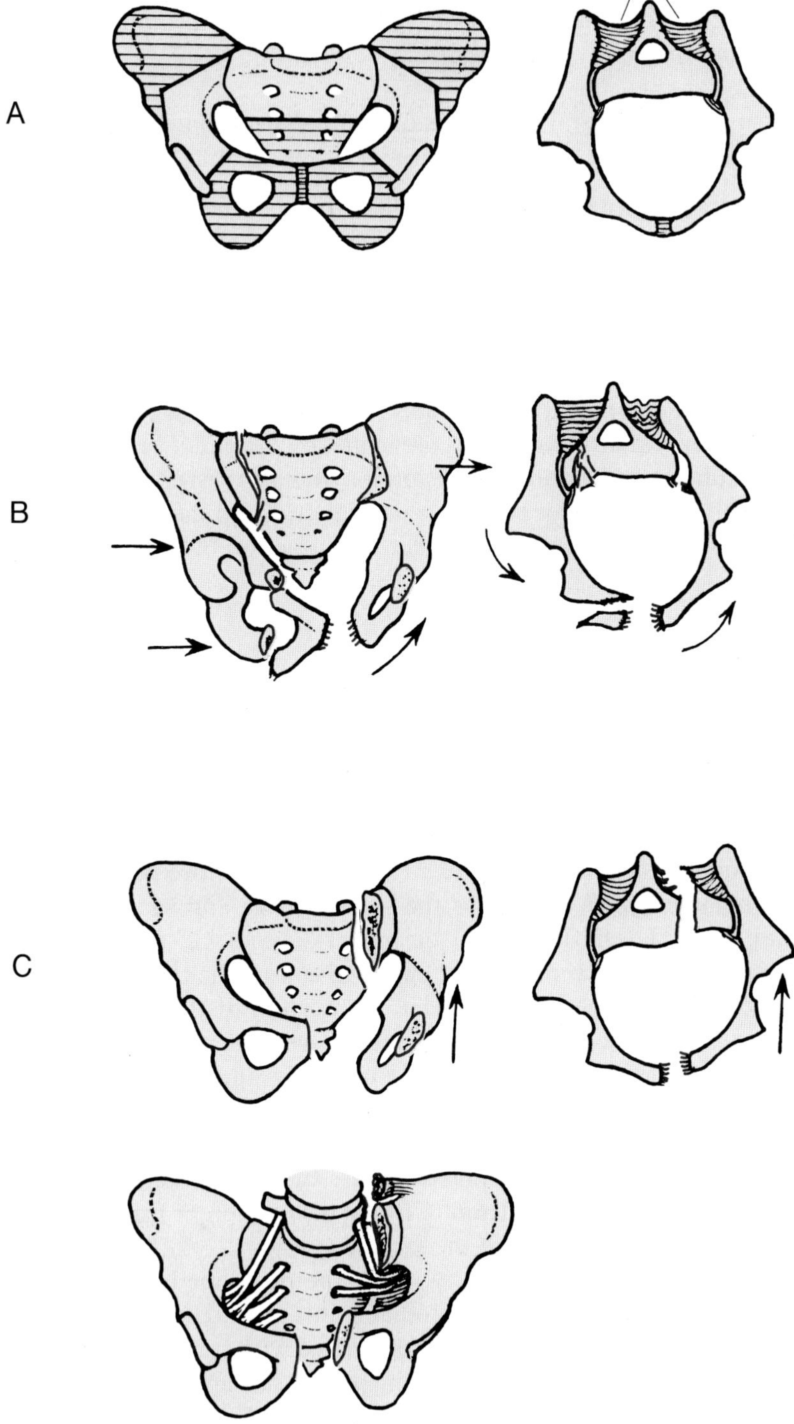

an overriding, locked symphysis or a superior ramus fracture tilted through a symphyseal disruption (tilt fracture). The posterior injury is a compression fracture of the anterior aspect of the sacrum. Again, the intact tension band of the pelvis as well as an intact pelvic floor do not allow vertical displacement in this injury type: therefore it has internal rotatory instability but is vertically stable.

Type B2.2 – Lateral Compression Injury, Contralateral Type (Bucket Handle)

A lateral compressive force applied to the ilium may result in a crush injury to the sacroiliac complex on one side and displacement of the anterior hemipelvis on the opposite side. The affected hemipelvis rotates internally by as much as 40°, and also anteriorly like the handle of a bucket. This particular type may cause a rotatory deformity of the hemipelvis as well as a leg length discrepancy. The posterior lesion is usually a sacral crush injury which may be associated with the anterior aspect of the sacroiliac joint akin to the compression type fracture of the vertebrae. The hemipelvis is displaced internally, but vertical displacement is prevented by the intact pelvic floor ligaments (sacrospinous, sacrotuberous). The anterior lesion may involve disruption of only one contralateral pubic ramus, all four rami or two contralateral rami and the symphysis pubis. Reduction requires derotation of the hemipelvis rather than traction in the vertical plane.

9.3.2.3 Type B3 – Bilateral B-Type Injury

9.3.3 Type C – Rotationally and Vertically Unstable (Vertical Shear) (Figs. 9.3, 9.6)

This injury is characterized by a rupture of the entire pelvic floor, including the posterior sacroiliac complex as well as the sacrospinous and sacrotuberous ligaments. The injury may be unilateral (type C1) or bilateral types C2 and C3. Posterior displacement of the hemipelvis by more than 1 cm, avulsion of the transverse process of the fifth lumbar vertebra, or detachment of the bony insertion of the sacrospinous ligaments from either the sacrum or ischial spine are presumptive evidence of vertical instability. The diagnosis of vertical instability is best made clinically and by computer tomography (CT). In all type C-injuries, the anterior lesion may be a disruption of the symphysis, a disruption of the inferior and superior pubic rami, a disruption of all four rami, or a disruption of two rami plus the symphysis pubis. In the unilateral type (C1), the posterior lesion may be a fracture of the ileum (C1.1), a dislocation or fracture-dislocation of the sacroiliac joint (C1.2) or a fracture of the sacrum (C1.3).

In the complete bilateral type C3, the posterior lesions may also be sacral fractures, fracture-dislocations of the sacroiliac joint, or fractures of the ilium.

Disruptions of the pelvic ring associated with fractures of the acetabulum are arbitrarily also called type C3 injuries, since the prognosis depends more upon the acetabular fracture than the pelvic ring disruption.

Figs. 9.4–9.6 Classification of pelvic fractures. For A subgroups, see text (Sect. 9.3.1).

Fig. 9.5 B1 open book injury. B2.1 and B2.2 lateral compression.

Fig. 9.6 C1.1 iliac fracture. C.1.2 sacroiliac dislocation. C1.3 sacral fracture.

Fig. 9.4

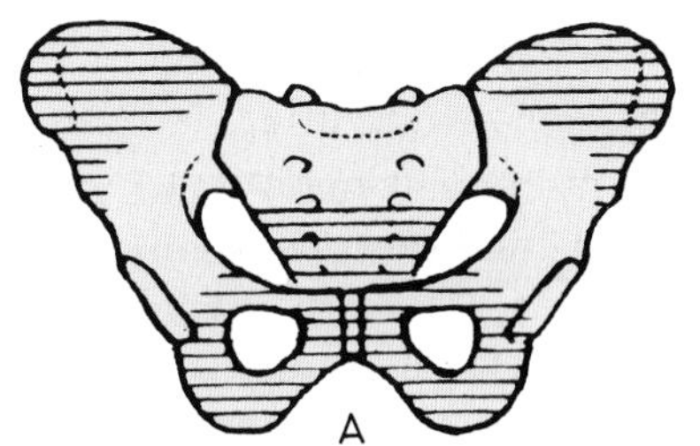

Fig. 9.5

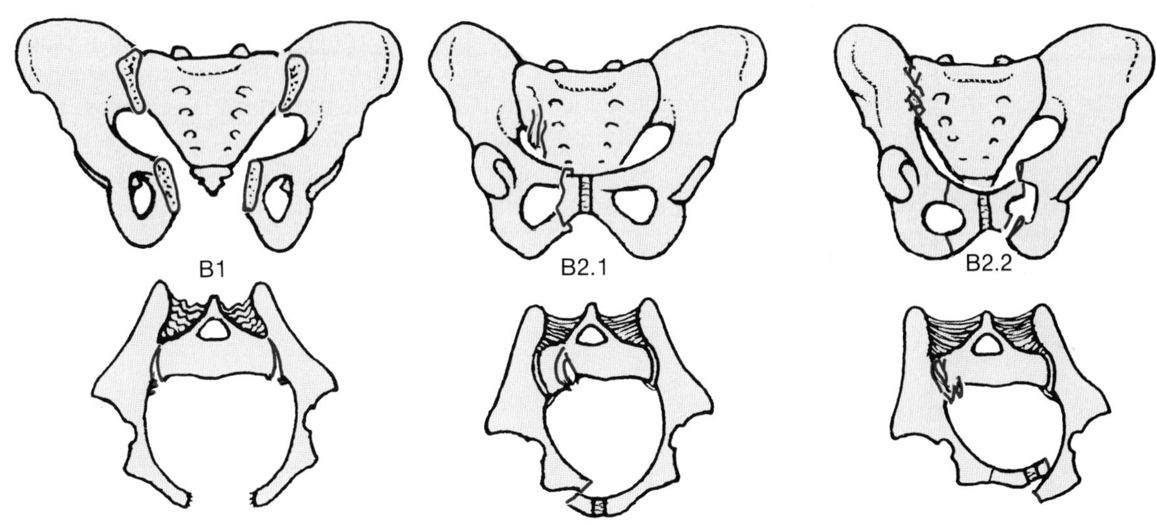

Fig. 9.6

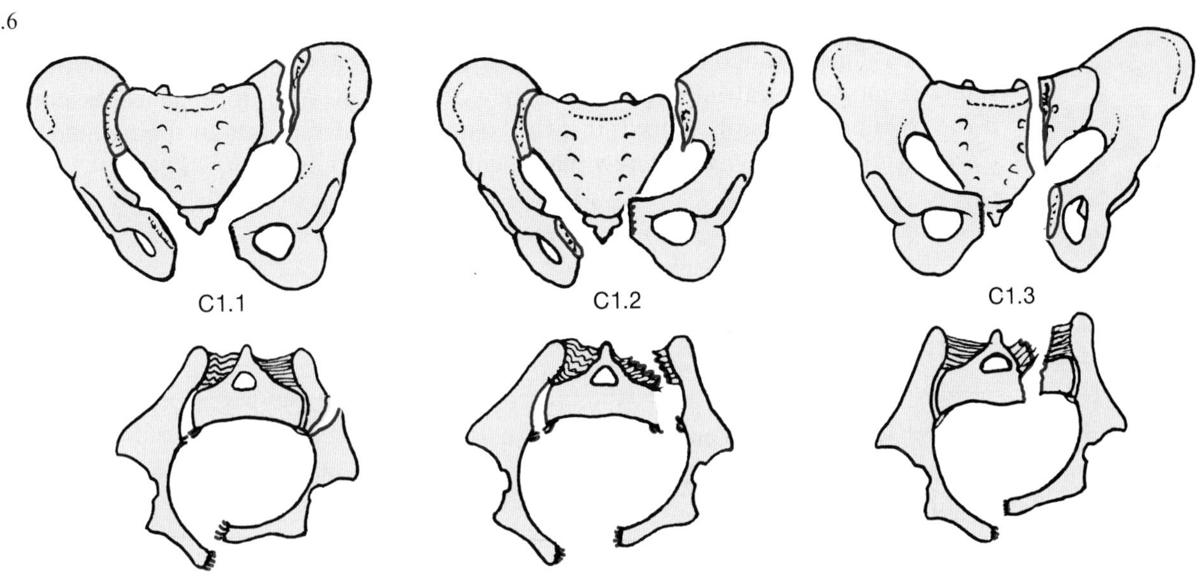

9.4 Decision-Making and Indications for Surgery

The vertically stable fractures types A and B rarely require either internal or external fixation. Indeed, type A fractures are usually managed nonoperatively.

Type B fractures are rotationally unstable but vertically stable. In the type B1 open book fracture, if the symphysis pubis is open more than 2.5 cm, stabilization may be achieved by either a simple external skeletal frame or a two-hole plate on the superior surface of the symphysis pubis.

The lateral compression type B2.1 injury is usually managed with bed rest alone and requires no external or internal fixation except in a polytraumatized patient, where external fixation offers many advantages. Type B3 injury is also vertically stable but may result in a leg length discrepancy. If this deformity is unacceptable to the patient, the pins of an external skeletal fixator may be used to help the surgeon externally rotate the hemipelvis and restore the leg length. If acceptable reduction is achieved, the external frame is completed. Internal fixation is rarely indicated.

Stabilization techniques are most useful in the vertically unstable types C1 and C2 injuries. These techniques may include external fixation, internal fixation anteriorly and/or posteriorly or a combination of both. Stabilization of the type C3 injury will depend on the configuration of the acetabular fracture and the pelvic ring disruption.

9.5 Approaches

9.5.1 Anterior Pelvis (Fig. 9.7)

The symphysis pubis is usually approached through a transverse Pfannenstiel incision. Occasionally, if the symphyseal stabilization is performed at the same time as laparotomy, it may be done through a paramedian or a midline abdominal incision. The pubic rami rarely require surgical intervention. If they do, they may be approached as above, but if the fracture is laterally placed, it must be approached through an ilioinguinal incision. Care must be taken to avoid screw placement in the hip joint (Fig. 9.7e).

Fig. 9.7 Approach to and fixation of anterior pelvis.

a Transverse suprapubic approach.

b Reduction of open book injury.

c Semi-tubular two-hole plate or a DCP fixed to both pubic rami by fully threaded large cancellous bone screws. This fixation is adequate for open book injuries without posterior instability, and immediate mobilization is possible.

d Double plating in cases where posterior stabilization in type C fractures cannot be carried out immediately. The anterior plate is a reconstruction plate.

e Reconstruction plate to stabilize a pubic ramus fracture.

Fig. 9.7

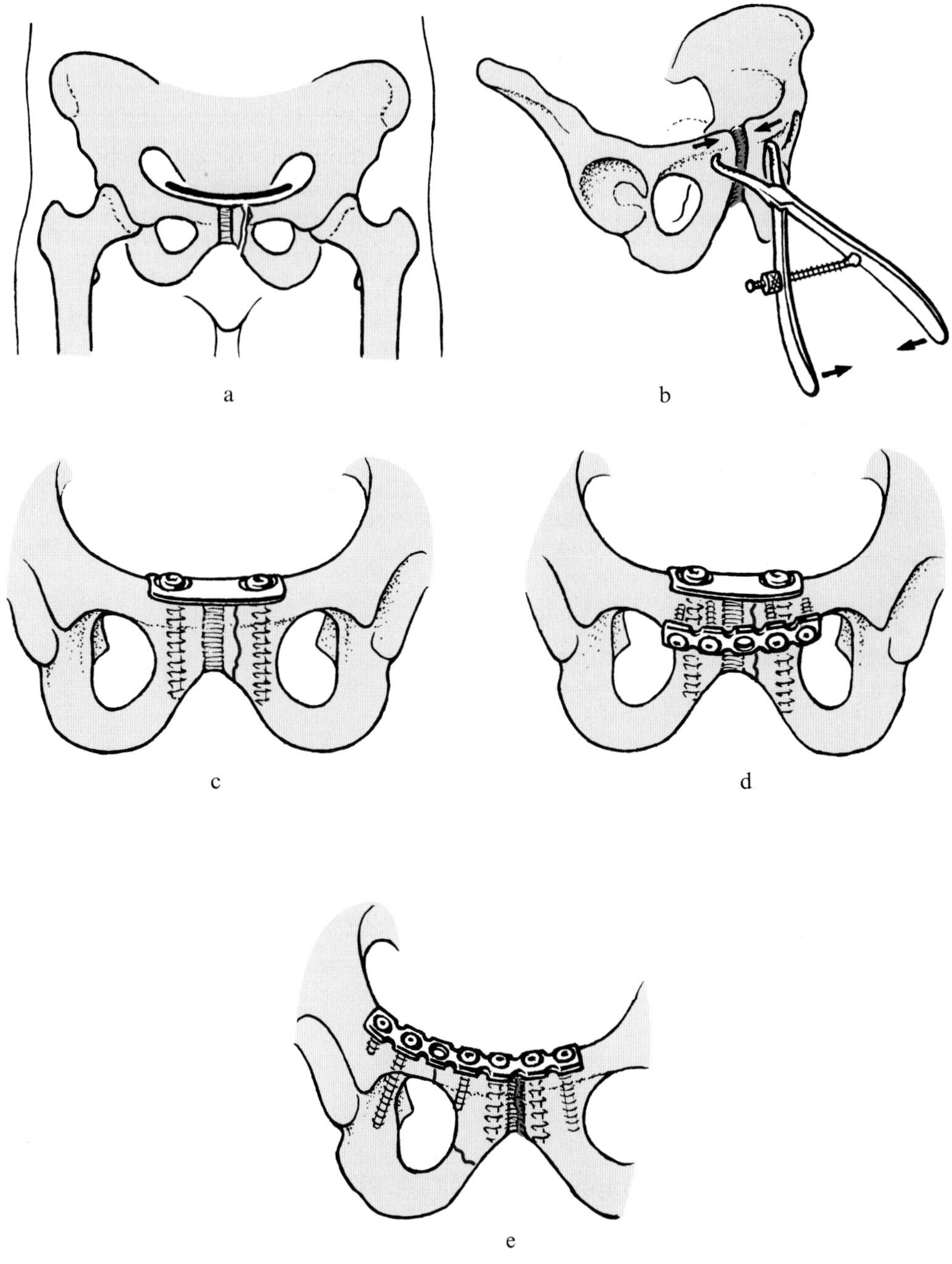

9.5.2 Posterior Pelvis

The sacroiliac complex may be approached anteriorly or posteriorly.

9.5.2.1 Anterior Approach

The anterior aspect of the sacroiliac joint or ilium may be approached through the posterior half of an ilioinguinal incision. The sacroiliac joint may be easily identified by stripping the iliac muscle from the inner wall of the ilium.

9.5.2.2 Posterior Approach

Fractures of the sacrum, fracture-dislocations of the sacroiliac joint and fractures of the ilium may also be approached posteriorly. Caution is advised in patients with crush injuries to the pelvis, as these posterior wounds have a tendency to necrose. For iliac fractures, the incision should be made in a vertical direction 1 cm lateral to the posterior superior iliac spine, avoiding the subcutaneous border of the bone.

9.6 Reduction

Even with a good surgical exposure, reduction of pelvic fractures may be difficult. Special equipment is desirable and should include pelvic reduction clamps, pointed fracture reduction clamps and special acetabular clamps (Fig. 9.11). Symphysis pubis disruptions may be reduced and held with either the pointed fracture reduction clamps or the pelvic reduction clamps. The pelvic reduction clamp is also useful in anterior approaches to the sacroiliac joint. The greater sciatic notch must be identified in all posterior approaches to check the adequacy of the reduction.

9.7 Methods of Internal Fixation

9.7.1 Anterior Pelvis: Symphysis Pubis (Fig. 9.7)

If the symphysis pubis disruption is part of a stable open book (B1) pattern, a two- or three-hole 4.5- or 3.5-mm dynamic compression plate (DCP) or a reconstruction plate placed along the superior aspect of the symphysis and fixed with fully threaded cancellous bone screws will suffice. If the symphysis disruption is part of a vertically unstable type C injury, and the posterior lesion cannot be stabilized, then the recommendation is to

---

Fig. 9.8 Safest method of stabilizing a sacral fracture by means of sacral bars, two bars going from one posterior iliac crest to the other to prevent rotation.

Fig. 9.8

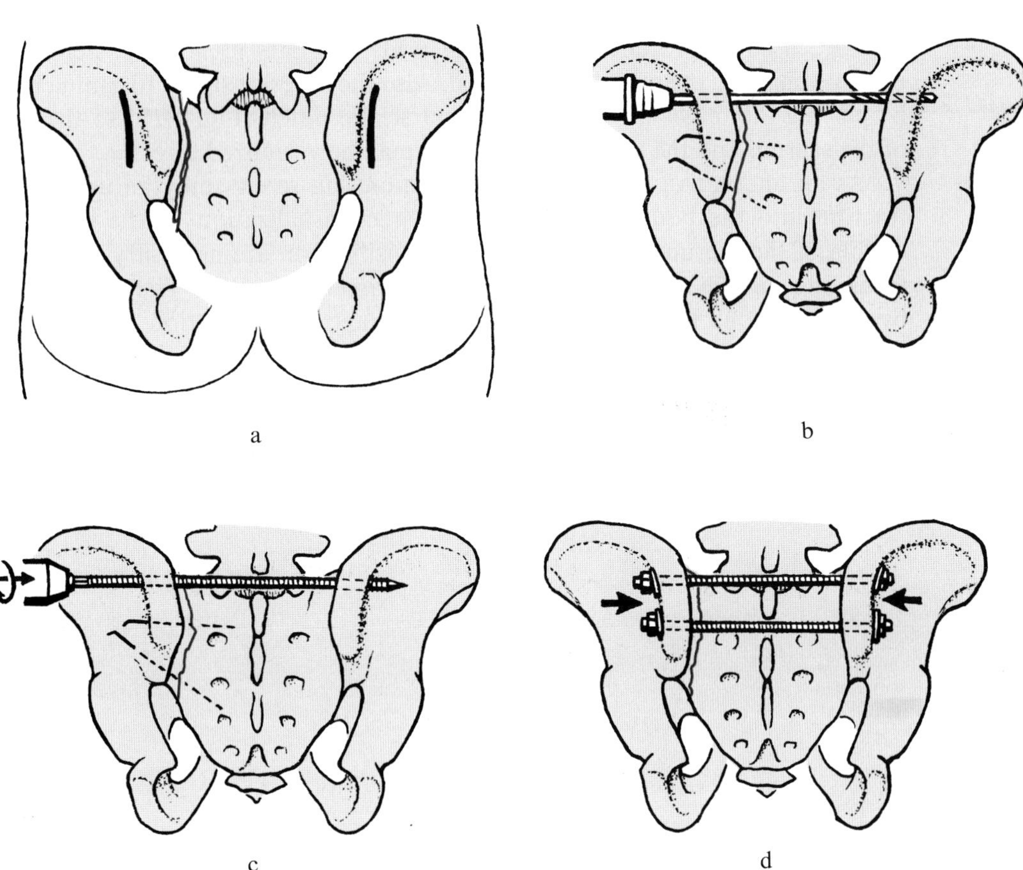

double plate the symphysis superiorly and anteriorly. The anterior plate is a 3.5- or 4.5-mm pelvic reconstruction plate contoured and fixed with the appropriate fully threaded cancellous screws.

9.7.2 Posterior Pelvis: Sacral Fracture

In vertically unstable (type C) injuries, the safest method of stabilizing a sacral fracture is to use sacral bars. These bars pass from one posterior superior spine to the other, thereby making direct fixation of the fracture with lag screws unnecessary. Two sacral bars are used to prevent rotation (Fig. 9.8). The bars must be posterior to the sacrum to avoid entering the sacral spinal canal. Also the anterior sacral foramina may be palpated by placing the finger through the greater sciatic notch (Fig. 9.9b) to the anterior surface of the sacrum and the posterior foramina may be visualized directly.

As an alternative, especially in non-union, lag screws may be used across the sacral fracture into the body of the sacrum. Direct visualization of the sacral foramina and the ala of the sacrum as well as image intensification are necessary to prevent the screws from entering the spinal canal or the S1 foramen (Fig. 9.9). The screws may be inserted by percutaneous techniques usually with image intensification. The use of cannulated cancellous bone screws greatly simplifies the technique.

Fig. 9.9 Fixation of sacroiliac dislocation by 6.5-mm cancellous bone screws. (According to Matta)

a Entry points of cancellous bone screws.

b Insertion of the index finger through the incisura ischiatica helps in aiming the drill.

c X-ray controls of screw position.

d, e Correct position of cancellous bone screws.

f Drilling directions to be avoided (sacral foramina, spinal canal, great vessels).

Fig. 9.9

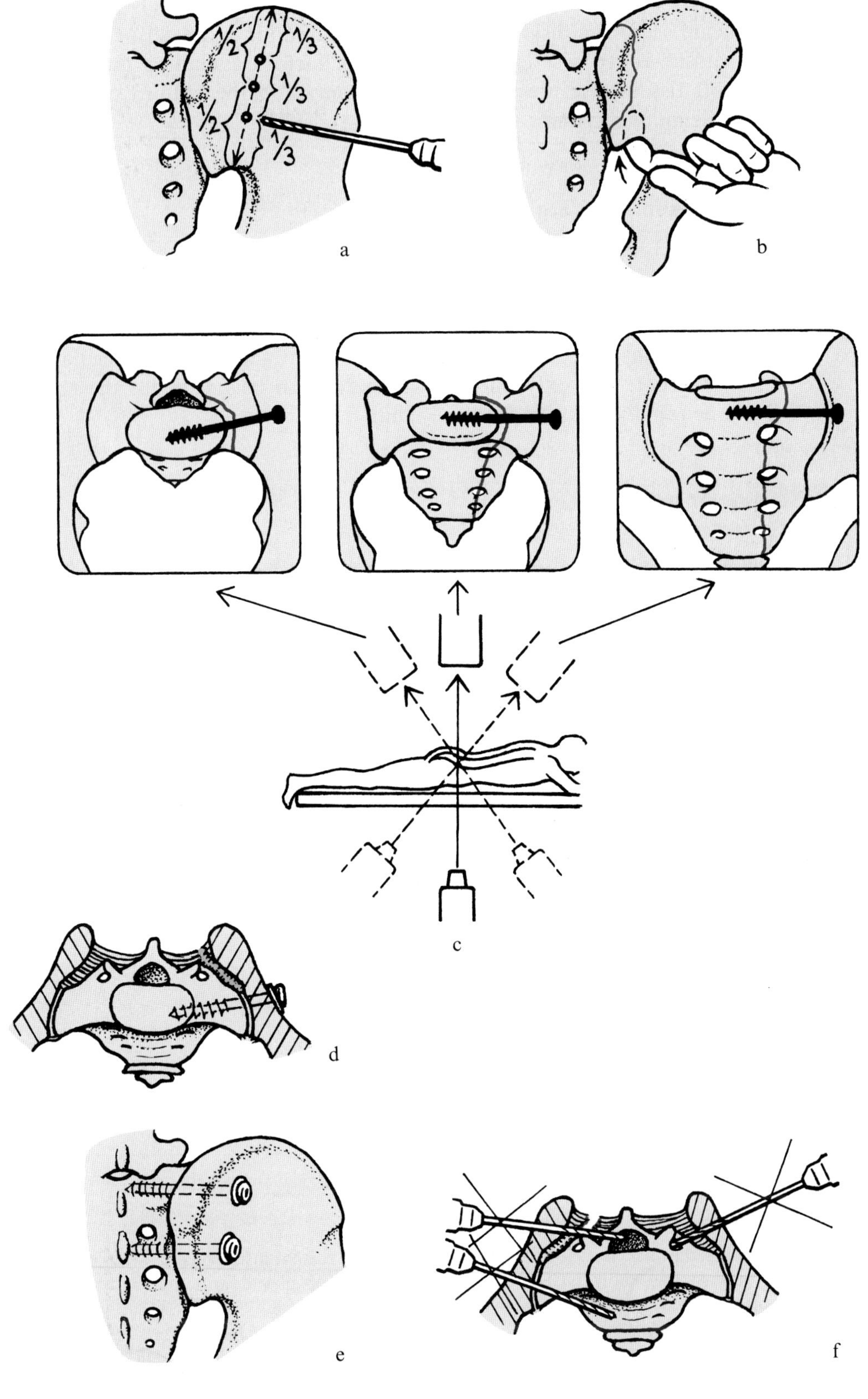

9.7.3 Sacroiliac Dislocation

For acute sacroiliac dislocations, either the anterior or posterior approach may be used. The chosen route will depend upon many factors, including the condition of the skin and soft tissues, the presence of a colostomy and the pattern of any adjacent fracture of the ileum or sacrum.

9.7.3.1 Anterior Approach (Fig. 9.10)

The anterior approach is favored over the posterior although posterior percutaneous techniques are gaining favour. Stable internal fixation is obtained by the use of two- or three-hole 3.5-mm DCPs fixed across the anterior surface of the sacroiliac joint. Only one screw can be placed into the sacrum since going too far medially may injure the L5 nerve root, and only one or two screws can be fixed into the adjacent ilium since the bone rapidly becomes extremely thin.

9.7.3.2 Posterior Approach (Fig. 9.9)

The sacroiliac dislocation may be stably fixed by posterior lag screws. In this case, the 6.5-mm lag screws need only enter the ala of the sacrum: the ala must, therefore, be exposed to allow direct palpation and accurate direction of the screw. Alternatively, percutaneous techniques using cannulated cancelleous bone screws may be applied.

9.7.4 Iliac Fractures (Fig. 9.11)

Iliac fractures are best stabilized by standard techniques of stable internal fixation using interfragmental compression with lag screws if possible, and 3.5- or 4.5-mm pelvic reconstruction plates with the appropriate fully threaded cancellous screws to neutralize the fracture. The plate should be placed near the iliac crest since the bone in the center of the pelvis is extremely thin.

Fig. 9.10
a Incision for anterior access to SI joint.
b Stripping the iliac muscle from the inner wall of the ilium exposes the SI joint, which is then fixed by at least two short DCPs. Only one screw can be placed into the sacrum lest the L5 nerve root be jeopardized.

Fig. 9.11 Reduction clamps, pusher and sciatic nerve retractor are useful in pelvic surgery.

Fig. 9.12 Iliac fractures fixed with cancellous bone screws in lag fashion (a), with DCPs (b) and with a reconstruction plate (c).

Fig. 9.10

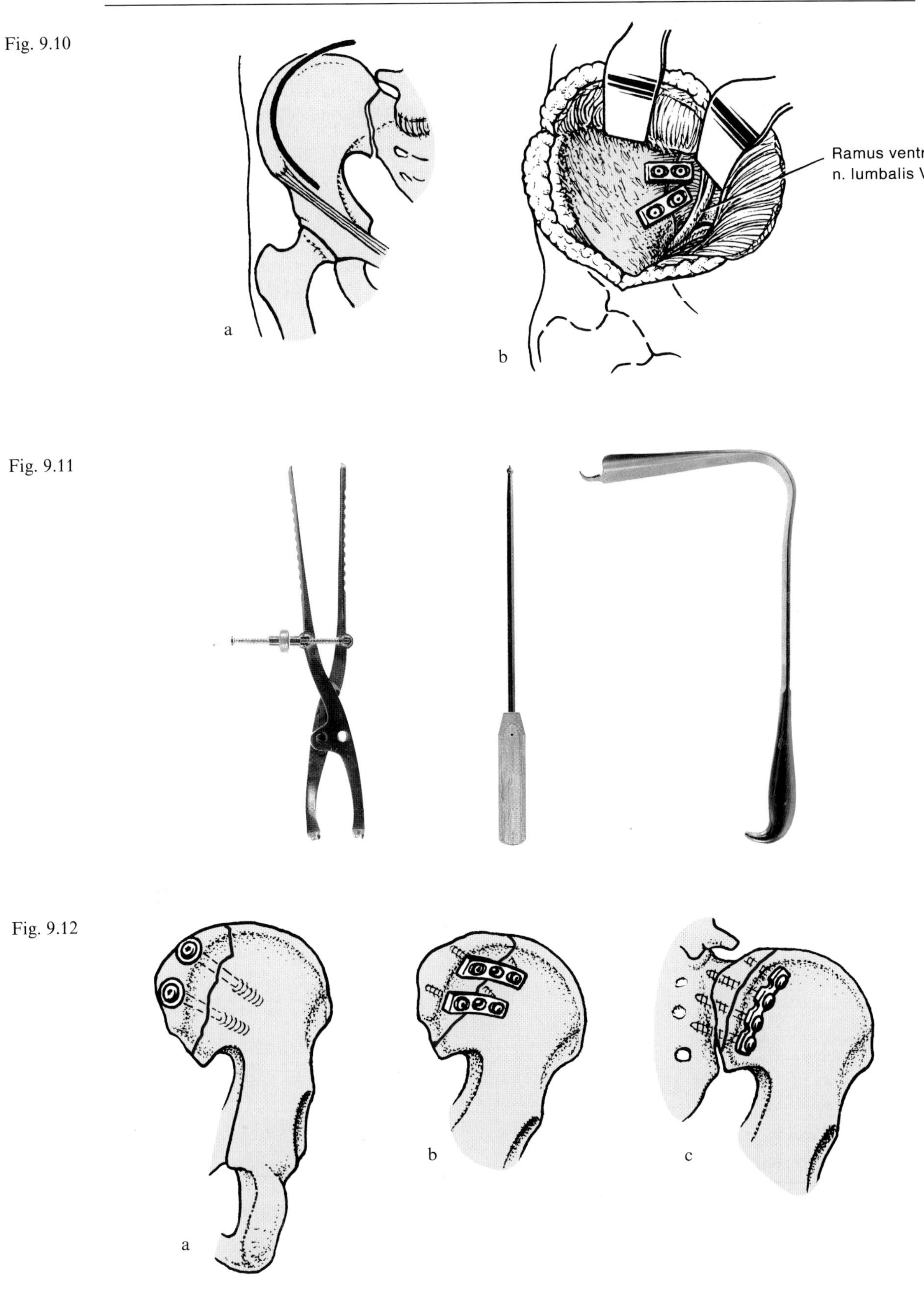

Fig. 9.11

Fig. 9.12

References

Matta J, Saucedo T (1989) Internal fixation of pelvic ring fractures. Clin Orthop 242:83–98
Pennal GF, Tile M, Waddell JP, Garside H (1980) Pelvic disruption: assessment and classification. Clin Orthop 151:12–21
Tile M (1984) Fractures of the pelvis and acetabulum. Williams and Wilkins, Baltimore
Tile M (1988) Pelvic ring fractures: should they be fixed? J Bone Joint Surg [Br] 70:1–12

10 ACETABULUM

10.1 Introduction

Displaced fractures of the acetabulum usually lead to disabling post-traumatic arthritis if the joint is not accurately reduced by open reduction and internal fixation (ORIF). For the fracture surgeon, acetabular fractures pose some of the most difficult technical problems. These difficulties include:

1. Correct characterization of the fracture type.
2. Selection of the surgical approach.
3. Performing the specialized surgical approaches that are necessary.
4. Obtaining a satisfactory reduction and fixation.

10.2 Diagnosis

An AP X-ray of the pelvis should be obtained in all patients with significant trauma (Fig. 10.1). Those with suspected or known acetabular fractures should additionally have the following radiological work-up:

1. An AP projection of the involved hip (Fig. 10.2).
2. A 45° oblique view of the pelvis with the involved hip rotated toward the X-ray tube (this projection is called the obturator oblique) (Fig. 10.3).
3. A 45° projection of the pelvis with the involved hip rotated away from the X-ray tube (this projection is termed the iliac oblique) (Fig. 10.4).
4. A computer tomography (CT) scan of the pelvis after evaluation of the four standard X-ray views. In most cases, this will further delineate the fracture lines and diagnose intra-articular free fragments. The dimensional imaging from the CT scan gives a composite overall picture of the fracture and facilitates planning.

Common associated lesions include significant intrapelvic hemorrhage, urological and neurological injuries, as well as pelvic ring disruptions and ipsilateral lower extremity fractures. All severe injuries to the pelvis are associated with a high incidence of pulmonary embolism and prophylaxis should be considered.

Fig. 10.1 The anterior and posterior columns of the acetabulum and their extent on the inner and outer aspects of the innominate bone.

Fig. 10.2 Radiographic lines as seen on the AP view of the hip.

1 Iliopectineal line; *2* ilioischial line; *3* roentgenographic "U;" *4* roof; *5* anterior rim; *6* posterior rim.

Fig. 10.3 Obturator oblique view of the innominate bone.

1 Anterior column; *2* posterior rim.

Fig. 10.4 Iliac oblique view of the innominate bone.

1 Posterior column; *2* anterior rim.

Fig. 10.1

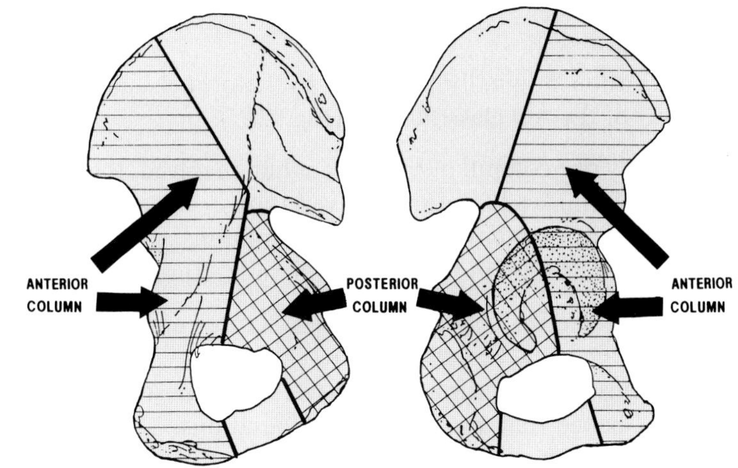

Fig. 10.2

Fig. 10.3

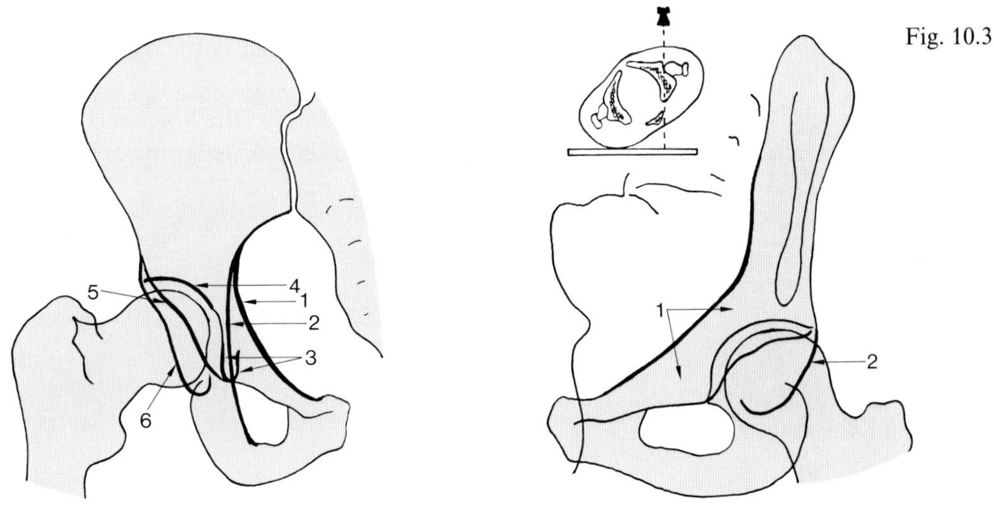

Fig. 10.4

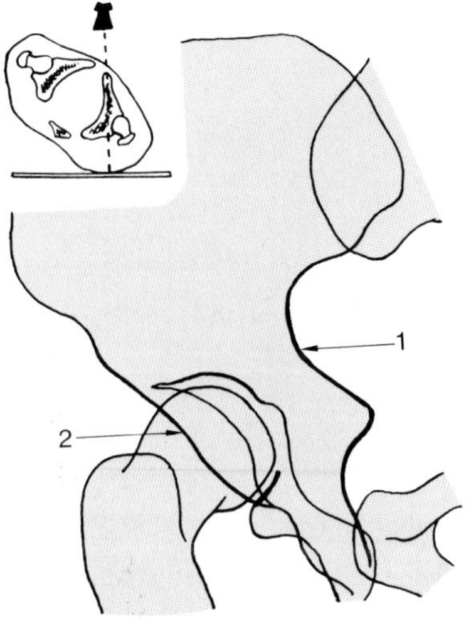

10.3 Fracture Classification

The classification originally proposed by Letournel has been modified to fit the groups A, B, and C of the AO classification (Fig. 10.5).

Type A Only one column of the acetabulum involved, the other column remaining intact.
- A1 Posterior wall fracture and variations.
- A2 Posterior column fracture and variations.
- A3 Anterior wall and anterior column fractures.

Type B Characterized by a transverse fracture component, where a portion of the roof remains attached to the intact ilium.
- B1 Transverse fracture and transverse plus posterior wall fracture.
- B2 T-shaped fracture with several variations.
- B3 Anterior wall or column plus posterior hemitransverse fracture.

Type C Fractures in both columns; characterized by fracture lines involving the anterior as well as the posterior column, but differs from type B in that all articular segments, including the roof, are detached from the remaining segment of the intact ilium.
- C1 Anterior column fracture line extending to the iliac crest.
- C2 Anterior column fracture line extending to the anterior border of the ilium.
- C3 Fracture lines which enter the sacroiliac joint.

Fig. 10.5. AO classification of acetabulum fractures.

Type A: Fractures involving only one of the two columns of the acetabulum.

Type B: Transverse fracture component present, a portion of roof remains attached to the intact ilium.

Type C: Anterior and posterior columns involved. No portion of roof remains attached to the intact ilium (fractures in both columns).

Fig. 10.5

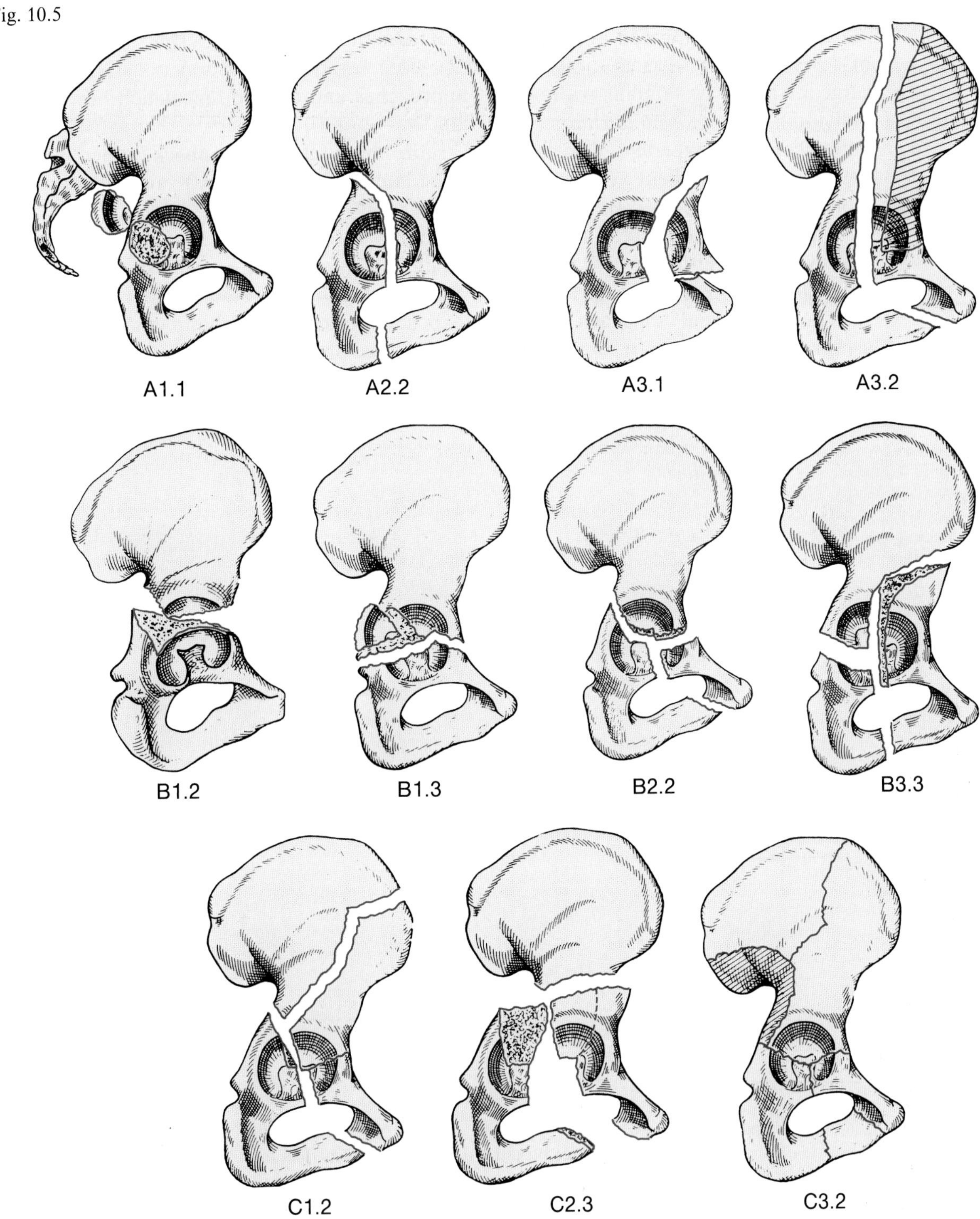

10.4 Surgical Approaches

No one surgical approach is ideal for all fractures of the acetabulum, but in the majority of cases, a single surgical approach can be used for both reduction and fixation. The surgeon should be familiar with several approaches and choose that which best fits the individual fracture configuration. There are four surgical approaches that satisfy the requirements of an experienced acetabular surgeon: the Kocher-Langenbeck (patient prone); the ilioinguinal (patient supine); the straight lateral (patient lateral); and the extended iliofemoral (patient lateral).

The Kocher-Langenbeck approach is primarily an approach to the posterior column. However, it can also give very useful though limited access to the anterior column through the greater sciatic notch (Fig. 10.6).

The ilioinguinal approach primarily exposes the anterior column and the internal aspect of the innominate bone. The posterior column may also be approached along its internal aspect beyond the pelvic brim (Fig. 10.7).

Fig. 10.6 Kocher-Langenbeck approach.

a Skin incision.

b Exposure of the retroacetabular surface by retracting the gluteus medius muscle anteriorly and proximally and the gluteus maximus, piriformis and obturatorius internus muscles posteriorly.

Fig. 10.7 Ilioinguinal approach.

a Skin incision.

b First window of approach exposing the internal iliac fossa by retracting the iliopsoas and abdominal muscles medially.

c Second window of approach exposing the pelvic brim and quadrilateral surface by retracting the iliopsoas and femoral nerve laterally and the external iliac vessels medially.

Fig. 10.6

Fig. 10.7

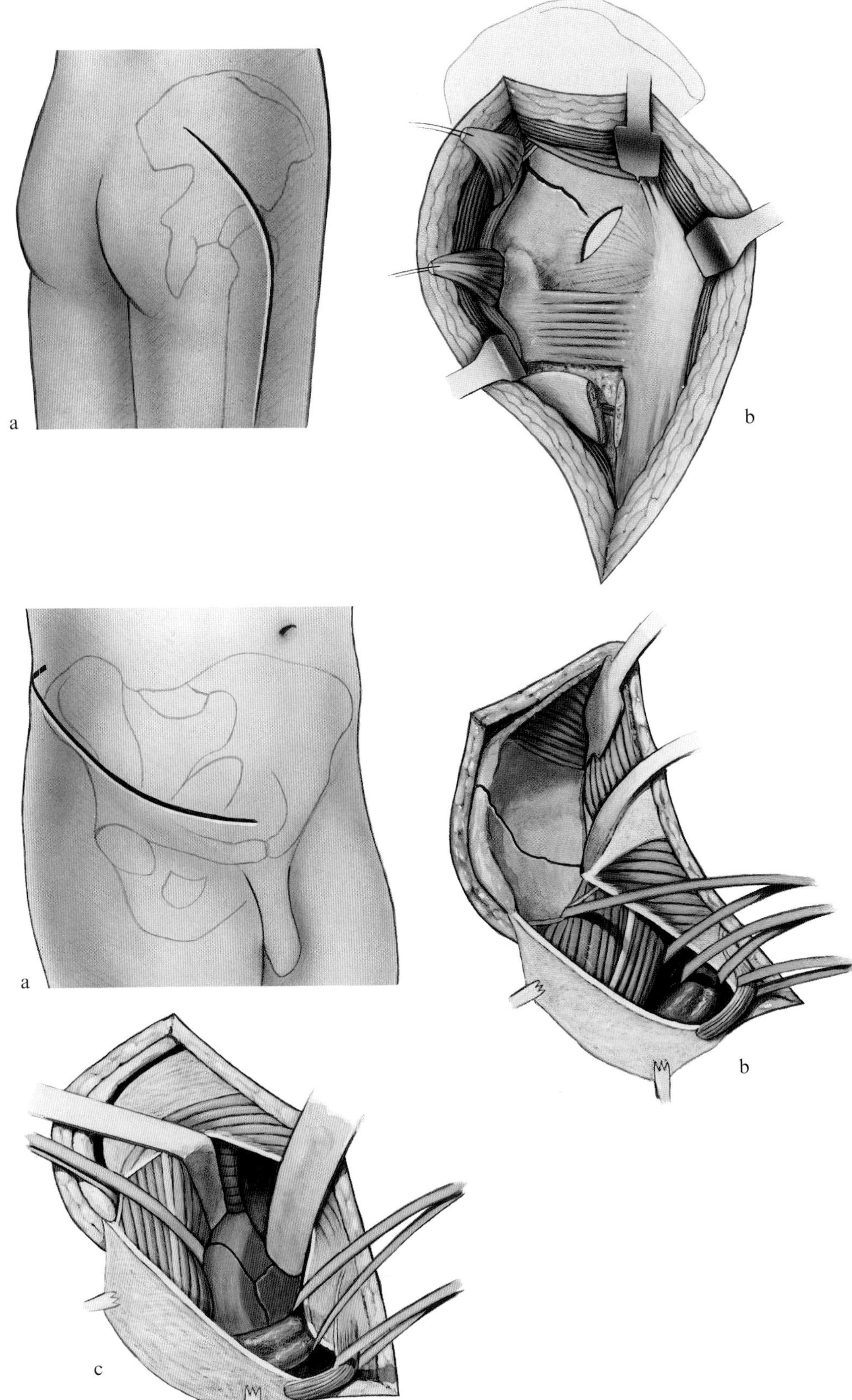

The extended iliofemoral approach primarily exposes the lateral aspect of the innominate bone and gives the best simultaneous exposure of both columns. Although access to the anterior column is more limited than with the ilioinguinal approach, elevation of the internal iliac fossa gives circumferential access to the bone. The extended iliofemoral approach with its commanding exposure is especially useful for older fractures in which bony callus must be excised or an osteotomy performed (Fig. 10.8).

Fig. 10.8 Extended iliofemoral approach.

a Skin incision.

b Exposure of the external aspect of the bone by retracting the glutei, piriformis and obturatorius internus muscles posteriorly.

c Exposure of the internal aspect of the bone by retracting the iliopsoas and abdominal muscles medially.

Fig. 10.8

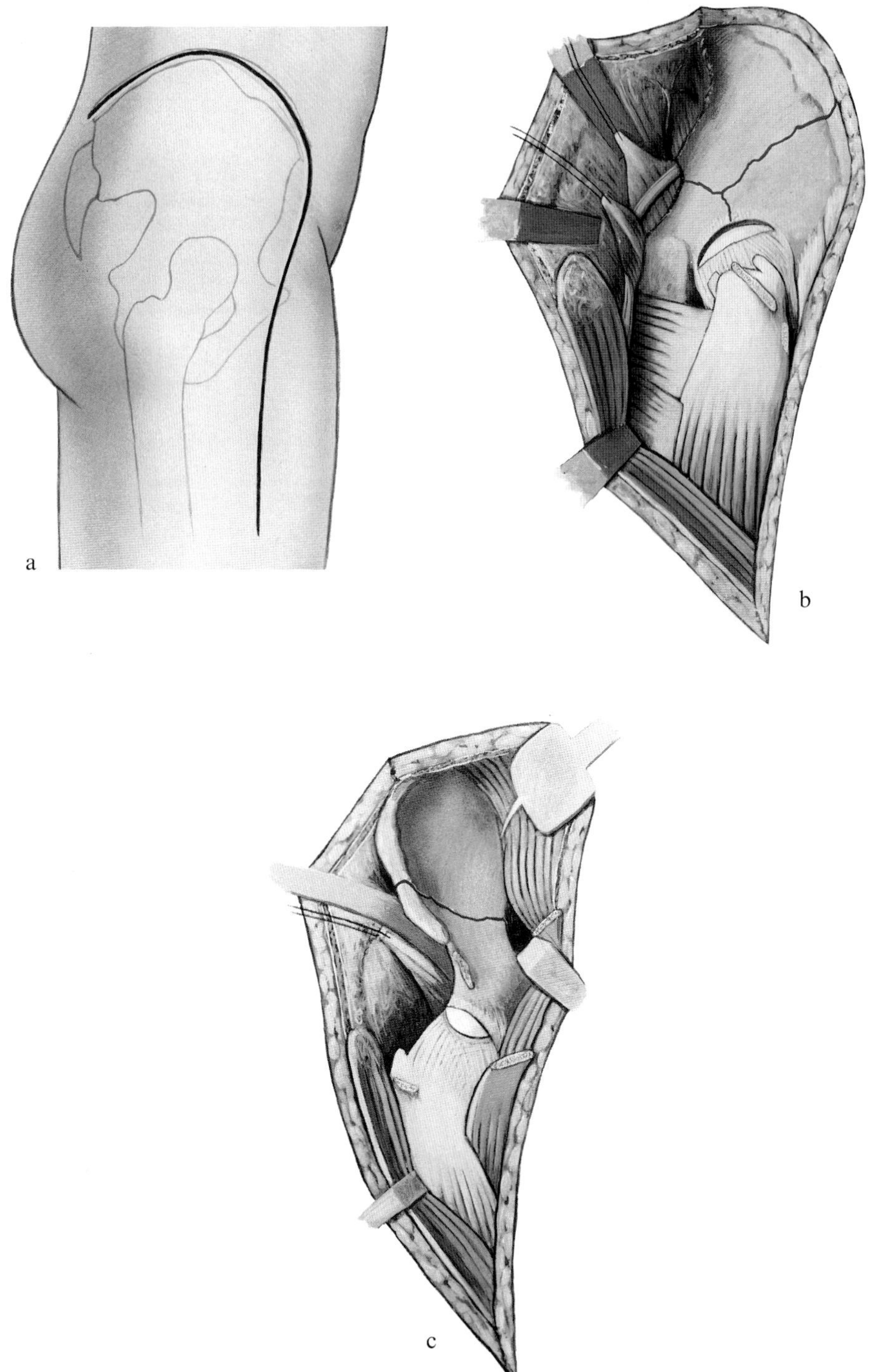

The straight lateral approach exposes the posterior column, the entire roof, and half of the iliac wing, and gives limited access to the anterior column (Fig. 10.9).

Fig. 10.9 Straight lateral approach. Skin incision and access to the bone.

a *1* "Supracristal point"; (highest point of iliac crest); *2* gluteal tuberosity; *3* anterior superior iliac spine; *4* posterior superior iliac spine; *5* greater trochanter; *6* sciatic nerve; *7* superior gluteal nerve.

b *1* Greater trochanter; *2* "supracristal point" (see Fig. 10.9a/1); *3* iliotibial tract; *4* tensor fasciae latae muscle.

c *1* Iliotibial tract; *2* gluteus medius muscle; *3* superficial branch of superior gluteal vessels; *4* piriformis muscle; *5* sciatic nerve; *6* inferior gluteal vessels; *7* gluteus maximus muscle; *8* vastus lateralis muscle; *9* "triceps coxae" (gemelli and obturatorius internus muscles); *10* quadratus femoris muscle; *11* tendon of gluteus maximus muscle.

d *1* Rectus femoris muscle, reflected head; *2* nerve of tensor fasciae latae; *3* gluteus medius and minimus muscles (reflected); *4* greater trochanter (after osteotomy); *5* tendon of piriformis muscle (cut); *6* sciatic nerve; *7* superficial branch of superior gluteal vessels; *8* origin of gluteus minimus; *9* superior gluteal nerve; *10* "triceps coxae" (gemelli and obturatorius internus muscles); *11* quadratus femoris muscle; *12* vastus lateralis muscle; *13* tensor fasciae latae muscle.

Fig. 10.9

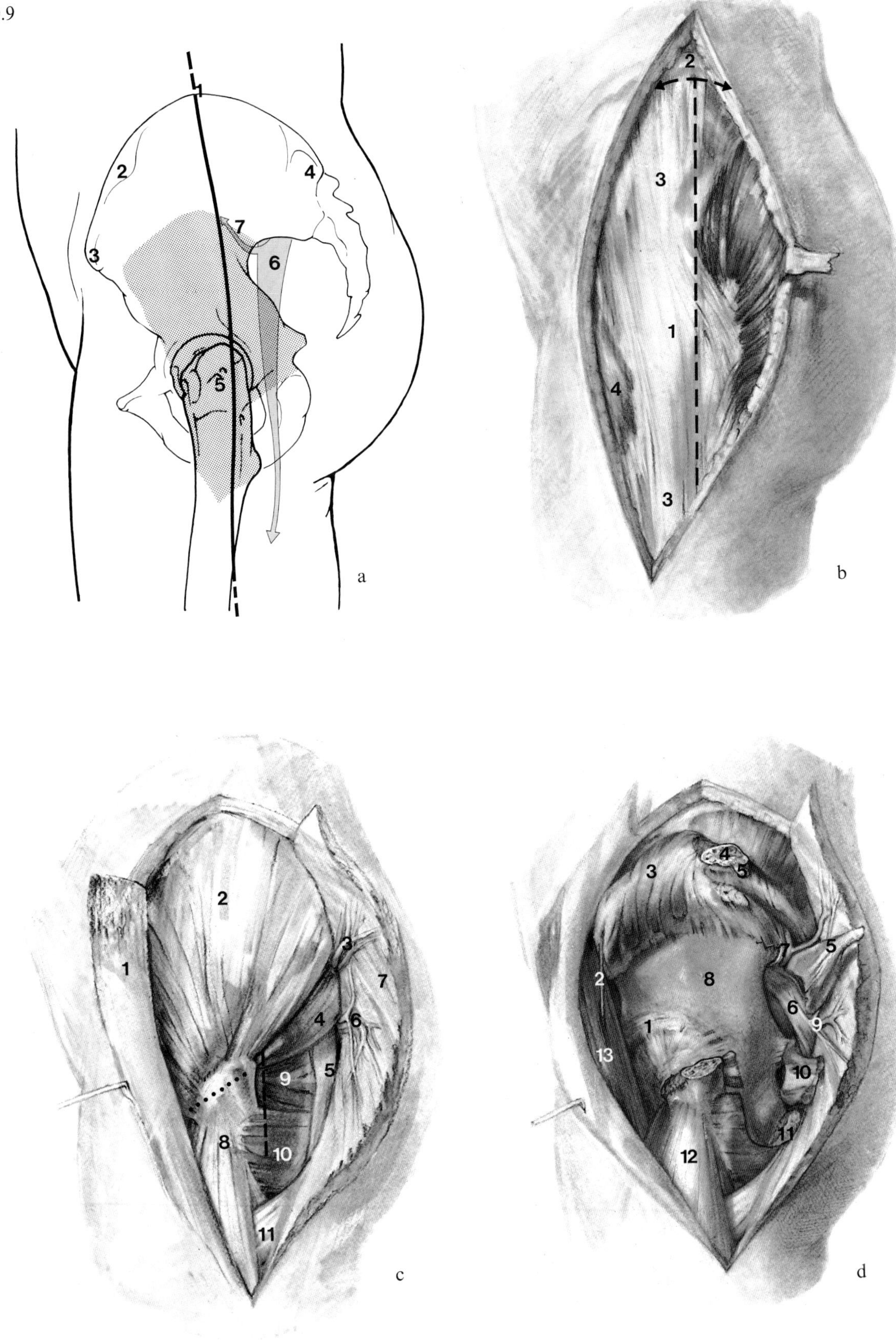

The use of a fracture table can be advantageous in positioning the extremity and in distracting the femoral head from the acetabulum, thus facilitating reduction and visualization of the articular surface (Fig. 10.10). Alternatively, the surgeon may choose to operate on a standard operating table and distract using the femoral distractor which is placed from the iliac crest to the femur (Fig. 10.11). The knee should be kept flexed at 45° to 60° throughout the operative procedure to prevent stretching the sciatic nerve. All four surgical approaches provide some exposure to both the anterior and posterior columns, but each has specific advantages and disadvantages.

Fig. 10.10 Use of the fracture table for distal and lateral traction.

Fig. 10.11 Use of the femoral distractor.

Fig. 10.10

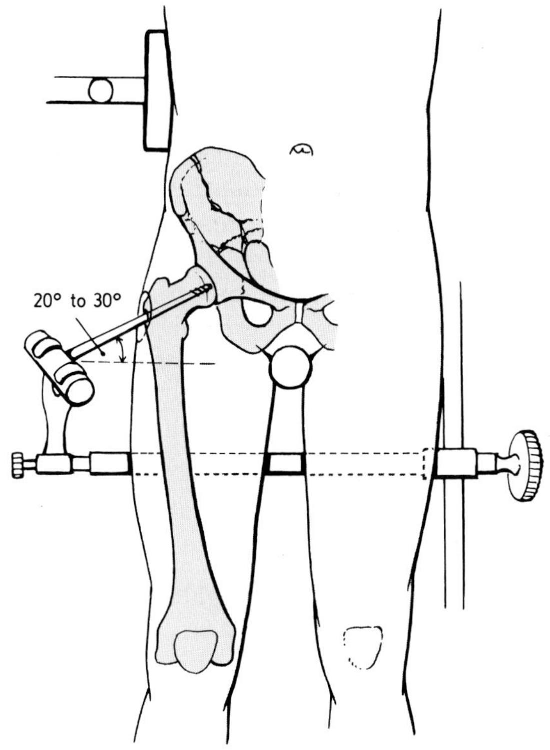

Fig. 10.11

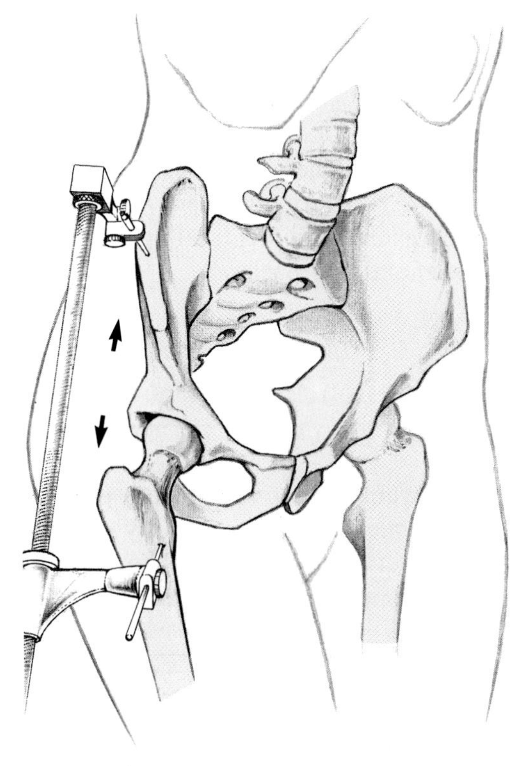

10.5 Timing and Planning

It is usually best to delay surgery until 2–3 days after the injury, when local bleeding has subsided and the patient's condition stabilized. Three weeks after the injury bony callus will be present, making any reduction much more difficult, so surgery should ideally be performed within 10 days of the injury.

The benefits of preoperative traction are very limited and it should never be applied to the proximal femur.

Posterior dislocation of the femoral head must be reduced immediately. Irreducible or unstable posterior dislocation is an indication for urgent surgery.

Antibiotics should be administered for a short pre- and postoperative period (24–48 hours).

For each fracture type, the following surgical approaches are suggested:

A1 Kocher-Langenbeck approach.
A2 Kocher-Langenbeck or straight lateral approach.
A3 Ilioinguinal approach.

B1 The Kocher-Langenbeck or straight lateral approach may be used effectively for the great majority of these fractures. The extended iliofemoral approach is useful for transtectal pure transverse fractures (B1.2) and difficult associated transverse and posterior wall fractures (B1.3).
B2 These fractures can usually be operated using the Kocher-Langenbeck approach, possibly with a subsequent ilioinguinal approach if the anterior column is not reduced. Alternatively, the straight lateral approach may be used, but if considerable difficulties are anticipated, the extended iliofemoral approach should be used initially.
B3 Ilioinguinal approach.

C1 These may be operated using the ilioinguinal approach. However, if there is complex involvement of the posterior column, the extended iliofemoral approach should be used.
C2 It is possible to operate these fractures using either the Kocher-Langenbeck or straight lateral approach. However, the best control of the fracture is obtained using the ilioinguinal and extended iliofemoral approaches.
C3 Extended iliofemoral approach.

10.6 Reduction and Fixation Techniques

The most useful instruments for acetabular surgery are the pelvic reduction clamp, the Farabeuf reduction forceps, and the variously sized pointed reduction forceps (Fig. 10.12). A ball-spike instrument is used to push bone fragments into place, and a Schanz screw with a handle or the femoral head corkscrew extractor is applied to the ischium to control

---

Fig. 10.12 Instruments for the reduction of acetabular fractures.

1 "King Tong" reduction forceps; *2* "Queen Tong" reduction forceps; *3* large-angled jaw reduction forceps; *4* small-angled jaw reduction forceps; *5* ball-spike; *6* large reduction forceps; *7* small reduction forceps; *8* pointed reduction forceps; *9* pelvic reduction forceps; *10* 6-mm Schanz screw; *11* universal chuck with T-handle; *12* sciatic nerve retractor.

Fig. 10.12

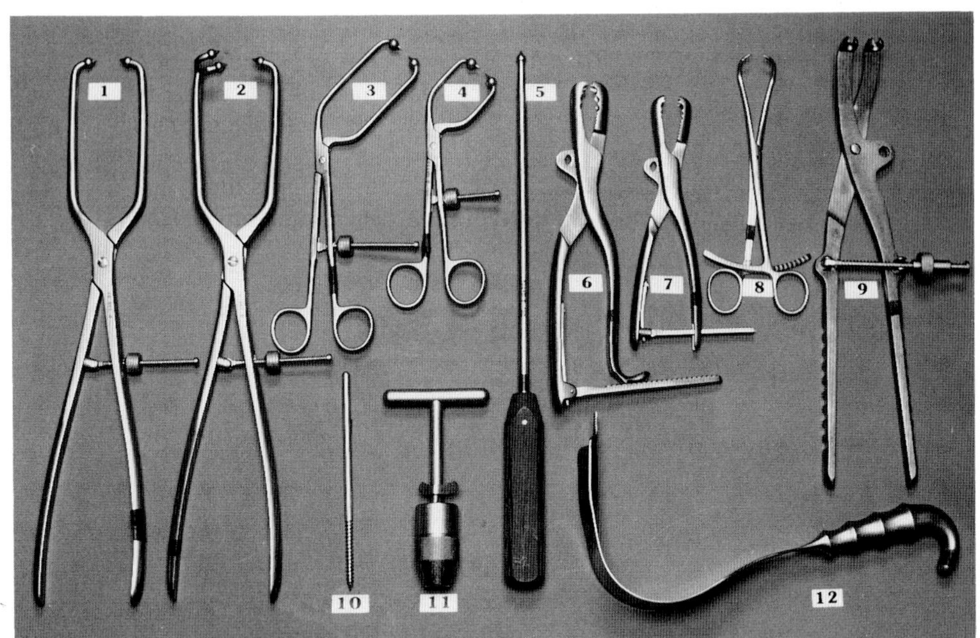

rotation of the posterior column. The pelvic reduction clamp and Farabeuf forceps are applied to screws inserted into different bone fragments. The pointed reduction forceps may be applied directly to a bone's surface, to shallow drill holes through the cortex, or to plastic rings and hooks. To reduce an acetabular fracture, it is often necessary to proceed in a stepwise fashion, first reducing and fixing single fragments, and then adding other fragments to the assembled parts. Precision in reduction is important at each step to ensure reduction of the articular surface. It is advisable to include all extra-articular fragments in the reconstruction. They are sometimes found along the iliac crest, the pelvic brim or within the greater sciatic notch, and they may provide a key to the eventual reduction and aid in achieving stability. The accuracy of reduction of the articular surface is ideally assessed by direct vision. In cases where this would require undesirable dissection of the soft tissue and the articular capsule, the degree of reduction is indicated by the reduction seen on the cortex of the innominate bone. A dislocated sacroiliac joint or displaced sacrum fracture must usually be reduced and fixed prior to the reduction of the acetabulum fracture. Initial fixation with lag screws (3.5-mm, 4.5-mm or 6.5-mm) usually allows reduction instruments to be removed so that plates, if required, can be applied. The straight, 3.5-mm reconstruction plate and the curved, 3.5-mm pelvic plate are the most useful for fixation. Precise plate contouring is essential.

Using the Kocher-Langenbeck approach, plates are normally applied to the retroacetabular surface. This is also the case with the extended iliofemoral and straight lateral approaches where plates are also applied to the iliac wing. Using the ilioinguinal approach, the most common position for the plate is along the superior surface of the pelvic brim. Occasionally a fracture may be stabilized by lag screws alone, but in the majority of cases, lag screw fixation must be supplemented by one or more plates. Long lag screws are very effective when placed between the two tables of the ilium or along the long axis of the anterior or posterior column (Figs. 10.14–10.17).

10.7 Postoperative Treatment

After careful soft tissue reconstruction and wound closure, suction drains are normally left in place for a period of 24–48 hours. Passive mobilization of the hip may be started within a few days. When the patient is comfortable enough, usually 5–10 days after surgery, gait training with active hip mobilization may be started allowing partial weight-bearing (15 kg) on the affected extremity. Full weight-bearing can normally be started 8 weeks after internal fixation.

Fig. 10.13 Implants for fixation of acetabular fractures, 3.5-mm and 4.5-mm curved and straight reconstruction plates. Extra long 3.5-mm, 4.5-mm and 6.5-mm screws.

Fig. 10.14 Internal fixation of posterior wall fracture (A.1.2) using the Kocher-Langenbeck approach.

Fig. 10.15 Internal fixation of a combined transverse and posterior wall fracture (B.1.3) using the Kocher-Langenbeck approach.

Fig. 10.16 Internal fixation of a combined anterior column and posterior hemitransverse fracture (B.3.2) using the ilioinguinal approach.

Fig. 10.17 Internal fixation of a both-column fracture (C.1.3) using the extended iliofemoral approach.

Fig. 10.13

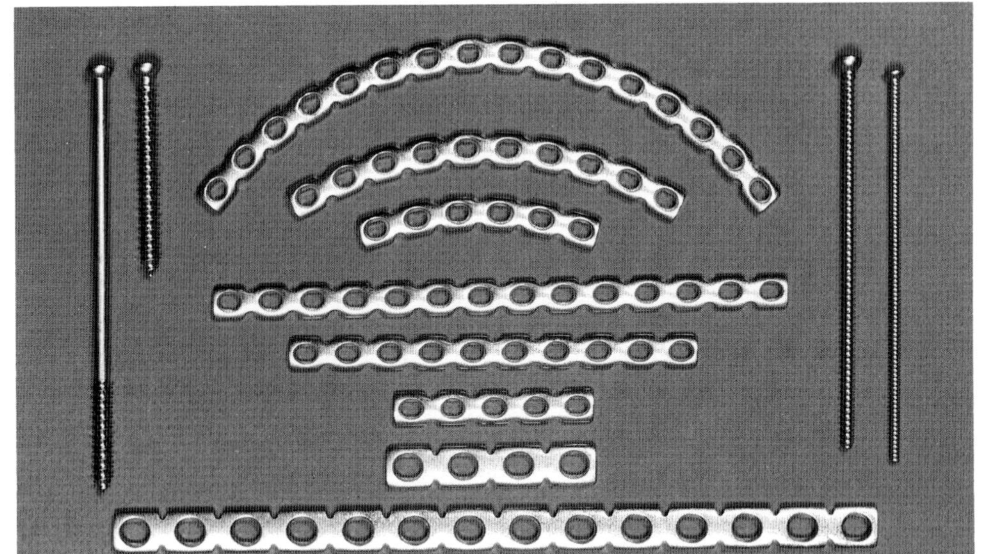

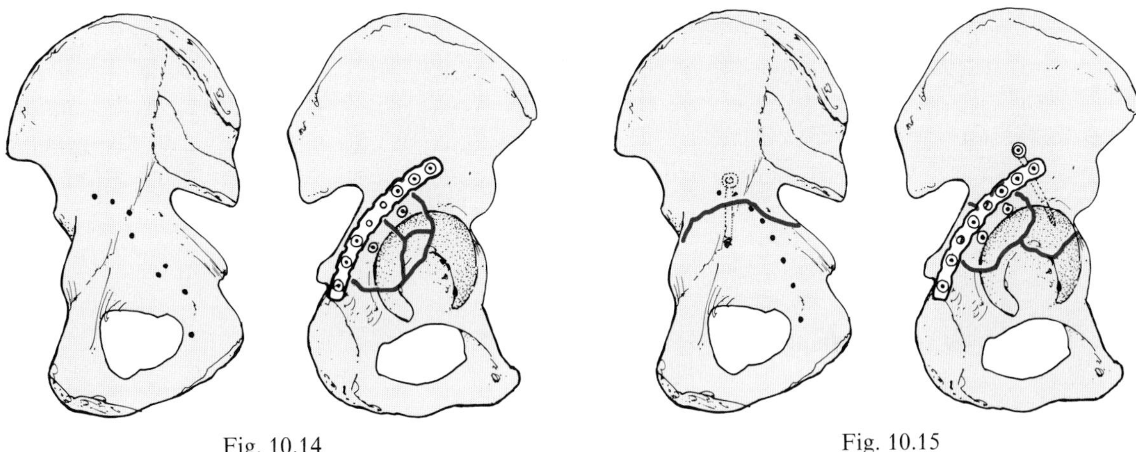

Fig. 10.14

Fig. 10.15

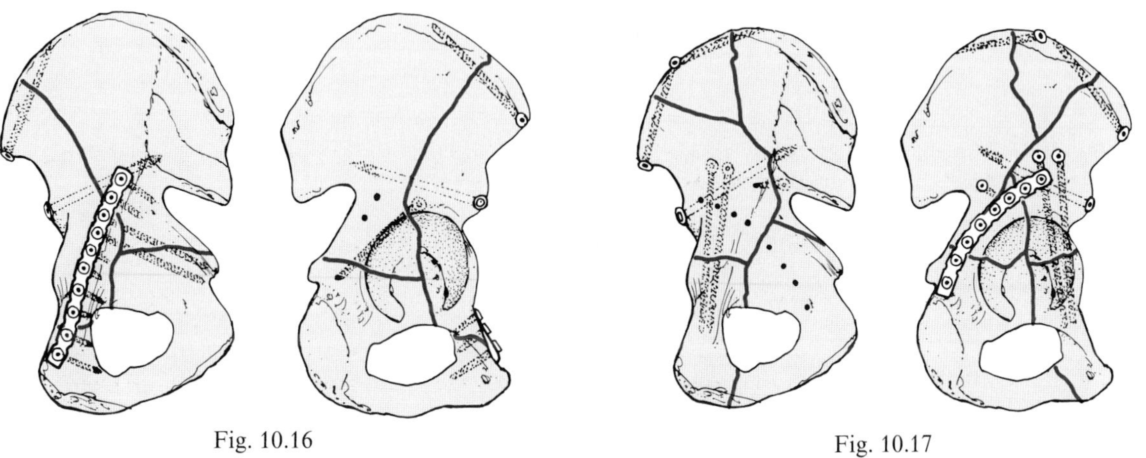

Fig. 10.16

Fig. 10.17

References

Epstein HC (1980) Traumatic dislocations of the hip. Williams & Wilkins, Baltimore

Judet R, Judet J, Letournel E (1964) Fractures of the acetabulum. Classification and surgical approaches for open reduction. J Bone Joint Surg [Am] 46:1615

Knight RA, Smith H (1958) Central fractures of the acetabulum. J Bone Joint Surg 40:1

Letournel E (1979) The results of acetabular fractures treated surgically: twenty-one years experience. In: The hip: proceedings of the Seventh Open Scientific Meeting of The Hip Society. Mosby, St. Louis

Letournel E (1980) Acetabulum fractures: classification and management. Clin Orthop 151:81

Letournel E (1981) Fractures of the acetabulum. Springer, New York Berlin Heidelberg

Matta JM, Merritt PO (1988) Displaced acetabular fractures. Clin Orthop 230:83

Matta J, Anderson L, Epstein H, Hendrick P (1986) Fractures of the acetabulum: a retrospective analysis. Clin Orthop 205:230

Matta J, Letournel E, Browner B (1986) Surgical management of acetabular fractures. Mosby, St. Louis (American Academy of Orthopaedic Surgeons Instructional Course Lectures, No. 35, p. 38)

Matta J, Mehne D, Roffi R (1986) Fractures of the acetabulum: early results of a prospective study. Clin Orthop 205:241

Mears DC, Rubash H (1986) Pelvic and acetabular fractures. Slack, Thorofare, NJ

Tile M (1984) Fractures of the pelvis and acetabulum. Williams & Wilkins, Baltimore

11 PROXIMAL FEMUR

11.1 Fractures of the Femoral Head

These are always part of a combined injury to the hip joint, often as a result of posterior and obturator dislocation or of fracture dislocation. Quite often they are associated with transverse fractures of the acetabulum.

Depression fractures are relatively frequent. They may be localized anteriorly, posteriorly or cranially. Besides this type we recognize shear fractures of a femoral head segment as well as avulsion fractures of ligamentum teres (especially in young adults) – shear fractures are quite often combined with depression of the head. If connected with ligamentum teres or the reflected part of the capsule, the fragment keeps its blood supply. The worst prognosis for a femoral head fracture results from a combination with a femoral neck fracture because in almost every case the main fragment of the femoral head loses its vascular supply (Brumback et al. 1987; Epstein et al. 1985; Roeder and De Lee 1980; De Lee et al. 1980; Pipkin 1957).

Relocation of the femoral head into the acetabulum must be performed as an emergency maneuver before further diagnostic steps are initiated. After reduction a standard AP view of the pelvis, contour views for detection of cranially located depressions and CT scans to visualize posterior and anterior depressions or shear fractures are taken. The congruency of the femoral head with the acetabulum can be checked by an AP X-ray of the pelvis taken under some axial load of the slightly abducted legs. The width of the joint space is compared with the opposite side. If the joint space is wider, the reason might be an interposed fragment, a folded ligamentum teres or an inverted labrum of the acetabular rim. A CT scan can visualize an interposed fragment but is less useful for soft tissue interpositions. The CT scan allows control of reduction of a shear fragment. Interpositions are best removed immediately by a posterior approach. However, sometimes their removal is easier by an anterior approach, particularly after posterior dislocations.

Small, infraligamentary shear fragments do not need to be reduced anatomically if they do not compromise motion of the joint. Bigger shear fragments normally end cranial to ligamentum teres and therefore include the weight-bearing area, which makes anatomic reduction mandatory. If this is not possible by closed methods, open reduction through a Smith-Peterson approach is necessary. The fragment is reduced avoiding further damage to the blood supply. Two-millimeter drill holes into the main fragment may produce bleeding as proof of maintained vascular supply. The fragment is fixed with small fragment screws buttressing the heads beneath the level of the cartilage. If additional depression is present, it may be elevated and the defect grafted with cancellous bone from the ipsilateral iliac crest. The same procedure may be considered for larger depression fractures. There is also the possibility of post-primary or secondary intertrochanteric corrections, in the direction of flexion, extension or abduction according to the localization of the lesion. Shear fractures of the femoral head combined with femoral neck fractures (see C3.2 and C3.3 fractures according to the AO classification) and a proven avascular main fragment of the head are best treated by either arthrodesis or joint replacement.

Fig. 11.1 The blood supply of the femoral head (according to Lanz and Wachsmuth 1972).

a As seen from in front.

b As seen from behind.

Most of the blood supply of the femoral head is derived from the medial femoral circumflex artery, which in the trochanteric fossa gives rise to three or four branches, the retinacular vessels. These run posterosuperiorly along the neck in a synovial reflection until they reach the cartilaginous border of the head, where they enter the bone to supply the head.
The obturator artery gives rise to the vessels within the ligamentum teres. These as a rule supply only a small portion of bone around the insertion of ligamentum teres. Additional blood supply to the head comes from intra-osseous vessels which run upwards from the metaphysis. In a neck fracture, of course, these are always interrupted.
The greater trochanter is supplied by an ascending branch of the lateral femoral circumflex artery. This branch anastomoses superiorly about the femoral neck with branches of the medial femoral circumflex artery.

Fig. 11.2 Fractures of the femoral head.

These are rare and always form part of a combined injury to the hip joint with, for example, posterior dislocation or fracture dislocation.

C1 Avulsion and shear.
C1.1 Avulsion of ligamentum teres.
C1.2 Shear fracture below ligamentum teres.
C1.3 Shear fracture above ligamentum teres.

C2 Depression.
C2.1 Posterosuperior.
C2.2 Anterosuperior.
C2.3 Superolateral.

C3 Combined fractures.
C3.1 Depression plus shear fracture.
C3.2 Shear plus subcapital fracture.
C3.3 Depression plus subcapital fracture.

Fig. 11.3 Fractures of the femoral head.

a Depression and shear fracture of the femoral head (C3.1).

b Elevation of the depression, cancellous bone graft and transchondral screw fixation of the shear fragment.

Fig. 11.1

Fig. 11.2

Fig. 11.3

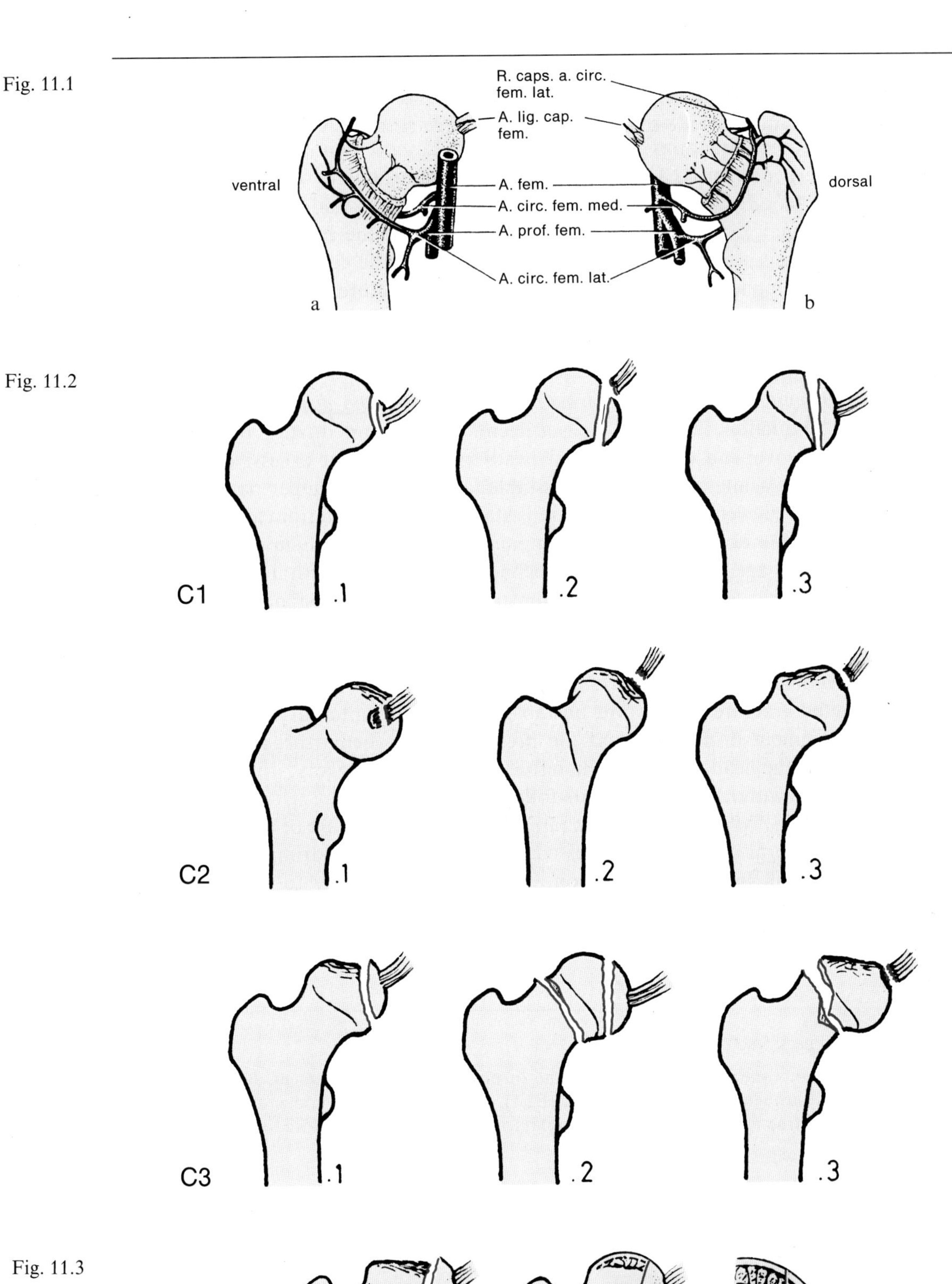

11.2 Femoral Neck Fractures

Femoral neck fractures are intra-articular. Lateral femoral neck fractures in children and elderly adults (B2.1), may be partially extra-articular.

The blood supply to the head can be damaged and various degrees of avascular necrosis may occur depending on the location of the head fracture. Stable subcapital, rarely transcervical fractures are recognized when the cervical cephalic cohesion is maintained by impaction (B1). In most transcervical fractures, there is partial contact between the fragments but a gap is visible in the superior part of the fracture (B2). The third group includes all displaced subcapital fractures (B3). Fractures in this group have the worst prognosis.

Subcapital or transcervial fractures with little or no displacement and impaction, also called abduction fractures, are sufficiently stable and do not require internal fixation if the retroversion of the femoral head fragment is not excessive. This retroversion is checked by a lateral X-ray ("cross-table lateral"). In younger patients, internal fixation is considered even when the fracture is stable. With an anterior capsulotomy, the hemarthros may be evacuated to prevent impairment of the blood supply of the head fragment. In the older age group, the risk of secondary dislocation with increased danger of femoral head necrosis can be accepted. Even under these circumstances, the evacuation of the hemarthros may be recommended since it also reduces the pain. If the stability is doubtful it can be checked under the image intensifier.

Transcervical neck fractures have a higher rate of avascular necrosis than the subcapital impacted fractures. They are unstable and require internal fixation. There is evidence that fragment dislocation and the pressure of the hemarthros can influence the blood supply of the head fragment. Therefore, we advocate surgery, if possible, as an emergency procedure within the first 6 hours following the fracture.

Displaced subcapital neck fractures have a very high rate of avascular necrosis. Vitality of the femoral head can be assessed intra-operatively by drilling the head fragment with a 2-mm drill bit before reduction. This technique is easy to apply, and provides more information than the more sophisticated techniques such as selective angiography and

---

Fig. 11.4 Femoral neck fractures.

B1 represents subcapital fractures with no or only minimal displacement. B2 fractures are transcervical fractures through the base of the neck (B2.1), mediocervical with adduction (B2.2) and shear fractures (B2.3). B3 fractures are displaced subcapital fractures and have therefore the worst prognosis.

B1 Subcapital with minimal displacement.
B1.1 With marked valgus.
B1.2 With slight valgus.
B1.3 Without displacement.

B2 Transcervical fractures.
B2.1 At the base of the neck.
B2.2 Mediocervical with adduction.
B2.3 Mediocervical with shear.

B3 Displaced subcapital fractures.
B3.1 With slight varus.
B3.2 With slight translation.
B3.3 With considerable displacement.

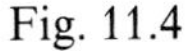

Fig. 11.4

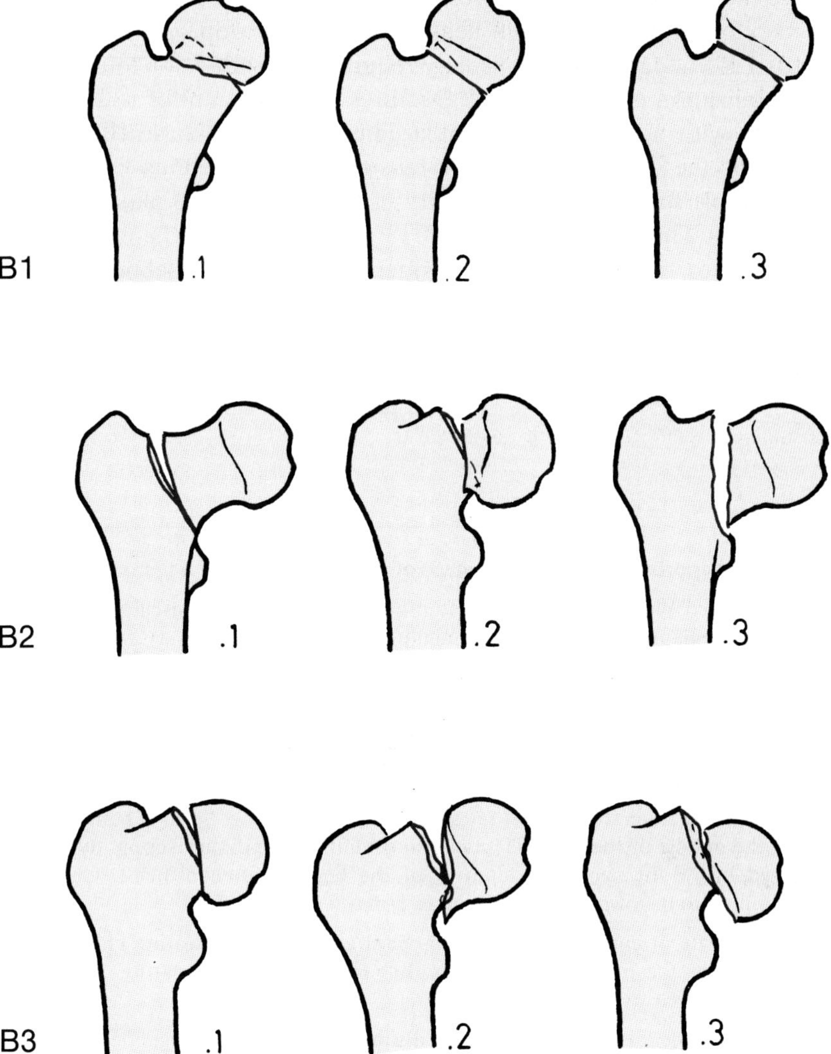

MRI, which are not available in the emergency unit at all times. Later, when avascularity of the femoral head is proven by further techniques like scintigraphy and MRI, revascularization procedures may be considered for younger patients, particularly with partial avascularity. The best time is 4–6 months after the accident, when the fracture is healed and before the femoral head collapses. In the older patient, primary femoral head replacement is indicated when the femoral head shows no intra-operative bleeding. Proven total head necrosis in younger patients usually requires arthrodesis or total hip replacement.

Stabilization of femoral neck fractures cannot be uniform. For the group of subcapital fractures with no or minimal displacement and impaction, the primary stability is quite good. For the others, fixation by two or three cancellous lag screws may be sufficient. It is possible to increase the stability using a 130° blade plate, but the technique is more demanding. The application of a DHS is also possible. Using this implant, it is especially important to transfix the two fragments with two Kirschner wires in order to prevent rotation of the neck fragment during the insertion of the screw. Rotational stability is finally secured by one additional screw (Bray et al. 1988; Madsen et al. 1987; Resch and Sperner 1987; Strömquist et al. 1984).

Fig. 11.5 The surgical approach and the main steps of internal fixation of a femoral neck fracture.

a Use a modified Watson-Jones anterolateral approach. Split the fascia lata in line with the skin incision. Develop the plane between gluteus medius and minimus on the one side and tensor fascia lata on the other. Preserve the nerve to tensor fascia lata. Expose the intertrochanteric region. This is done by making an L-shaped incision in the insertion of vastus lateralis and by reflecting the muscle downwards and forwards.

b The capsule is then opened anteriorly in line with the neck axis, and with the aid of three retractors the fracture is exposed. The tip of the first 16-mm-wide long-tipped retractor is passed over the anterior lip of the acetabulum. The second retractor must have a short tip. It is hammered superiorly into approximately the middle of the neck. Here it cannot damage the blood supply to the head. The third retractor is passed below the neck. The control of the head is often difficult. One can stabilize the head by hammering into its lower half the tip of an 8-mm retractor.

c Prepare the site of entry for the seating chisel and insert the seating chisel and two 2.5-mm Kirschner wires as far as the fracture. Remember that the blade of the seating chisel should be as close to the calcar as possible.

d In order to reduce the fracture, first of all disimpact the fracture by gentle external rotation and adduction. Then, with careful traction, internal rotation and abduction, carry out an exact anatomic reduction. The reduction is greatly facilitated by having gained control of the head by means of the 8-mm retractor mentioned in b above. Stabilize the fracture by driving into the head the two 2.5-mm-thick Kirschner wires, which serve also as guide wires for the insertion of the seating chisel.

e Flex the hip to 90° and check the accuracy of the reduction inferiorly and medially.

f The next important step is the impaction of the fracture. The leg is abducted and internally rotated. The internal rotation is important to prevent retroversion of the head as impaction occurs. Take the slit hammer, apply it to the base of the greater trochanter and strike it firmly with a mallet to impact the fracture. This will convert the adduction fracture into a stable abduction fracture with the head in slight valgus and anteversion.

g Flex the hip again to 90° and check the reduction at the level of the calcar. If all is well, hammer in the seating chisel a further 20 mm. This will drive it into the head. Check the hip for freedom of motion.

h Remove the seating chisel and replace it with a four-hole 130° angled plate. The blade of the plate should as a rule be 20–25 mm longer than the length of the seating chisel, measured from its point of entry to its point of exit at the fracture. Check the reduction once again, and the freedom and range of movement of the hip joint.

Fig. 11.5

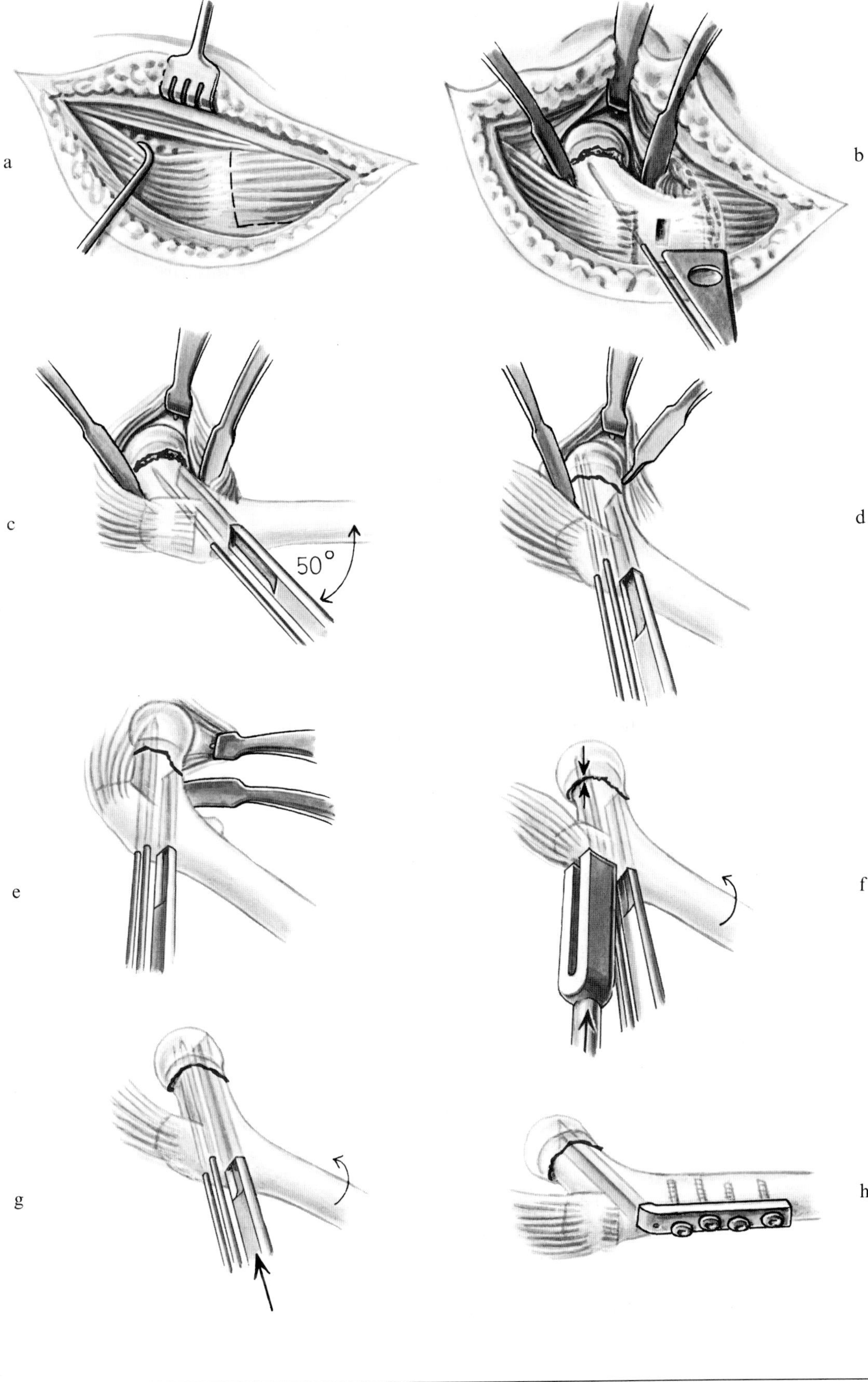

All femoral neck fractures in the younger age group with solid cancellous bone are reduced anatomically and fixed by large cancellous bone screws. Only in the rare instance of a vertical fracture in osteoporotic bone is valgus osteotomy and a fixation using the 120° angle blade plate considered. Inserting the seating chisel, the fragments should not be distracted. This complication can be avoided by predrilling the slot for the seating chisel.

In the older age group, optimal fixation is achieved using the 130° blade plate after having reduced the fracture anatomically and impacted the head on the neck. After this maneuver, the femoral head looks on the neck "like a hat on a hook" (Weber) and the implant has only the function of load sharing.

The steps of the technique using a 130° plate are described in Chap. 3. The recommended anterior arthrotomy in the direction of the long axis of the neck does not impair the blood supply to the head but gives a perfect view of the fracture and permits removal of the intracapsular hematoma. The DHS gives the weakest rotational stability. If used for femoral neck fracture it should be combined with an additional lag screw.

In patients with a life expectancy of less than 5 years, as well as in the rare association of femoral neck fracture and ipsilateral osteoarthritis of the hip joint, prosthetic replacement is preferred (femoral head prosthesis in the first case, total joint replacement in the second).

Fig. 11.6 Displaced subcapital fracture (B3.2).

a The fragments have been impacted with slight overcorrection into valgus and without retroversion. Fixation has been carried out with the four-hole 130° angled plate and two screws.
The blade of the plate has been inserted into the lower half of the head beneath the intersection of the tension and pressure trabecular systems.

b The same fracture treated with a DHS in combination with an additional cancellous bone screw. The function of this screw is only to block rotation. One may observe some backing out of the screw as sintering occurs and further impaction of the fragment takes place. This screw should, if possible, be inserted parallel to the large screw of the DHS.

Fig. 11.7

a A similar fracture treated with three large cancellous bone screws. Cannulated screws can also be used.

b In the presence of a vertical fracture plane, the shearing forces can be transformed into compressive forces carrying out an intertrochanteric valgus osteotomy of some 30°–40° and fixation with the double-angled 120° plate.

c Fractures of the base of the femoral neck in younger patients are best treated with two or three cancellous bone screws or large cannulated (cancellous) screws.

Fig. 11.6

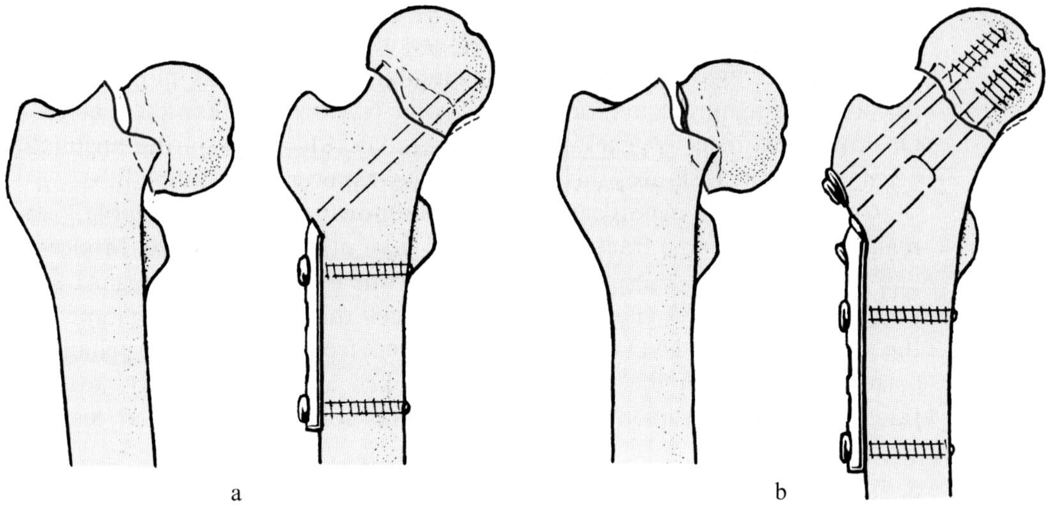

Fig. 11.7

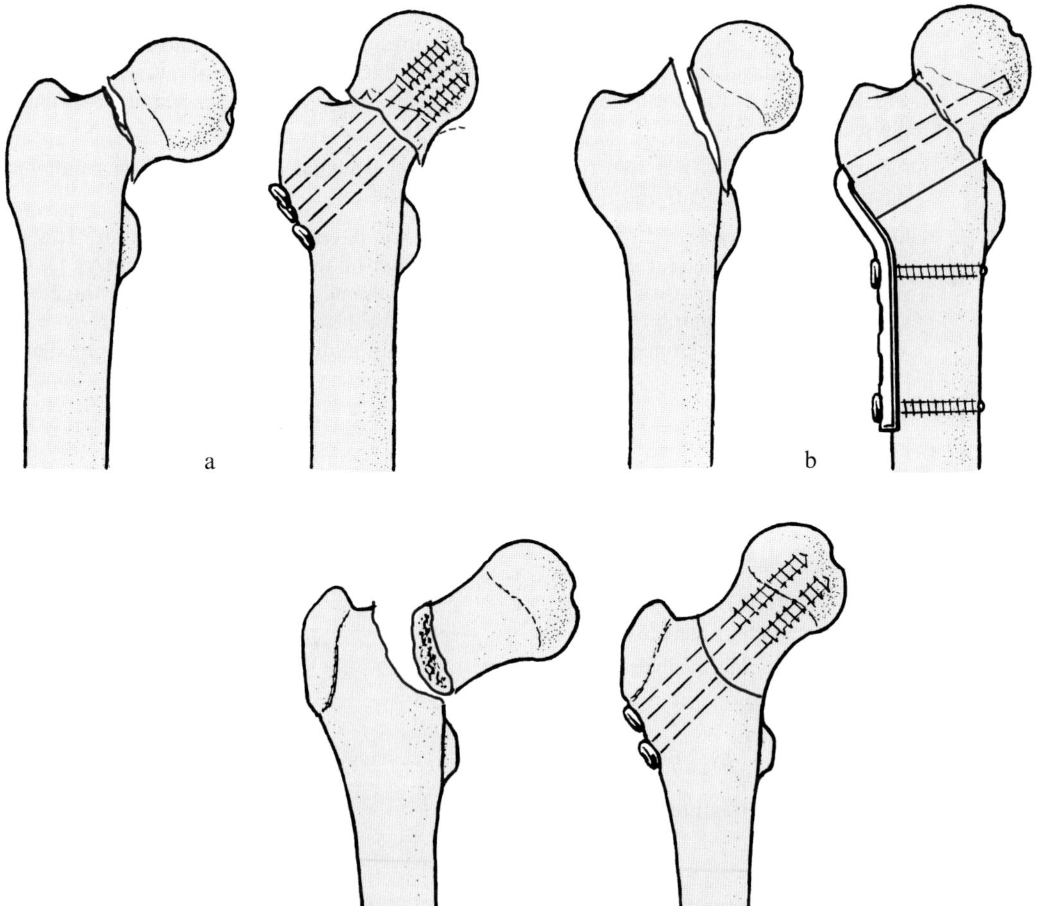

a

b

c

11.3 Fractures of the Trochanteric Region

Unlike the subcapital fractures, these are almost always extra-articular and therefore not associated with the danger of avascular necrosis. This most frequent fracture of the proximal femur occurs, on average, some 6 years later than the femoral neck fracture. Operative treatment is generally accepted today. Mortality during hospitalization is high because in many instances this fracture is the last event in a fading life.

Concerning the classification, the well-known definitions "stable" and "unstable" really mean that some fractures are easier than others to stabilize. Modern classifications aim at combining a descriptive and a prognostic evaluation with regard to actual fixation possibilities. The AO classification subdivides the trochanteric fractures as follows: In the simple fractures (A1) the fracture line runs from the greater trochanter to the medial cortex distally, with the medial cortex broken at one level only. In A2 fractures the fracture direction is identical but the medial cortex is broken at least on two levels.

Fig. 11.8 Trochanteric fractures.

Group A1 represents the simple two-part fractures. Subgroup A1.1 includes the fractures ending on the medial side just above the lesser trochanter. Subgroup A1.2 embraces all two-fragment fractures with impaction of the calcar into the distal fragment. Type A1.3 is in principle a two-part trochanterodiaphyseal fracture.

A2 fractures extend over two or more levels of the medial cortex. They are subdivided according to the number of fragments and the posterior fragmentation.

Group A3 is characterized by a fracture through the lateral cortex of the femur. The so-called reversed fracture runs from lateral distal to medial proximal of the lesser trochanter (A3.1). Quite often there is an undisplaced fracture separating the greater trochanter from the neck-head fragment. A3.2 fractures are true intertrochanteric fractures, occasionally with a lateral fracture of the proximal main fragment. A3.3 fractures are in principle A3.1 fractures with an additional fracture of the medial cortex including the lesser trochanter.

A1 Trochanteric, simple.
A1.1 Cervicotrochanteric.
A1.2 Pertrochanteric.
A1.3 Trochanterodiaphyseal.

A2 Pertrochanteric, multifragmentary.
A2.1 One intermediate fragment.
A2.2 Two intermediate fragments.
A2.3 More than two intermediate fragments.

A3 Intertrochanteric.
A3.1 Reversed, simple.
A3.2 Transverse, simple.
A3.3 With additional fracture of medial cortex.

Fig. 11.9

a Trochanteric two-fragment fracture.

b This fracture can be fixed with a condylar plate. The tip of the plate should be inserted into the lower portion of the femoral head, below the intersection of the tension and pression trabecular systems. The proximal cortex screw has been inserted as a lag screw into the calcar.

c This fracture can also be treated with a DCS.

Fig. 11.8

Fig. 11.9

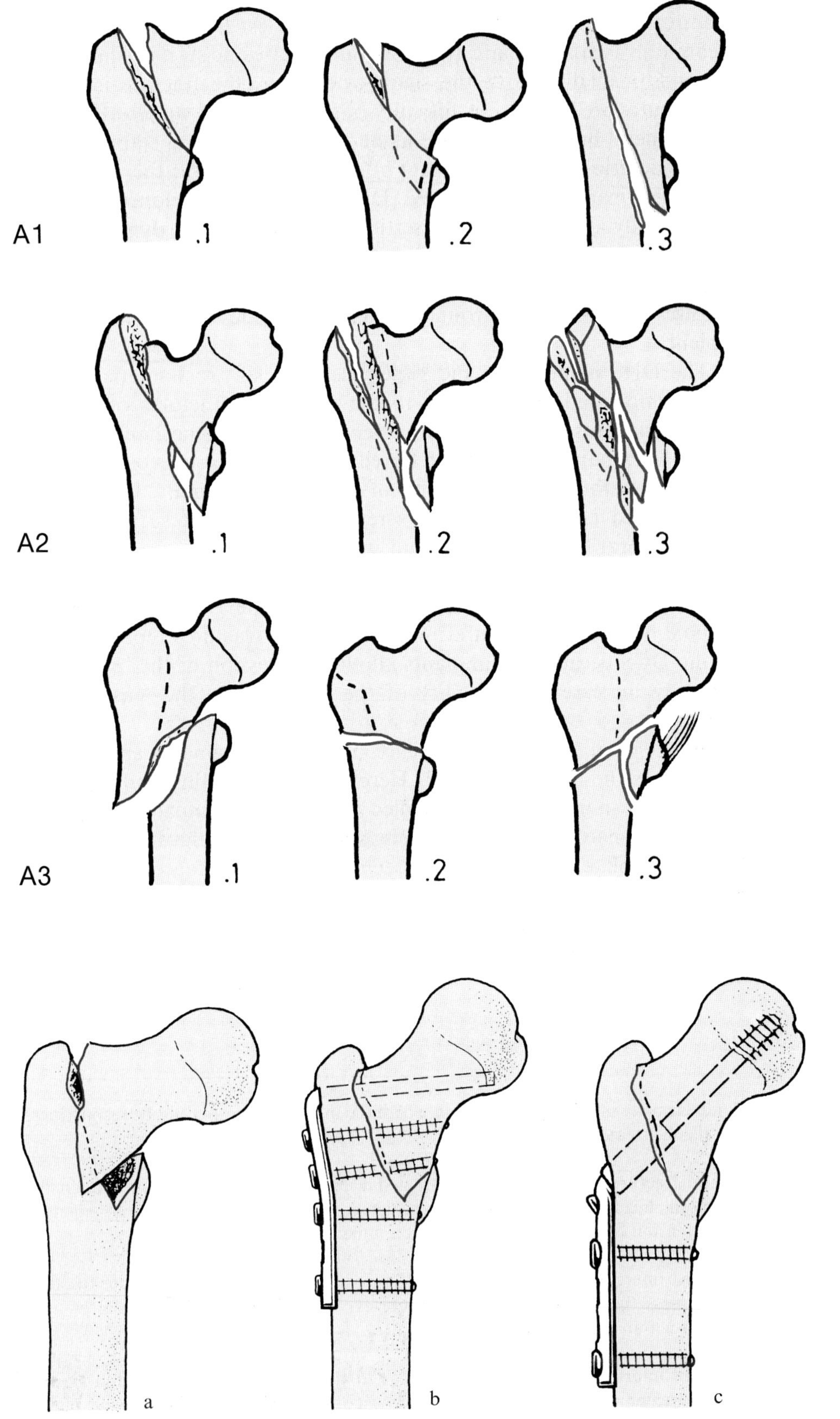

A3 fractures are those with a fracture of the lateral cortex. They are called intertrochanteric fractures when the fracture plane is more or less horizontal, the small trochanter being in continuity with the shaft. If the lateral fracture line starts distally to the small trochanter and ends medially above the small trochanter, the fracture is referred to as reversed. A3 fractures are known for difficulty of reduction and stabilization.

In general high demands are made on the mechanical stability of the internal fixation of trochanteric fractures. The AO offers three implants: the well-known 95° or condylar plate, the dynamic condylar screw (DCS), a recently developed implant similar in function to the condylar plate and in insertion technique to the dynamic hip screw (DHS), and finally the DHS itself, which allows controlled secondary impaction along the axis of the sliding screw. The 130° blade plate is no longer recommended for fresh trochanteric fractures on mechanical grounds, in view of the less favorable results obtained with this implant.

The DHS is indicated and widely used for all trochanteric fracture types, but there exists a more refined approach to the variety of fractures of the trochanteric area: in younger patients with bigger fragments and better mechanical quality of the femoral bone, the condylar plate is preferred, allowing a solid complex of implant and bone and thus anatomic reconstruction of the proximal femur. In principle, this can also be accomplished by the DCS. The screw of this implant sacrifices somewhat more bone in the femoral head and neck, and without an additional screw provides less rotational stability (against flexion or extension of the leg), but the application is somewhat easier. Suitable fractures for the condylar plate and the DCS are the A1.1 and A1.3 as well as some of the A2.1 fractures. Most of the A3 fractures represent very good indications for the DCS because the implants allow compression of the broken lateral cortex, which markedly increases the stability of the montage by the tension band function of the plate.

In older patients, in the presence of smaller fragments and more osteoporotic bone, the DHS is the favored implant. Here increased stability and early function at the price of some leg shortening by controlled axial fracture impaction are rated higher than leg length and anatomy. The previously recommended valgus resection osteotomy using the 130° blade plate for fixation has been abandoned because of its very high complication rate. Today such fractures are best treated with the DHS. In the presence of a short head-neck fragment, especially in A2.3 fractures, a femoral head prosthesis has to be considered (Delvaux and Putz 1987; Jensen 1980; Kyle et al. 1979; Larsson et al. 1988).

Fig. 11.10 Condylar plate in a fracture situation where the medial buttress could be reconstructed. The same fracture can also be treated with a DCS.

Fig. 11.11 Typical fracture morphology to be treated with a DHS. If the proximal main fragment is very short, a femoral head prosthesis can be considered. The main trochanteric fragment is fixed by means of a wire tension band. (The screw should be somewhat more distal.)

Fig. 11.12 Reversed intertrochanteric fracture (A3.1), fixation with DCS plate. Note the tension in the side plate to compress the fracture of the lateral cortex. For this reason the head screw is placed higher to gain distance within the proximal fragment.

Fig. 11.13 Reversed intertrochanteric fracture similar to that in Fig. 11.12 but with a typically displaced fracture of the greater trochanter. Fixation using a condylar plate. Again the side plate has to be tensioned. The fixation becomes more difficult when the fracture line of the greater trochanter runs more in the frontal plane. Note that again the blade is placed high in the proximal fragment.

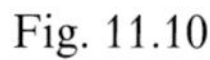

Fig. 11.10

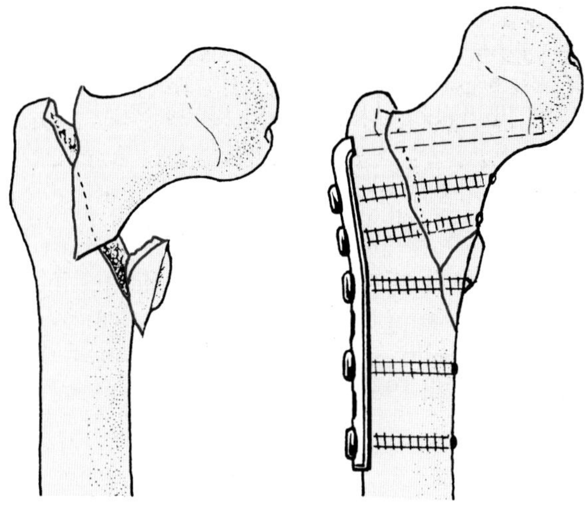

Fig. 11.11

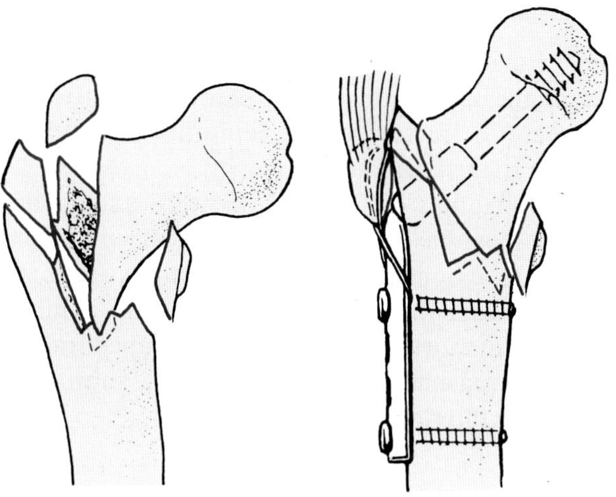

Fig. 11.12

Fig. 11.13

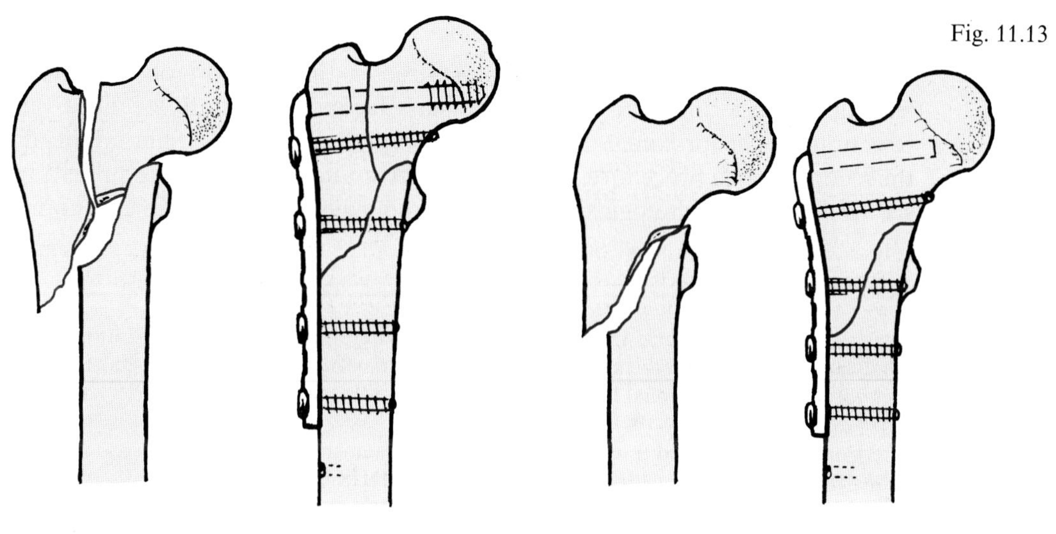

11.3.1 Subtrochanteric Fractures

Although the subtrochanteric fractures are classified as femoral shaft fractures, for some types, especially when the fracture extends into the trochanteric area, the condylar plate or the DCS are indicated. The current management of subtrochanteric fractures is representative for the change in the technique of internal fixation, namely the preference of indirect reduction techniques over the former anatomic reduction and careful medial reconstruction. Intramedullary nails and condylar plates are used as interlocking implants. In every case where the condylar plate is used, it must be tensioned using the articulated tension device. The AO distractor greatly facilitates indirect reduction without additional damage to the blood supply of the fracture area. With respect to the blood supply of the fragments, a cancellous bone graft is no longer required routinely as recommended previously (Kinast et al. 1989).

11.3.2 Fractures of the Proximal End of the Femur Combined with Ipsilateral Shaft Fractures

Femoral shaft fractures can be combined with neck fractures (shear type) or subtrochanteric fractures of the same side. The proximal fractures should be treated first, especially in the presence of a fracture of the femoral neck with its potential implications for the blood supply of the femoral head.

When screw fixation of the neck fracture and nailing of the femoral shaft fracture are planned, the possible interference of the two implants has to be anticipated.

Intertrochanteric or subtrochanteric fractures are treated either together with the shaft fracture, using a condylar plate or a DCS with a long side plate (up to 24 holes), or separately, using a short side plate for the upper fractures and a straight plate for the shaft fracture. Increasingly, combinations of a subtrochanteric with a shaft fracture are stabilized using an interlocking nail.

11.3.3 Metastatic Fractures of the Proximal Femur

The majority of these fractures are localized in the trochanteric-subtrochanteric region, leaving the neck and head of the femur unaffected. If they are localized very proximally, resection of the proximal fragment and replacement by a femoral head prosthesis is the recommended procedure. More distal metastatic involvement requires a tumor prosthesis. In certain morphological conditions, and especially when life expectancy is relatively

---

Fig. 11.14 Intertrochanteric transverse fracture with a small anterolateral fragment. Fixation with a tension band condylar plate, the blade being introduced high. Very often the separate fragment can be locked firmly and does not need additional fixation.

Fig. 11.15 Intertrochanteric reversed fracture with additional fragment of the medial cortex. Note the short fracture zone. If this is combined with severe osteoporosis, a DHS is the best implant.

Fig. 11.16 Same fracture with large fracture zone and good bone quality. This condition is best treated with a tension band condylar plate or DCS.

Fig. 11.14

Fig. 11.15

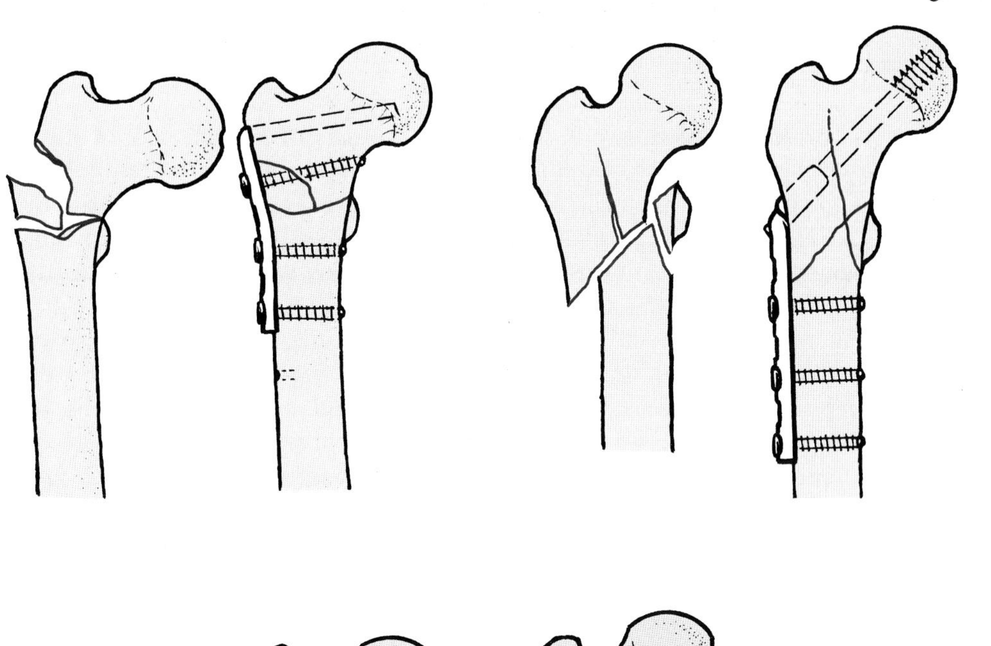

Fig. 11.16

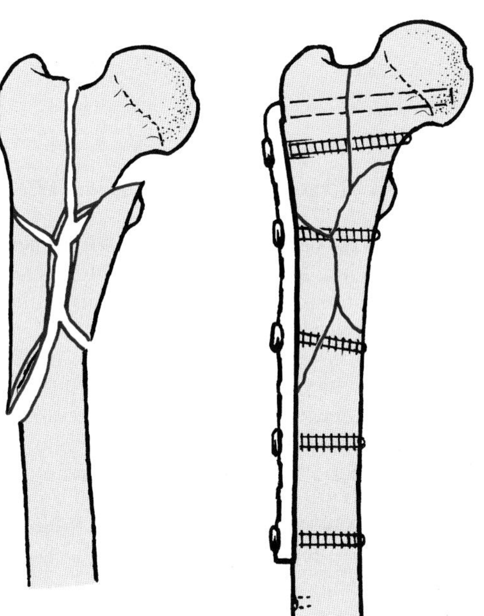

high, as in metastatic breast cancer, a reconstruction using a plate-cement complex with a condylar plate and a small intramedullary straight plate replacing the medial cortex may be considered.

11.4 Aftercare of Proximal Femur Fractures

A correct postoperative X-ray control consists of an AP view of the operated area and a cross-table lateral view of the most proximal part of the femur showing the position of the implant in the neck and head. The entire leg receives a slightly compressive dressing and is placed in a rubber foam splint to keep it in neutral position. Remobilization is normally started on the first postoperative day with bedside sitting, followed by walking first in a frame and then on crutches. Partial weight-bearing is allowed according to the stability achieved in the individual fracture; this decision also depends largely on the compliance of the patient. The patient begins isometric muscle exercises as soon as possible. Active straight leg raising should be avoided for the first 6 weeks. After this period, a second X-ray control and a clinical check-up are recommended. Special attention is then paid to the abductor musculature and exercises are recommended to strengthen it. Further control X-rays should be obtained at 12 weeks, if necessary at 24 weeks and finally at 52 weeks after surgery. Proximal femur fractures normally take 3–5 months to heal.

References

Bray TJ, Smith-Hoefer E, Hooper A, Timmermann L (1988) The displaced femoral neck fracture. Clin Orthop 230:127

Brumback RJ, Kenzora JE, Levitt LE, Burgess AR, Poka A (1987) Fractures of the femoral head. In: Brand RA (ed) The hip. Proceedings of the 14th open scientific meeting of the Hip Society

De Lee JC, Evans JA, Thomas J (1980) Anterior dislocation of the hip and associated femoral head fractures. J Bone Joint Surg [Am] 62:960

Delvaux D, Putz P (1987) L'ostéosynthèse des fractures de l'éxtremité proximale du fémur par vis-plaque à compression (DHS). Acta Orthop Belg 53:40

Epstein HC, Wiss DA, Cozen C (1985) Posterior fracture dislocation of the hip with fractures of the femoral head. Clin Orthop 201:9

Jensen JS (1980) Trochanteric fractures. An epidemiological, clinical and biomechanical study. Acta Orthop Scand [Suppl]:188

Kinast C, Bolhofner BR, Mast JW, Ganz R (1989) Subtrochanteric fractures of the femur: results of treatment with the 95° condylar blade-plate. Clin Orthop 238:122

Kyle RF, Gustilo RB, Prennar RF (1979) Analysis of 622 intertrochanteric hip fractures. J Bone Joint Surg [Am] 61:216

Larsson S, Elloy M, Hansson LJ (1988) Fixation of unstable trochanteric hip fractures. Acta Orthop Scand 59:658

Lanz T, Wachsmuth W (1972) Bein und Statik. Springer, Berlin Heidelberg New York, p 164 (Praktische Anatomie I/4)

Madsen F, Lunde F, Andersen E, Birke H, Hvass J, Poulsen TD (1987) Fixation of displaced femoral neck fractures. Acta Orthop Scand 58:212

Pipkin G (1957) Treatment of grade IV dislocation of the hip: a review. J Bone Joint Surg [Am] 39:1027

Resch H, Sperner G (1987) Vergleichende Ergebnisse komprimierender und nicht komprimierender Operationsmethoden nach medialer Schenkelhalsfraktur. Unfallchirurgie 13:308

Roeder LF, De Lee JC (1980) Femoral head fractures associated with posterior hip dislocations. Clin Orthop 147:221

Strömquist B, Hansson LJ, Nilson LT, Thorngren KG (1984) Two-year follow-up of femoral neck fractures. Acta Orthop Scand 55:521

12 FEMORAL SHAFT AND DISTAL FEMUR

12.1 Introduction

The advantages of early stable internal fixation have been particularly well demonstrated in the treatment of femur fractures. Not only is permanent impairment of knee function prevented by adequate aftertreatment, but fixation of femur fractures greatly reduces the pathophysiological sequelae of this severe injury, particularly if sustained by high energy impact. Nonoperative treatment requires traction for several weeks followed by a cast or brace. At the end of this time, full restoration of function in the knee joint may take months, if it succeeds at all, and malunion or delayed union is not a rare occurrence.

As a rule, therefore, we consider every fracture of the femur as an urgent indication for operative treatment. In femoral shaft fractures intramedullary nailing is the preferred method. Indications for medullary nailing have been extended by the introduction of the universal nail which may be used either conventionally or with the interlocking feature. The locked universal nail makes it possible to stabilize fractures extending beyond the "classical" middle third both proximally and distally, and is particularly indicated in complex fractures.

Where it is not possible to stabilize a fracture by medullary nailing, angle blade plates, broad dynamic compression plates (DCP and LC-DCP), dynamic hip screws and dynamic condylar screws may be indicated. As grade 2 and especially grade 3 open fractures should not be reamed, they are considered indications for either plating or stabilization by external fixation. Straight plates are placed on the dorsal lateral aspect of the bone, thus acting as tension bands, provided there is bony support opposite to the plate. To accelerate union, medial bone grafting is recommended in all cases because even well reduced and adapted cortices will undergo micromovements which may lead to bone resorption and also cause fatiguing of the plate.

For open as well as closed reduction of femoral shaft fractures, the AO distractor has proven particularly useful in both nailing and plating. It helps to gently reduce the fragments "indirectly" and to minimize additional soft tissue stripping. In plating, the vastus lateralis muscle should only be detached from the bone as far as necessary to place the plate onto the femur. Once correct axial and rotational alignment is obtained, the plate has only to maintain this position. Within about 6–8 weeks after such "gentle" plating, undisturbed medial fragments will be integrated into a large callus mass in a very similar way to that which occurs with closed locked nailing.

For both intramedullary nailing and plating, we prefer the patient to be positioned on his side. The supine position may be preferable for the multiply injured patient or for treatment of bilateral lesions to the lower limbs, as it allows two teams to work simultaneously.

As explained in Chap. 6, stabilization of femur fractures should be carried out as early as possible after injury, especially in polytraumatized patients. In rare instances of unavoidable delay, the patient may be kept in traction until conditions are satisfactory for surgery. Traction should be skeletal through the distal condyles or, preferably, the tibial tubercle. The weight used should not exceed one-tenth of the body weight. Some overdistraction of the fragments may be useful prior to surgery.

12.2 Subtrochanteric Fractures of the Femoral Shaft

Subtrochanteric fractures may be treated by use of the condylar blade plate, the condylar screw or the universal nail with interlocking. To use the interlocking nail, the most proximal fracture line must be at least 2 cm distal to the lesser trochanter.

12.2.1 Technique of Condylar Plate Fixation of the Proximal Femoral Shaft

A 20-cm lateral incision is made as shown in Fig. 12.1 and the soft tissues are entered posteriorly to vastus lateralis, reflecting this muscle forward. A Kirschner wire is placed on the anterior surface of the femoral neck which indicates both the neck-shaft angle and the anteversion of the femoral neck and helps to appropriately place the seating chisel for the condylar plate.

Fig. 12.1 The surgical approach to the femur.

1 The straight incision for intramedullary nailing begins at the tip of the greater trochanter and is extended upwards.

2 The proximal straight lateral incision is the standard approach to the proximal femur with reflection of vastus lateralis. It is used for fractures or intertrochanteric osteotomies.

3 The straight lateral incision for the shaft follows an imaginary line from the tip of the greater trochanter to the lateral epicondyle. It is sometimes referred to as the mailbox incision because vastus lateralis is lifted upwards and forwards like a lid. All perforators are carefully ligated to keep the blood loss to a minimum. An anterior transmuscular approach leads to scarring and binding down of the quadriceps and may damage the blood supply and nerve supply to vastus lateralis.

4 The approach to the distal femur. If in addition there is a tangential fracture of the medial condyle, then a second medial parapatellar incision (5) is necessary.

Fig. 12.1

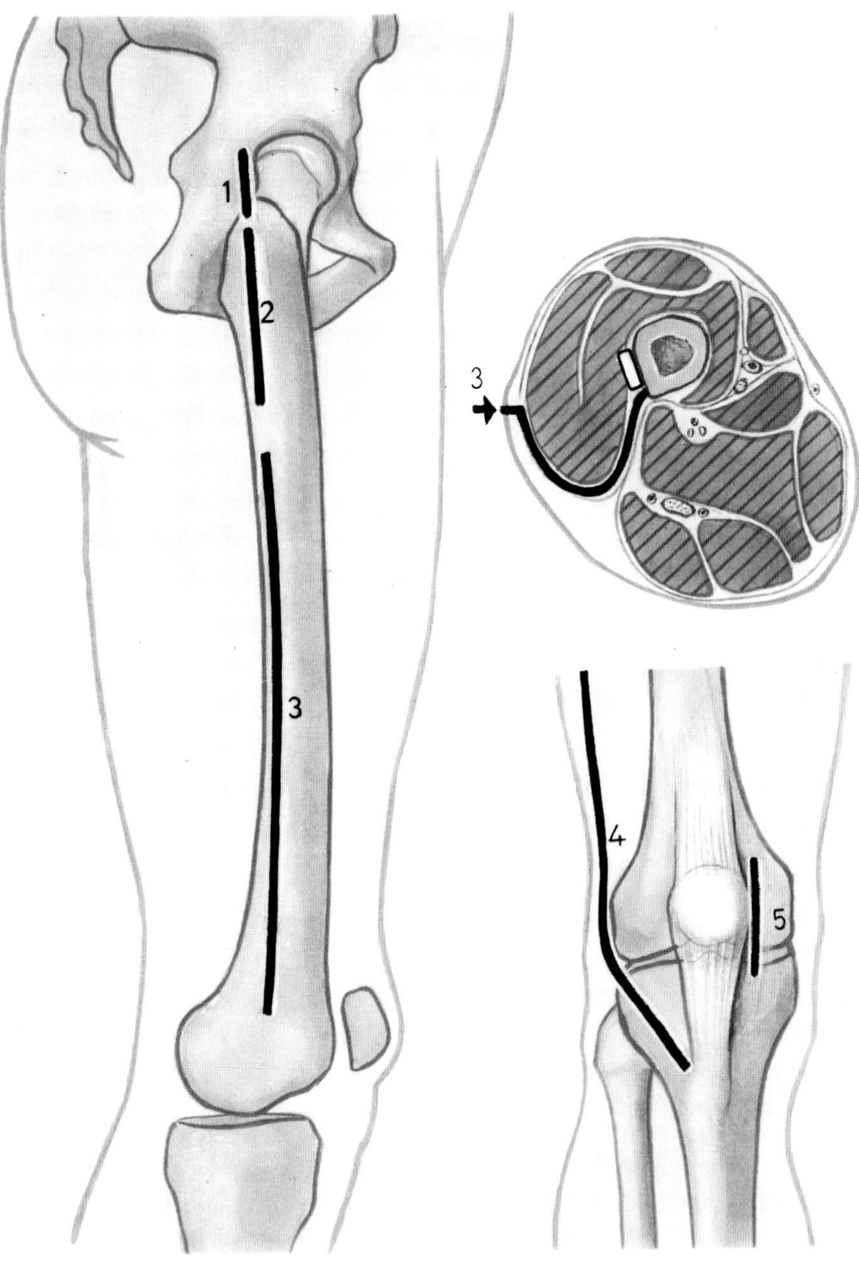

The proximal fragment should be fixed by the blade and additionally by one or two proximal screws which should go into the calcar (Fig. 12.2). Before a hole is drilled into the calcar, the 3.2-mm drill guide should be inserted deep into the 4.5-mm hole to prevent the drill bit from sliding along the slope of the calcar. The additional screw(s) in the proximal fragment very significantly improve(s) the proximal fixation of the condylar plate. Once the reduction of the fracture is complete, axial compression is applied either by using the self-compressing principle of the DCP or LC-DCP or, better, by first using the articulated tension device at the distal end of the plate.

In simple fractures, a plate-independent lag screw in the AP direction will already have secured reduction prior to axial compression, but this reduction has to be checked before inserting all necessary remaining screws as determined by the preoperative planning. In fractures with butterfly fragments, the major fragments are first reduced, for example with a temporary cerclage wire, and then fixed with one or two lag screws before axial compression is applied.

Fig. 12.2

a Internal fixation of a 32-A2 fracture: reduction, insertion of lag screw (1), insertion of the Kirschner guide wires (see Chap. 3), opening of the cortex for the condylar plate, insertion of the condylar plate (2), insertion of cortex screw into calcar (3), and axial compression (4).

b Internal fixation of a 32-B2 fracture: reduce the butterfly and fix it to either the proximal or the distal fragment with a lag screw (1). Reduce the main fragments and maintain temporary reduction with bone clamps. Insert the seating chisel and the blade of the condylar plate (2) into the neck. Triangulate the fixation in the calcar with cortex screws (3) and apply compression either with the articulated tension device or with the DCP (4). Insert the proximal screw (5) and then complete the fixation by inserting the remaining screws.

b′ Internal fixation of a 32-B3 fracture with medial butterfly: note the two plate-independent lag screws.

General remark on all three cases illustrated: Axial compression has been instituted by means of the articulated tension device putting the condylar plate under preload, counteracting the anticipated bending stresses on the plate from muscular activity and weight-bearing.

It has to be noted that these subtrochanteric fractures would have also lent themselves to the application of the DCS.

Fig. 12.2

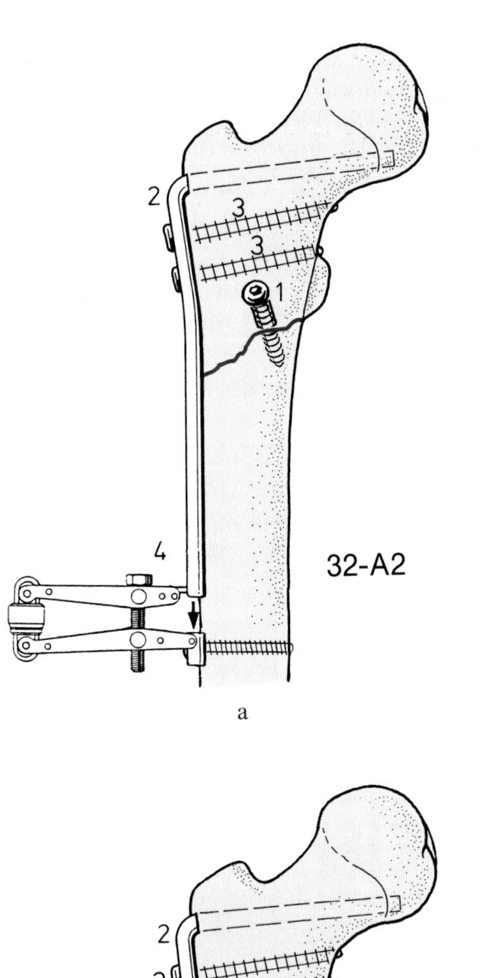

a

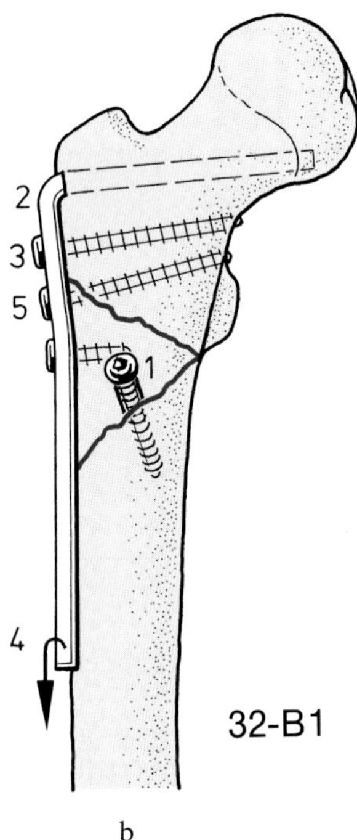

b

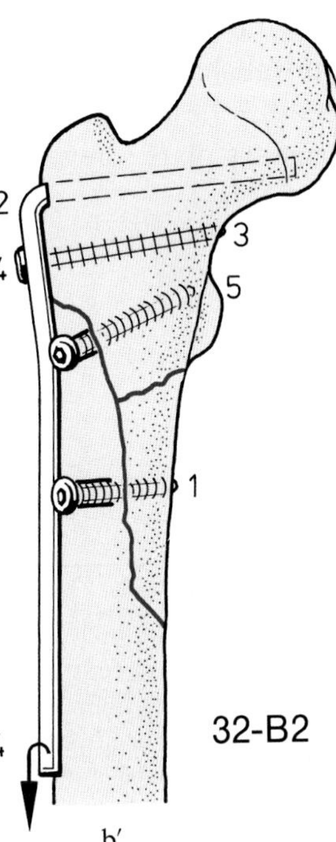

b′

12.2.2 Fixation of Subtrochanteric Fractures with the Dynamic Condylar Screw (DCS)

For illustration of step-by-step procedure, see Fig. 3.51.

The patient is in a supine position. The approach is the same as for the condylar plate, dorsal to vastus lateralis. If necessary, the insertion of vastus lateralis at the innominate tubercle is partly cut, leaving about 1 cm of the tendinous insertion for the subsequent reattachment. The fracture is exposed and reduced. In simple two-part fractures, a lag screw can be inserted in the AP direction and used as a first means of fixation. The axis of the femoral neck in terms of anteversion and neck-shaft angle is determined by placing the Kirschner wire on the anterior aspect of the femoral neck.

The guide pin is inserted using the DCS angle guide at the entry point determined preoperatively using templates on the AP X-ray. This lies at the intersection of the anterior and the middle third of the trochanteric bulge.

In the axial view, the guide pin is parallel to the Kirschner wire placed on the femoral neck. The tip of the guide pin lies about 2 cm away from the articular surface in the lower half of the femoral head, and the drill hole is made with the triple DCS reamer to the corresponding depth. If the guide pin is inadvertently withdrawn, it must be reinserted in the manner described for the dynamic hip screw technique in Chap. 3.

In hard cancellous bone, the screw thread is precut with the tap using the shorter of the two centering sleeves. To avoid rotation of the head, the proximal fragment must be firmly secured by a small Steinmann pin during tapping and lag screw insertion. The DCS is then inserted using the longer of the two centering sleeves. The T handle of the wrench must be parallel to the femoral shaft at the end of the screw insertion to allow the plate barrel to slip correctly over the screw shaft. The plate is aligned to the femoral shaft. The two proximal screws are inserted across the calcar using the same technique as described for the blade. The distal part of the side plate is then fixed with the necessary plate screws, whereby compression may be added.

Fig. 12.3

a This 32-C1 fracture is first reduced by means of the distractor and then fixed either by a condylar plate (illustrated in the figure) or with a DCS.

If at all possible begin by reducing and fixing the proximal lateral butterfly with a lag screw (1). Insert the seating chisel and then the condylar plate (2), insert the cortex screws into the calcar (3) and drill the 4.5-mm hole through the second hole of the condylar plate and insert the connecting bolt (4). Insert the distractor (5) and begin the distraction (6). Reduce the fracture. As soon as you have achieved axial continuity either medially or laterally, place the plate under tension. Fix the plate to the shaft with a short screw (7) and check the axial alignment. Insert the lag screw, if this has not already been done (8), and then the short and long screws (9) to fix the plate to the shaft and complete the fixation. A medial cancellous onlay graft is recommended.

b Fixation of this 32-C3 fracture does not aim at complete anatomic reconstruction but leaves the medial fragments as undisturbed as possible. Again the reduction is facilitated by the use of the distractor. If medial fragments remain in continuity with muscle, a cancellous onlay graft is not necessary.

Fig. 12.3

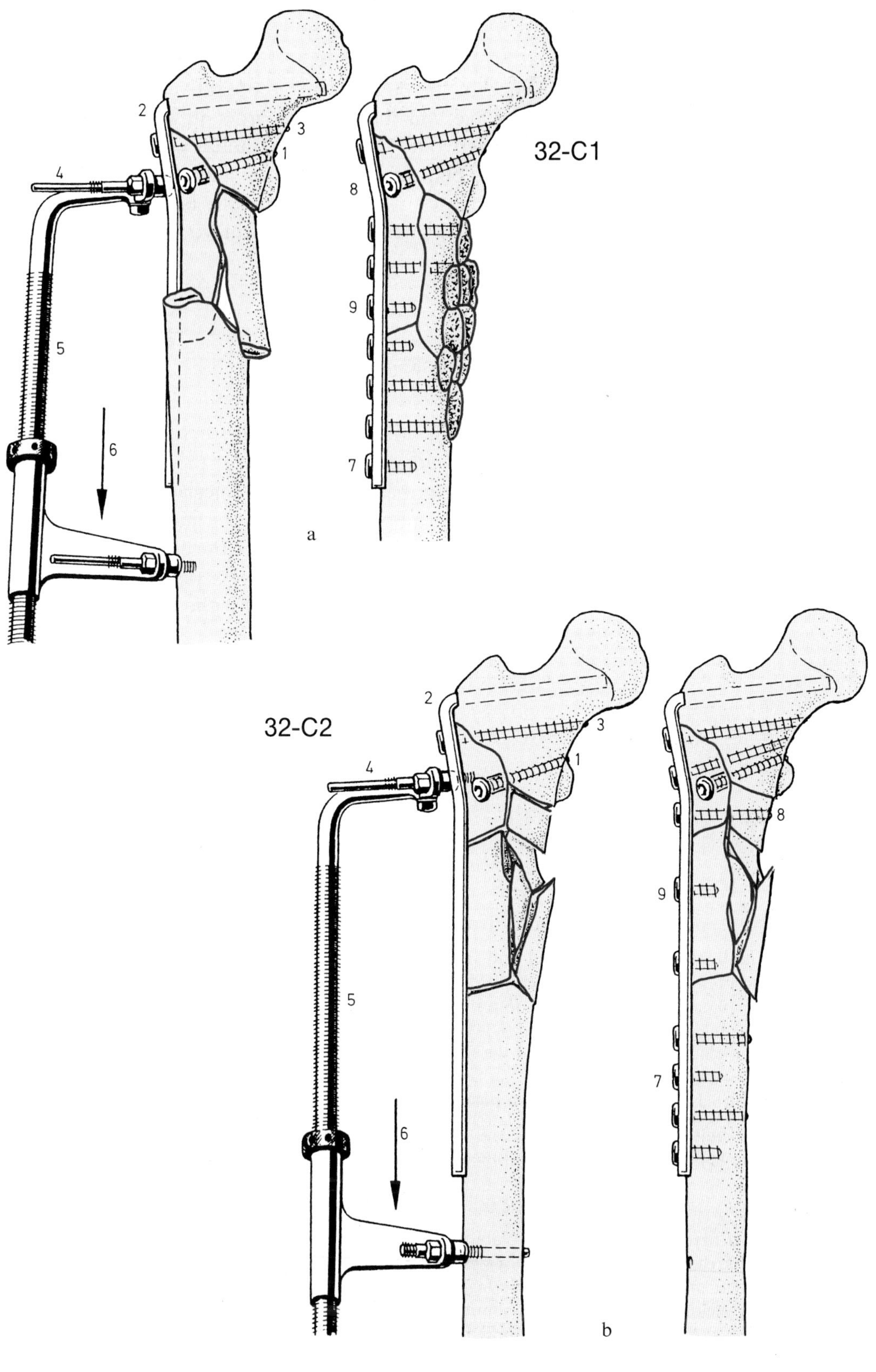

In very complex fractures, the condylar blade plate or the condylar screw is inserted into the proximal fragment prior to reduction. Gentle reduction without disturbing any additional fragments may then be undertaken with the aid of the femoral distractor. The reduction should be planned on a drawing of the femur made from an X-ray of the normal side. As outlined in the chapter on preoperative planning, one should draw the different fragments in place and indicate the order in which the reduction and the internal fixation will be carried out. In complex fractures, length and rotation should be carefully restored with the help of the distractor and the fragments should then be bridged by either a condylar plate or condylar screw. It is more important to maintain soft tissue attachments to all fragments than to achieve perfect anatomical reduction in this situation.

12.2.3 Technique of Inserting the Universal Interlocking Nail

Subtrochanteric fractures in which the most proximal fracture line is at least 2 cm distal to the intact lesser trochanter are suitable indications for the universal nail with interlocking. The general technique is described in Chap. 4. Special attention must be given to the positioning of the patient. In most institutions, the patient is placed on a fracture table suitable for intra-operative fluoroscopy in either the supine or the lateral decubitus position. Alternatively, the patient may be placed on a regular operating table and the large femoral distractor used for reduction, whereby the fragments usually "fall into place".

Fig. 12.4 Simple subtrochanteric fracture fixed with a condylar plate.

The fracture is first reduced and fixed with a lag screw. The blade of the plate must be inserted into the neck at a point pre-determined from the preoperative drawing. A cortex screw is inserted through the plate into the calcar to improve the fixation of the plate in the proximal fragment. The second proximal cortex screw functions as a lag screw. This second screw is inserted only after the plate has been placed under tension and the fracture under axial compression.

Fig. 12.5 Subtrochanteric fracture with a butterfly.

The butterfly is first reduced and fixed with lag screws to the main fragment. The condylar plate is then applied. Note that some of the screws are short.

Fig. 12.6 A very complex subtrochanteric fracture with a deficient medial buttress.

As a first step, the condylar plate is inserted into the proximal fragment and fixed with cortex screws to the calcar. The distractor provides indirect reduction of the different fragments. These should preferably be left undisturbed but may be lagged across the plate. Finally an extensive cancellous graft is carried out medially. Weight-bearing should be kept at 8–10 kg for the first 6–8 weeks. During this time, the bone graft will usually form a bridge medially. Weight-bearing can then increase.

General comment on Figs. 12.4–12.6: These subtrochanteric and high femoral shaft fractures would lend themselves to fixation by a DCS but application of the condylar plate gives adequate fixation.

Fig. 12.4

Fig. 12.5

Fig. 12.6

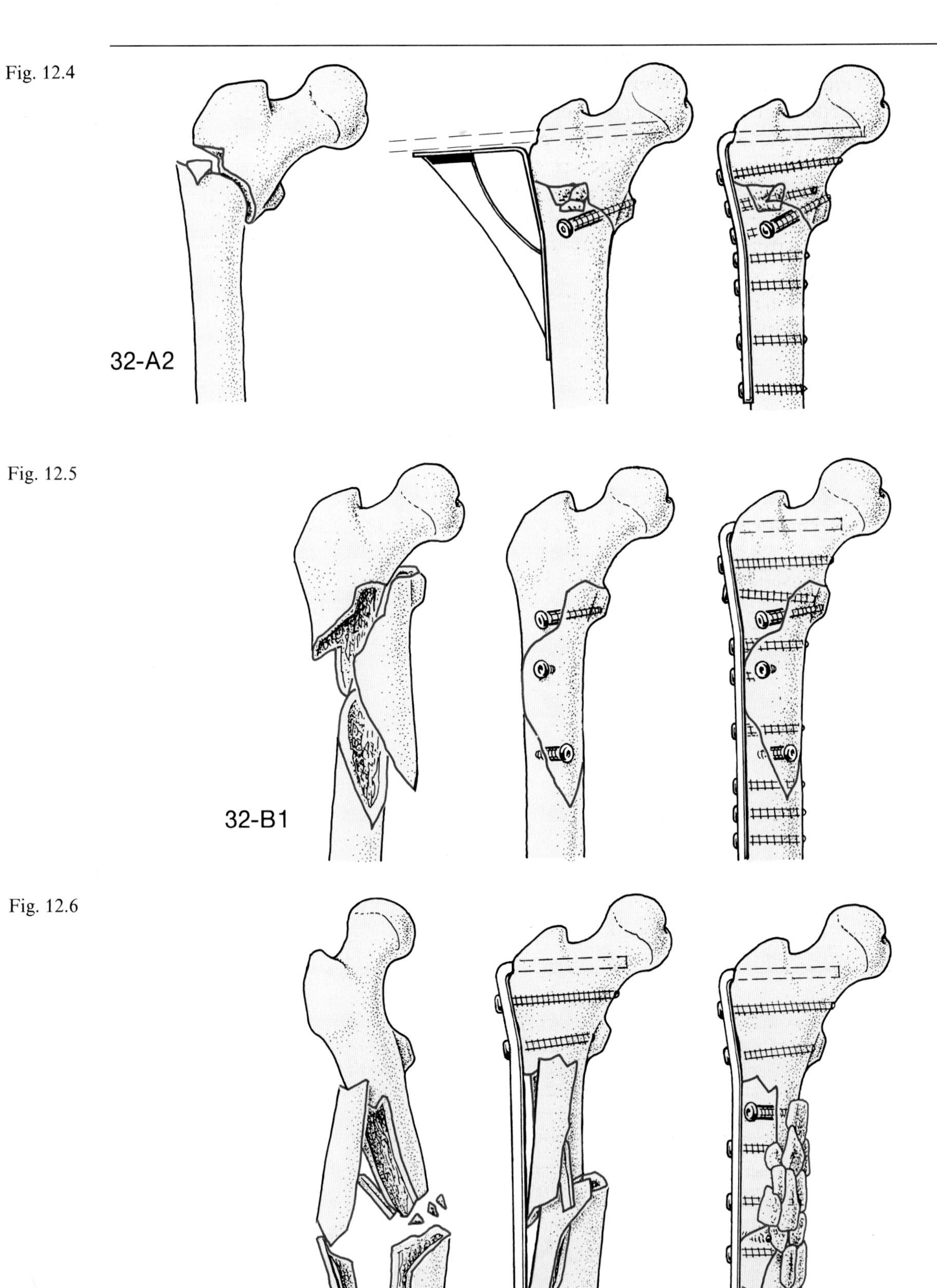

Fig. 12.7 A 32-C3 fracture.

a Such complex fractures should not be approached with anatomic reconstruction in mind because the blood supply of the main fragments must be carefully respected.

b Reduction of length and axis should be carried out by means of the articulated tension device, which is used in this particular case for distraction. Very careful introduction of a preliminary circular wire may be carried out without interfering too much with the blood supply of the fragments, but it only provides good axial positioning of the proximal main fragment.

c, d The rest of the fragments are left undisturbed and screws are only inserted where either the proximal or the distal main fragment offers good hold. In this particular case there is very rapid formation of a large mass of callus thanks to the preservation and/or rapid restoration of blood supply to the cortical fragments. This case shows the successful application of the DCS.

Fig. 12.7

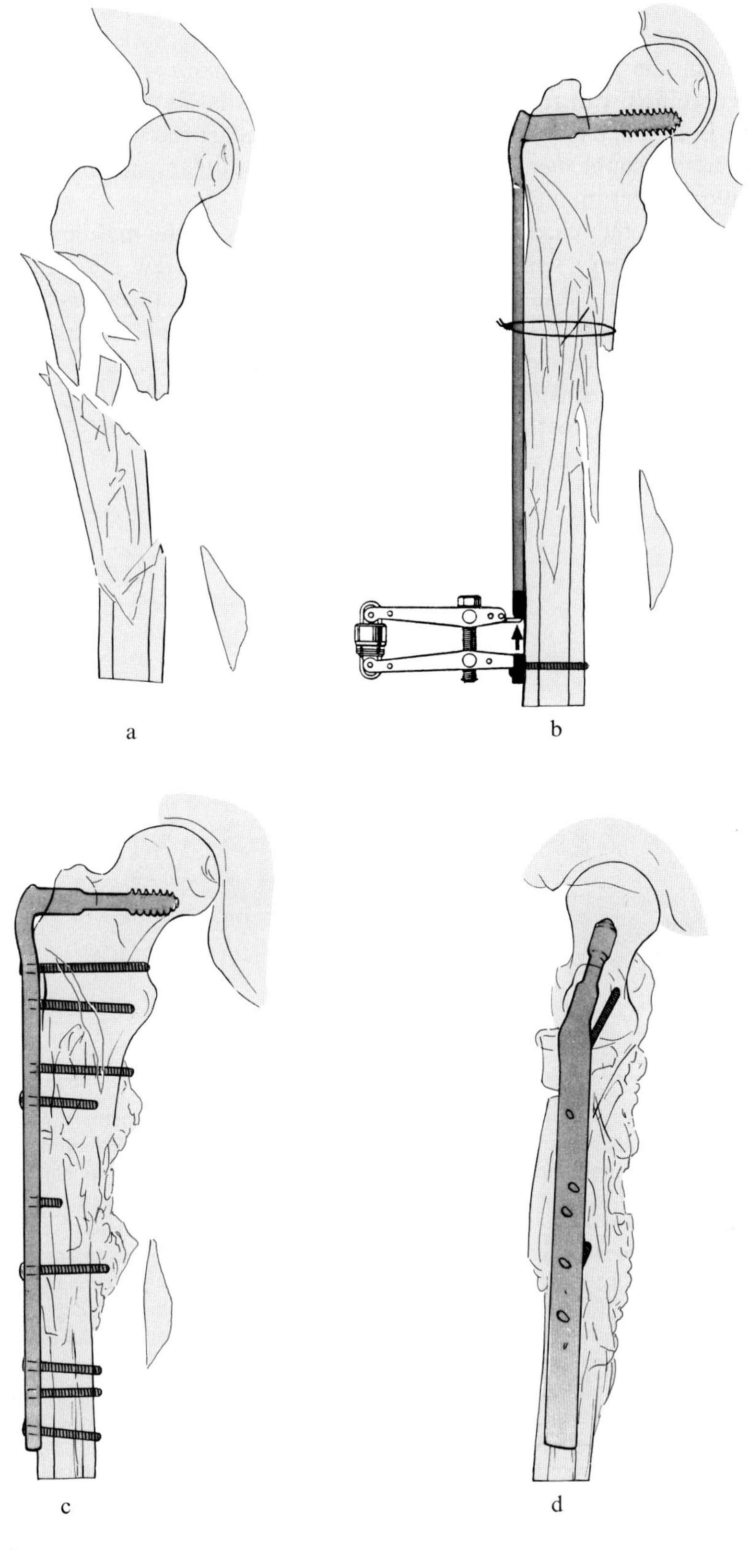

12.3 Fractures of the Middle Third of the Femoral Shaft

The middle third of the femur is the real domain of the intramedullary nail. Nailing is combined with reaming of the medullary canal as described in Chap. 4. The universal nail is used in its locked mode to stabilize complex fractures. We therefore now discourage the use of supplementary plating with intramedullary nailing as advocated in the second edition of this manual.

If for some reason, types A and B fractures of the middle third are fixed with plates, interfragmentary application of at least one lag screw across the plate or independent of the plate is recommended and an autogenous cancellous bone graft on the medial aspect of the femur is mandatory (Fig. 12.8). In type C fractures, the different fragments should not be denuded in an attempt to reduce them anatomically or by adding bone grafts. Length and rotation are restored using only the distractor, and a bridging plate is then applied to the posterolateral aspect of the femur. Any major fragment should be stabilized by a lag screw, preferably across the plate.

Fig. 12.8 There will always be indications for plating in short oblique fractures which in themselves would be ideal for medullary nailing, as there are circumstances which make nailing difficult or time consuming, particularly in polytrauma patients. A sound knowledge of how to plate such fractures is therefore necessary. In this particular case, a broad DCP has been applied with *one* interfragmentary lag screw. A 4.5-mm shaft screw, if available, will give the best interfragmentary compression and stability and should therefore be used. A cancellous onlay graft to the opposite cortex is strongly recommended even if the latter appears completely restored, as is still likely that some resorption of the opposite cortex may lead to minimal interfragmentary instability. Resulting repeated bending stresses of the plate might lead to plate fatigue. This should be prevented by a rapid build-up of periosseous callus on the opposite cortex induced by the onlay graft.

Deposit of cancellous bone when treating femoral shaft fractures by plating is particularly advocated in the rare cases where such a procedure is chosen for 32-A2 and 32-A3 fractures. If resorption occurs between the fragment ends, bending stress on the plate is concentrated on a very small area and fatigue fracture is much more likely to occur than if the bending stress on the plate is distributed over a long distance, such as in a bridge or wave plate. Application of such modifications in very short fractures is, however, not recommended, and therefore the alternative is the onlay graft!

Fig. 12.9 This 32-B3 fracture with comminution of the distal fragment is best treated by closed intramedullary nailing by means of the universal interlocking nail.

Fig. 12.8

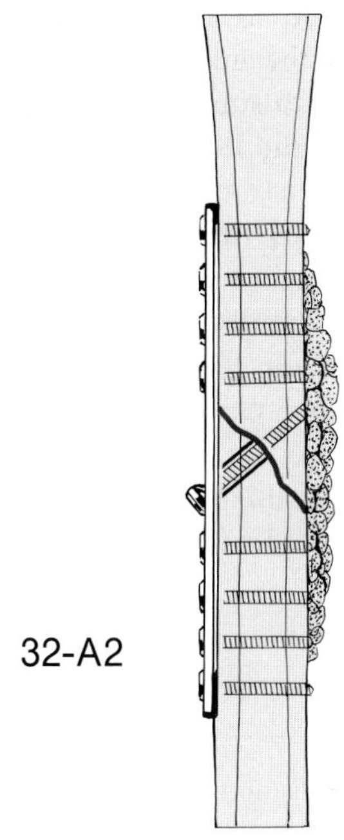

Fig. 12.9

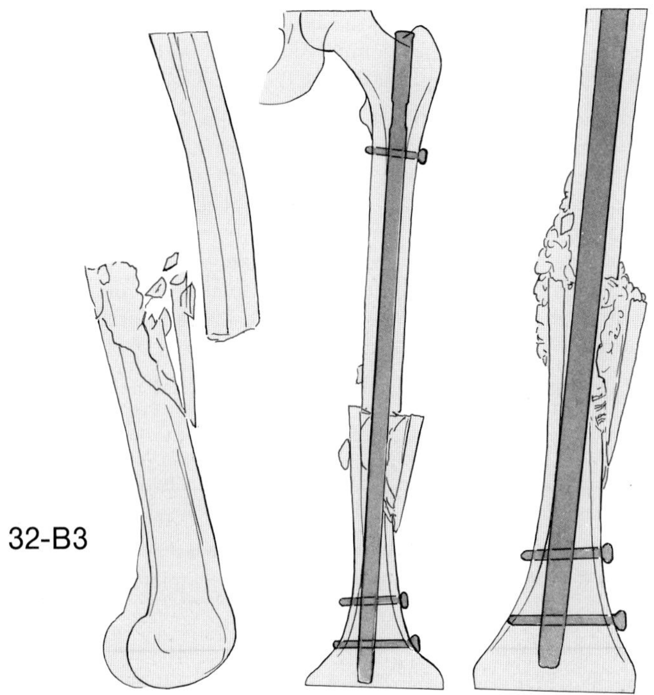

12.4 Extra-Articular Fractures of the Distal Femur

In the distal femur, the medullary canal flares like a trumpet. A regular nail fails to provide sufficient hold on the distal fragment even if the canal is not reamed. These fractures are, therefore, an indication for the use of the interlocking mode of the universal nail. As a rule, the nail used should be one that fits the isthmus without reaming. Restricted reaming is only indicated if the isthmus of the femur is very narrow.

A condylar blade plate (95°) or the DCS may be preferred in a number of cases, particularly in very distal fractures with medial fragmentation, and if intra-articular extension is suspected. It should be combined with lag screws in spiral fractures.

The use of the condylar blade plate together with the necessary instruments and the correct insertion of the seating chisel parallel to the knee joint and in line with the long axis of the femur is described in Chap. 3. The use of the distractor may often facilitate fracture reduction. Restoration of the medial cortex by this indirect reduction is very often successfully achieved without damage to the blood supply.

Fig. 12.10 Internal fixation of fractures of the distal femur illustrating various 33A and 33B fractures.

A1: An avulsion fracture of the proximal insertion of the medial collateral ligament has been fixed with a 4.0-mm cancellous bone screw with a washer.

A2: Simple supracondylar fracture. Reduction and fixation with Kirschner wires. Open the cortex for the insertion of the seating chisel. With the aid of the condylar guide, insert the Kirschner guide wires and then insert the seating chisel. Use the five-hole condylar blade plate with a 50- or 60-mm blade. Be sure to supplement the fixation of the blade in the distal fragment by the insertion of one or two cancellous bone screws. Apply axial compression either with an articulated tension device or by making use of the self-compressing principle of the DCP or LC-DCP.

A3: Supracondylar fracture combined with a complex fracture of the distal shaft. Do not attempt a reduction; position the patient supine with the knee at 90°. Insert the guide wires. Open the lateral cortex for the insertion of the seating chisel and then insert the seating chisel parallel to the knee joint with the seating chisel guide parallel to what is taken as the long axis of the femur. Insert a 9- or a 12-hole condylar plate. Forcibly bend the knee over the knee support. This applies traction to the shaft. While this traction is maintained, fix the plate with one screw to the proximal fragment. Check the rotational alignment. Do not attempt an anatomic reduction of the multiple fragments but leave them alone with their soft tissue attachments intact. Instead of reduction carry out very extensive cancellous bone grafting.

Note: For these examples of 33-A2 and 33-A3 fractures, the DCS would have been a very adequate alternative implant.

B1 (left): Fracture of the lateral condyle. In the young adult, carry out anatomic reduction and temporary fixation with a Kirschner wire. Then fix the fracture with two cancellous bone screws with long threads. The washers are used to prevent the sinking of the screw heads through the cortex.

B1 (right): If the bone is osteoporotic use a T plate as a buttress plate. Reduce the fracture, fix it temporarily with Kirschner wires, carefully contour the T plate and then fix the fracture with two cancellous bone screws.

B2: Fracture of the lateral condyle with a long proximal extension. If the bone is very osteoporotic, reduce the fracture, keep it reduced with a reduction clamp and then carefully contour a long T plate and use it as a buttress plate. Insert whichever screws you can as lag screws.

B3: Tangential posterior fracture of one or both condyles (Hoffa fracture). Fix the fracture with 6.5-mm cancellous bone screws with 16-mm threads. Insert the screws in the AP direction at right angles to the femoral shaft axis. Insert the screws as far laterally as possible to avoid the articular cartilage. If this is impossible, countersink the heads below the articular cartilage.

Fig. 12.10

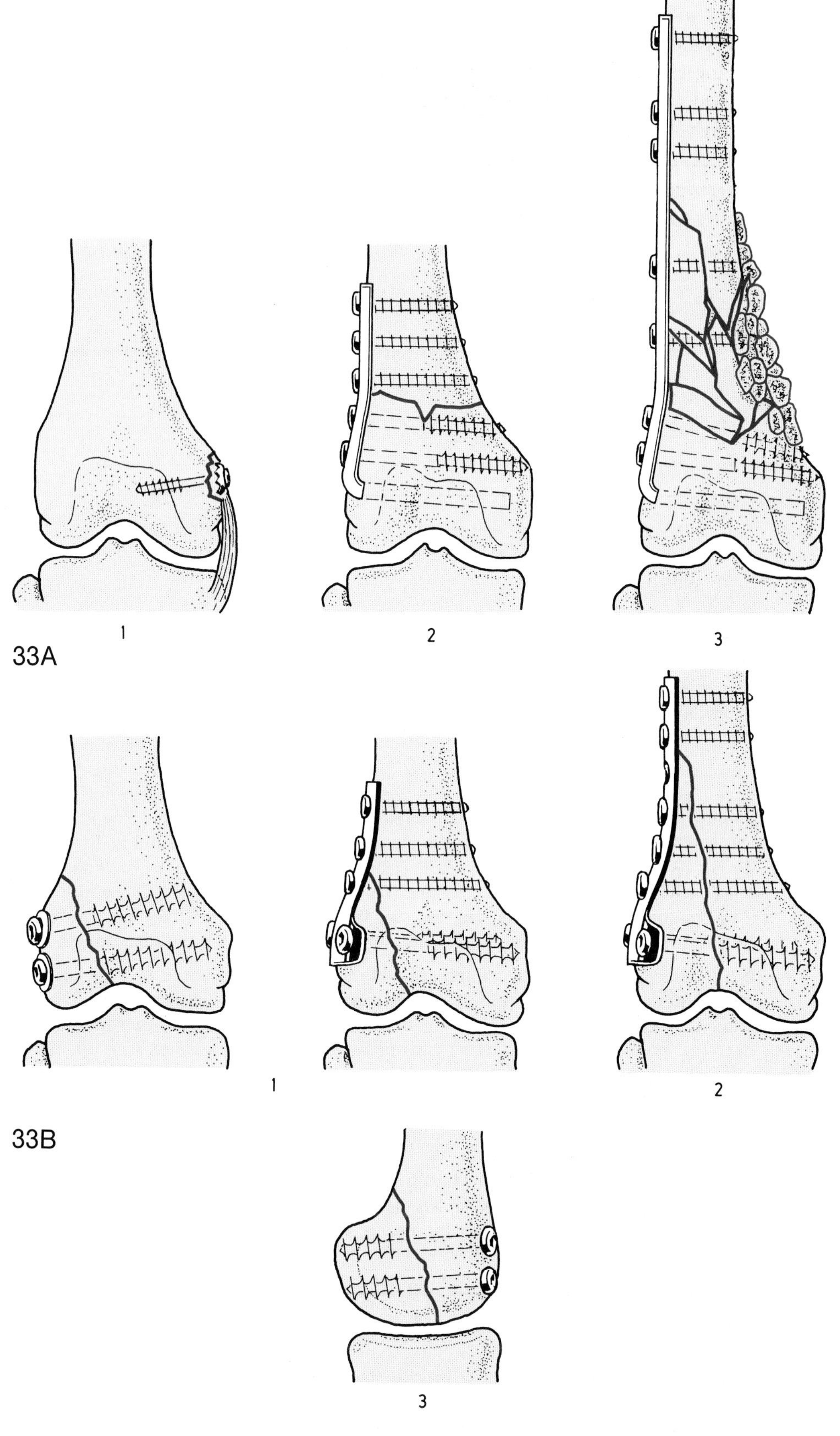

The DCS is a very good alternative to the condylar blade plate. Provided the entry point of the screw is correctly chosen, it allows easier alignment of the side plate with the femoral shaft. In fractures with condylar fragmentation (types C1 and C2), the use of a DCS is particularly recommended. The lag screw effect of the dynamic condylar screw provides interfragmentary compression and thus increased stability. The application of the DCS is detailed in Fig. 3.50.

For condylar fractures (types B1, B2 and B3), screw fixation, occasionally with a buttressing 4.5-mm T plate, is sufficient. For very complex condylar fractures (type C3), the use of the heavy condylar buttress plate is recommended (Fig. 11.12).

Fig. 12.11 This 33-A3 fracture has been successfully treated by application of a DCS.

Fig. 12.12 Internal fixation of examples of 33-C fractures.

For C1 and C2 fractures, the condylar plate as well as the dynamic condylar screw are very suitable implants. Very hard, young bone presents problems when hammering in the seating chisel and the condylar plate. Both implants, if placed correctly, allow immediate mobilization and give very good results if the patient is placed in the 90/90/90 position immediately after internal fixation. An alternative is the immediate institution of continuous passive motion for such cases.

C1: Supracondylar fracture or so-called T or Y fracture. Determine the point of entry for the seating chisel. Reduce the condyles with the knee flexed to 90°. Occasionally a few comminuted cortical fragments have to be disimpacted and elevated out of the metaphysis. Temporarily fix with Kirschner wires and then carry out the fixation of the intercondylar fracture with two long threaded cancellous screws with washers. Take care not to obstruct the site of entry for the seating chisel and make sure that the threads do not cross the fracture. As the seating chisel is driven in parallel to the knee joint axis, the assistant must provide counter-pressure medially. This fracture can also be treated in a manner similar to the simple supracondylar fracture, i.e., the supracondylar component of the fracture can be reduced prior to the insertion of the seating chisel. This makes it possible to use the condylar guide.

C2: Bicondylar fracture with comminution of the distal shaft. Operate with the knee bent to 90°. Carefully reduce the joint fragments and elevate all depressed metaphyseal fragments. The condyles are reduced and fixed with lag screws as in C1 fractures. The condylar screw of appropriate length is then inserted over the guide wire which is strictly parallel to the sagittal knee axis. With the knee forcibly flexed to apply traction, the barrel of the side plate is slid over the screws and then fixed to the reconstituted condylar block by one or two cancellous bone screws. Rotational alignment and range of movement of the knee joint are checked after preliminary fixation of the side plate. If there is bone loss medially, an extensive cancellous graft must be performed.

C3: Bicondylar fracture combined with complex fracture of the distal femur and anterior tangential fracture of one or both condyles. An additional medial parapatellar incision becomes unavoidable whenever there is a tangential fracture of the medial condyle. Whenever there are tangential fractures of both condyles, one can run into problems with the insertion of the seating chisel because of the AP lag screws necessary to fix the anterior tangential fragments. In these cases, we use the long condylar buttress plate. Take great care to avoid frontal or sagittal malalignment. If the medial buttress is deficient, carry out an extensive cortico-cancellous bone graft. Prior to the fixation of the fracture with the lateral condylar buttress plate, reduce the tangential fractures and fix them with lag screws. Then reduce the condyles and fix them temporarily with three or four Kirschner wires. Cannulated large cancellous bone screws can conveniently be placed over these wires. Apply the plate and insert additional lag screws through the plate. Then reduce the shaft and fix it to the plate. Finally carry out an extensive cancellous graft as already indicated.

Fig. 12.11

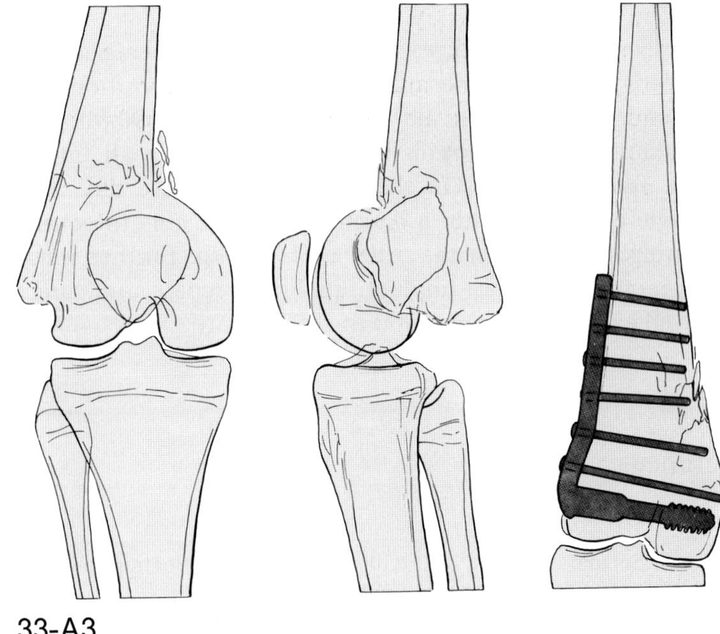

Fig. 12.12

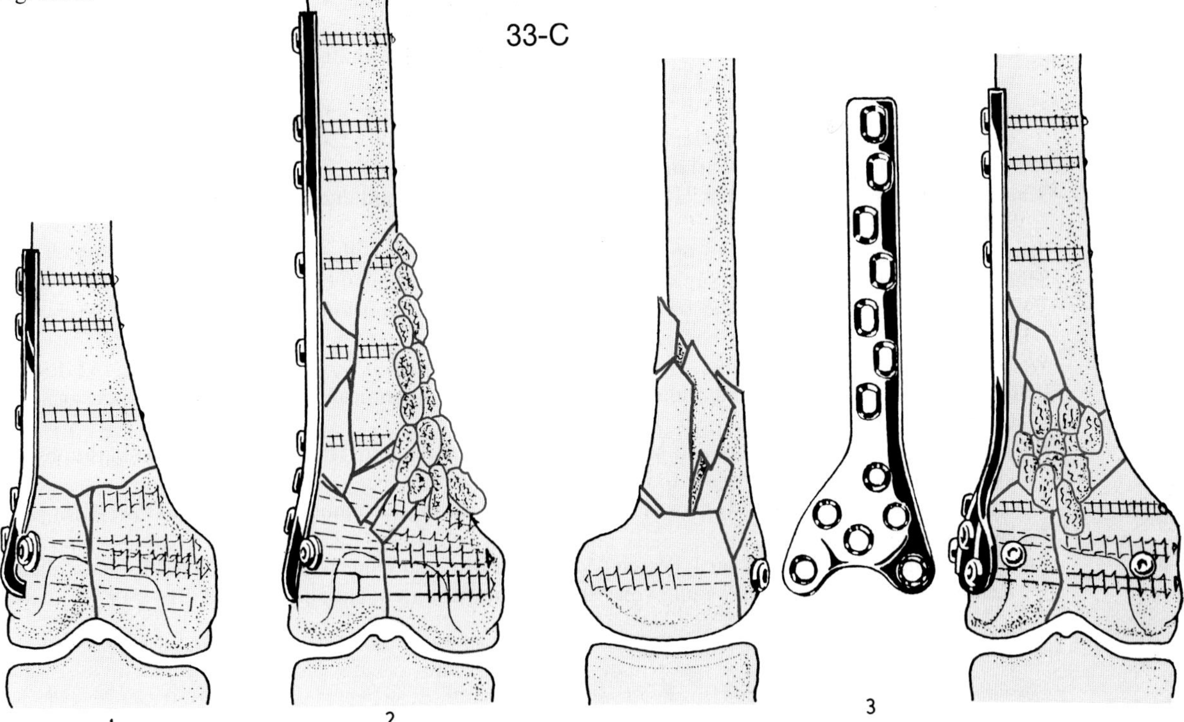

12.5 Postoperative Treatment

All fractures of the middle and distal femur are positioned for the first 4–5 days with the hip and knee flexed at 90° in the so-called 90/90/90 position. If available, the use of continuous passive motion is very beneficial in all intra-articular fractures, and is therefore recommended. On the fifth postoperative day, the patient is allowed to sit and dangle his legs. Within a day or two, he is able to get up using crutches and begin partial weight-bearing on the order of 10–15 kg. Further weight-bearing depends on the type of fracture, choice of implant, quality of repair, and clinical and radiological follow-up, as well as on the co-operation of the patient.

References

Bansal VP, Singhal V, Mam MK, Gill SS (1984) The floating knee. 40 cases of ipsilateral fractures of the femur and tibia. Int Orthop 8:183–187

Browner BD (1986) Pitfalls, errors, and complications in the use of locking Küntscher nails. Clin Orthop 212:192–208

Haas N, Tscherne H, Krettek C (1986) Kombinationsfrakturen von Oberschenkelschaft und proximalem oder distalem Femurende. Unfallheilkunde 182:307–310

Hansen ST, Winquist RA (1979) Closed intramedullary nailing of the femur. Clin Orthop 138:56–61

Healy WL, Brooker AF (1983) Distal femoral fractures. Clin Orthop 174:166–171

Johnson KD, Tencer AF, Sherman MC (1987) Biomechanical factors affecting fracture stability and femoral bursting in closed intramedullary nailing of femoral shaft fractures, with illustrative case presentations. J Orthop Trauma 1:1–11

Kinast C, Bolhofner BR, Mast JW, Ganz R (1989) Subtrochanteric fractures of the femur. Results of treatment with the 95° condylar blade-plate. Clin Orthop 238:122–130

Küntscher G (1962) Praxis der Marknagelung. Schattauer, Stuttgart

Maatz R, Lentz W, Arens W, Beck H (1983) Die Marknagelung und andere intramedulläre Osteosynthesen. Schattauer, Stuttgart

Schatzker J (1987) The rationale of operative fracture care. Springer, Berlin Heidelberg New York

Schatzker J, Lambert DC (1979) Supracondylar fractures of the femur. Clin Orthop 138:77–83

Tscherne H, Trentz O (1977) Die frischen Verletzungen der Femurkondylen. Langenbecks Arch Chir 345:395–401

Weller S (1975) Die Marknagelung – gute und relative Indikationen, Ergebnisse. Chirurg 46:152–154

Weller S, Renne J (1973) Grundsätzliche Fehler und Komplikationsmöglichkeiten der Marknagelung. Chirurg 44:533–539

Willenegger H (1975) Verplattung und Marknagelung bei Femur- und Tibiaschaftfrakturen: Pathophysiologische Grundlagen. Chirurg 46:145

Winquist RA, Hansen ST (1984) Closed intramedullary nailing of femoral fractures. J Bone Joint Surg [Am] 66:529–539

Zuber K, Schneider E, Eulenberger J, Perren SM (1988) Form und Dimension der Markhöhle menschlicher Femora in Hinblick auf die Passung von Marknagelimplantaten. Unfallchirurg 91:314–319

13 PATELLA AND TIBIA

13.1 General Considerations

In the surgical treatment of tibia fractures, particularly fractures in the diaphysis, there are three possible methods of surgical treatment: medullary nailing; external fixation; and compression fixation using lag screws, most often in combination with a neutralization plate (protection plate).

Examples of all three methods will be illustrated. However, the technical aspects of medullary nailing and of external fixation are dealt with in two chapters (Chaps. 4, 5) devoted to these treatment modalities. Plate application to the tibia varies according to the location and "anatomy" of the fracture. These details could not be included in Chap. 3 and are therefore emphasized here. This chapter may, therefore, appear biased in favor of plate application. We consider, however, all three methods as complementary, although we are aware of the increasing preference for medullary nailing, not only in the femur, but also in the tibia. Chapter 1 demonstrates how modern plates (e.g. the LC-DCP) minimize cortex necrosis and plate osteoporosis. This, in our view, will – with good reason – increase the indication for the precision osteosynthesis made possible by lag screw techniques in combination with neutralization plates, particularly in fractures close to the proximal and distal tibial metaphysis.

13.2 Surgical Approach to the Patella

Position: Supine, leg straight, tourniquet applied.

Skin incision: Patella fractures are approached through a straight longitudinal midline incision (Fig. 13.1).

13.3 Surgical Approach to the Tibia

13.3.1 Surgical Approach to the Tibial Plateau

Tibial plateau fractures are approached either through a straight longitudinal midline incision or, for the lateral condyle, through a curved incision whose upper part starts laterally halfway between the patella and the tibial plateau and which then curves downwards to run straight just lateral to the anterior crest of the tibia. If both plateaus are to be approached simultaneously, a long, straight, longitudinal midline incision is standard (exceptionally, a lateral and a medial incision separated from each other by at least 7 cm are used).

A transverse incision has always been advocated, for the reason that the Langer's lines are transverse and an incision parallel to them leads to the best cosmetic result. However, complex lesions of the patella and of the meta- and epiphyseal part of the proximal tibia may need later extensive procedures, including total knee prosthesis, which requires extensive straight approaches. A previous transverse scar may jeopardize wound healing in such cases.

When working with type B and C tibial plateau fractures, it is necessary to expose the lateral and/or the medial tibial condyle in such a way that it is possible to see both its articular cartilage and the cortex where it joins the shaft. To achieve such exposure on the lateral side, the proximal insertion of the extensor muscles must be reflected and the anterior lateral tibial surface exposed. In order to expose the articular cartilage of the tibial plateau, it is necessary to divide the capsule below and parallel to the meniscus. A cuff of tissue must remain on both to permit subsequent resuturing of the meniscus to the tibia.

Once the capsule has been incised, the meniscus is retracted upwards to provide adequate exposure of the articular surface (Fig. 13.2).

Fig. 13.1 Approach to the patella and the tibial plateau.

1 Nervus peroneus superficialis. *2* Caput fibulae. *3* Ligamentum collaterale laterale. *4* Patella. *5* Ramus infrapatellaris nervi sapheni. *6* Ligamenta cruciata genus. *7* Ligamentum collaterale mediale. *8* Tuberositas tibiae.

Fig. 13.2 Exposure of the lateral tibial plateau elevating the meniscus.

1 Musculi extensores cruris (musculus tibialis anterior). *2* Ramus muscularis nervi peronei profundi. *3* Arteria recurrens tibialis anterior. *4* Ligamentum collaterale laterale. *5* Meniscus lateralis articulationis genus (elevated). *6* Fascia cruris. *7* Corpus adiposum infrapatellare genus (Hoffa). *8* Condylus lateralis tibiae. *9* Rami infrapatellares nervi sapheni. *10* Tuberositas tibiae.

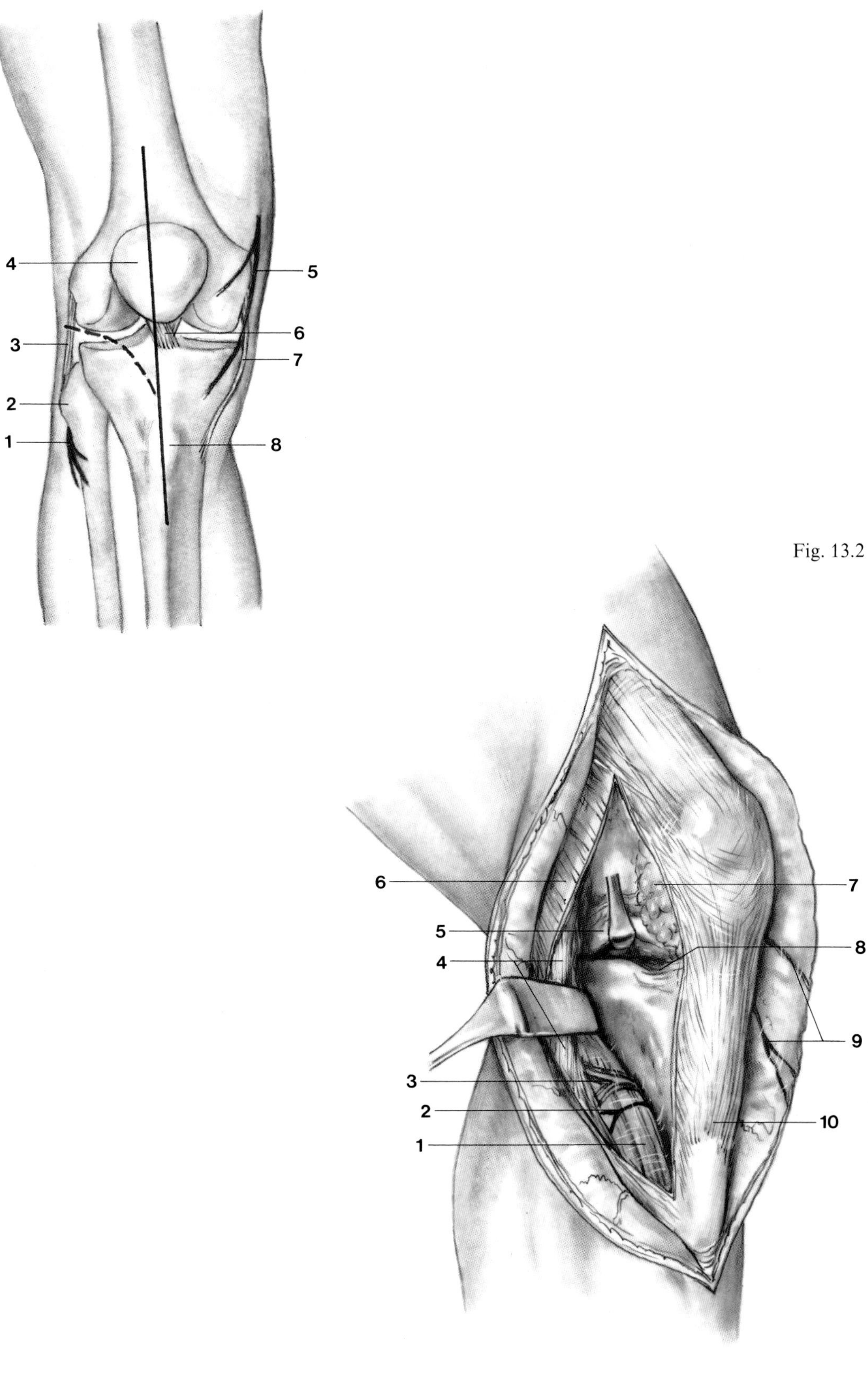
Fig. 13.1
4
5
3
6
7
2
1
8
Fig. 13.2
6
7
5
8
4
9
3
2
10
1

13.3.2 Surgical Approach to the Shaft of the Tibia

The skin incision lies 1 cm lateral to the anterior crest of the tibia. In order to correspond to Langer's lines, it must be perfectly straight (Figs. 13.3, 13.4). Exceptionally, a posteromedial approach can be chosen, mostly to deposit cancellous bone. In the supramalleolar region, the incision is curved medially and posteriorly so as to describe a gentle arch around the front of the medial malleolus (Fig. 13.5).

Long incisions are recommended to get adequate exposure. A straight incision in the lower leg, if carefully closed, leaves a barely visible scar.

The fracture surfaces are cleaned cautiously using a small periosteal elevator with a suction tip. The periosteum is reflected only 1 or 2 mm from the fracture. The fractures, once exposed, should be carefully examined and compared with both the X-ray and the preoperative drawing of the internal fixation.

The posterior medial incision is hardly ever used in fresh fractures, but more commonly in secondary bone grafting (Fig. 13.6).

The approach to open fractures is determined by the location of the injury. Minimal additional devascularization of both the soft tissues and the bone is paramount (see Chap. 17).

Fig. 13.3 The standard approach to the shaft of the tibia for screw fixation and plating: straight incision over the diaphysis curved around the medial malleolus.

Fig. 13.4 The two approaches to the tibia.

1 Nervus suralis and vena saphena parva. *2* Musculus soleus. *3* Musculus gastrocnemius, caput laterale. *4* Musculus flexor hallucis longus. *5* Arteria peronea. *6* Musculus peroneus brevis. *7* Nervus peroneus superficialis. *8* Musculus peroneus longus. *9* Musculus extensor digitorum longus. *10* Musculus extensor hallucis longus. *11* Musculus tibialis anterior. *12* Nervus peroneus profundus and arteria tibialis anterior. *13* Nervus saphenus and vena saphena magna. *14* Musculus tibialis posterior. *15* Musculus flexor digitorum longus. *16* Nervus tibialis and arteria tibialis posterior. *17* Musculus plantaris. *18* Musculus gastrocnemius, caput mediale.

Fig. 13.3

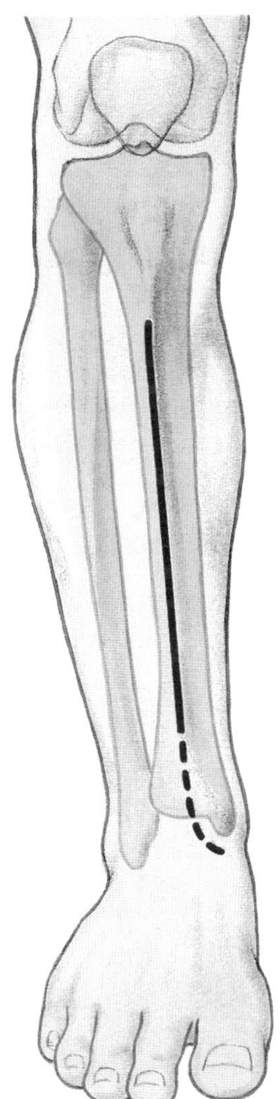

Fig. 13.4

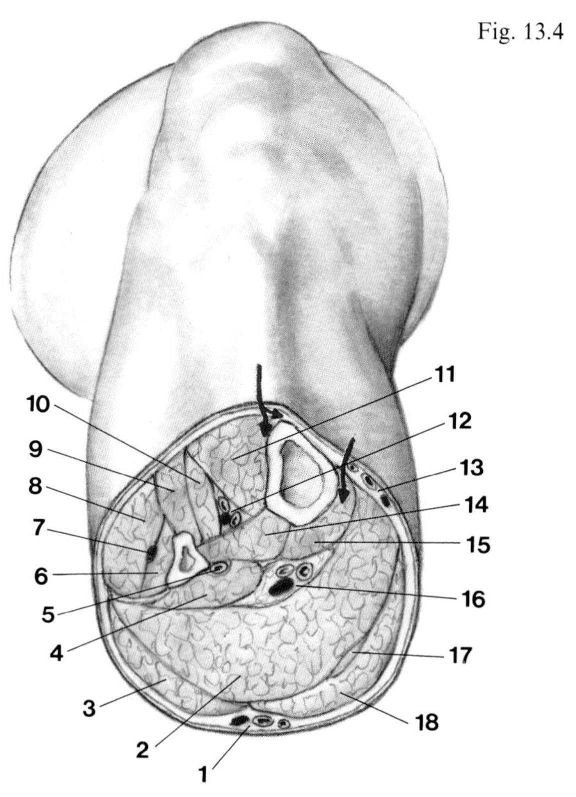

Fig. 13.5

a The approach to the distal tibia.

1 Articulatio talocruralis. *2* Margo anterior tibiae. *3* Nervus saphenus. *4* Malleolus medialis.

b Exposure of the talotibial joint.

1 Fascia cruris and retinaculum extensorum (divided). *2* Articulatio talocruralis. *3* Ligamentum mediale (ligamentum deltoideum).

Fig. 13.5

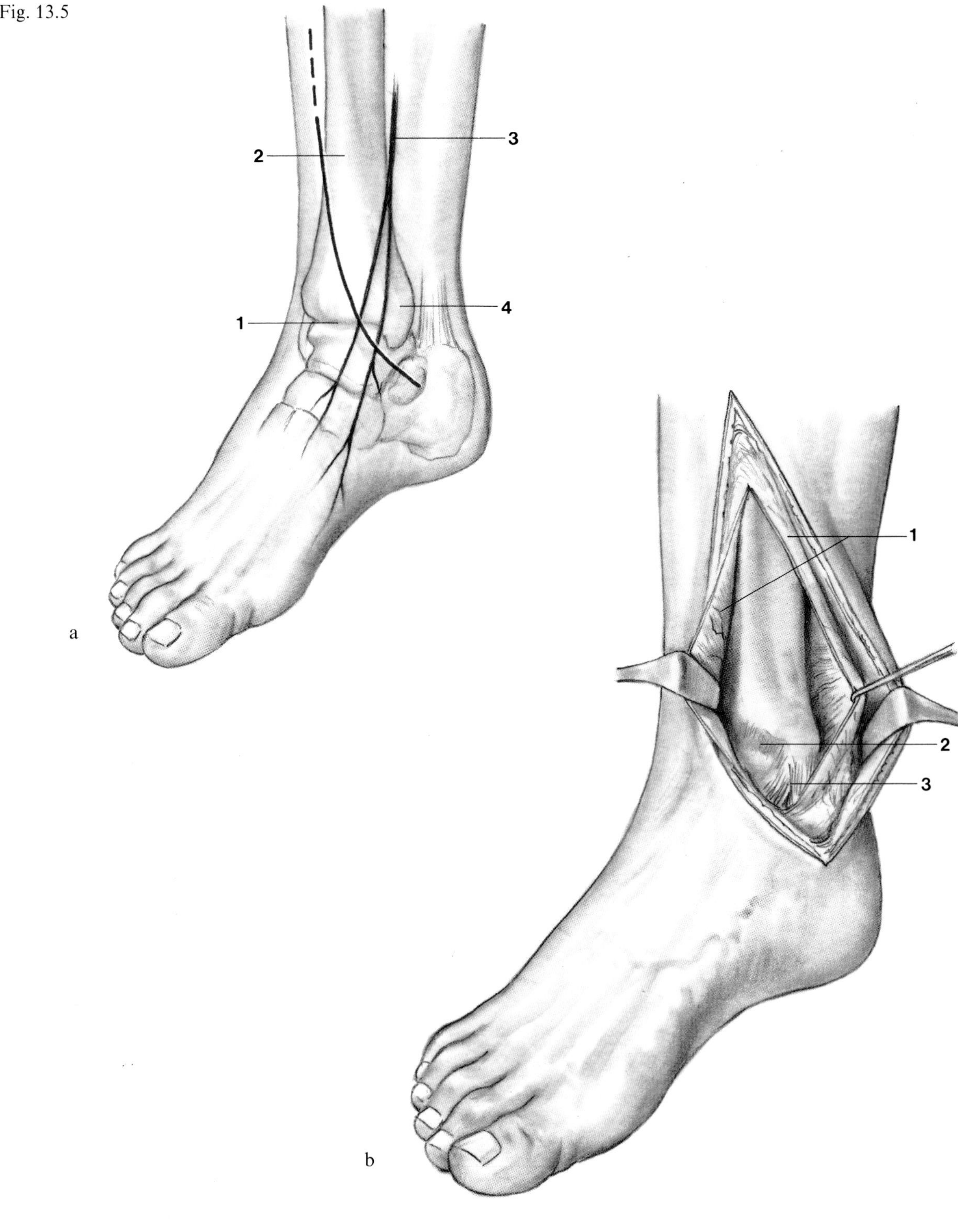

Fig. 13.6

a The approach to the posterior aspect of the tibia.

1 Malleolus medialis. *2* Musculus soleus. *3* Condylus medialis tibiae. *4* Musculus gastrocnemius, caput mediale. *5* Tendo calcaneus (tendo Achillis).

b Deep layers of the approach to the posterior tibial shaft.

1 Fascia cruris (lamina superficialis, edge of incision). *2* Vena saphena magna. *3* Musculus gastrocnemius, caput mediale. *4* Facies medialis tibiae. *5* Fascia cruris (lamina profunda over musculus flexor digitorum longus). *6* Venae perforantes.

Fig. 13.6

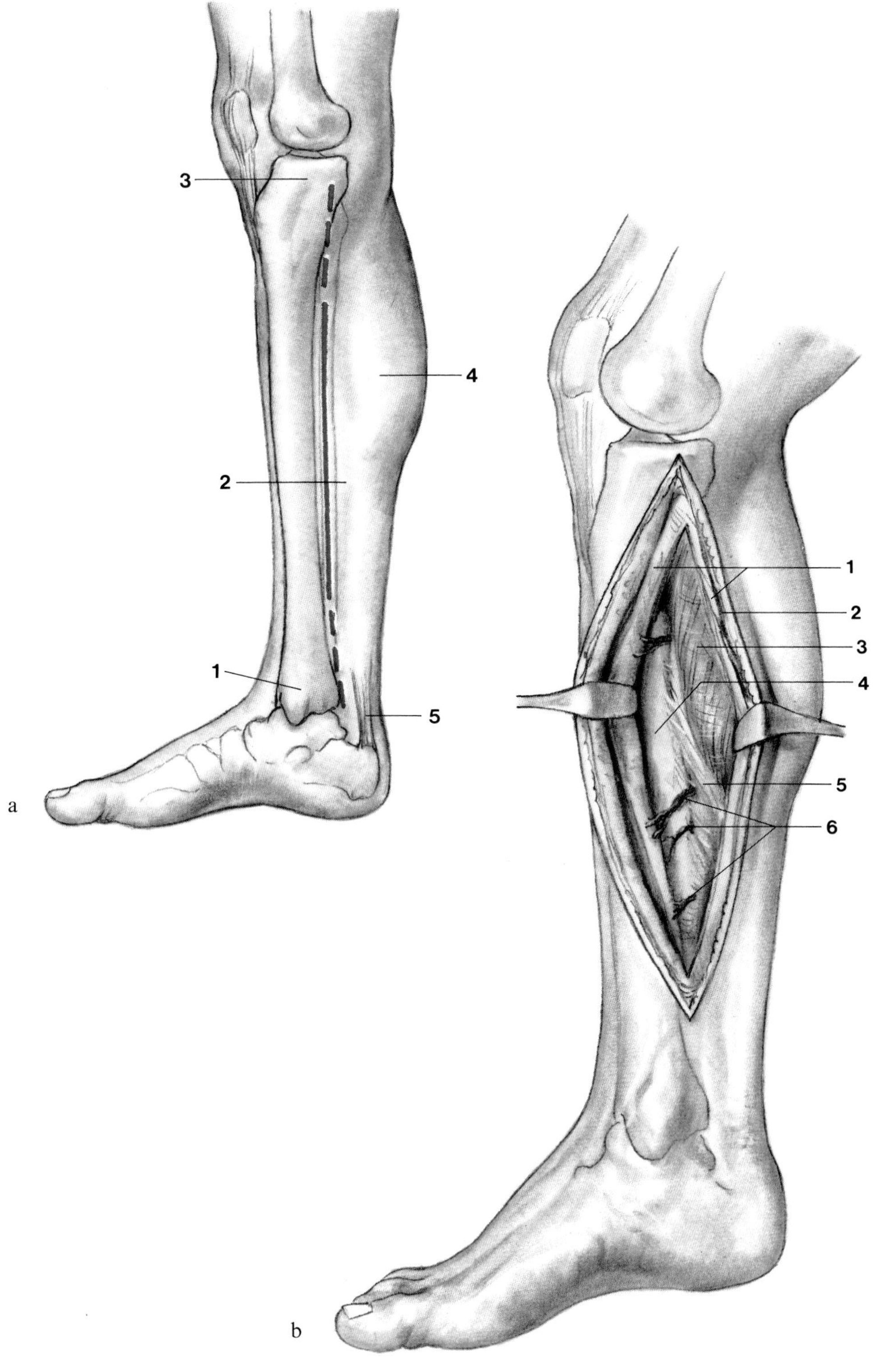

13.3.3 Surgical Approach to the Distal Third of the Tibia Including Pilon Fractures

Whenever there is a concomitant fibula fracture, two incisions are required with a bridge of skin at least 7 cm in width. The medial incision exposing the distal tibia lies just lateral to the anterior crest of the tibia down to the joint level and then curves medially around the medial malleolus (Fig. 13.5). The lateral incision starts behind the posterior edge of the fibula and turns gently around its distal end (Figs. 13.7, 13.8).

Fig. 13.7 Approach to the fibula.

1 Rami calcanei laterales nervi suralis. *2* Nervus cutaneus dorsalis lateralis pedis (nervus suralis). *3* Nervus cutaneus dorsalis intermedius (nervus peroneus superficialis). *4* Nervus cutaneus dorsalis medialis. *5* Nervus peroneus superficialis. *6* Malleolus lateralis. *7* Ligamentum talofibulare anterius. *8* Ligamentum talocalcaneare laterale. *9* Ligamentum calcaneofibulare.

Fig. 13.8 Deep layers of the approach to the fibula.

1 Ligamentum calcaneofibulare. *2* Retinaculum musculorum fibularium. *3* "Facies subcutanea fibulae." *4* Musculi peronei. *5* Musculus extensor digitorum longus (musculus peroneus tertius). *6* Ramus perforans arteriae peroneae over front syndesmosis. *7* Ligamentum talofibulare anterius.

Fig. 13.7

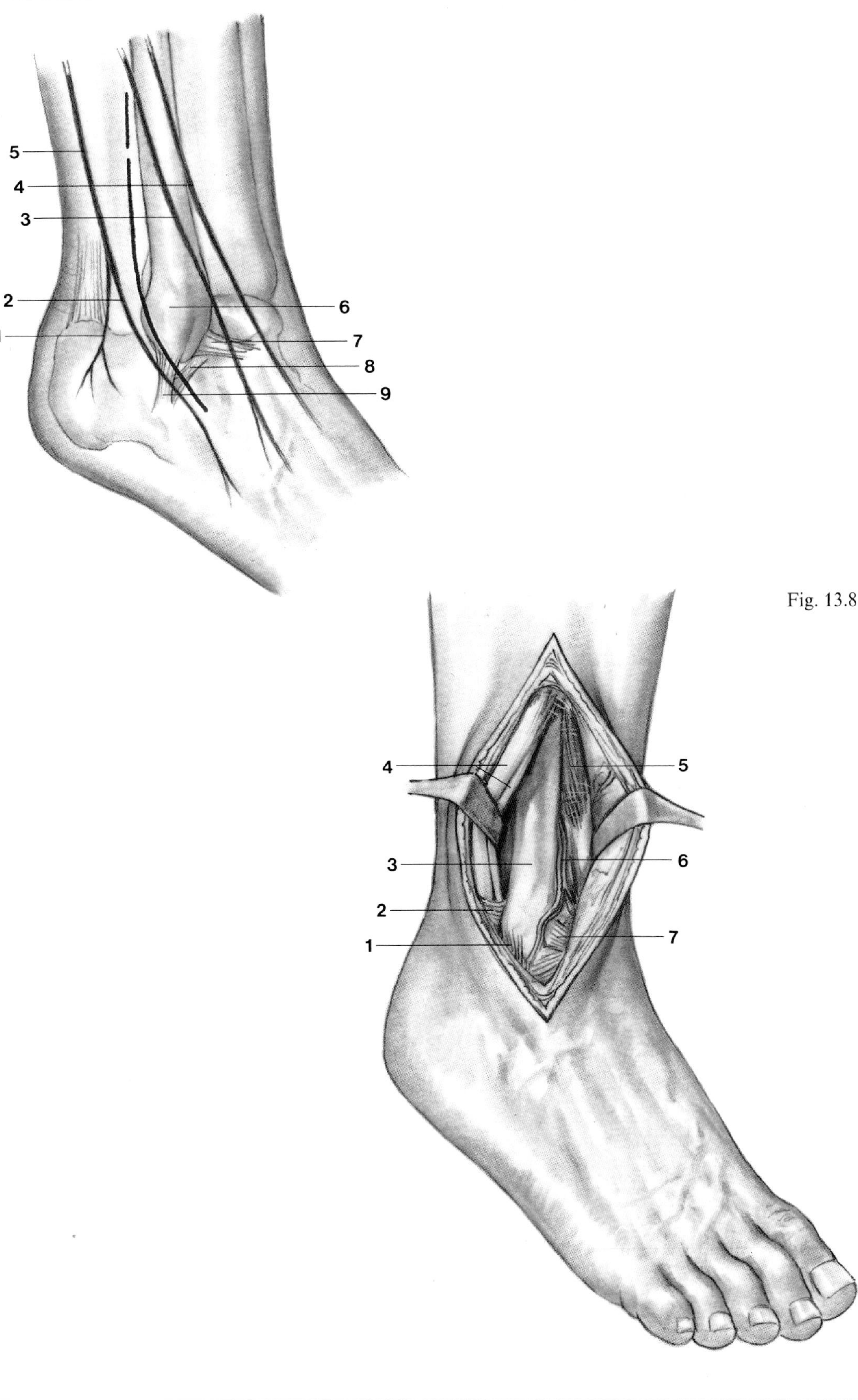

Fig. 13.8

13.4 Fractures of the Patella

Pauwels used an anterior wire suture for a fractured patella, thus successfully applying the principle of tension band fixation. Tension band wiring has since become the preferred method of internal fixation for fractures of the patella.

Pauwels also showed that even very complex fractures of the patella could be treated with immediate mobilization if the joint capsule and the retinacula were not ruptured or, if ruptured, carefully repaired and the reduced fracture protected with a tension band wire. The results of such treatment were surprisingly good, even though some patellae ended up longer than normal. Primary patellectomy is not recommended and should be considered only in the case of severe articular incongruity.

Vertical fractures of the patella without displacement are treated nonoperatively. If displaced, they should be reduced and fixed using two transverse lag screws.

Avulsion fractures of the inferior pole of the patella are best first fixed with a small cancellous bone screw which is then supplemented with a tension band wire (Fig. 13.9).

The repaired infrapatellar tendon must be protected by a tension band wire. In an osteoporotic tibia, the traction-absorbing wire may be passed around a screw inserted transversely through the tibial tubercle (Fig. 13.10). Using this technique, great care must be taken not to produce a patella baja. A preoperative X-ray of the opposite knee will indicate the correct position of the patella.

13.4.1 Tension Band Wiring of the Patella

Tension band wiring is particularly suitable for simple transverse fractures of the patella. The fracture and the articular surfaces of the patella and of the femoral condyles are carefully examined. The Sharpey fibers and the prepatellar expansion of the quadriceps tendon are reflected 2–3 mm on each side of the fracture. Anatomical reduction is carried out and maintained temporarily using the pointed reduction clamps. The first tension band wire is inserted through the quadriceps tendons close to the bone. The passage of the wire through the tendon is made very much easier by passing a curved large-bore needle through the tendon close to the bone at exactly the desired location. The wire is then pushed into the lumen of the needle and the needle is withdrawn leaving the wire in place. Using a similar procedure, the other wire end is placed through the patella tendon, close to the distal fragment. During tightening, palpation of the articular surface allows evaluation of the reduction and permits optimal wire tension to be applied.

Fig. 13.9 An avulsion of the distal pole.

Tension band wiring alone tends to tilt the inferior pole into the joint. The fragments should therefore be first fixed with a lag screw. The fixation is then completed with a tension band wire.

Fig. 13.10 Rupture of the infrapatellar tendon.

The ruptured infrapatellar tendon is repaired with resorbable sutures. The suture line is then protected with a figure-of-eight tension band wire which is passed through the quadriceps insertion and the tibial tubercle. If the tibial tubercle is osteoporotic, a screw is inserted transversely through bone and the tension band wire is wound around the screw. The figure-of-eight tension band protects the repair of the tendon and makes early mobilization possible. The tension band wire should be removed after about 6 months.

Fig. 13.9

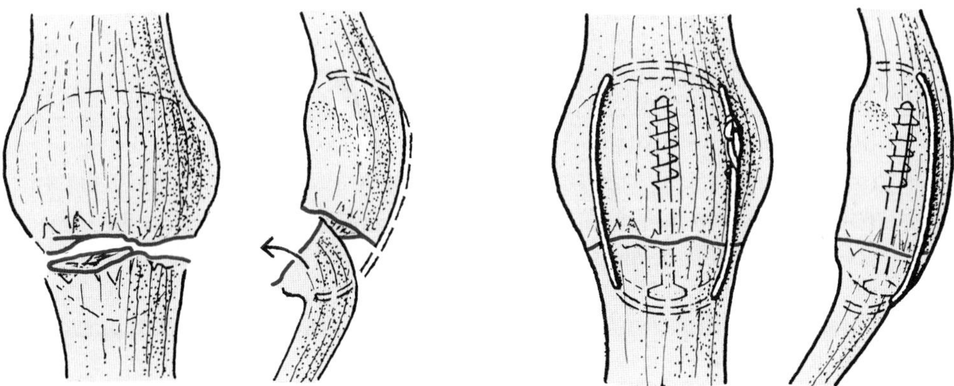

Fig. 13.10

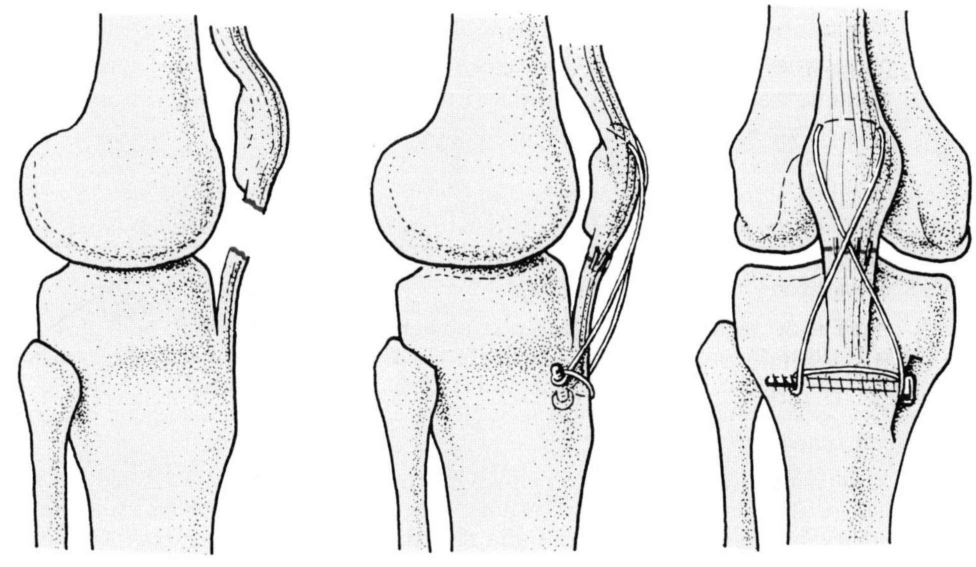

The second wire must be inserted more ventrally and is passed through the Sharpey fibers. Note that when the knee is flexed, the fracture surfaces come under compression and should remain so not only during flexion but also during extension.

13.4.2 Internal Fixation of the Patella with Two Kirschner Wires and Tension Band (Fig. 13.11)

If pure tension band wiring does not retain the reduction because of shearing, two Kirschner wires should be applied. They anchor the tension band wire and prevent tilting of the fragments. The tension band wire is passed posterior to the vertical Kirschner wires using either a wire passer, a curved large-bore needle, or a curved Redon (Hemovac) needle with the wire in the Redon tube.

This method, using Kirschner wires and tension band fixation, can be used not only for transverse fractures but also for complex fractures of the patella (if necessary combined with lag screws or additional oblique Kirschner wires).

13.4.3 Postoperative Treatment

A soft, comfortable dressing is applied and if the fixation is satisfactory when the range of motion is tested intraoperatively, both active and passive exercises (CPM!) should begin immediately after operation. If the fixation lacks stability, it must be redone because a lengthy period of plaster immobilization will be deleterious to the knee.

Fig. 13.11 Tension band fixation of the patella.

Position the patient supine with the knee slightly flexed over a roll. Note that only when the knee is flexed to 90° or more (110°–120°) does the articular surface of the patella come into contact with the intercondylar notch. Make a straight longitudinal incision directly over the middle of the patella. Expose the fracture and clean its edges. Elevate any articular depressions and if necessary fill the defects with cancellous bone.

a About 5–6 mm from the anterior surface of the patella, drill with the 2-mm drill bit two parallel drill holes in the proximal fragment. The distance between the two drill holes should be 20–25 mm. To ease drilling, hold the patellar fragment with the reduction clamps and tilt the fragment so that the fracture surface faces you. Once the first hole is drilled, the drill bit is removed and is replaced with a Kirschner wire. This Kirschner wire then serves as a guide for the second drill hole. This ensures that the two drill holes will be parallel to one another. For direction control, insert two 1.6-mm-thick and 15-cm-long Kirschner wires into the two drill holes.

b Replace the Kirschner wires with 2-mm drill bits inserted in a proximodistal direction. Reduce the fracture and keep it reduced with the reduction clamps with tips. Check the accuracy of reduction.

c If reduction is perfect, drill with the 2-mm drill bits the holes in the distal fragment.

d Replace drill bits by Kirschner wires, bent 180° at proximal end.

e, f Tighten and secure the wire using the AO wire-tightener. Hammer the Kirschner wires with their bent end into the bone, then cut their distal end.

g An alternative possibility: form one wire loop on the opposite side, use wire twister on the near side and tighten. The loop (eye) on the opposite side allows secondary tightening.

h A second wire in a "figure-of-eight" form may be added to improve the tension band effect.

Fig. 13.11

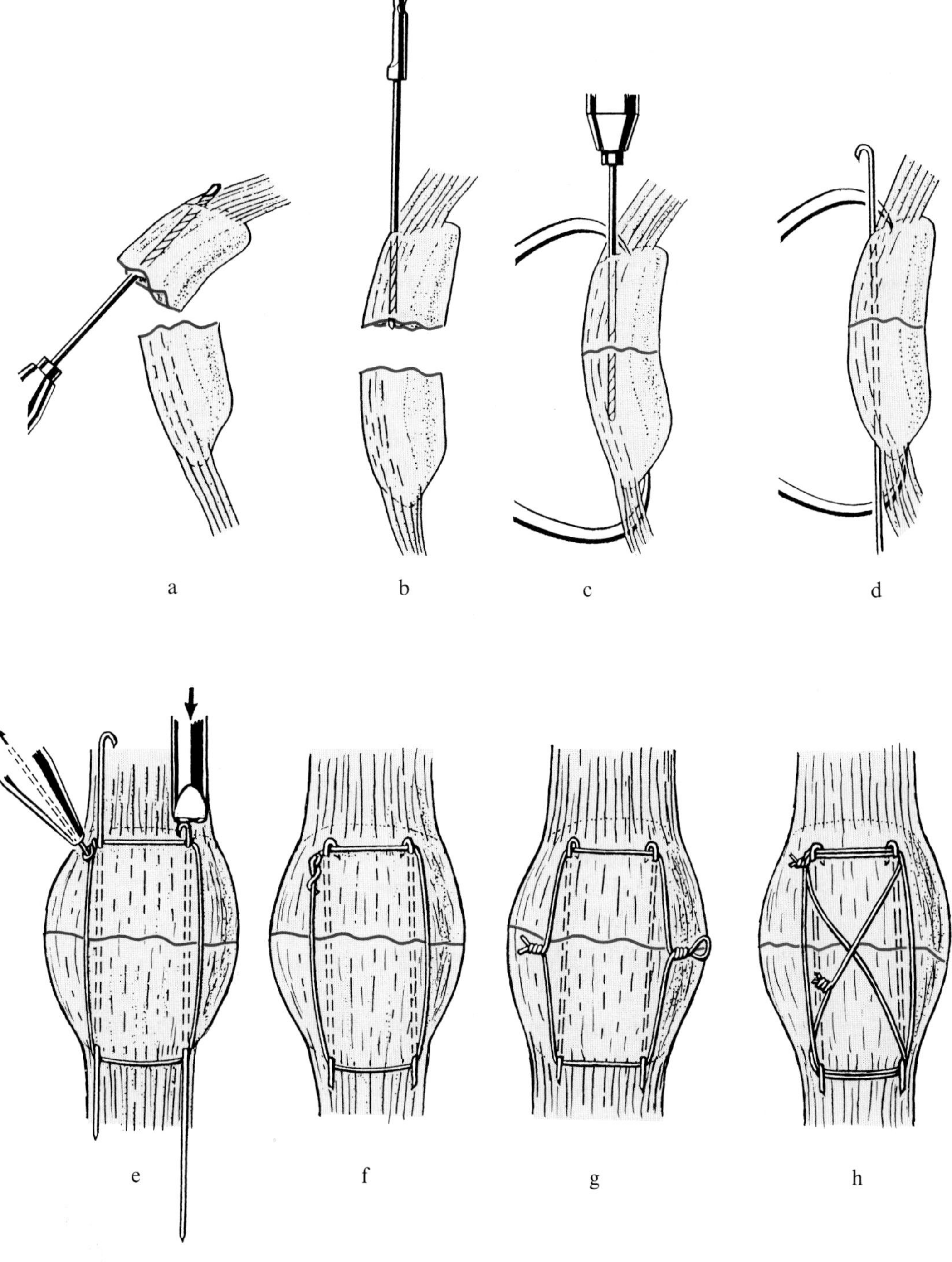

13.5 Fractures of the Tibia

13.5.1 Tibial Plateau Fractures

Rüedi et al. (1975b) and Schatzker and Tile (1987) have clearly demonstrated by late follow-up that any significant dislocation of the joint surface across the various B and C fractures requires open reduction and adequate internal fixation.

13.5.1.1 Concomitant Injuries

Tibial plateau fractures are often combined with concomitant injuries of vessels, nerves, capsule, collateral and crucriate ligaments as well as the menisci.

The vast majority of tibial plateau fractures concern the lateral condyle. For compression fractures of the lateral tibial plateau to be produced, the medial collateral ligament and capsule must remain intact throughout the initial phase of the deforming forces. Once the ligaments have been torn, a valgus deformation cannot exert any compressive force on the lateral tibial plateau. It is important to recognize that a combination of lateral plateau fractures and disruption of the medial collateral ligaments occurs in about one third of all cases. Therefore, once the lateral plateau has been reconstructed, it is important to test the integrity of the medial collateral ligament and capsule by applying a valgus force first with the knee in full extension, and then in various degrees of flexion. The knee must also be examined and tested for injuries to the menisci and cruciate ligaments.

13.5.1.2 Internal Fixation of Different Types of Tibial Plateau Fracture

The basic goals and principles for all types of tibial plateau fracture are:

- Reconstruction of joint congruity.
- Re-establishment of the tibial alignment.
- An adequate buttress to maintain congruity and alignment, with bone graft and internal fixation acting as a buttress.
- Repair of meniscus and ligaments.

We wish to re-emphasize here the necessity of using a buttress with adequate implants. Lag screws alone rarely provide adequate stability against shearing. A plate used for buttressing not only supports the cortex but also holds up the proximal plate screws.

Another possibility which may be successful is ligamentotaxis by means of a bridging external fixator which is anchored in the tibia and femur and left in place for 6 weeks. Immediate checking by X-ray will tell whether the reduction by ligamentotaxis has been successful enough to continue this form of treatment. If not, ORIF may be necessary. Subsequent mobilization by active movement (and possibly by CPM) leads to full functional recovery, provided that the reduction is maintained.

13.5.1.3 Monocondylar Fractures (Type B)

In wedge fractures (type B1) fixation is carried out using two cancellous bone screws with washers (Fig. 13.12a, b) or, if axial overload is to be expected, by a plate to further buttress the lateral fragment (Fig. 13.12c, d). A buttress can be provided by a narrow dynamic compression plate (DCP), an L plate or a T plate. A posterior wedge fragment can be reduced and fixed with two lag screws (Fig. 13.12e, f).

Impaction fractures with central depression (type B2) (Fig. 13.13a, b) can be reduced by fenestrating the anterior cortex of the tibia just in front of the fibula. Through this window, a bone punch reduces the depressed articular surface from below. The elevation of the depressed joint surface results in a defect in the metaphysis which must be packed with cancellous bone. It is usually enough to stabilize and protect the reduction with one or two transverse cancellous bone screws provided with washers (Fig. 13.13c).

In depression wedge fractures with split and impaction (type B3) (Fig. 13.14a–d), the fracture permits direct visualization of the impacted fragments. Every large lateral fragment should be left in periosteal connection and should be rotated laterally. After reduction of the joint surface, temporary fixation of the lateral cortex is carried out with one or more Kirschner wires. The resultant defect in the metaphysis must be carefully filled with a cancellous bone graft which aids in supporting the elevated joint surface. Finally internal fixation is completed by adding a buttress plate. The T or L plates fit the lateral contour of the tibia very well. Fixation using L plates requires less exposure dorsally than fixation with T plates and allows placement of the posterior screw through a separate stab incision.

Fig. 13.12 Options of internal fixation for different type B1 wedge fractures.

a, b A lateral wedge fracture fixed under compression with a proximal lagged cancellous bone screw and buttressed at its tip with a lower cortex screw.

c, d Internal fixation with a buttress plate.

e, f Internal fixation of a posterior wedge fracture (rare).

Fig. 13.13

a Type B2 fracture depressed lateral tibial plateau.

b Fenestration of the lateral tibial condyle and reduction of the depressed fragments.

c The end result after grafting the metaphyseal defect and stabilizing the fracture with one or two cancellous lag screws.

Fig. 13.14

a Type B3 fracture. Combined wedge and depression fracture.

b Reduction and temporary fixation with Kirschner wires.

c Bone grafting with cancellous bone.

d Insertion of the buttress plate (the regular DCP, T plate or L plate can be used).

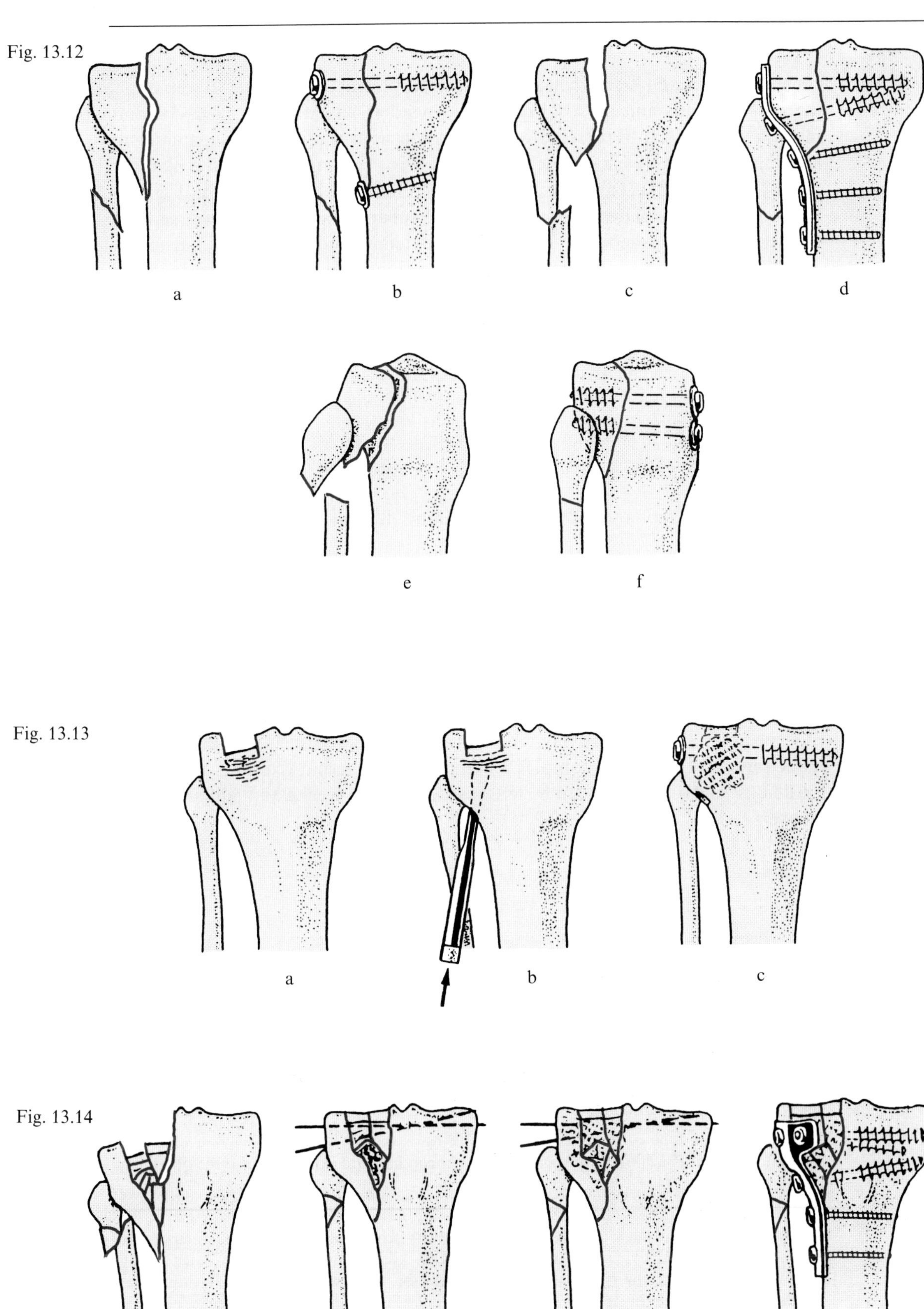
Fig. 13.12
a
b
c
d
e
f
Fig. 13.13
a
b
c
Fig. 13.14
a
b
c
d

13.5.1.4 Bicondylar Fractures (Type C)

Usually the medial tibial condyle escapes any joint depression. It remains attached to the pes anserinus and mostly breaks out together with the intercondylar eminence. This makes it possible to repair the whole condyle with the inserting ligaments and tendons. Laterally, we usually encounter a more extensive comminution of the plateau. The reduction of this portion is carried out as described for type B3 fractures in Fig. 13.15a–c.

If exposure is inadequate and the tibial tubercle is fractured as a separate fragment, then it may be elevated together with the patellar tendon. If the tibial tubercle is intact, an alternative option is to sever the patellar tendon in a Z form and to move it upwards with the infrapatellar fat pad and menisci.

Everything possible must be done to preserve both menisci. Peripheral detachments are carefully resutured with resorbable sutures.

The steps for the reconstruction and fixation are the same as for all other intra-articular fractures:

- The first step is to reconstruct the plateau and to fix it temporarily using pointed reduction forceps and/or Kirschner wires which may then be replaced by cannulated screws.
- The second step is to fill up the remaining defect under the plateau with a cancellous bone graft.
- The third step is to join it to the shaft again using pointed reduction forceps or Kirschner wires.
- The last step is the definitive stabilization using one or sometimes two buttress plates, one laterally and the other medially. The plates have to be contoured very precisely and fixed with screws (Fig. 13.15c).

The skin flaps of the extensive exposure must be handled very gently to prevent wound-edge necrosis. Intraoperatively, the distractor or an external fixator greatly facilitates reduction and fixation of complex fractures. The external fixator – in combination with local lag screw fixation – can be left in place for 3–4 weeks and still allows full functional recovery!

Fig. 13.15

a, b Type C3 fracture.

c The final result of an open reduction and internal fixation with a small medial and a larger lateral buttress plate. Beware of doing any damage to the usually intact medial tibial plateau.

d An example of a type of a 41-C3 injury requiring a special approach because of compromised bone and soft tissues. It is a complex proximal tibial plateau fracture extending into the tibial diaphysis.

e, f The approach is one of articular reconstruction and fixation with a simple lag screw followed by bridging the knee with an anterior unilateral frame providing moderate distraction in order to stabilize the soft tissues by ligamentotaxis. Half-pins are utilized away from the tibial fracture focus, so as not to limit possible more definitive fixation in the future. One additional advantage of such a construct is that is allows elevation of the limb, as the frame may be utilized to support the injured extremity in a position higher than chest level. When the soft tissues have healed, in 2–3 weeks, either the frame may be broken down and reapplied beneath the knee joint so as to allow motion, or internal fixation may be employed as a delayed secondary procedure.

Fig. 13.15

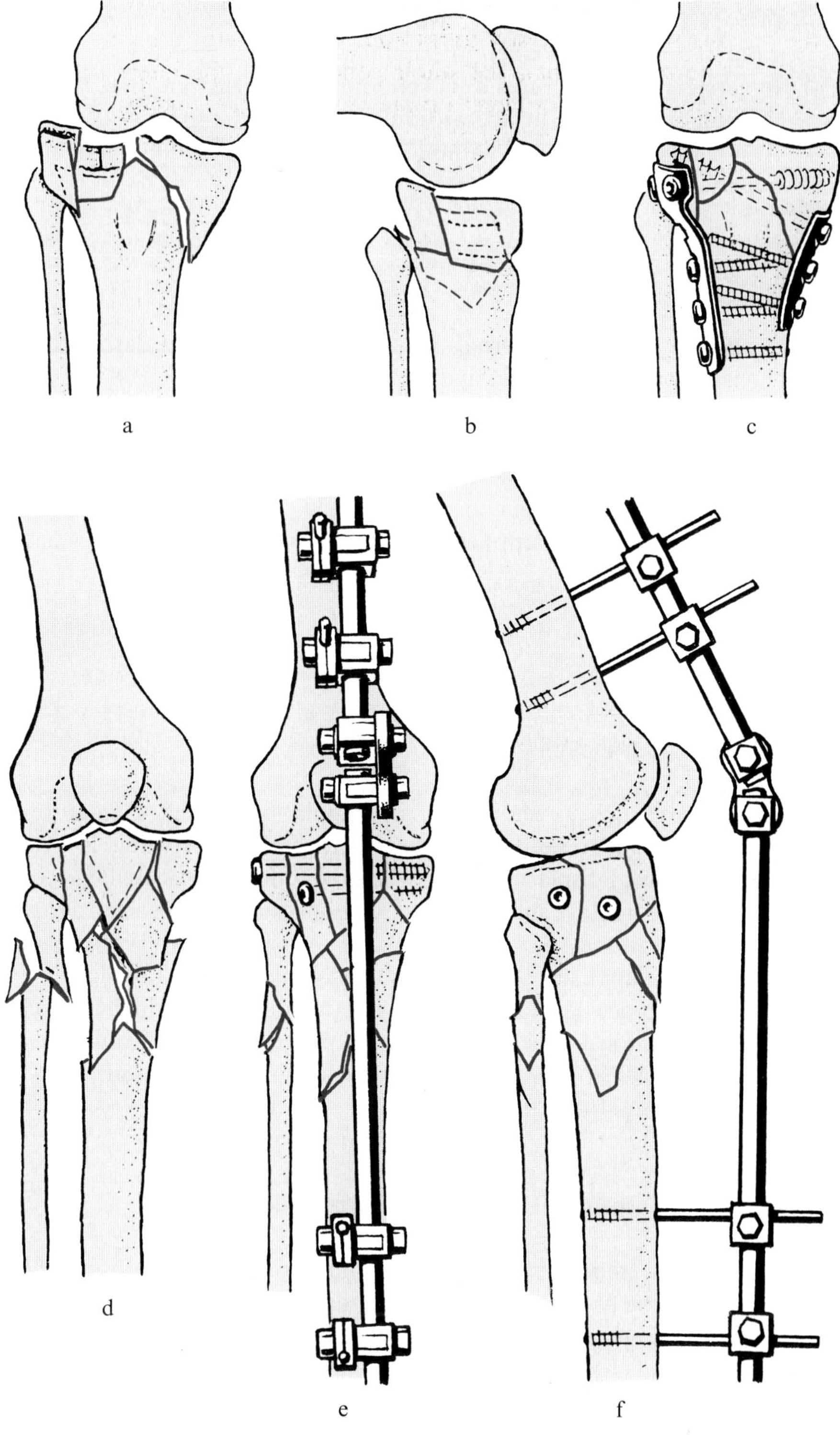

An external fixator which bridges the joint with some degree of distraction (Fig. 13.15d–f) may be considered postoperatively under three sets of conditions:

- In very complex, open or unstable fractures as a temporary fixation, especially in a polytrauma patient when internal fixation must be delayed.
- In very complex fractures in which joint reconstruction must be restricted to lag screw fixation of the joint surface without fixation to the shaft.
- As a reduction technique without open exposure through ligamentotaxis as an alternative to a plaster cast.

13.5.1.5 Postoperative Treatment

Postoperative care after internal fixation is similar to that described for patella fractures and consists of active and passive motion, making use of CPM. For the first 3–4 months, weight-bearing must be limited to 10 kg, depending on the severity of the fracture type and the degree of osteoporosis and cartilage damage.

If ligaments, tendons and menisci have been resutured, intraoperative testing of tolerable flexion and extension has to be performed. Hinged splints which allow predetermined degrees of movement are applied for 4–6 weeks until the structures have healed.

13.5.2 Tibial Shaft Fractures

13.5.2.1 Principles of Treatment

The problems, such as shortening or angulation, which a fracture of the tibial shaft presents, are evident right from the start: if the shortening is between 0.5 and 1 cm with minimal axial displacement or when reduction can easily be accomplished and maintained, then the fracture should be treated nonoperatively in accordance with the guidelines initially laid down by Böhler (1929) and Watson-Jones (1955), and a long leg plaster cast should be applied. Dehne (1969) recommends a PTB plaster and Sarmiento and Latta (1981) a brace. Unstable fractures of the tibial shaft which are treated nonoperatively require traction for 3 weeks followed by a plaster or brace fixation, usually for 3 months. This often results in permanent impairment due to malunion, joint stiffness, and postthrombotic edema formation.

13.5.2.2 Indications for Open Reduction and Internal Fixation

Open reduction and internal fixation should be considered only if the staff and environment meet all the prerequisites outlined (see Chap. 6).

The following are our indications for open reduction and internal or external operative fixation of tibial shaft fractures in adults and, in rare instances, in children:

Absolute indications

- Concomitant vessel or nerve injuries.
- Compartment syndrome.

Recommendable indications

- Shaft fractures in polytrauma patients who require intensive care treatment.
- All grade 2 and 3 open fractures (see p. 151, 684).
- Unstable fractures with interposition of muscle, tendon or tilted bone fragments.
- Unstable fractures with displacement of the main fragments of more than one half of the shaft diameter, especially in nonspiral fractures.
- Fractures with shortening of more than 1 cm.
- Fractures initially treated closed which have slipped into unacceptable positions.
- Segmental fractures.
- Ipsilateral fractures of the femur or severe knee or ankle injuries.
- Varus deformity exceeding 8° in isolated tibia fractures.
- Short oblique fractures associated with a comminution zone.
- Half rotation fractures (Jahna and Wittich 1985), especially when the dorsal spike of the distal fragment is posteriorly displaced.

Very complex fractures of the tibia may present tremendous technical problems for internal fixation. Such fractures, if they are not combined with displacement in the adjacent joints, are best treated nonoperatively or with an external fixator. If, during subsequent treatment, problems arise such as delayed union or non-union, they usually involve only one fracture line in one segment of the bone, rather than the whole extensive area of comminution: technically, therefore, they have become a very much simpler problem to treat.

13.5.2.3 Guidelines for the Selection of Stabilization Procedures for Shaft Fractures

Intramedullary nailing is the best treatment for closed short oblique and transverse fractures at the middle third of the tibia. Interlocking devices for intramedullary nails have to be used if the fractures are located in the proximal or distal third. Tibia shaft fractures which are not suitable for intramedullary nailing may be treated either by a combination of lag screws with a neutralization plate or by an external fixator. All short oblique fractures which are plated should have a lag screw inserted across the fracture either independent of the plate or – if feasible – across the plate.

13.5.2.4 Fracture Types

Transverse and Short Oblique Fractures of the Middle Third of the Tibia

Short oblique fractures are defined as measuring less than twice the diameter of the fractured bone. These fractures, together with transverse fractures, are ideal indications for conventional intramedullary nailing (see Chap. 4).

Transverse and Short Oblique Fractures of the Proximal and Distal Thirds of the Tibia

In the *proximal third*, these fractures need special fixation in view of the very strong lever arms. Lag screws should be inserted between the major fragments, preferably through the plate which is fixed to a minimum of six cortices. A tension band plate should be added on the anterior crest of the tibia to neutralize the bending forces in the sagittal plane. This tension band plate may be a short semi-tubular or a one-third tubular plate and represents one of the few indications for double plating (Fig. 13.16). As a preferable alternative, an interlocking nail may be considered.

Fig. 13.16 High short oblique fractures.

a Two semi-tubular plates or one semi-tubular and one DCP (or, better, LC-DCP) are fixed with short screws to the anterior and posteromedial edge of the tibia, respectively. The anterior plate acts as a tension band (note that its proximal limit is the tibial tubercle). The surgical approach is an incision down the middle of the medial surface of the tibia.

b Cross section.

c Proximal interlocking is a very good alternative, using the interlocking universal tibia nail.

Fig. 13.16

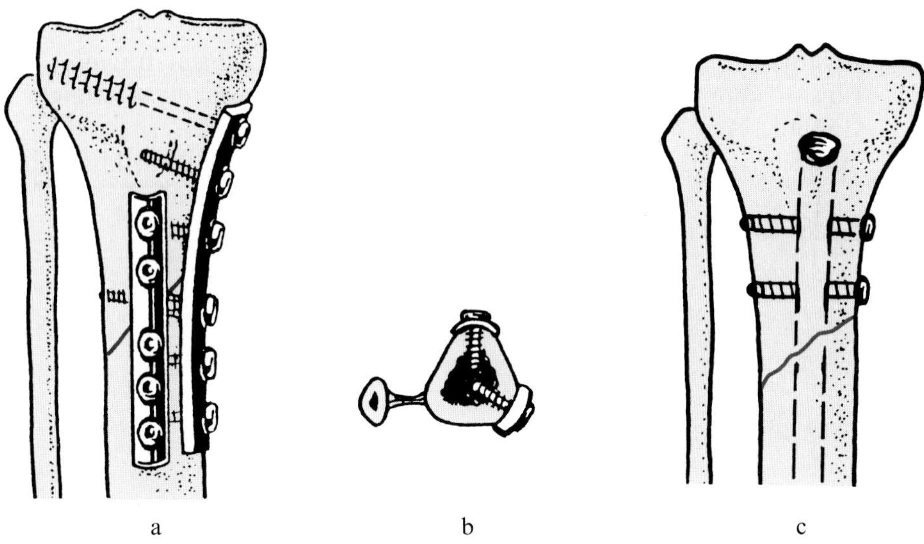

In the distal third, a short oblique fracture may be stabilized with an interlocking tibia nail, by an external fixator or by a combination of lag screws, which exert interfragmental compression, and a neutralization plate (Fig. 13.18). Optimally compressing lag screws cannot always be inserted across the plate. This should be anticipated during preoperative planning. In this case, lag screw fixation will be carried out first and the neutralization plate added afterwards.

Torsion Fractures

Relatively pure torsional forces result in a two-fragment fracture. The incipient crack runs at about 45° to the long axis and the ends join by a straight longitudinal split (Fig. 13.17).

If torsion is combined with bending, this gives rise to a third fragment: the torsion butterfly. We distinguish three torsion butterfly fragments: an anterior (Fig. 13.19); a posterolateral (Fig. 13.20); and a posteromedial (Fig. 13.21).

Fig. 13.17

a Simple torsion fracture: look for incomplete fracture line and hidden torsional butterflies (*dotted lines* indicate the typical location of the hidden fracture lines). Reduction is easy with the help of the reduction clamp.

b The screws are inserted at right angles to the shaft and are staggered, since they follow the spiral of the fracture.

Fig. 13.18 Short spiral fracture of the distal third of the tibia.

a Fixation using the interlocking universal tibia nail. Note that the proximal interlocking screw is in a sagittal direction, the distal one in a transverse direction.

b Fixation with a lag screw independent from the plate in combination with a neutralization plate (Note: any screws which cross the fracture line, even though they are used to fix the plate, should be inserted as lag screws).

Fig. 13.19 Fracture with anterior torsional butterfly.

a, b Such a fracture type seen in the AP and lateral projections.

c The torsional butterfly is fixed to each of the main fragments with a lag screw. A six-hole neutralization plate completes the fixation. Note that the third screw from the top of the plate has been inserted as a lag screw and adds to the interfragmental compression of the fracture.

d Side view.

e Cross section showing the main fracture line crossed by a lag screw inserted through the plate as well as by a lag screw inserted from in front and used to fix the torsional butterfly.

Fig. 13.17

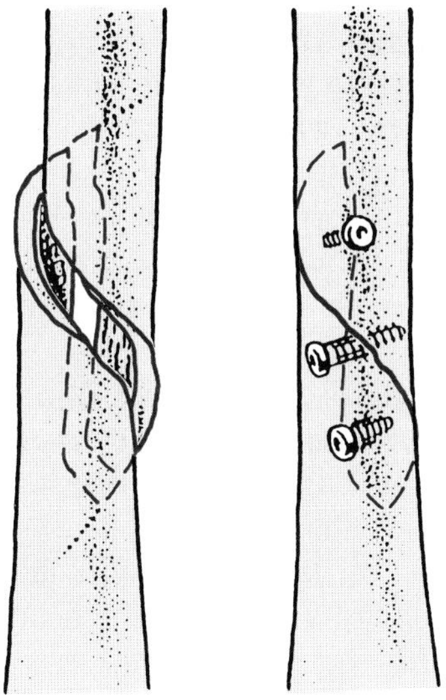

a b

Fig. 13.18

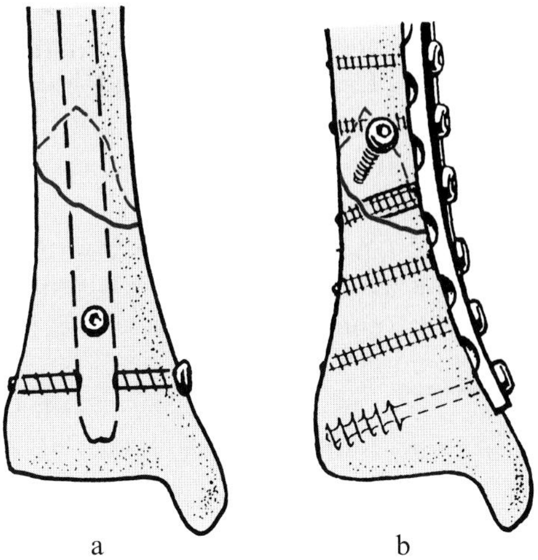

a b

Fig. 13.19

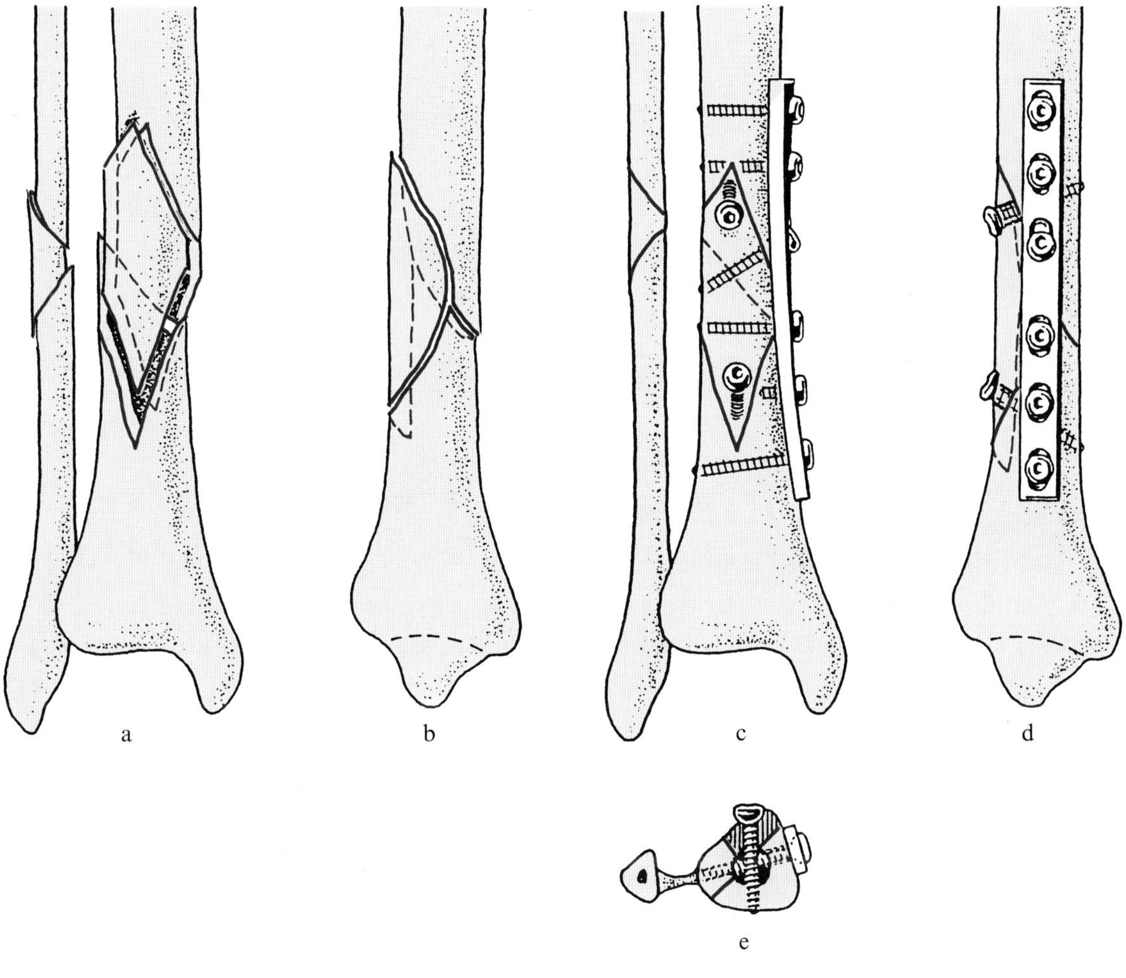

a b c d

e

Operative technique: cleanse and carefully inspect the fracture lines. Pure spiral fractures and fractures with an anterior torsional butterfly are very easy to reduce. Once reduced, they are held with a reduction clamp. Fractures with a posterior torsional butterfly are more difficult and at times require temporary cerclage wiring for reduction. Treatment alternatives are illustrated in Figs. 13.20–13.25.

Usually the internal fixation is carried out first with 3.5-mm or 4.5-mm cortex lag screws. The neutralization plate is added later. Depending on the preoperative planning and drawing, if a lag screw can be placed through the plate, fixation is carried out as described in Chap. 3.

Screw fixation alone is not usually advisable and screw fixation in combination with a neutralization plate is generally preferable to screw fixation alone. The latter may only be considered in extremely long spiral fractures whose length is three to four times the diameter of the bone (Fig. 13.17). The technique of inserting lag screws is reviewed in Chap. 3. The "half rotation fracture" described by Jahna and Wittich (1985) is often an indication for open reduction and internal fixation to prevent delayed union and non-union.

The tibia does not have a constant tension side. Load distribution varies during the different phases of the gait. Neutralization plates can therefore be applied to the most accessible medial surface of the tibia. Exceptions to this rule and therefore to placement of the plate on the lateral cortex of the tibia are:

- Damage to the soft tissue envelope on the medial side.
- Pseudarthroses of the tibia with varus deformity.
- A posteromedial torsional butterfly fragment (Fig. 13.21).
- Small or multiple fragments medially.

Fig. 13.20 Posterolateral torsional butterfly.

a, b Representation of the fracture type.

c Temporary fixation with a cerclage wire permits reduction of the "invisible butterfly" as traction is applied to the limb.

d, e The completed internal fixation.

f Cross section showing the lag screws between the main fragment and the butterfly across the plate.

g Application of a unilateral one-tube external fixator in a sagittal plane, leaving the fracture undisturbed.

Fig. 13.21 Posteromedial torsional butterfly.

a, b Representation of the fracture type.

c The torsional butterfly is fixed to each of the main fragments with a lag screw which does not cross the plate. The medially applied neutralization plate joins the two main fragments.

d The torsional butterfly is fixed with lag screws inserted in an AP direction. The main fragments are joined with a laterally applied neutralization plate. This allows one to use a shorter plate and one does not have to drill such large holes in the butterfly fragment, since all the gliding holes are drilled through the main fragments.

e Lateral view of the internal fixation.

Fig. 13.20

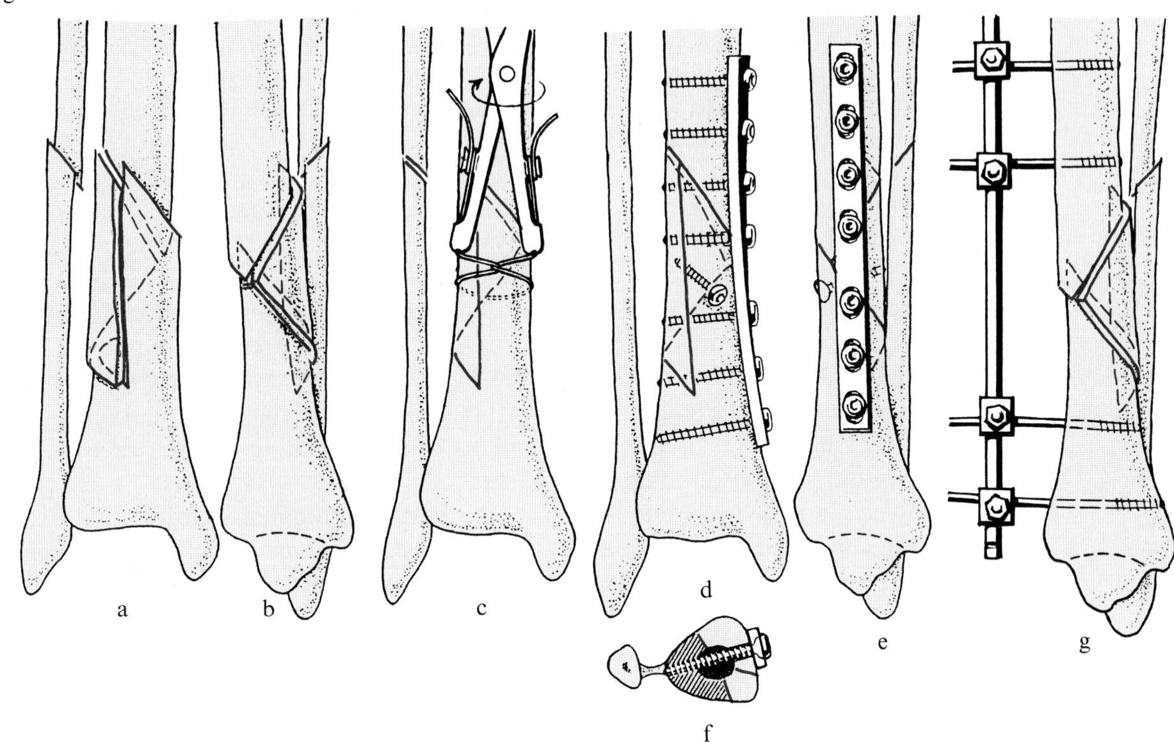

Fig. 13.21

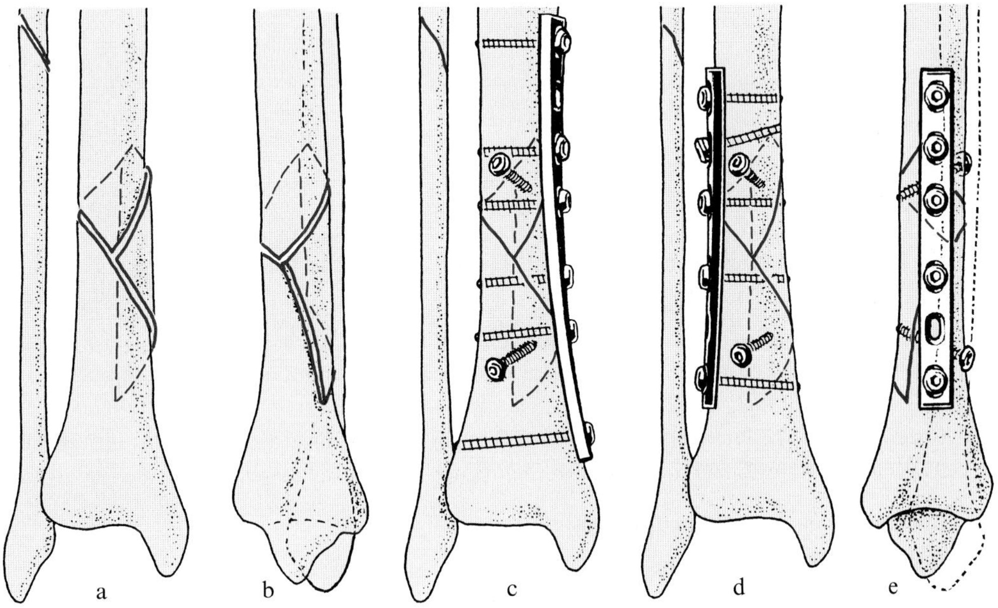

a b c d e

Bending Fracture with a Burst (Bending) Butterfly

Bending fractures are usually more severe injuries, because they occur as a result of direct force. Butterfly fragments which are the result of bending forces are hazardous because they often lose their blood supply and break out easily during reaming for intramedullary nailing. If this happens during open intramedullary nailing, such a fragment should be replaced by a primary cancellous bone graft.

If internal fixation with a plate is performed, the burst butterfly should be fitted and fixed with two 3.5-mm cortex screws used as lag screws (Fig. 13.22). To facilitate the reduction without stripping the butterfly fragments, temporary distraction can be helpful. With an area of avascular cortex longer than 1 cm or over a comminuted zone, a primary cancellous onlay bone graft is indicated to speed up callus formation. In second and third degree open fractures, it is safer to perform this graft after wound healing.

If the plate bridges the butterfly fragment, biomechanically useless screws should be left out of the plate. In the unhappy event that a screw hole lies over a fracture line, the near cortex should be drilled to 4.5 mm to avoid spreading of the fracture. The screw will then only bite into the opposite cortex.

Alternatively, in closed bending fractures with butterfly fragments, an external fixator can be used in combination with lag screws and a cancellous bone graft. This is especially recommended in closed fractures associated with severe muscle and skin trauma with a potential for compartment syndrome where prophylactic fasciotomy appears to be indicated. A valid fixation of such fractures can be achieved with the interlocking universal tibia nail (Fig. 13.22f).

In bending fractures with two butterfly fragments, one of the solutions shown in Fig. 13.23 (or an external fixator) may be chosen. With more butterfly fragments, the number of complications will increase. The greater the complexity of the fracture, the more we are inclined to recommend nonoperative treatment or closed manipulation and insertion of an external fixator. Sometimes, limited internal fixation can be performed

---

Fig. 13.22 Bending fracture.

a, b Representation of the fracture.

c Reduction and internal fixation of the burst butterfly by means of two small cortex lag screws which do not go through the plate. The neutralization plate joins the two main fragments. One lag screw has been inserted through the plate in such a way that it lags the two main fragments together.

d Side view.

e Alternative: replacement of the devitalized burst butterfly by a primary cancellous bone graft. This technique is also recommended if in open intramedullary nailing of the tibia the burst butterfly breaks out.

f Fixation using the interlocking universal tibia nail. At the distal end, note the sagittal position of the proximal interlocking screw.

Fig. 13.23 Complex (comminuted) fracture of the tibia.

a, b Representation of the fracture.

c The situation after reduction and temporary fixation with a cerclage wire and two lag screws.

d The internal fixation has been completed with a long plate and three separate lag screws. All screws traversing the fracture have been inserted as lag screws!

e Fixation using the interlocking universal tibia nail.

f Reduction (indirect) using distractor and secondary plating, avoiding exposure of the many fragments. Anatomic reduction as shown in the illustration is not mandatory as long as length and rotation are perfect. Alternatively, an external fixator is used instead of a long plate.

Fig. 13.22

Fig. 13.23

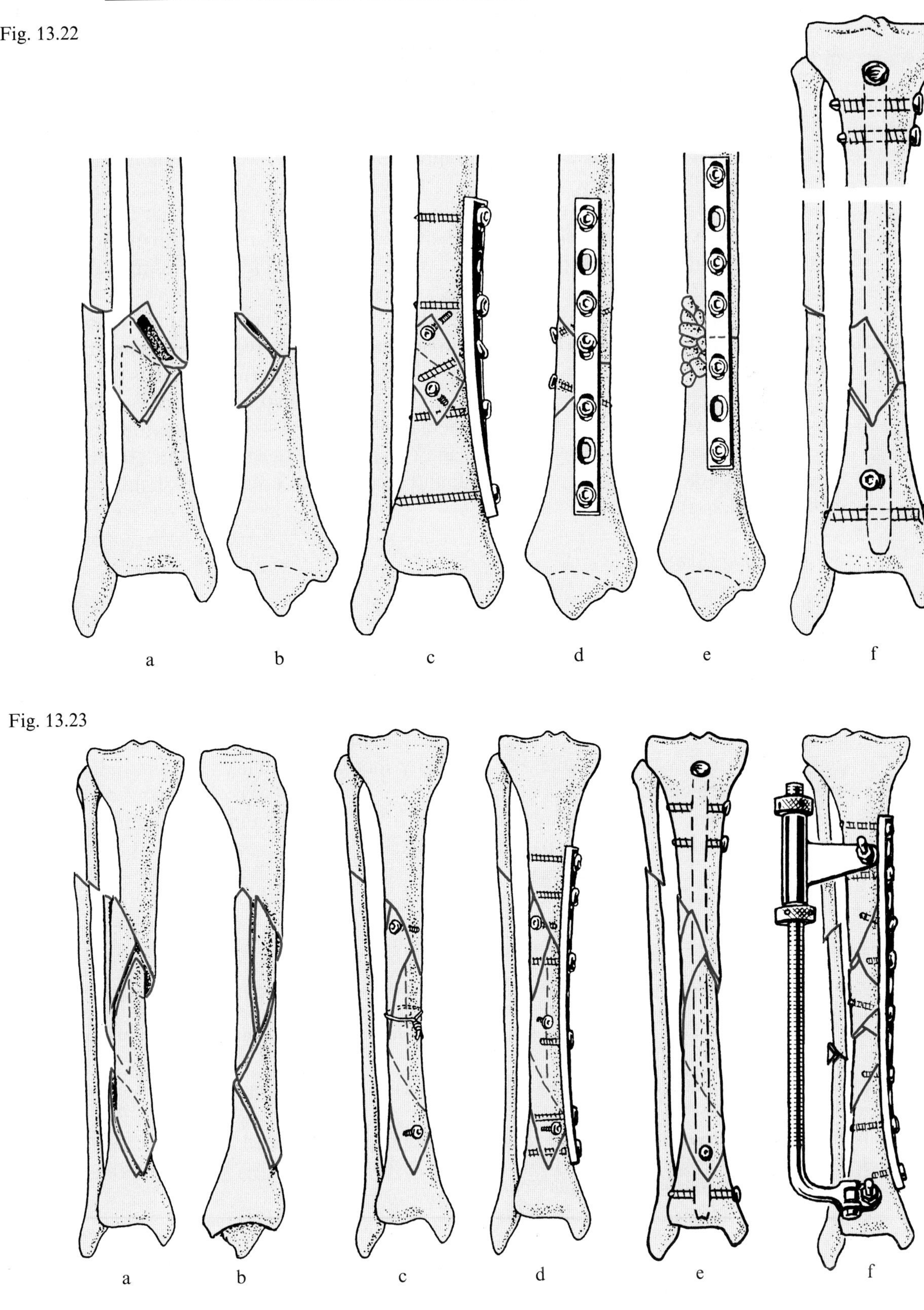

using lag screws to build up the proximal and distal main fragment without stripping and devascularization of these fragments. Secondary bone grafting after 6–12 weeks is often indicated, particularly after primary fixation by means of an external fixator.

Segmental Fractures

A segmental fracture has one or more fragments including the full circumference of the bone.

In simple segmental fractures, the DCP and the LC-DCP allow each fracture to be placed under axial compression independently from the others. The fragments have to be reduced accurately, but exposure should be minimal to avoid unnecessary devascularization (Fig. 13.24a–d).

An intramedullary nail may also be used to good advantage. It should be combined with interlocking bolts to provide rotational stability and avoid shortening. Reaming has to be done very cautiously – if at all – to avoid spinning the fragments (Fig. 13.24e, f). A valid alternative method – especially if the soft tissue envelope is not reliable due to acute or old damage (post-thrombosis syndrome) – is the sagittal double bar external fixator or the unilateral, two-plane (V-shaped) external fixator. Additional lag screws in oblique fractures may be added, and a cancellous onlay graft should be considered (Fig. 13.24g).

Short, Highly Complex Tibia Shaft Fractures

Localized areas of extensive comminution of the shaft make reconstruction of the cortical diaphysis very difficult. If such fractures are associated with damage to the soft tissue envelope, the leg is best stabilized by a unilateral one- or two-plane (V-shaped) external fixator. Primary or delayed cancellous bone grafting may be indicated. Open reduction can be facilitated by the distractor letting the fragments "fall into place" without additional devitalization. A cancellous bone graft should be added (Fig. 13.25). A one-third tubular plate to fix the fractured fibula very markedly increases stability. An alternative is the unreamed interlocking nail.

Compartment syndrome may occur more often in very complex fractures and can be easily missed in unconscious patients! Secondary plating or nailing might be considered later.

Fig. 13.24 Segmental fractures of the tibia.

a, b Representation of the fracture type and its fixation with a medially applied plate and separate lag screws inserted across the main fracture lines. This type of fixation can be carried out only if the soft tissue envelope is intact. Low fibular fractures, if fixed by a one-third tubular plate, in many instances greatly add to the stability of low tibia fractures!

c, d The internal fixation of an open fracture or of a fracture with a damaged soft tissue envelope. The plate is applied laterally under muscle cover.

e, f The use of an intramedullary nail with slight or no reaming to regain axial alignment of the fragments. Additional rotational stability is obtained by means of interlocking. Cancellous bone may have to be added in a second operation if not done primarily.

g Application of an anteromedian external fixator may be chosen as a good alternative.

Fig. 13.25 Short, shattered segment of the tibial shaft.

a, b Small shattered and denuded cortical fragments are best removed and replaced by cancellous bone graft. In such cases, it is best to bridge the zone of comminution by means of an anteromedial external fixator and to fix the fibula with a one-third tubular plate. (However, never sacrifice fragments with soft tissue attachment which can be fitted into place by indirect reduction!).

Fig. 13.24

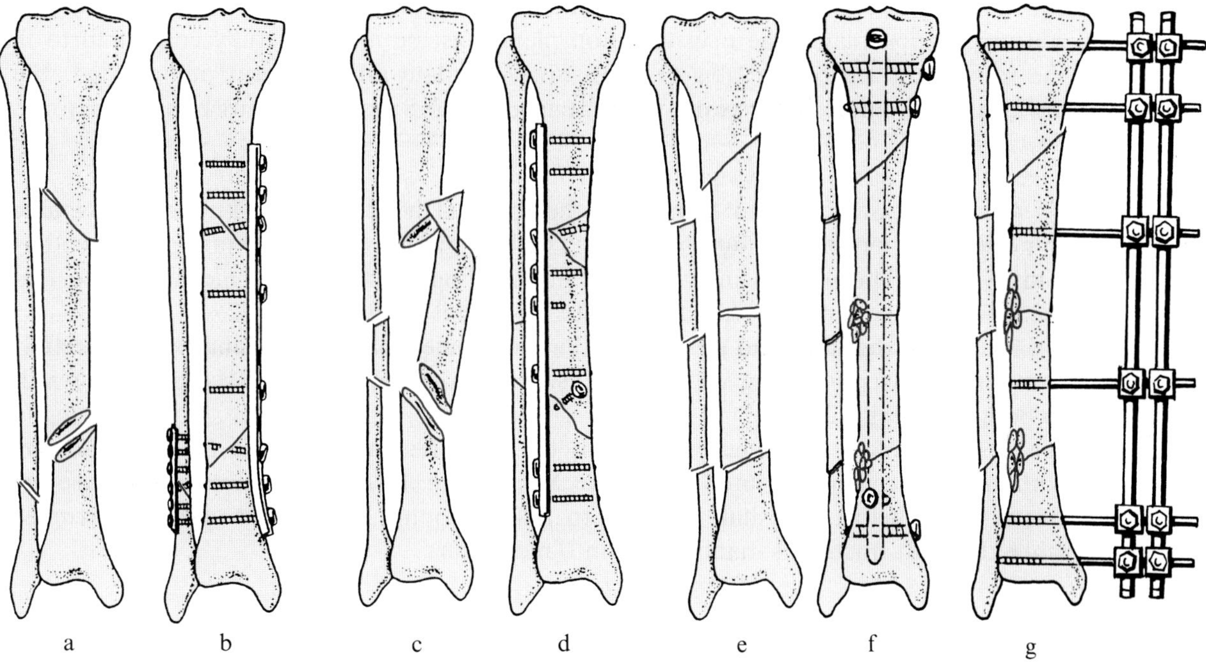

Fig. 13.25

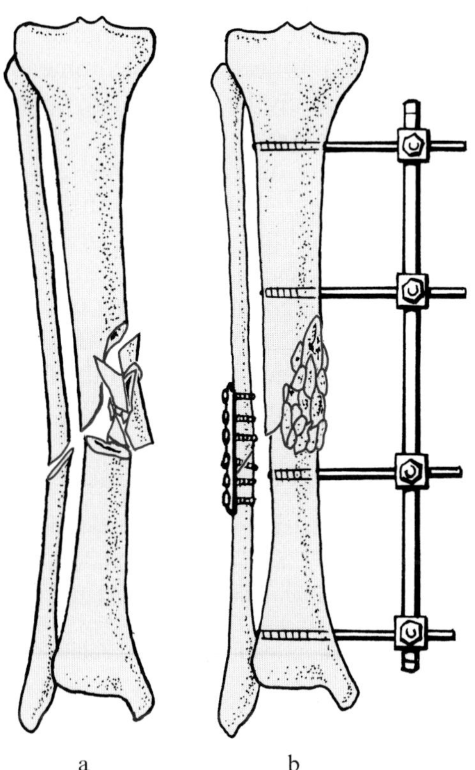

Torsional Fractures of the Distal Third of the Tibia Without Either an Extension into the Joint or an Undislocated Fissure Line into the Joint

Fractures with torsional butterfly fragments require the combination of a lag screw with a neutralization plate. The neutralization plate must be most carefully contoured to fit the medial surface of the tibia (Fig. 13.26). The plate must be bent and twisted. For distal screw fixation of the plate, the fully threaded 6.5-mm cancellous bone screws may be chosen, but normally 4.5-mm cortex screws can be anchored very solidly. (See also Fig. 13.18b.)

A bending press is used to achieve the required bend, and bending irons are used to achieve the required amount of twist. The bending pliers allow simultaneous bending and twisting. The plate is inserted into the bending pliers at an angle of 45°, so that the anterior edge is proximal and the posterior edge is distal (Fig. 13.27).

The use of the DCP and the LC-DCP allows some axial compression by the carefully contoured plate proceeding with screw insertion from the middle of the plate outwards to both ends (Fig. 13.26).

In spiral fractures of the distal tibia, the fractures can extend into the ankle joint without displacement (fissure lines of the X-ray) (Fig. 13.17). A lag screw should secure this fracture before the shaft is fixed so that the joint is not inadvertently disrupted when the shaft fracture is manipulated into reduction.

13.5.3 Fractures of the Distal Third of the Tibia with Extension into the Ankle Joint: "Pilon Fractures"

Very complex fractures with little dislocation and preserved anatomy of the joint surface obviously feature an intact joint capsule and should be treated conservatively. Control tomography in AP and lateral projections is recommended. Fragment dislocation extending to the joint surface can rarely be reduced by ligamentotaxis and therefore requires open reduction and internal fixation.

These are extremely delicate operations. They are carried out in a skin territory – the distal part of the lower leg – which has the most precarious microcirculation of the whole body. Any rough handling or kinking of skin flaps, especially with a tourniquet in place, easily leads to catastrophe.

There are five important diagnostic elements which determine the operative strategy in dealing with the 43B and 43C type fractures of the distal tibia – the classical tibial pilon fractures. Three of these elements concern the fibula and two the distal tibia. These five elements occur in six combinations.

Fig. 13.26 Fracture of the distal tibia without extension into the ankle joint.

a, b Lag screw fixation combined with a neutralization plate which was contoured to fit exactly the shape of the bone. Screw 1 is applied after fixation of the butterfly fragment. It is placed as a lag screw between the two main fragments, across the plate. Screw 2 provides additional fixation for the plate to the tibia, and screw 3 is inserted in load position to achieve axial compression. The remaining screws are inserted in neutral positions.

Fig. 13.27

a, b The bending pliers allow simultaneous bending and twisting of the plate which is necessary in contouring the plate to fit the distal third of the tibia. To this effect, the plate is introduced at an angle of 45° (Fig. 13.27b).

Fig. 13.26

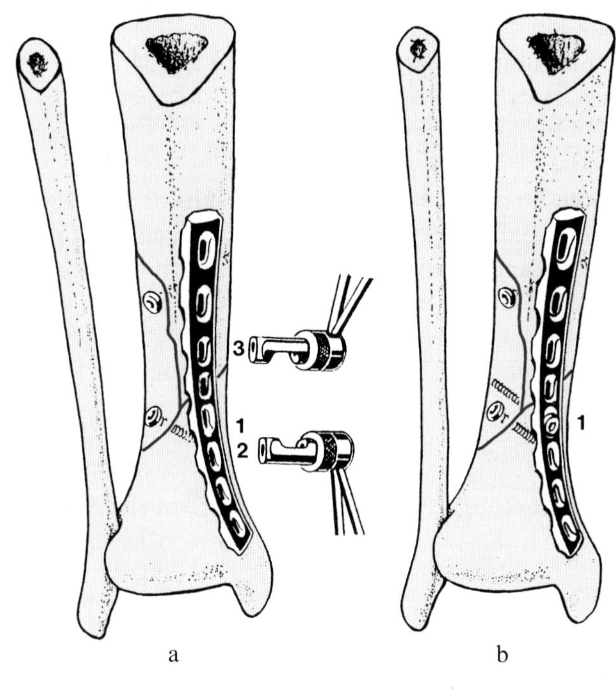

Fig. 13.27

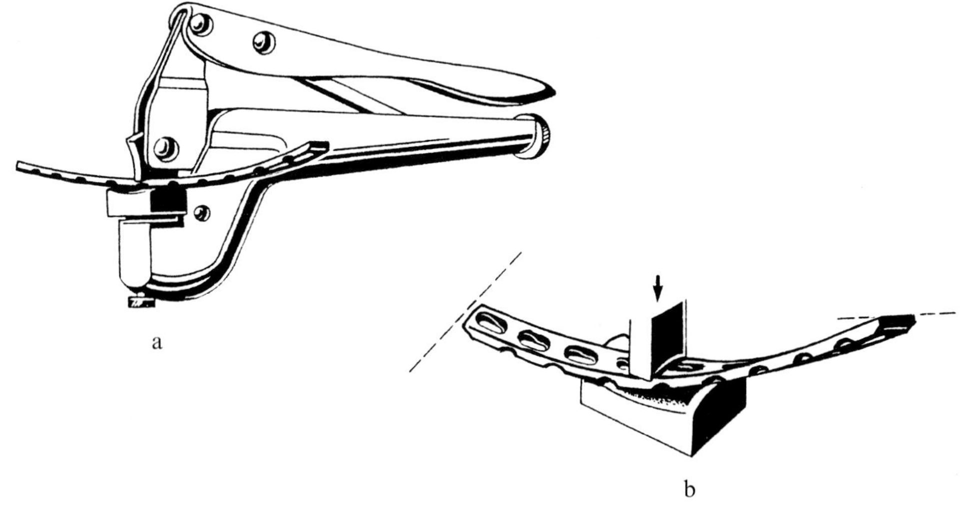

Evaluation of Fibula

- The fibula is fractured (about 80% of pilon fractures)
  - Simple fibula fracture
  - Complex fibula fracture
- The fibula is intact (about 20% of pilon fractures)

Evaluation of Distal Tibia

- Explosion fractures with no loss of substance (very characteristic for young, hard bone and usually sustained under the influence of moderate energy)
- Impacted fractures with loss of substance by compression of the involved cancellous bone (more likely to occur in osteoporotic bone or when high energy is absorbed)

The steps of operative reduction and fixation consider the following six fracture situations:

Fibula intact	Explosion fracture of the distal tibia Impacted fracture of the distal tibia
Simple fibula fracture	Explosion fracture of the distal tibia Impacted fracture of the distal tibia
Complex fibula fracture	Explosion fracture of the distal tibia Impacted fracture of the distal tibia

Occasionally the external fixator or the distractor may be used to facilitate reconstruction by ligamentotaxis. With very precarious skin, the external fixator may also be used as a buttress device to prevent secondary deformity (Fig. 13.28e, f).

13.5.3.1 Operative Procedures with Fibula Fracture Present

Reduction and fixation of the fibula is carried out as the first step. This is easy with a *simple fibula fracture* (Fig. 13.28) but considerably more difficult in a *complex fibula fracture* where one wants to be sure that length and rotation are correctly reconstituted. The first act of fibular reconstruction greatly helps in reducing the distal tibia fracture.

Reconstruction of very complex fibula fractures (or with intact fibula but complex fractures of the distal tibia) require X-ray comparison with the intact side for control of reduction!

With a fibula fracture present, two incisions with a skin bridge of at least 7 cm between them are necessary (see Sect. 13.3.3).

Fig. 13.28 The four steps in the reconstruction of the distal tibia.

a Fracture type C2 with simple fibula fracture.

b First step: fibular reconstruction.

c Second step: reconstruction of the articular surface and its temporary fixation with Kirschner wires.

d Third and fourth steps: bone grafting of the defect with cancellous bone and then buttressing medially or anteriorly to prevent subsequent varus deformity. Whether bone grafting is done before or after application of the buttress plate depends on the accessibility of the bone defect.

e Indirect reduction using the distractor and temporary fixation of joint fragments with Kirschner wires. Internal fixation can then be applied to the fibula.

f Fixation using an external frame if the soft tissues do not permit primary internal fixation of the tibia. Most of the fine fracture fragments of the joint can be stabilized with 3.5-mm cortex screws.

Fig. 13.28

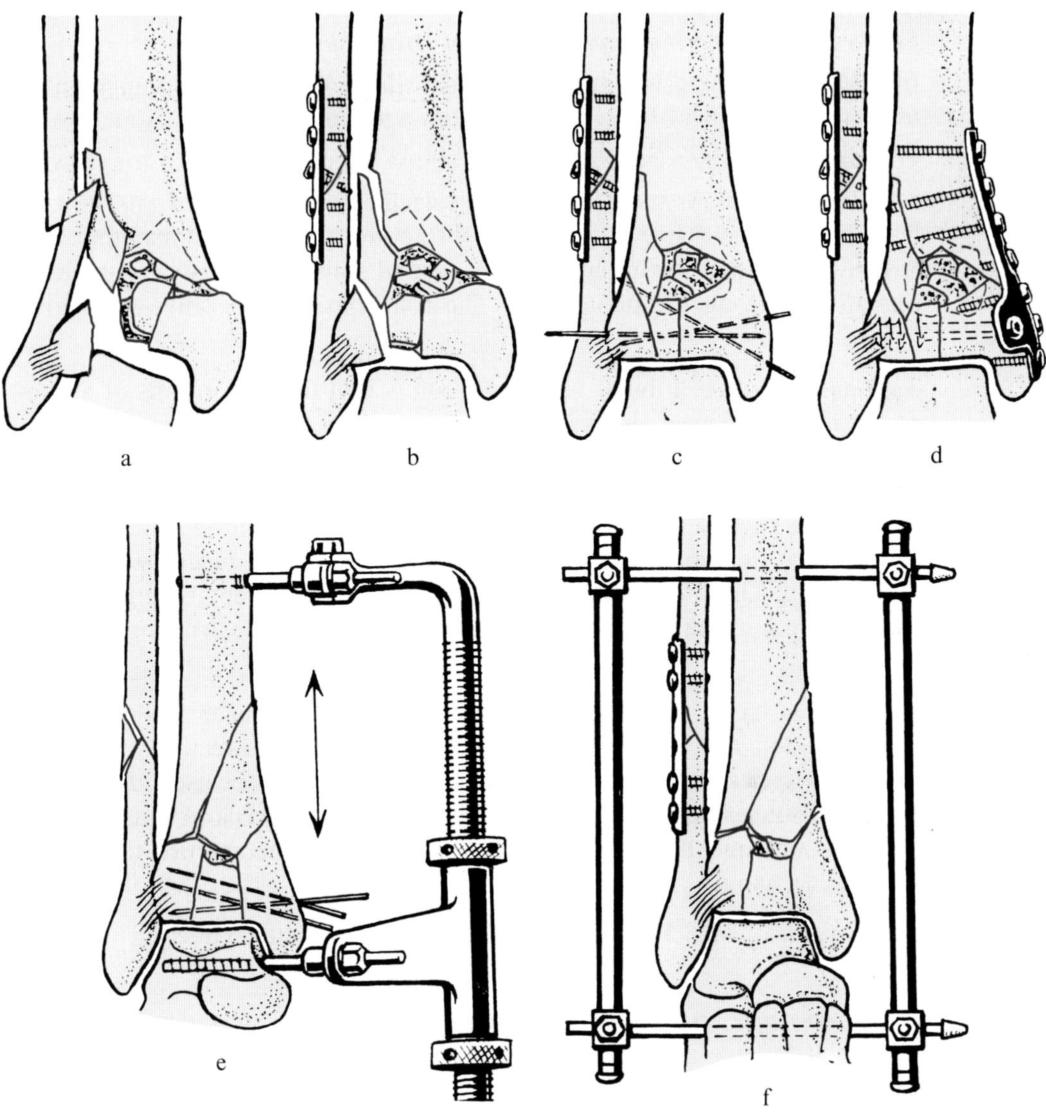

Fibula Fracture and Explosion Fracture of Distal Tibia

Simple and, if at all possible, also complex fibula fractures should be reduced in a first step. As there is no or only minimal loss of substance, lag screw fixation of the reduced tibia fragments is adequate in young bone, and healing occurs rapidly in the metaphyseal area. In osteoporotic bone, prevention of secondary varus deformity by applying a medial buttress plate is recommended.

Fibula Fracture and Impacted Fracture of Distal Tibia

In cases where there is a fibula fracture, whether simple or complex, and an impacted fracture of the distal tibia, a preparatory and four "classical" operative steps have to be performed, as advocated by Rüedi et al. (1968).

Preparatory step. As the necessity of replacing the compressed and impacted cancellous bone is clearly anticipated, harvesting of good quality cancellous bone before the reconstructive operation (or in parallel by a second team) is strongly recommended to shorten operating time on the pilon itself. The four classical operative steps are illustrated in Fig. 13.28b–d.

First operative step. Fibular reconstruction is best done by means of a one-third tubular plate. This maneuver alone in most cases brings about a surprisingly good reduction of the distal tibia fracture. In about 20% of cases, a primary fibular reconstruction is not possible because of extensive comminution, or it does not help in the reduction of the tibia because the fracture is high and the syndesmotic ligaments and interosseous membranes are ruptured. In these cases, the operation begins with the reconstruction of the tibia. One must search for the key main fragment because it will indicate the correct length of the tibia and allow one to begin the reconstruction.

Second operative step. Reconstruction of the joint surface. Quite often, the articular surface of the talus has to be used as a template for the articular reconstruction. Temporary fixation is obtained with Kirschner wires or occasionally directly by inserting small cancellous bone screws. Cannulated cancellous bone screws can be useful for replacing optimally placed Kirschner wires! Kirschner wires as well as screws can be inserted from the medial side and subsequently from the lateral side, through the anterior tibial tubercle (tubercle of Tillaux-Chaput).

Third operative step. Filling in the bony cavity left after reduction with cancellous bone graft.

Fourth operative step. Medial buttress plate. T plates, cloverleaf plates or occasionally simple DCPs give adequate support. The cloverleaf plate is the thinnest and the most easily contoured plate, but it accepts only 3.5-mm or 4.0-mm screws. It can easily be cut to the desired shape and is therefore very flexible in its application. If the main fracture lines are in a frontal plane, the T or cloverleaf plate is placed on the anterior surface of the distal tibia (Fig. 13.29).

Primary arthrodesis is rather controversial because a good final result can be achieved even in severe complex fractures as long as the cartilage is not badly damaged. Furthermore, if arthrodesis should become necessary, it is much easier to perform if the metaphyseal area has consolidated into a solid block.

Fig. 13.29

a, b If the main fracture lines are in a frontal plane, the T plate or the cloverleaf plate is placed on the anterior surface of the distal tibia. The cloverleaf plate can be tailored by removing the middle leaf if necessary.

Fig. 13.29

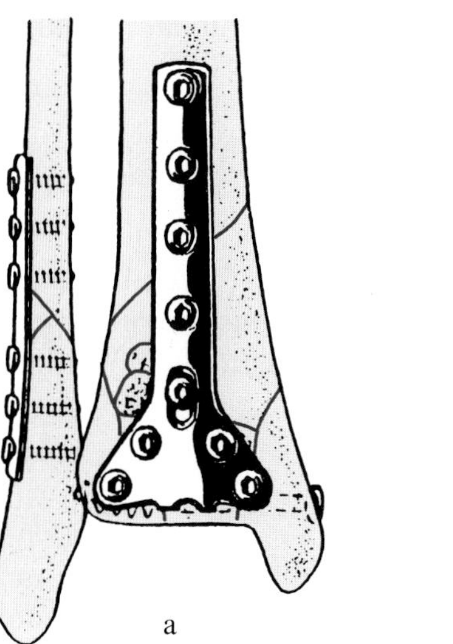

a

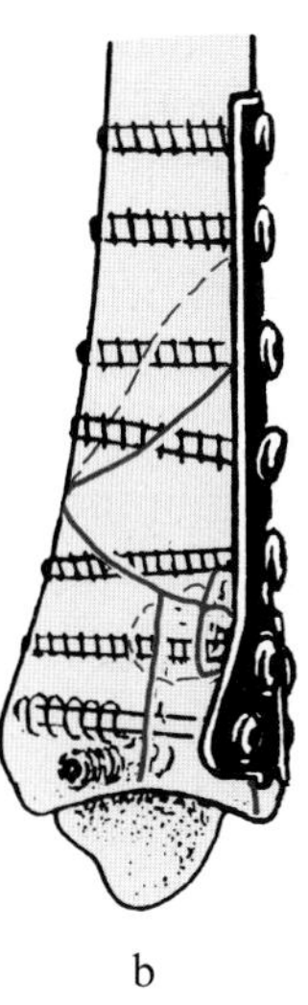

b

13.5.3.2 Operative Procedure with an Intact Fibula

In the majority of cases there is one major tibia fragment which, after reduction, indicates the length and the axis of the distal tibia. Often this tibia fragment is still fixed to the fibula by the tibiofibular ligaments of the syndesmosis.

Intact Fibula and Explosion Fracture of Distal Tibia

The primary operative act is directed to the reconstruction of the joint surface. Preliminary fixation with Kirschner wire is very helpful. Stabilization of a well-reduced explosion fracture in young bone is perfectly adequate and fully compatible with early active mobilization. Osteoporotic bone needs an additional medial buttress, preferably using the relatively thin cloverleaf plate.

Intact Fibula and Impacted Fracture of Distal Tibia

Good exposure of the distal joint surface is particularly important. Therefore, the incision over the tibia is somewhat more to the lateral side but still curves around the medial malleolus. It is in these cases that the talus can often be used as a mold to return impacted, cartilage-bearing fragments to their anatomic position. The resulting metaphyseal cavity has to be filled in with cancellous bone.

Open Pilon Fractures

Most of the time, the soft tissue injury lies on the medial side. Reconstruction of the fibula can be performed without undue risk and in most cases restores length, axis and to some extent even joint alignments. Secondary anatomic reconstruction of the distal tibia is thus greatly facilitated. Temporary medial stabilization can be achieved with a triangular unilateral external fixator anchored in the calcaneus, metatarsal I and the midshaft tibia.

Postoperative Care of Pilon Fractures

The principle is early movement with emphasis on dorsiflexion and delayed weight-bearing! The comminuted intra-articular component of the fracture must be allowed to heal with firm union, and weight-bearing can therefore only start after 4 weeks and then gradually increase over the next 1–2 months. A U splint is used for the first few days, keeping the ankle joint at 90° to prevent equinus deformity. For the relatively long period of non-weight-bearing and partial weight-bearing, we recommend a tibial walking caliper (Fig. 13.30), which takes the weight off the pilon. A set of exchangeable springs supports the foot and increasingly puts weight onto the fracture.

Fig. 13.30 The tibial walking caliper.

This is available in four sizes. It allows early motion but delayed weight-bearing. With a little practice, the patient can resume walking without the help of crutches. Weight is transmitted to the tibial condyles and to the patellar tendon. The foot is kept out of equinus by means of a spring. This relieves most of the weight from the distal tibia. The patient must begin gradually with the use of the weight-relieving caliper, because initially its use results in some obstruction to venous return.

Fig. 13.30

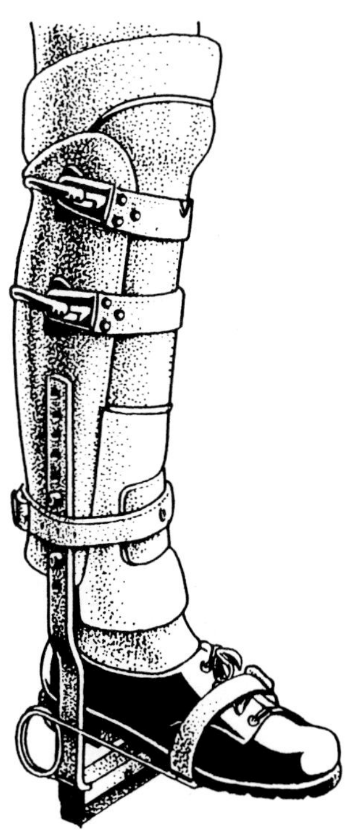

References

Allgöwer M (1967) A healing of clinical fractures of the tibia and rigid internal fixation. Reprint from "The healing of osseous tissue". Natl Acad Sci – Natl Res Council, pp 81–89

Bandi W (1974) Die distalen intraartikulären Schienbeinbrüche des Skifahrers. Aktuel Traumatol 4:1–6

Böhler L (1929, 1963) Die Technik der Knochenbruchbehandlung. Maudrich, Vienna

Dehne E (1969) Treatment of fractures of the tibial shaft. Clin Orthop 66:159

Ganz R, Allgöwer M, Ehrsam R, Matter P, Perren SM (1969) Clinical experience with a new compression plate DCP. Acta Orthop Scand [Suppl] 125

Hansen ST Jr, Veith RG (1987) Closed Küntscher nailing of the tibia. In: Browner BD, Edwards CC (eds) The science and practice of intramedullary nailing. Lea and Febiger, Philadelphia

Herzog K (1960) Die Technik der geschlossenen Marknagelung des Oberschenkels mit dem Rohrschlitznagel. Chirurg 31:465

Jahna H, Wittich H (1985) Konservative Methoden in der Frakturbehandlung. Urban and Schwarzenberg, Vienna

Küntscher G (1962) Die Marknagelung. Springer, Berlin Göttingen Heidelberg

Küntscher G, Maatz R (1945) Technik der Marknagelung. Thieme, Leipzig

Mast J, Jakob R, Ganz R (1989) Planning and reduction technique in fracture surgery. Springer, Berlin Heidelberg New York

Müller ME, Allgöwer M, Willenegger H (1963) Technik der operativen Frakturenbehandlung. Springer, Berlin Göttingen Heidelberg

Pauwels F (1965) Gesammelte Abhandlungen zur funktionellen Anatomie des Bewegungsapparates. Springer, Berlin Heidelberg New York

Perren SM, Russenberger M, Steinemann S, Müller ME, Allgöwer M (1969) A dynamic compression plate. Acta Orthop Scand [Suppl] 125

Rüedi T, Matter P, Allgöwer M (1968) Die intraartikuläen Frakturen des distalen Unterschenkelendes. Helv Chir Acta 35:556–582

Rüedi T, Matter P, Allgöwer M (1973) Frakturen des Pilon Tibial: Ergebnisse nach 9 Jahren. Arch Orthop Unfallchir 76:248–254

Rüedi T, Kolbow H, Allgöwer M (1975a) Erfahrungen mit der dynamischen Kompressionsplatte (DCP) bei 418 frischen Unterschenkelschaftbrüchen. Arch Orthop Unfallchir 82:247–256

Rüedi T, Hell K, Müller C (1975b) Nachkontrolle von 50 operativ behandelten Tibiakopffrakturen. Helv Chir Acta 42:27–29

Rüedi T, Hochstetter AHC, Schlumpf R (1984) Operative Zugänge der Osteosynthese. Springer, Berlin Heidelberg New York

Sarmiento A, Latta LL (1981) Closed functional treatment of fractures. Springer, Berlin Heidelberg New York

Schatzker J, Tile M (1987) The rationale of operative fracture care. Springer, Berlin Heidelberg New York

Schenk RK, Willenegger H (1964) Histologie der primären Knochenheilung. Langenbecks Arch Klin Chir 308:440–452

Schneider R (1961) Die Marknagelung der Tibia. Helv Chir Acta 28:207

Schneider R (1963) Komplikationen bei der Marknagelung der Tibia. Helv Chir Acta 30:95–97

Schweiberer L, Hofmeier G (1967) Die Bündelnagelung bei Unterschenkel- und Oberarmfrakturen. Zentralbl Chir 92:48, 2903

Schweiberer L, Van de Berg A, Dambe LT (1970) Das Verhalten der intraossären Gefässe nach Osteosynthese der frakturierten Tibia des Hundes. Therapiewoche 20:1330

Szyszkowitz R, Reschauer R, Seggl W (1981) Gefahren der Plattenosteosynthese und Möglichkeiten des Fixateur externe in der Frakturversorgung. Hefte Unfallheilkd 153:183–189

Szyszkowitz R, Fellinger M, Passler J (1986) Spongiosaplastic oder Verfahrenswechsel. Hefte Unfallheilkd 200:280–284

Szyszkowitz R, Fellinger M, Passler J (1987) Verzögerte Frakturheilung. In: Schmit-Neuerburg KP, Stürmer KM (eds) Die Tibiaschaftfraktur beim Erwachsenen. Springer, Berlin Heidelberg New York

Szyszkowitz R, Reschauer R, Seggl W (1988) Pilon fractures of the tibia. In: Chapman MW et al. (eds) Operative orthopaedics, vol 3. Lippincott, Philadelphia

Tscherne H, Lobenhoffer H, Russe O (1984) Proximale intraarticuläre Tibiafrakturen. Unfallheilkunde 87:277

Watson-Jones R (1955) Fractures and joint injuries. Livingstone, Edinburgh

Weber BG (1972) Die Verletzungen des oberen Sprunggelenks. Huber, Bern

Weber BG, Cech O (1976) Pseudarthrosis. Pathophysiology, biomechanics, therapy, results. Huber, Bern

Weller S (1965) Die Marknagelung von Ober- und Unterschenkelbrüchen. Dt Med Wochenschr 16:681–684

Weller S (1974) Die Marknagelung von Unterschenkelschaftbrüchen. Hefte Unfallheilkd 117:98–102

Willenegger H (1975) Verplattung und Marknagelung bei Femur- und Tibiaschaftfrakturen: pathophysiologische Grundlagen. Leitthema: Nagelung oder Plattenosteosynthese? Chirurg 46:145

14 MALLEOLAR FRACTURES

14.1 Introduction

Although the ankle joint may be damaged by a direct force, such as a blow to the malleolus or a gunshot, the majority of malleolar fractures are indirect injuries resulting from subluxation or dislocation of the talus out of the ankle mortice. Certain fracture patterns are always associated with distinct ligamentous disruptions or their equivalent avulsion fractures of the ligamentous attachments.

14.2 Significant Anatomic and Functional Features

There are two groups of ligaments:

1. The inferior tibiofibular ligamentous complex guarantees a tight elastic ankle mortice and consists of three elements:

- At the level of the ankle joint, the anterior syndesmotic ligament joins the anterior tibial tubercle (tubercle of Tillaux-Chaput) to the lateral malleolus (Fig. 14.1a).
- The stronger posterior syndesmotic ligament joins the lateral malleolus to the posterior tibial tubercle, which is the lateral extension of Volkmann's triangle (Fig. 14.1b).
- The interosseous membrane joins the fibula to the tibia proximal to the syndesmosis.

2. The collateral ligaments prevent any tilting movement of the talus in the ankle mortice and include the following:

- The lateral collateral ligament has three divisions: the anterior talofibular ligament, the calcaneofibular ligament and the posterior talofibular ligament (Fig. 14.2a).
- The medial collateral, or deltoid, ligament has two main parts, the tibiotalar and the tibiocalcaneal (Fig. 14.2b).

The talus is in close contact with the entire articular surface of the mortice in all positions of dorsiflexion and plantar flexion of the foot. This intimate contact is the principal mechanism for load distribution at the ankle and must, therefore, be perfectly restored after injury. Normal motion between the distal tibia and fibula at the syndesmosis is an essential part of the mechanism for maintaining this contact.

Exact anatomic reconstruction of the ankle mortice is necessary for perfect congruity with the talus. The integrity of the ankle mortice depends upon:

1. The correct length of the fibula and its exact position in the fibular notch of the tibia (Fig. 14.3).

2. The integrity of the tibiofibular bond, which consists of three elements: the anterior syndesmotic ligament, the posterior syndesmotic ligament and the interosseous membrane (Fig. 14.1a, b).

Reconstruction of the lateral complex, i.e., the fibula with its tight elastic connection to the tibia (the fibulo-syndesmotic complex), has biomechanical priority over the reconstruction of the medial malleolus. Nevertheless, the medial malleolus and the posterior tibial margin are important stabilizing articular structures. Even minimal displacements of joint fragments will result in incongruity between the talus and the ankle mortice, resulting in secondary traumatic arthritis.

The diagnosis of a malleolar injury demands identification of all the fractures and ligamentous injuries. The level of the fibular fracture allows one to deduce the injury to the tibiofibular ligamentous connections in all indirect injuries. The various patterns are a reflection of the direction and energy of the applied force.

- If a transverse fracture of the lateral malleolus is at the level of, or distal to, the tibiotalar articulation, then the tibiofibular ligamentous connections (the anterior and posterior syndesmotic ligaments and the interosseous membrane) are intact.
- If an oblique fracture of the distal fibula passes upwards and backwards from the level of the ankle joint, then some degree of disruption of the anterior portion of the tibiofibular ligamentous complex is usual.
- If a fibular shaft fracture does not extend below the syndesmotic ligamentous connections, then there is always disruption of this complex. This may be either ligamentous disruption or avulsion with a bony attachment, or a combination of the two. Such an injury will always result in major instability of the ankle mortice. On this basis, ankle fractures may be classified according to the level of the fibular injury: type A, type B, and type C.

Fig. 14.1 The anatomy of the tibiofibular ligaments.
a Seen from the front.
b Seen from the back.

Fig. 14.2 The collateral ligaments, the "guide ropes" for the talus.
a The three divisions of the collateral ligament.
b The deltoid ligament.

Fig. 14.3 Cross section at the level of the syndesmotic ligaments. The lateral malleolus fits snugly into the fibular notch of the tibia and is held in place by the tight elastic syndesmotic ligaments.

Fig. 14.1

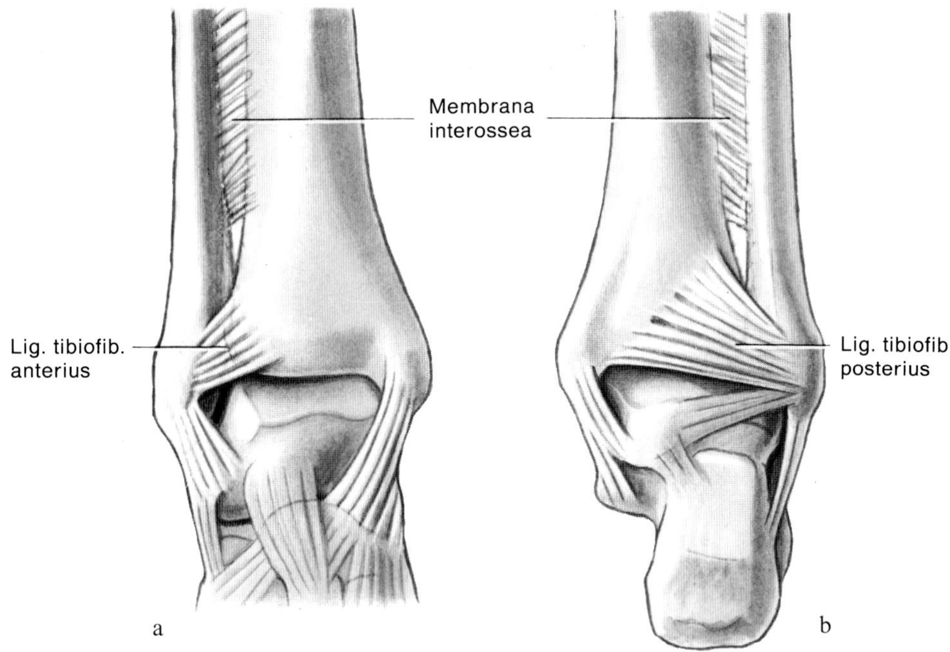

Fig. 14.2

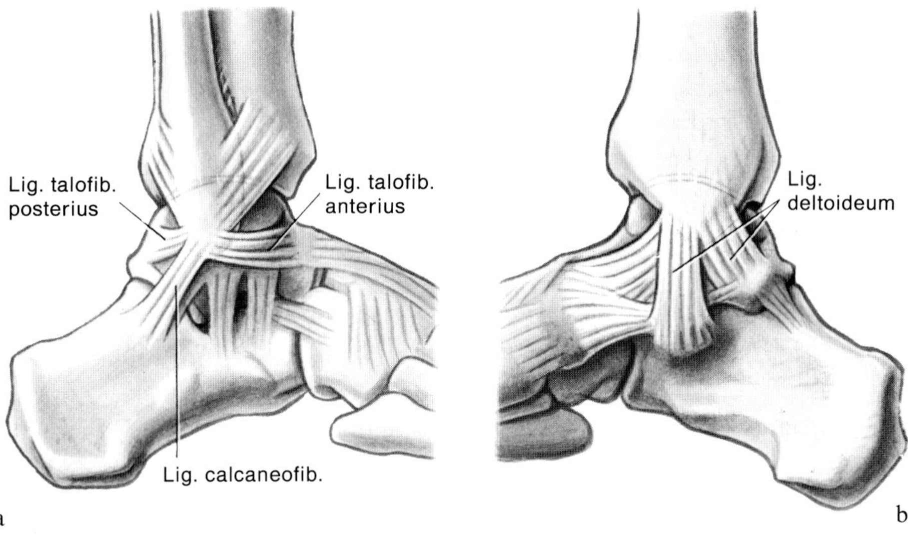

Fig. 14.3

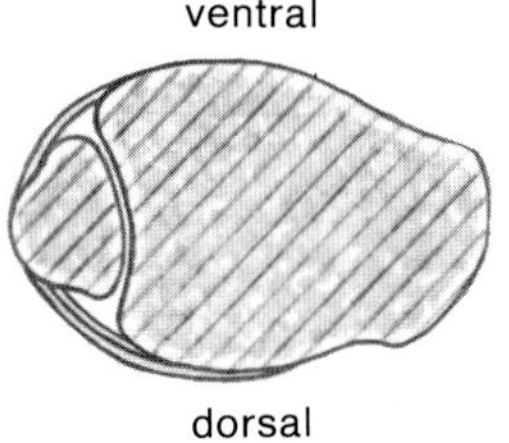

14.3 Classification of Malleolar Fractures According to Weber and Danis

The higher the fibular fracture, the more extensive is the damage to the tibiofibular ligaments and thus the greater the danger of ankle mortice insufficiency. There are three patterns of injury according to the level of the fibular fracture (Fig. 14.4).

14.3.1 Type A (44-A1–3)

Fibula: Transverse avulsion fracture at or below the level of the ankle joint (Fig. 14.4a), or rupture of the lateral ligament complex (Fig. 14.4a′).

Medial malleolus: Intact or sheared, with the fracture line somewhere between the horizontal and the vertical. Not infrequently there is also a localized compression fracture of the medial articular surface of the tibia.

Posterior edge of tibia: Usually intact. Occasionally, there is a posteromedial fragment which is sometimes connected with the medial malleolar fragment.

Tibiofibular ligamentous complex: Always intact.

14.3.2 Type B (44-B1–3)

Fibula: Oblique fracture of the distal fibula passing upwards and backwards from the level of the ankle joint (Fig. 14.4b). The fracture line may be smooth or complex depending upon the forces involved.

Medial malleolus: Avulsion fracture of varying size, or rupture of the deltoid ligament.

Posterior edge of tibia: Either intact or sheared off as a posterolateral fragment, the so-called Volkmann's triangle.

Tibiofibular ligamentous complex: The interosseous membrane is, as a rule, intact. The posterior syndesmotic ligamentous complex is either intact or detached with a fracture of the posterior tibial lip (Volkmann's triangle).

The anterior syndesmosis is intact if the oblique fracture of the lateral malleolus is below the level of the ankle joint. If, however, the fracture line begins at the level of the ankle joint, then the anterior syndesmosis is either partially or completely torn, or alternatively there may be avulsion of the ligament with either its tibial or fibular insertion.

Fig. 14.4 The three types of malleolar fracture patterns.

Fig. 14.4

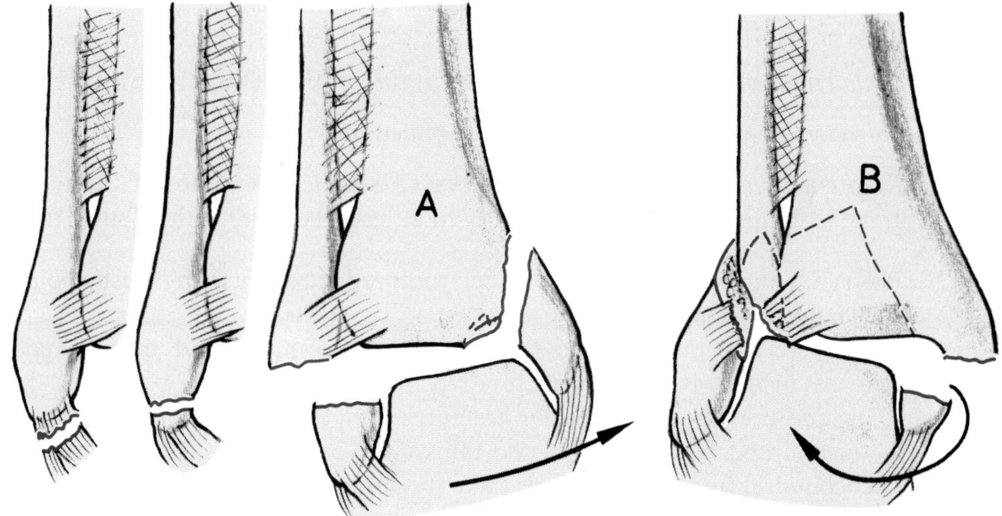

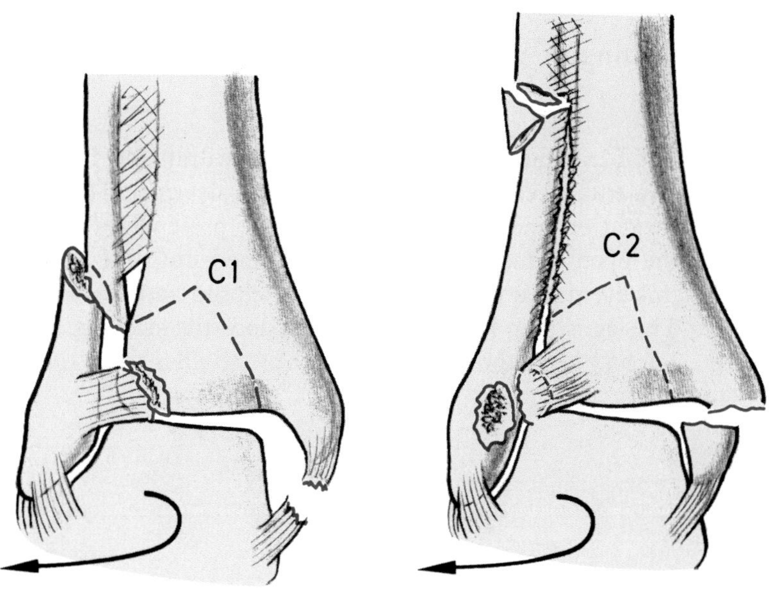

14.3.3 Type C (44-C1–3)

Fibula: Shaft fracture anywhere between the syndesmosis and the head of the fibula (Fig. 14.4c, d).

Medial malleolus: Avulsion fracture or rupture of the deltoid ligament.

Posterior edge of tibia: Either intact or pulled off.

Tibiofibular ligamentous complex: Always disrupted. Rupture of the interosseous membrane from the ankle joint proximally to at least the level of the fibular fracture.

The syndesmotic ligaments are either ruptured through their substance or avulsed with their bony attachments.

The *severity* of injury to the ligamentous complex and of the malleolar fracture increases progressively from fracture type A to B to C.

In addition to the malleolar fractures and ligamentous injuries, shear fractures of the medial and lateral edge of the talus must be recognized. These may be fairly large osteochondral fragments, or pure flake fractures. As many of these injuries are not readily evident radiologically, their presence should carefully be sought at the time of surgery.

In order to achieve the principal aim of restoration of both the stability and the anatomic congruity of the ankle joint, surgical reconstruction is frequently indicated. Careful preoperative assessment of the soft tissues and circulation is an essential prerequisite of this surgery (Fig. 14.5).

14.4 Timing of Surgery

The ideal time for the procedure is within the first 6–8 hours following injury, before any true swelling or fracture blisters develop. The initial swelling is due to hematoma formation and not to edema. In the presence of severe edema and/or fracture blisters, the open reduction must be postponed until the soft tissue condition has improved. In this event, the fracture is reduced, closed and immobilized in a well-padded plaster cast. The leg is then kept elevated to reduce the swelling before open reduction is undertaken. Surgery is postponed 4–6 days until the edema has subsided.

Fig. 14.5 The radiological technique and clinical examination.

a For an AP view of the ankle joint the leg is internally rotated 20° to bring the transmalleolar axis parallel to the X-ray plate.

b Clinical stress varus AP view of the ankle to demonstrate varus tilting of the talus in the mortice.

c Testing for the anterior drawer sign. The sole of the foot is held onto a firm surface with the ankle in some plantar flexion. With one of the examiner's hands behind the heel to stabilize the foot, the other hand presses backwards on the tibia to elicit any AP instability of the talus in the ankle mortice.

Fig. 14.5

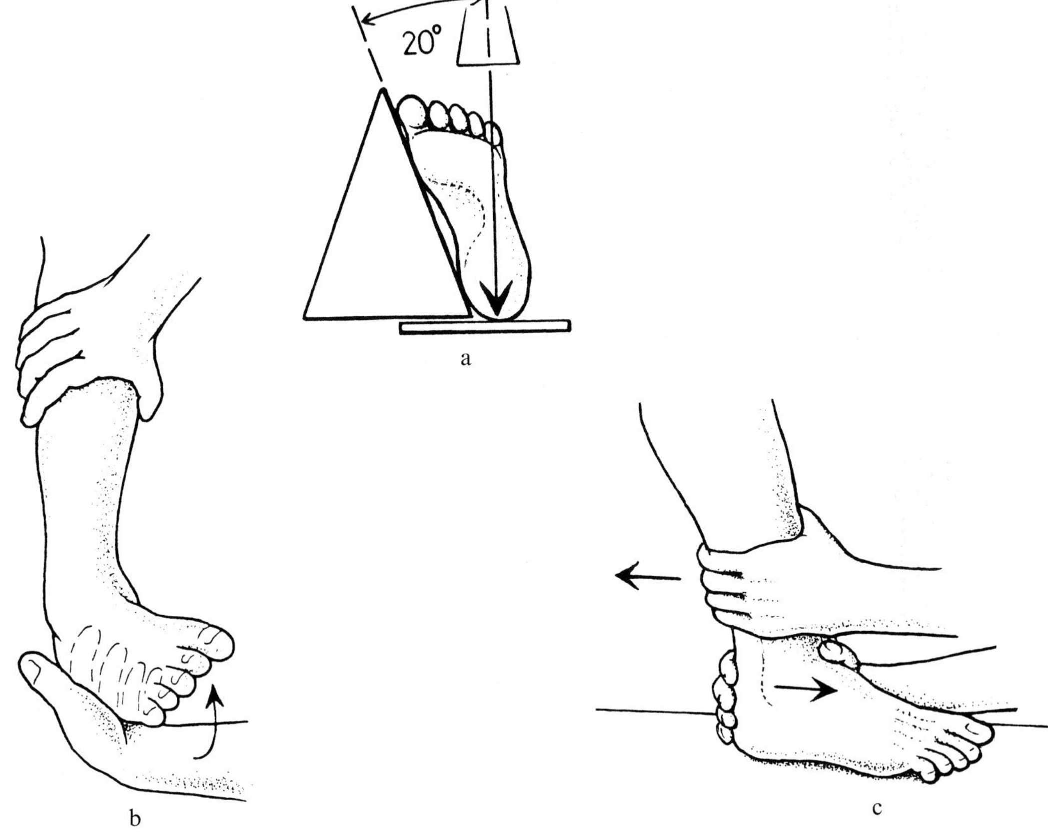

14.5 Technique of Radiological Diagnosis of Ankle Injuries (Figs. 14.5, 14.6)

AP and lateral projections, with the X-ray beam centered carefully on the ankle joint, are essential. For the AP and the lateral projection the leg must be in 20° of internal rotation. This position brings the transmalleolar axis parallel to the X-ray plate (Fig. 14.6a, c). Oblique fracture of the shaft of the fibula, which is often mistakenly judged to be an isolated injury, is almost always a type C malleolar fracture. In such cases, careful radiographic study of the ankle joint is necessary in order to demonstrate the concomitant injuries to the mortice. If an injury to the anterior tibial tubercle (tubercle of Tillaux-Chaput) is suspected, then an additional X-ray is taken with the leg in 45° of external rotation. If clinical features indicate a major ankle injury but ankle X-ray is apparently normal, a type C injury with a proximal or even subcapital fibular fracture should be suspected and the appropriate X-rays should include both the ankle and the entire length of the fibula.

Stress AP and stress lateral X-rays are used to demonstrate lateral ligamentous injuries (Fig. 14.6b). Isolated ruptures of the anterior talofibular ligament do not necessarily result in varus tilt of the talus on the AP stress view, but will result in anterior instability of the talus which is seen on a lateral stress view (Fig. 14.6c′). Only with additional disruption of the lateral collateral ligament complex will the talus tilt into varus. Stress studies of the injured ankle will be valid only if undertaken under local, regional or general anesthesia and then compared with the uninjured ankle.

Fig. 14.6 Evaluation of the X-rays.

a The ankle articulation with the leg in 20° of internal rotation: the joint space is of equal width throughout. The subchondral bone plates of the talus and the tibia are parallel. The line of the subchondral plate of the tibia, projected over the gap, is continuous with the subchondral line of the lateral malleolus without a step.

a′ Even the slightest shortening of the fibula can be recognized radiologically as a step in the alignment of the subchondral plates of the tibial plafond and the lateral malleolus. Lateral shift of the talus and consequent widening of the medial joint space are seen.

b An AP stress X-ray of the ankle joint. Note the 10° varus tilt of the talus. This denotes that the important calcaneofibular ligament is injured, in addition to the anterior talofibular ligament.

c An AP stress X-ray as seen from the side, without subluxation of the talus.

c′ Anterior subluxation of the talus. A difference between the injured and uninjured ankles of 3 mm or more in the width of the joint space is pathognomonic of an injury of the anterior talofibular ligament.

Fig. 14.6

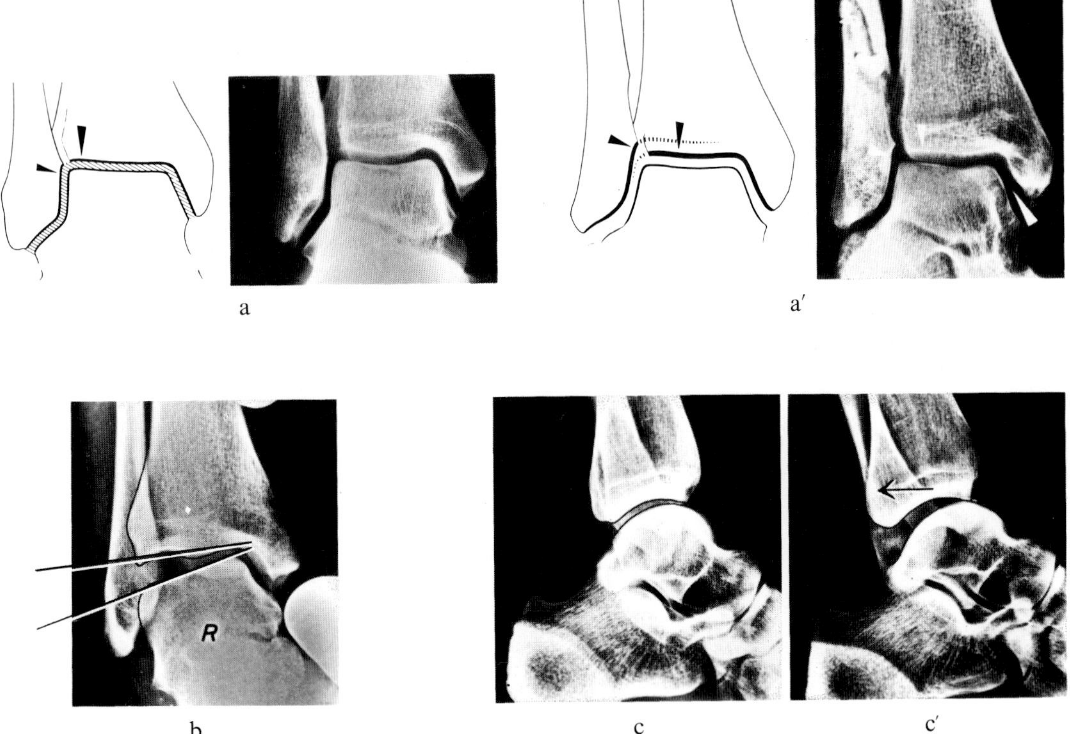

14.6 Steps in Open Reduction and Internal Fixation

For approaches, see Fig. 14.7a–c. Reconstruction of the fibula has priority. It is worthwhile, therefore, to begin the operation with the reduction and provisional fixation of the fibula. Occasionally, the anatomic reduction of the fibula is impeded by soft-tissue interposition on the medial side, such as a torn deltoid ligament, the tendon of tibialis posterior or of flexor hallucis longus, or the periosteum. In such cases, before the fixation of the fibula can be completed, the medial malleolus must be exposed, the joint surfaces inspected, and the malleolus reduced and internally fixed.

After any anatomic reduction, it is always necessary to secure temporary stabilization. For the provisional stabilization of the lateral malleolus, the pointed reduction clamps or the self-centering bone clamps are used. Depending upon the size of the fragment, use either the pointed reduction clamps or Kirschner wires for provisional fixation of the medial malleolus. The definitive internal fixation is then carried out, either using lag screws or with a one-third tubular plate.

In the firm, cortico-cancellous metaphyseal regions of young and active patients, light countersinking of lag screws is permitted. If there is any doubt about the quality of the bone in these metaphyseal regions, then it is generally advisable to use an appropriate washer with the lag screw, rather than to countersink.

Fig. 14.7 Surgical approaches for malleolar fractures.

a The exposure of the lateral malleolus and the anterior syndesmosis. The skin incision runs more or less parallel to the superficial fibular nerve, which must not be damaged. The anterior syndesmosis and the anterior edge of the fibula come into view only after transection of the extensor retinaculum. The distal malleolar fragment should be denuded as little as possible.

b The standard incision for the exposure of the medial malleolus, avoiding division of the saphenous vein. Once the capsule is opened, one can judge the accuracy of the reduction and the state of the articular surface.

c Incision for the simultaneous exposure of the medial malleolus and a large Volkmann's triangle.

d Incision for placement of posterior "anti-glide" plate as suggested by Weber (see also Fig. 14.9d).

Fig. 14.7

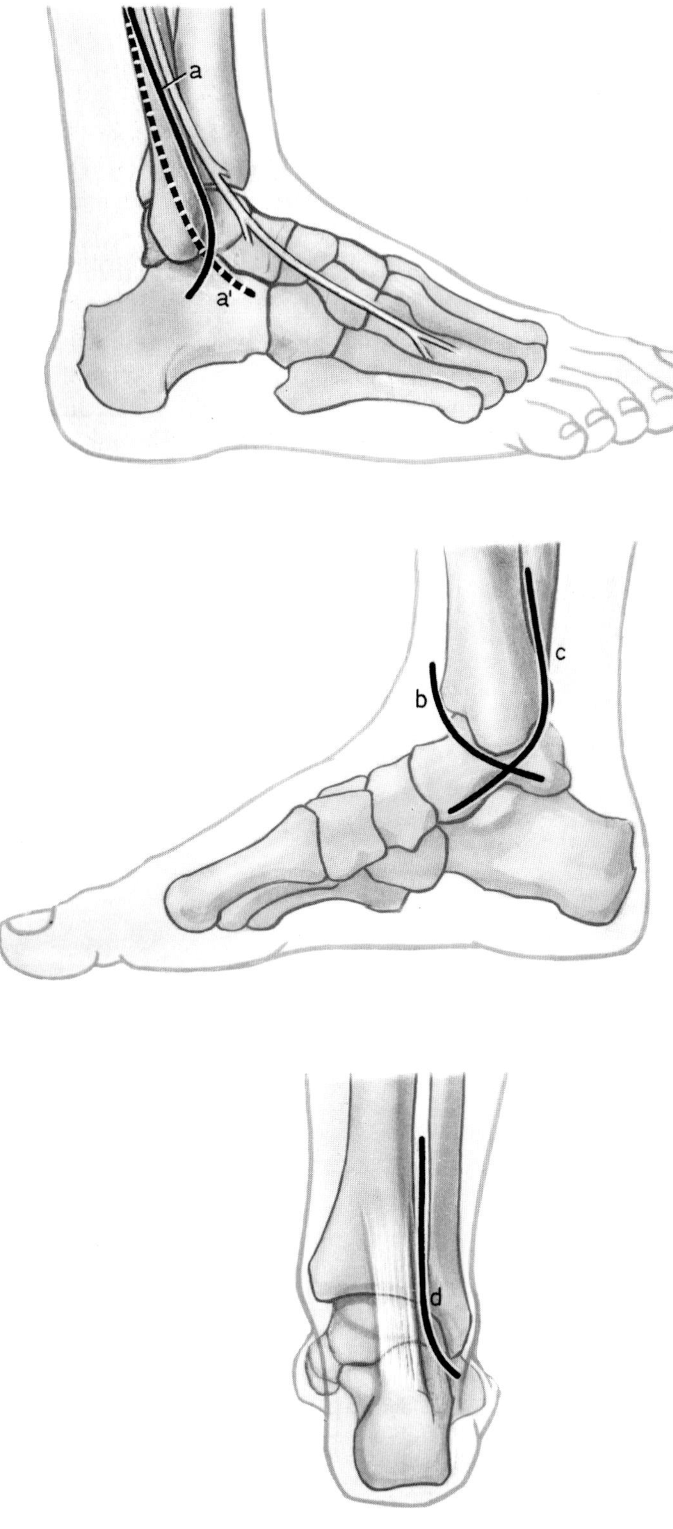

14.6.1 Type 44-A1–3 Malleolar Fractures (Fig. 14.8)

If the lateral malleolus is avulsed it is fixed as shown in Fig. 14.8a, b, using either a one-third tubular plate or a tension band wiring technique.

Next the fracture of the medial malleolus is exposed and any trapped periosteum is carefully reflected to expose the fracture edges. The anterior capsule is always torn, affording a good view of the intra-articular portion of the fracture. Small bone splinters from the anterior edge of the tibia may be removed, but larger pieces should be reduced. If an impaction fracture of the articular surface of the tibia is reduced, the resulting cancellous bone defect should be grafted.

Provisional stabilization is achieved with Kirschner wires and definitive fixation is then carried out according to the principles of interfragmentary compression (Fig. 14.8c, d). As this medial malleolar fracture has been caused by an adduction force, the medial tibial cortex is the compression rather than the tension side of the fracture, and so tension band wiring is unsuitable for a type A medial malleolar injury. The torn capsule need not be sutured.

A posteromedial fragment must be carefully reduced and fixed from the posteromedial aspect (Fig. 14.8e).

Fig. 14.8 Type A fracture: typical ORIF.

a The ruptured lateral collateral ligament and capsule may be sutured as one layer.

b An avulsion fragment of the lateral malleolus is first stabilized with two Kirschner wires and then fixed under compression by means of a tension band wire loop.

c Where the bone is of good quality, a large lateral malleolar fragment may be fixed with a well-contoured one-third tubular plate, functioning as a tension band.

d A large shear fragment of the medial malleolus is fixed with a Kirschner wire and a 4-mm cancellous bone screw.

e Posteromedial fragments associated with type A fractures are rare. They always lie next to the medial malleolar fragment. Such fragments may be exposed, reduced and fixed with small cancellous bone screws from a posteromedial direction.

Fig. 14.8

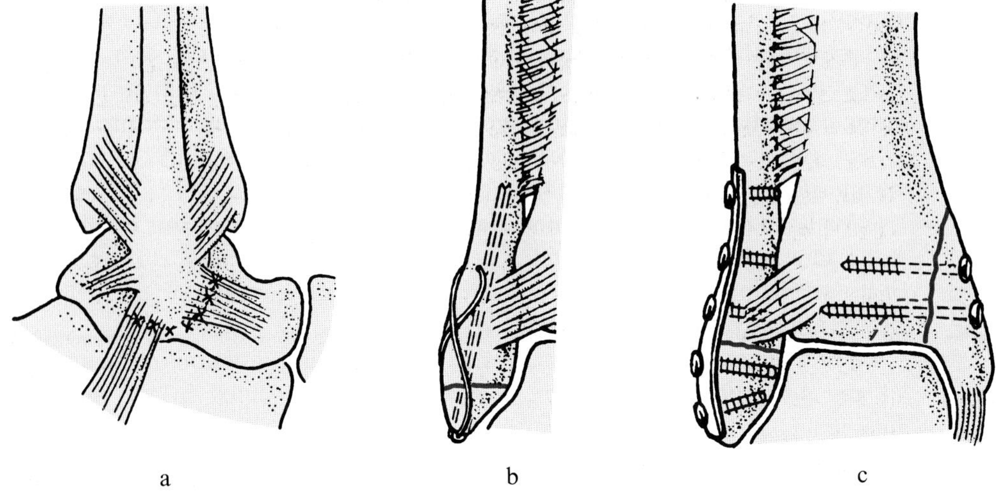

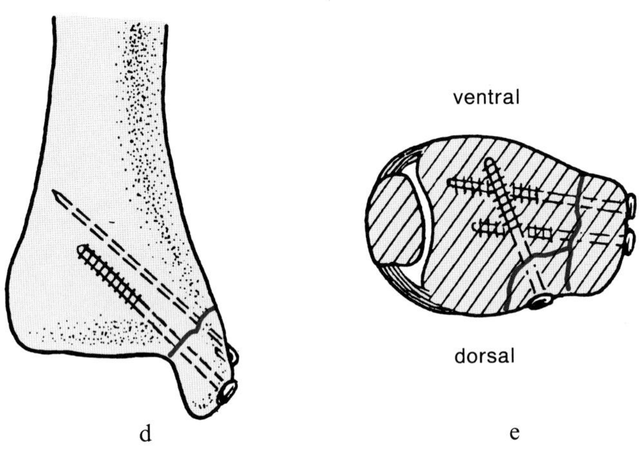

14.6.2 Type 44-B1–3 Malleolar Fractures (Fig. 14.9)

The exposure of the fibula comes first. By careful external rotation of the foot, the dome of the talus can be exposed through the fibular fracture site. If flake fractures are present, these are removed. The lateral malleolus is usually shortened, displaced posteriorly and laterally and is externally rotated. Anatomic reduction is best carried out using a pointed reduction clamp which also serves as a means of provisional stabilization. Check the accuracy of the reduction along the posterior edge of the fibula (for details of internal fixation, see Fig. 14.9a–d).

Avulsion fractures of the medial malleolus are fixed by means of either small cancellous bone screws or a tension band wire, depending upon the size of the fragment. If there is no suspicion of any soft tissue interposition, a rupture of the deltoid ligament may not require exposure and suture (Fig. 14.9e–g).

Exact reduction of the lateral malleolus results in reduction of the upward displacement of any posterolateral fragment, as the two are connected by the posterior syndesmotic ligament. The fracture gap, however, remains open. Thin, nonarticular, posterior tibial fragments need not be fixed. Larger posterior tibial fragments, bearing articular cartilage, must be carefully reduced through a posteromedial exposure. All that is usually required to achieve this is to introduce a narrow instrument and press downwards and forwards with its tip. Temporary fixation is then accomplished with a Kirschner wire which is inserted anteromedially. Definitive fixation is then carried out with a cancellous bone screw, which is inserted in an anteroposterior direction (Fig. 14.9h–h‴).

Fig. 14.9 Type B fracture: typical ORIF.

a The short oblique fracture of the fibula is fixed with a 3.5-mm cortex lag screw. This fixation is supplemented with a one-third tubular plate functioning as a neutralization plate.

b, c, d Different methods of internal fixation of the lateral malleolus in accordance with the different fracture patterns.

d Posterior placement of a one-third tubular "anti-glide" plate according to Weber.

e, f The different types of internal fixation of the medial malleolus.

g If exposure of the deltoid ligament becomes necessary because of soft tissue interposition, then it should be sutured (for exposure, see Fig. 14.7).

h A large posterolateral fragment of the tibia is carefully reduced and then fixed with a 4-mm cancellous bone screw inserted in an AP direction.

h′, h″, h‴ Lag screw fixation of the posterolateral Volkmann's triangle as seen from the side, from behind and in cross section.

Fig. 14.9

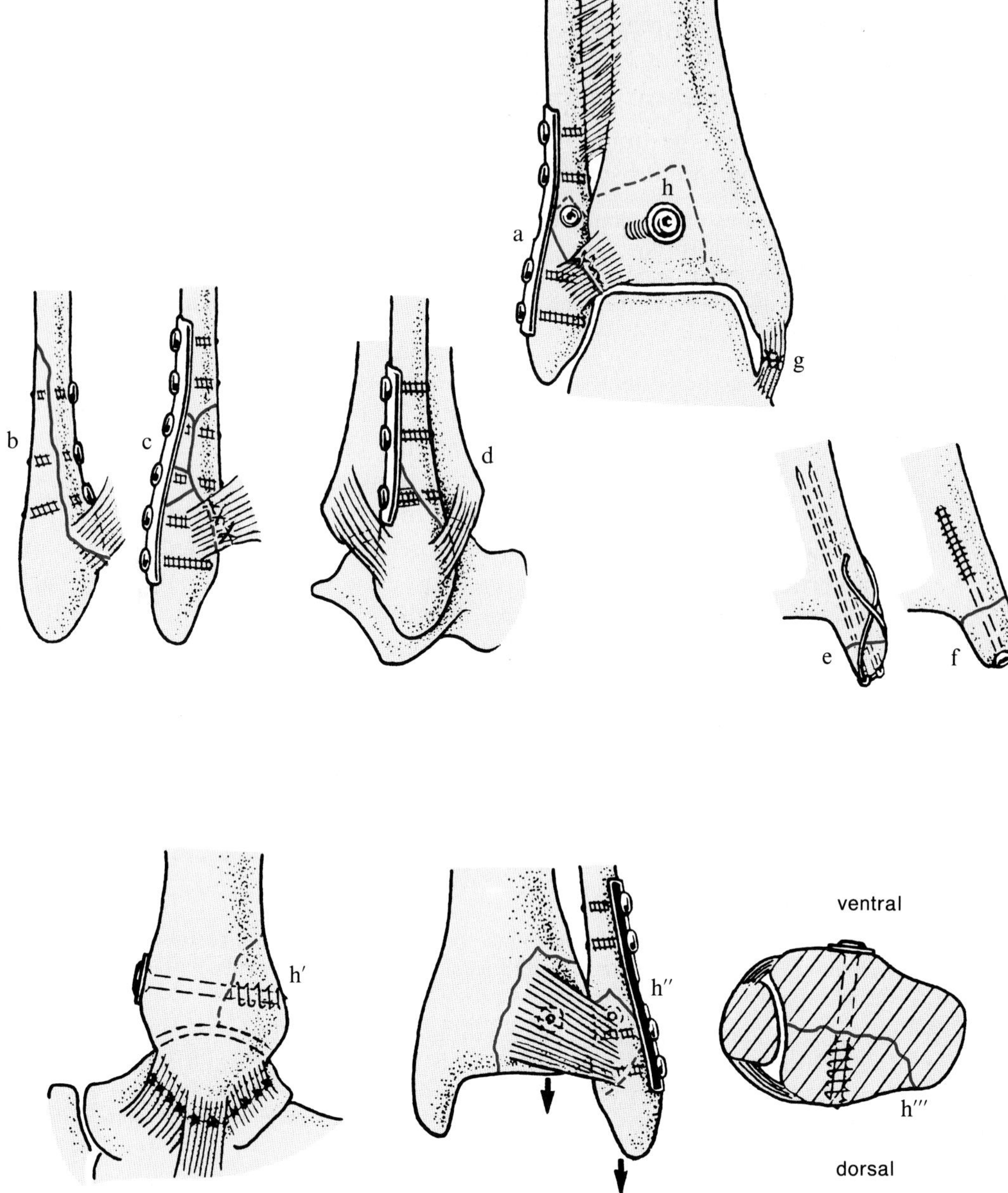

14.6.3 Type 44-C1–3 Malleolar Fractures (Fig. 14.10)

The operation begins with the exposure of the fibular shaft fracture. The restoration of the exact length of the fibula is essential. The shaft fracture is reduced and stabilized with lag screws either alone or, more usually, in combination with a one-third tubular plate.

Next, the anterior syndesmosis is exposed. If avulsed from the tibia (tubercle of Tillaux-Chaput) or from the fibula, it is reduced and fixed with a small (3.5-mm or 2.7-mm) lag screw. If the anterior syndesmosis to torn in its substance, it may be sutured.

Very high fractures of the fibula, through the fibular neck, need not, as a rule, be exposed, but the fibula must be reduced down into its normal position in the fibular notch by traction using a hook or a towel clip. Next, stabilize the fibula at this location with a Kirschner wire and take an X-ray to check the alignment of the subchondral plate of the distal tibia with that of the lateral malleolus (Fig. 14.6a).

Whether any further fibular fixation is necessary depends upon the stability of the syndesmosis (this is best tested with a hook, Fig. 14.10a), the degree of damage to the interosseous membrane, the rigidity of the internal fixation of the fibula, and on any repair of the syndesmosis. If, upon testing with a hook, residual instability can be demonstrated, then stability is restored by the insertion of a positioning screw 2–3 cm above the ankle joint. This should be a 3.5-mm cortex screw, which is inserted through the fibula into both cortices of the tibia. The screw must be inserted obliquely from back to front at an angle of 25°–30°, starting posterolaterally and aiming anteromedially. The 3.5-mm thread should be tapped into both the fibula and the tibia, as this screw is not intended to act as a lag screw, but purely to maintain the correct position of the fibula in relation to the tibia (Fig. 14.10c).

The medial malleolus and the posterolateral fragments are fixed as discussed under type B fractures.

Fig. 14.10 Type C fracture: typical ORIF.

a The fibular shaft fracture is reduced and stabilized with a one-third tubular plate. The torn anterior syndesmotic ligament is then tested with a small hook. The small avulsion fracture of the medial malleolus is fixed with two Kirschner wires and a tension band wire loop.

b, b′ A fracture of the midshaft of the fibula is fixed with a plate. The anterior syndesmosis is avulsed from its attachment to the lateral malleolus. This is reduced and fixed with either a small cancellous bone screw or a transosseous wire suture. The ruptured deltoid ligament may be sutured. A large posterolateral fragment is carefully reduced and then fixed with a large cancellous bone screw. This restores stability to the ankle mortice.

c, c′ Not infrequently, the subcapital fibular shaft fracture is not shortened and does not need open reduction. It is most important, however, to check very carefully for any shortening on an AP X-ray of the ankle. Look for any step in the alignment of the subchondral plates of the tibial plafond and the lateral malleolus. Any shortening must be corrected. A small avulsion fracture of the anterior syndesmotic ligament from the tibia is reduced and fixed with a small cancellous bone screw.

c″ Since this injury involves almost the full extent of the interosseous membrane, the fixation of the anterior syndesmotic ligamentous origin may not provide sufficient stability to the ankle mortice and a positioning screw is necessary. It is introduced obliquely from back to front at an angle of 25°–30°, the thread being tapped into both the fibula and the tibia. The avulsion fracture of the medial malleolus is fixed under compression using one or two 4-mm cancellous bone screws.

d Exact anatomic reduction of the fibula into the fibular notch of the tibia guarantees a normal ankle mortice. Imperfect reduction with shortening of the fibula leads to widening of the ankle mortice and valgus tilt of the talus. Even small degrees of malreduction and of valgus talar tilt are likely to lead to post-traumatic degenerative arthritis.

Fig. 14.10

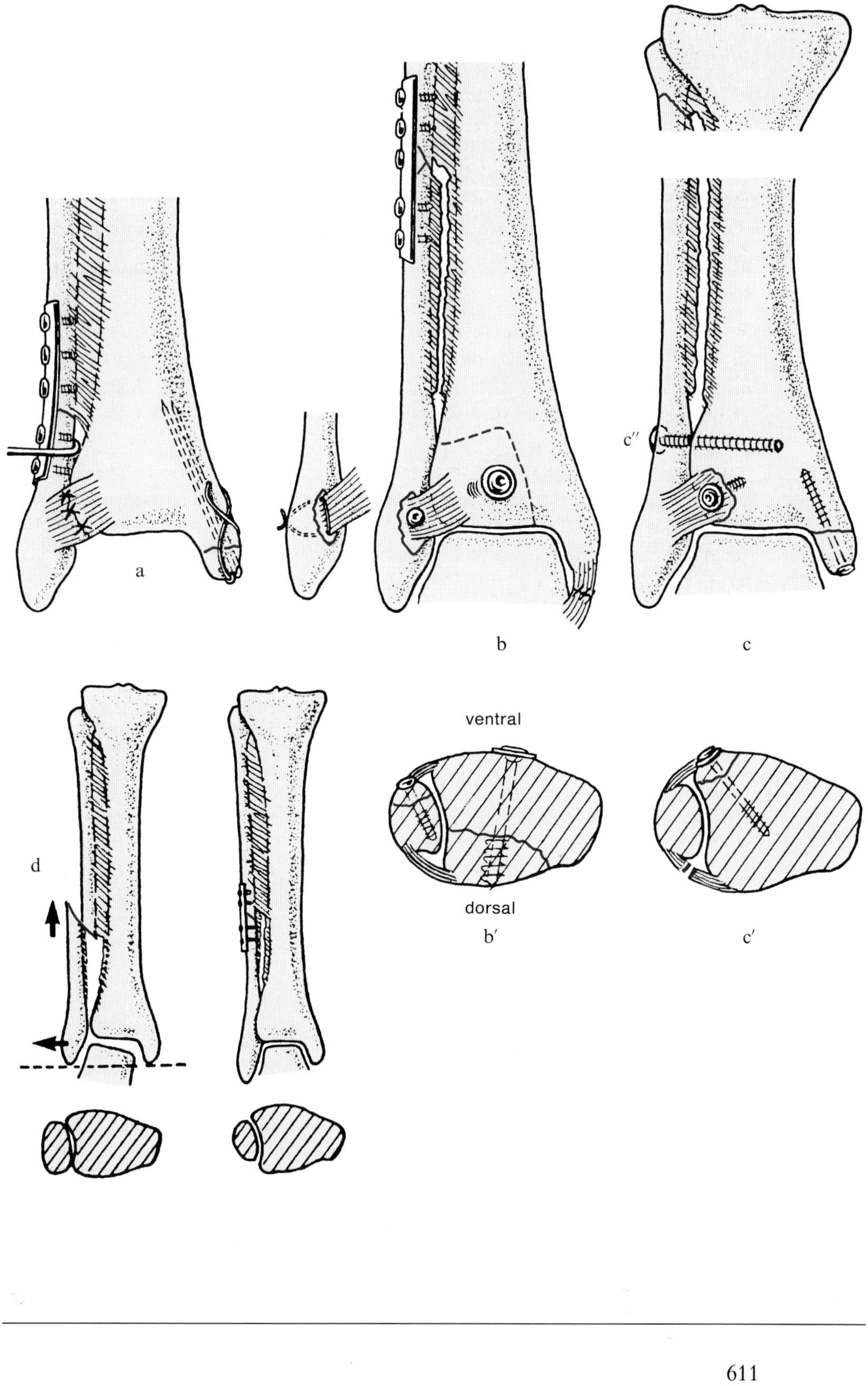

a

b

c''

c

d

ventral

dorsal

b′

c′

14.7 Postoperative Treatment

As in all cases of internal fixation, suction drainage is employed in malleolar fractures for the first 24–48 hours. In order to prevent an equinus deformity, the ankle is splinted at 90° by means of a plaster of Paris back-slab applied while the patient is under anesthesia (see Fig. 6.2). The patient is encouraged to begin early active dorsiflexion of the toes and ankle, under supervision, with the plaster splint temporarily removed. Once painless motion can be performed and swelling has subsided, the plaster splint is abandoned, usually between the 4th and the 10th postoperative day, depending upon a number of clinical factors, including pain, swelling and wound healing.

See Chap. 6 for details concerning the starting of early walking exercise, partial weight-bearing and implant removal.

References

Hughoo JL, Weber H, Willenegger H, Kuner EH (1979) Evaluation of ankle fractures: non-operative and operative treatment. Clin Orthop 138:111–119

Lamprecht E, Ochsner PE (1984) Spätprobleme nach konservativ und operativ behandelten "pilon-tibial" Frakturen. Helv Chir Acta 51:629–631

Lindsjo U (1981) Operative treatment of ankle fractures. Acta Orthop Scand 52 [Suppl]:189

Mast JW, Teipner WA (1980) A reproducible approach to the internal fixation of adult ankle fractures: rationale, technique and early results. Orthop Clin North Am 11:661–679

Phillips WA, Schwartz HS, Keller CS, Woodward HR, Rudd WS, Spiegel PG, Laros GS (1985) A prospective, randomized study of the management of severe ankle fractures. J Bone Joint Surg [Am] 67:67–78

Weber BG, Simpson LA (1985) Corrective lengthening osteotomy of the fibula. Clin Orthop 199:61–67

Yablon IG, Segal D, Leach RE (1983) Ankle injuries. Churchill Livingstone, Edinburgh

15 FOOT

15.1 Introduction

As pointed out by Inman (1976), the major joints in the hindfoot work in conjunction with the ankle to provide normal gait. Fractures of the talus, calcaneus, and the navicular and cuboid bones frequently involve the ankle joints, and, as in other major intra-articular fractures, it is desirable to achieve stable anatomic fixation and early motion whenever possible.

Similarly, motion in the metatarsophalangeal joints is also essential to normal gait and needs to be maintained. The length and angulation of the metatarsal shafts determine the distribution of weight-bearing in the forefoot. If fractures in these bones result in a significant shortening or an angulation, normal weight distribution can be altered enough to cause very symptomatic forefoot weight concentration, and the bones may need to be treated with internal fixation to regain their anatomic position.

15.2 Individual Bones

15.2.1 Talus Fractures

In addition to restoring articular surfaces, we believe that anatomic compression fixation decreases the rate of avascular necrosis anticipated by the Hawkins (1970) criteria and classification. It also allows earlier motion without danger of displacement (Fig. 15.1). Although some low-energy grade I talar neck fractures may prove stable with closed reduction, we believe that better results will be achieved in almost all other fractures with open reduction and stable fixation.

A grade I fracture that has been reduced closed in anatomic position can be stabilized with one or two screws placed from a posterior direction. A transverse skin line incision can be made for cosmetic reasons, and after the extreme posterior portion of the talus has been located, drills, positioned using an image intensifier, can be used. We use a 4.5-mm drill through the body of the talus, and insert the 3.5-mm drill guide and the 3.5-mm drill into the neck and head before pretapping. Then a 6.5-mm cancellous bone screw is placed across the fracture. When tightened securely, this screw will usually allow early motion. In a larger bone two screws can be used, and even in small bones two 4.5-mm cortex screws with appropriate gliding holes might be preferred (Fig. 15.1 a, b).

When grade I fractures are complex or cannot be reduced anatomically, open reduction is preferred. In grades II and III, open reduction is essential. We make two incisions: the first is linear (medial) and parallel to the normal alignment of the talus and talonavicular joint; the second is placed laterally and can be linear or in the skin line, e.g., an Ollier incision (Mann 1986). The fracture needs to be observed from both sides to control anatomic alignment, especially in rotation, and any stripping of soft tissues across the dorsum of the neck and head region must be avoided. The problem is to expose enough of the fracture to allow good visibility without damaging the blood supply.

Any gaps resulting from comminution should be filled with cancellous bone graft. The (new) 3.5-mm cortex screw is placed from the medial side after the appropriate gliding hole has been driven into the head and then countersunk under the articular surface. A small notch can be made in the navicular bone to allow the best positioning of the medial screw. Kirschner wires can be used for provisional fixation but must be kept out of the area of screw fixation. If the fracture includes a portion of the lateral flare (shoulder) of the talus along with the head and neck fragment on the lateral side, it can be easily fixed with a second screw. We prefer the 3.5-mm screws with gliding holes, but a 4.0-mm cancellous bone screw or a 4.5-mm screw may be used in very large bones or for large patients (Figs. 15.1 c).

Splinting may be needed postoperatively if the quality of the fixation or the bone stock is less than ideal. In this case, early union may need to be determined before any stressful mobilization is initiated. During the day and beginning 48 h postoperatively, gentle, active motion may take place with the splint or cast removed, but at night, the fracture should be kept in a right-angle position to prevent loss of dorsiflexion.

15.2.2 Calcaneus Fractures

It is becoming increasingly common to internally fix intra-articular fractures of the calcaneus. There is usually a medial fragment including the sustentaculum tali together with varying widths of the medial portion of the posterior facet. This fragment is split from the remaining calcaneus by a vertical (sagittal plane) fracture line. The remaining posterior

---

Fig. 15.1 Fractures of the talus.

a A 6.5-mm cancellous bone lag screw and a Kirschner wire provide ideal fixation for undisplaced fractures of the talar neck or those that can be reduced anatomically by closed means. The posterior talus is approached from a posterior lateral direction and the body of the talus is predrilled with a 4.5-mm drill bit, while the neck is drilled with a 3.5-mm drill bit. A Kirschner wire placed parallel to the central drill hole prevents rotation as the screw is inserted. A cancellous bone screw may be inserted using the image intensifier for guidance or a cannulated screw may be used after preliminary Kirschner wire fixation. Large, 4.5-mm drill bits are used in the talus because the bone is usually much denser than metaphyseal cancellous bone, and a larger drill hole prevents the 6.5-mm screw from binding or splitting the body of the talus.

b Two 3.5-mm cortex screws provide fixation for a posterior body fragment. Again, the first screw is placed through a 3.5-mm gliding hole, drilled as perpendicular as possible to the fracture line to compress the fracture, and the second screw is placed either parallel or at another angle to prevent rotation.

c Fixation with two 3.5-mm cortex screws is ideal for talar neck or distal body fractures. The screws are placed through bilateral anterior incisions after open reduction of the talus. The first screw is placed through a 3.5-mm gliding hole in the proximal fragment perpendicular to the fracture line, and the second is placed from the opposite side at the best angle that can be obtained to prevent rotation. If one of the screws is placed in or near the cuneonavicular articular surface, countersinking the screw will prevent irritation to the joint.

Fig. 15.1

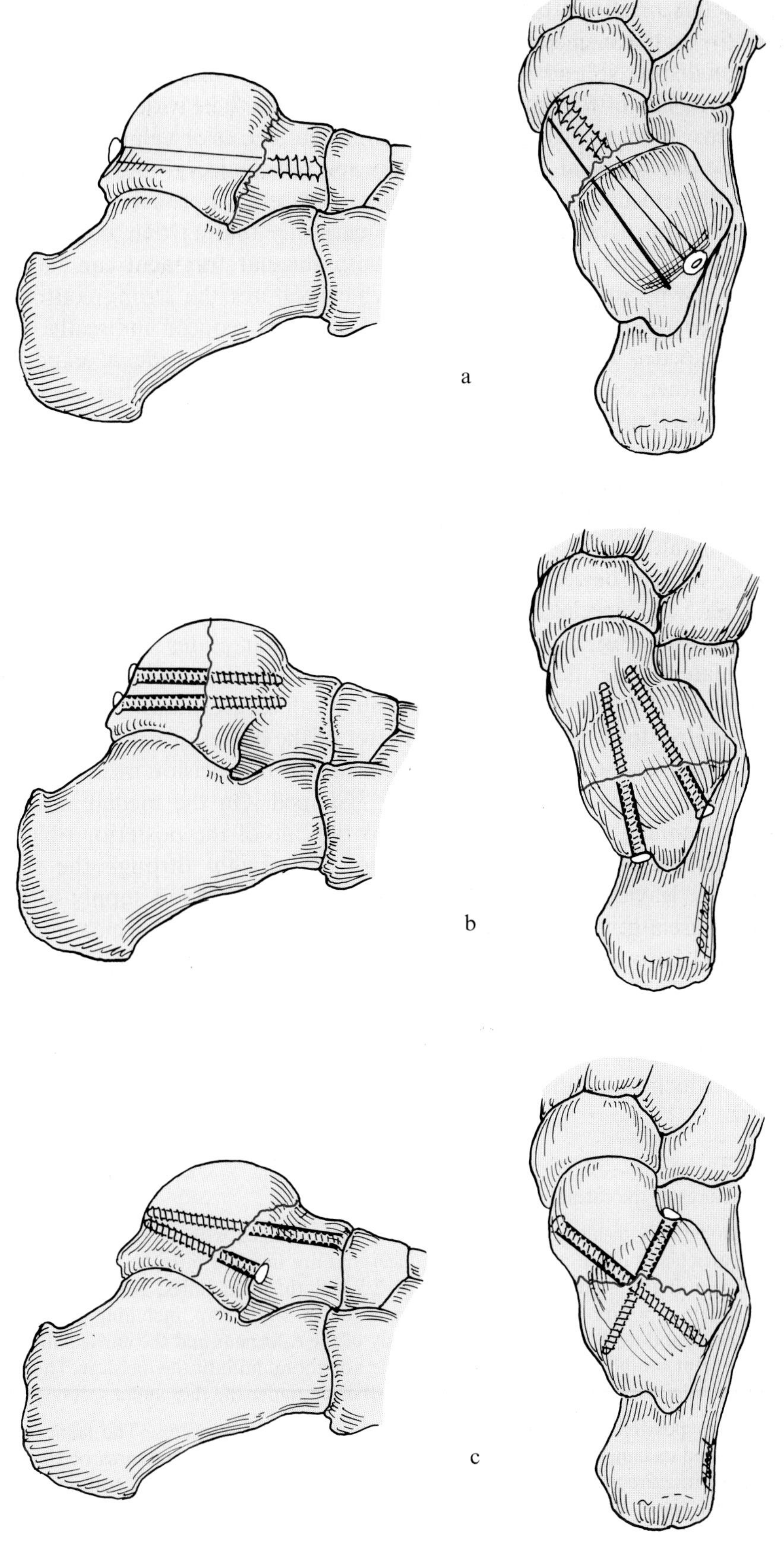

facet is generally crushed down into the posterior body of the calcaneus in various patterns and this results in bulging of the lateral wall with various fracture lines. The posterior body of the heel is usually angled into varus in relation to the subtalar joint but is often displaced laterally, in which case it appears to be in valgus in relation to the weight-bearing line of the leg. Post-traumatic arthritis, heel widening, a shortened leg, shortened triceps surae, lateral malleolar impingement, varus or valgus, and later secondary anterior ankle impingement result from more severe fractures if these are not reduced.

Both medial and the more common lateral approaches have been used in the past. Advocates of both approaches are currently finding that both are needed on occasion. On the medial side, the constant sustentacular fragment can be elevated by backward and downward pulling the body which restores the strong contour of the medial wall. The posterior facet and lateral wall are thus reduced indirectly. From the lateral side, the widened lateral wall is visualized and moved aside to expose the posterior facet. It can then be reduced under direct vision while the medial sustentacular fragment and the medial wall are held and reduced indirectly.

Computed tomography (CT) scans should be taken of a calcaneus fracture. A recommended cutting plane is at right angles to the superior surface of the calcaneus, giving a clear view of the fracture lines in the posterior and middle facets and into the calcaneocuboid joint.

Fixation devices for calcaneus fractures vary. In addition to standard screws (Fig. 15.2a), special reconstruction plates and one-third tubular plates (possibly flattened) work well (Fig. 15.2b). Two one-third tubular plates or one Y plate may be used on the lateral side. Bèzes points out that the screw in the area under the sinus tarsi must be angled up to catch the sustentaculum tali securely and the more posterior screw should be angled down into the denser matter of the posterior calcaneus (Bèzes et al. 1984).

There are several proven approaches for the incision on the lateral side, varying from straight to gently curved to L- or J-shaped. On the medial side, a straight incision is used running about 1 cm inferior to the line of the posterior tibial tendon. In all cases, soft tissue demands that the incision go straight through the skin and subcutaneous tissues, leaving them attached so as to maintain blood supply to the skin. The surgeon must use a gentle retraction technique and good timing, which means that these fractures should be operated on either immediately following the injury or after the swelling has subsided.

Postoperatively, the foot should be kept elevated for 3–5 days and gentle, active mobilization should be allowed if fixation is good. The patient should sleep in a bivalved cast which holds the foot in a right-angle position, avoiding going into equinus. During

---

Fig. 15.2 Fractures of the calcaneus.

a A moderately displaced calcaneus fracture may be fixed with screws only. The screws are placed under the articular surface of the posterior facet and are inserted into the sustentacular fragment under direct vision using 3.5-mm gliding holes and 2.5-mm threaded holes. Note the recommended approach for adequate exposure. This incision elevates a full-thickness flap, including the sural nerve and the peroneal tendons, and exposes both the lateral body of the calcaneus and the entire subtalar joint. The calcaneocuboid joint can be exposed by extending the horizontal limb of the incision. The incision is closed carefully using Allgöwer-Donati sutures with a small drain under the flap and a soft compressive dressing.

b Various possibilities for fixation of complex calcaneus fractures. The same approach that is used for displaced calcaneus fractures may be used for more complex fractures of the calcaneus but, depending on the fracture pattern, the screws may have to be placed from different angles or other fixation devices may be more suitable. Alternative fixation that adequately supports the fracture and still meets the biomechanical demands of the calcaneus are a single reconstruction plate or a reconstruction plate used together with a flattened one-third tubular plate.

Fig. 15.2

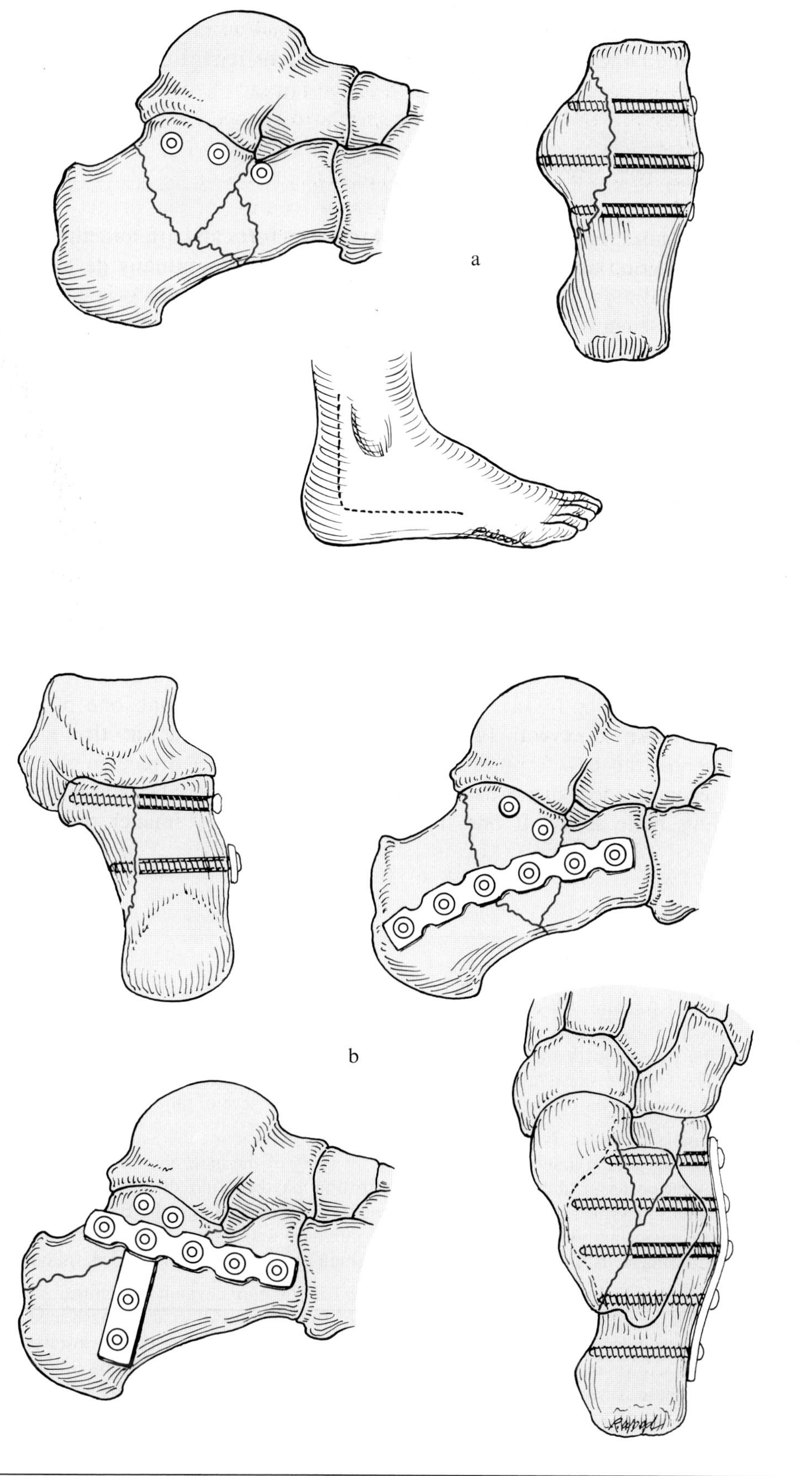

the day, if a cast is not used, the patient should wear elastic hose and be allowed touch-down weight-bearing with frequent elevation and inversion/eversion exercise. The patient should be warned to have limited expectations regarding the recovery of subtalar motion.

15.2.3 Navicular Fractures

Navicular fractures often occur as stress fractures and are sometimes initially misdiagnosed as anterior tibial tendinitis. The navicular bone eventually develops a vertical split near the midbody. Fractures of the navicular bone may also originate as traumatic fractures with elements of both crushing and avulsion. Traumatic navicular fractures are much more difficult to reduce and treat and often have accompanying cartilage damage from a crushing injury. For reduction of complex navicular fractures, a small distractor placed between the base of the first metatarsal and the calcaneus may be very helpful.

The proximal joint of the navicular bone (talonavicular joint) is part of the crucial joint complex that includes the calcaneocuboid and talocalcaneal joints. It is needed for pronation and supination in gait and should be anatomically reconstructed if at all possible. The distal joint of the navicular bone (the cuneonavicular joint) has little motion and may be sacrificed if necessary.

Reducing and fixing stress fractures is generally quite easy. A small incision is made over the medial tubercle and over the lateral side of the navicular bone, allowing a large sharp-pointed clamp to be placed transverse to the fracture to reduce it anatomically. Starting laterally, two lag screws are placed across the fracture perpendicular to the fracture line (Fig. 15.3a). In a very large-boned individual, one of these screws might be a 6.5-mm screw with 16-mm threading, which gives a very firm compression. In smaller bones, the new 3.5-mm screw with a gliding hole drilled in the proximal fragment is recommended since it has a stronger shank than the older, commonly used 4.0-mm cancellous bone screw. If one fragment is considerably smaller than the others, it may be

---

Fig. 15.3 Fractures of the navicular bone.

a Stress fracture. Classic navicular stress fractures are usually undisplaced or minimally displaced and occur in a sagittal plane near the midbody. A very small incision may be made medially to reduce the fracture with the point of a Weber forceps. The main incision is located lateral to the fragment. The fracture site is compressed with 3.5-mm cortex screws inserted through 3.5-mm gliding holes. If the bone appears to be sclerotic, perforating the area several times with a small drill is recommended.

b Simple fractures. For a dorsal avulsion of the navicular, a 3.5-mm cortex screw is placed through a 3.5-mm gliding hole and is secured into the body of the navicular bone. If the medial tubercle is avulsed by the posterior tibial tendon, stronger fixation may be required. A 3.5-mm cortex or a 4.0-mm cancellous bone screw placed into the row of cuneiform bones through the fracture line and across the body of the navicular bone provide satisfactory purchase and withstand the distraction force of the tendinous attachment. Although not shown here, a small plastic washer may be helpful on this longer screw.

c Complex fractures. Similar fixation is used for complex navicular fractures. A distractor may be applied from the medial malleolus to the base of the first metatarsal to accomplish indirect reduction. A complex navicular fracture caused by compressive forces will not securely grip intrafragmental screws by itself. The screws are placed across the fractures lines and through the row of cuneiform bones for better purchase. Since motion of the talonavicular joint is essential for normal gait, restructuring the talonavicular joint as anatomically as possible is critical, while maintaining motion between the distal navicular bone and the row of cuneiform bones is less important. Again, 3.5-mm cortex screws are placed through 3.5-mm gliding holes in the proximal fragment and washers may be added if desired.

Fig. 15.3

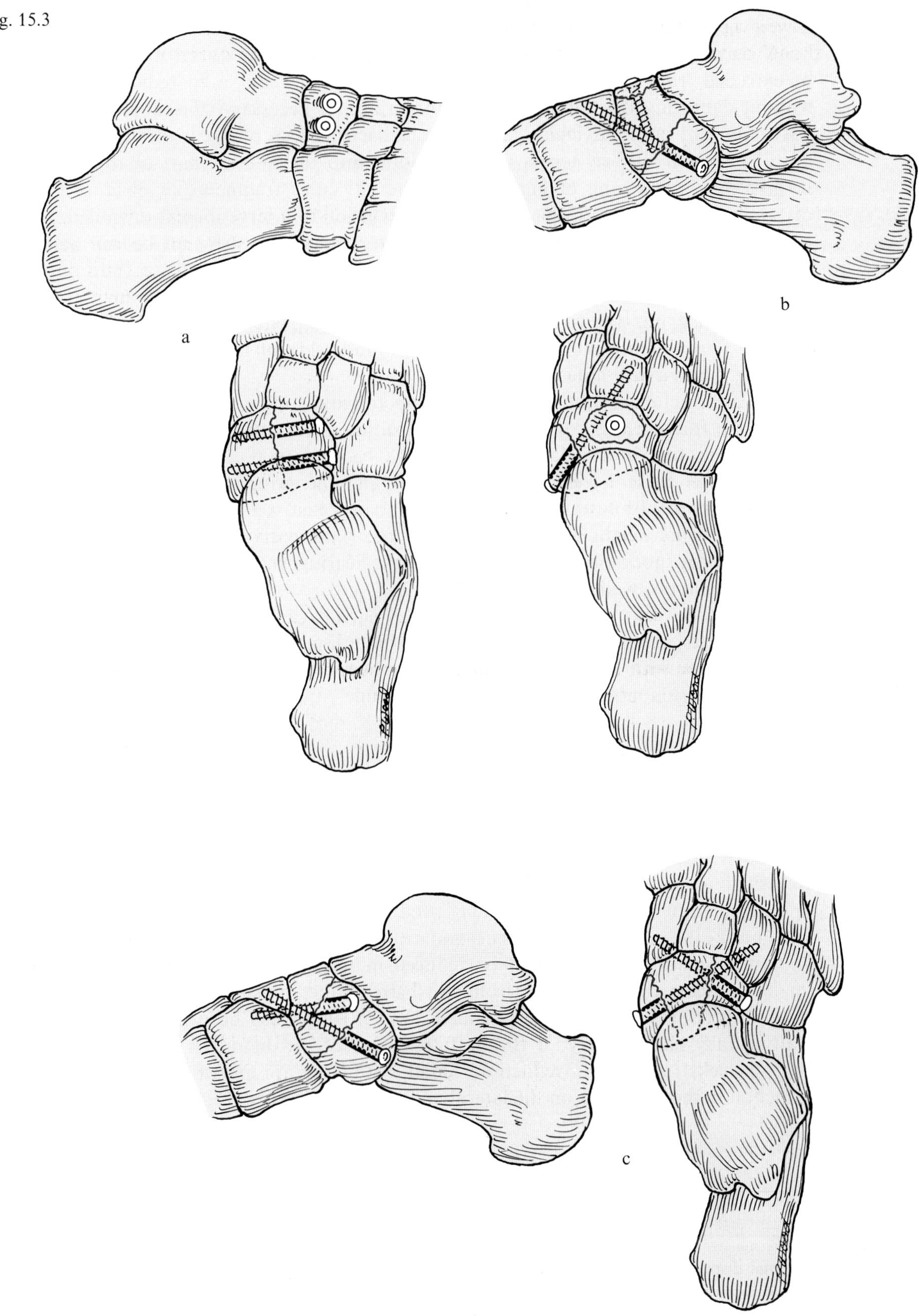

advisable to start in the smaller and fix to the larger. In this case, a gliding hole is driven very carefully into the smaller fragment.

A crushing or axial load fracture may cause a dorsal or dorsal medial fragment to be extruded from the body of the navicular bone. The aim is to reduce the navicular without damaging the talonavicular joint surface. If necessary, the more immobile and less important cuneonavicular joint may be sacrificed. Screws can be drilled from the dorsal proximal surface across the distal joint into the inferior part of the cuneiforms to give purchase strong enough to hold the navicular fragments in place (Fig. 15.3b, c). Similarly, when part of the fracture is an avulsion of a large medial tubercle fragment, a lagging 4.0-mm cancellous bone screw with a plastic washer can be run across the tubercle fragment perpendicular to the fracture and into the second or third cuneiform bone to give good purchase. If the posterior tibial tendon has had a major purchase on the tubercle, it is wise to supplement or augment the posterior tibial tendon by transferring the flexor digitorum communis into the underside of the first cuneiform bone by inserting it into a drill hole in the bone.

As with fractures of the calcaneus, postoperative casting is done immediately, particularly if the fracture was complex or if the fixation is tenuous. The cast may be bivalved for active motion in the daytime but should be kept in position at night for at least 14 days. After these 2 weeks, the initial cast and the sutures can be removed and the swelling is hopefully resolved. A very well-molded cast is then applied and the patient can begin partial weight-bearing of some 10 kg or alternatively, crutch walking in elastic hose with early motion but very guarded weight-bearing. In both cases, the patient should be in a neutral bivalved cast at night.

About 6–8 weeks after the operation, the patient can start full weight-bearing with a well-molded cast for the first 2 weeks. Rehabilitation continues with the patient wearing a support shoe with a firmly molded orthotic support. Physiotherapy should emphasize inversion/eversion mobilization and strengthening.

15.2.4 Cuboid Fractures

Isolated fractures of the cuboid bone are quite uncommon. When they do occur, they are usually either an impaction or a crushing fracture. Some may not be severe enough to warrant open reduction; others may need to be distracted and even grafted. If actual splits occur, they can be fixed in the standard manner with lag screws.

Crush fractures may have to be reduced indirectly with the aid of a distractor. A small distractor can be placed from the base of the midshaft of the fifth metatarsal to the posterior portion of the calcaneus. When length has been gently restored, bone grafting may be necessary; if the graft remains soft, a distractor can be left in place for 3–5 weeks to maintain reduction. Small distractors are extremely useful for indirect reduction in the foot both on the lateral and medial sides (Fig. 15.4).

Fig. 15.4 External distraction may be used to reduce ordinary compression cuboid fractures, but distracting the cuboid bone may produce a gap, which should be filled with cancellous bone. The distractor may be left in place for 3–4 weeks to maintain position. If external distraction is used, a Schanz screw may be inserted at each side of the fracture. Internal fixation may be added in the cuboid bone.

Fig. 15.4

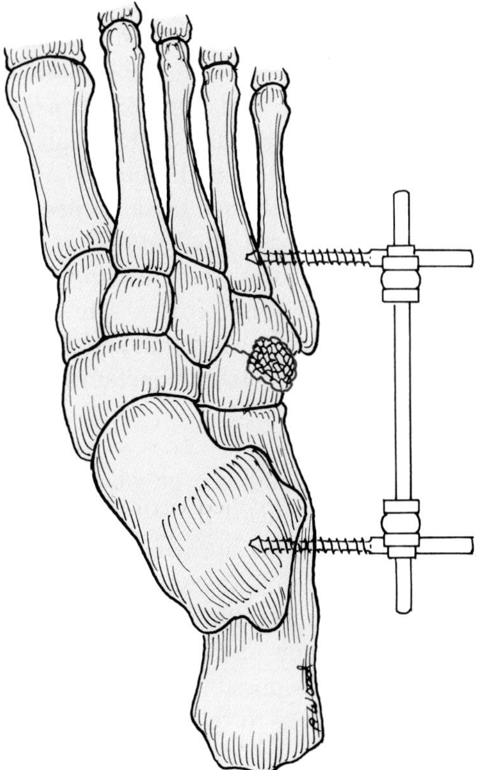

15.2.5 Tarsometatarsal Fracture Dislocations

Injuries at the tarsometatarsal level are significant both for their immediate disabling consequences and for directly related delayed problems such as pronation/abduction of the forefoot, post-traumatic arthritis and lack of stability in individual metatarsals with subsequent disordered forefoot weight-bearing. Following a review of numerous cases, our opinion is that it is essential to achieve anatomic position with good stability in these fractures to ensure normal foot function.

When displacement is minimal or fractures occur at one or more metatarsal bases, closed reduction and casting with or without Kirschner wire fixation may be adequate for an optimal result. If moderate to marked displacement or isolated dislocation occurs without fracture, anatomic open reduction and screw fixation is necessary if optimal function is to be expected.

Depending on the location and number of metatarsals involved, one to three linear incisions, each 3–4 cm long, are made centered about 1 cm distal to the joint line. These are made between the first and second metatarsal bases, the third and fourth metatarsal bases, and laterally over the fifth metatarsal as needed.

The joints are reduced and a small notch is cut into the dorsum of the metatarsal about 1–1.5 cm distal to the joint where an appropriate screw is applied perpendicularly across the joint. The new 3.5-mm cortex screw with a gliding hole in the metatarsal is ideal and in larger individuals, a 4.5-mm screw can be used in the same way. Kirschner wires are used in the third and fourth metatarsals and when there is a fracture in the proximal metatarsal base (Fig. 15.5).

Note that the drill holes should not be placed in the base of the notch made in the metatarsal but at the upper end of the notch. The reason is that the screw head should be kept from striking the inclined surface and splitting the base of the metatarsal.

Postoperative management is the same as for navicular fractures. Screws should be removed after 12–14 weeks since the joint is not fused and motion will eventually cause the screw to fatigue. Although screw fracture is not particularly significant, the patient should be forewarned of this possibility, and if any symptoms occur, the proximal half of the screw should be removed to relieve the problem.

Fig. 15.5 Displaced fractures of the proximal metatarsal metaphysis (Lisfranc's fractures) are best treated by open reduction and anatomic repositioning. A screw may be placed easily from the dorsum of the first metatarsal but screw placement in the second metatarsal may present difficulties. Angling the second screw from the lateral side of the proximal second metatarsal into the first cuneiform may be more effective. Screws are difficult to place in the third and fourth metatarsals, but these fractures may be fixed with Kirschner wires because stability here is not crucial. Either a screw or a Kirschner wire may be placed in the cuboid fifth metatarsal joint. Placing 3.5-mm cortex screws through gliding holes made in the proximal fragment is recommended.

Fig. 15.5

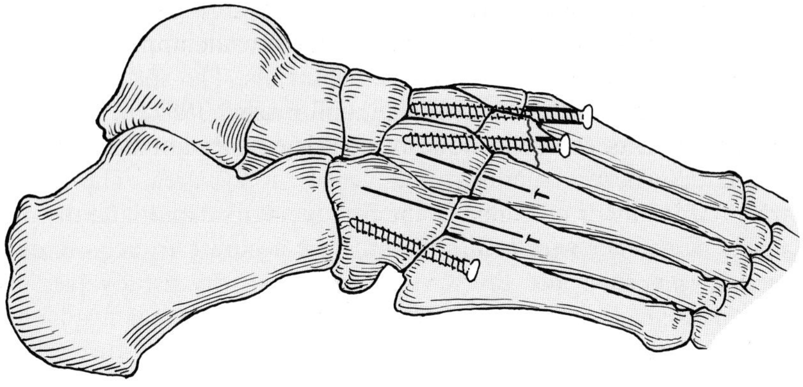

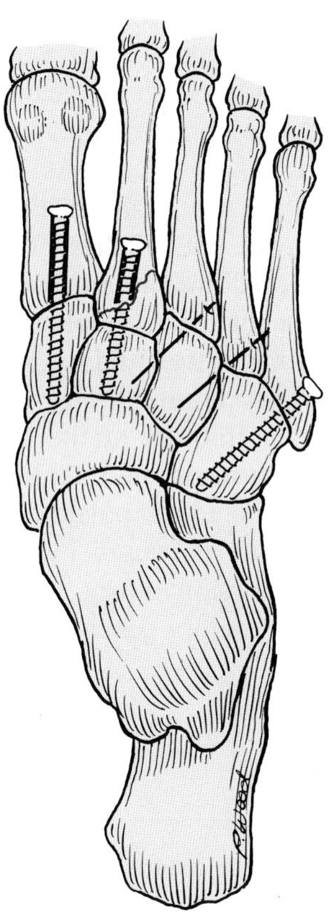

15.2.6 Metatarsal Fractures

Displaced metatarsal shaft fractures should be reduced anatomically to re-establish equalized weight-bearing across the metatarsal heads. This is done with either intramedullary Kirschner wires or one-third tubular plates. In smaller patients and in the lateral metatarsals, the 2.7-mm plate system may be preferable. In general, however, the plates are used most commonly on the first metatarsal while appropriately placed Kirschner wires are usually adequate for the lesser metatarsals. The special Büchler plate might be used on the distal first metatarsal (Büchler and Fischer 1987).

Reduction is generally done by making a straight dorsal incision linearly, avoiding the multiple nerves, tendons, and vessels in the area. The plates may then be placed straight dorsally or medially on the first metatarsal and laterally on the fifth metatarsal.

The Kirschner wire technique must be accurate to achieve anatomic alignment. The fracture is opened and the Kirschner wire is run distally just under the dorsal cortex parallel to the axis of the bone, across the metatarsal head and through the inferior portion of the base of the proximal phalanx, then out through the plantar skin under the toes. The fracture is then anatomically reduced and the Kirschner wire is driven retrogradely beneath the dorsal cortex: if necessary, it may be driven more proximally into the tarsal region. This is especially good if there is any question of tarsometatarsal instability.

There is a tendency to angulate the wire from dorsal to plantar across the distal fragment to avoid the metatarsophalangeal joint. This must be avoided because when the fracture is reduced, this position produces an extension deformity that results in decreased weight-bearing of the metatarsal head, which is exactly what we attempt to avoid by carrying out an internal fixation (Fig. 15.6).

The Kirschner wires are left in place for approximately 4 weeks and the patient is kept in a cast with touch-down weight-bearing during that time. The wires are then removed and the patient is placed in a molded walking cast for another 2–4 weeks, depending on evidence of callus formation and union. During this time, the metatarsophalangeal joints are actively and passively mobilized.

A special problem is a fracture at the base of the fifth metatarsal – the so-called Jones fracture at the junction of the metaphysis and diaphysis and the more proximal avulsion fractures which include a portion of the metaphyseal base (Kavanaugh et al. 1978). This avulsion fracture is caused by the peroneus brevis in conjunction with the plantar fascia after an inversion injury. A proximal shaft or a Jones fracture may be a stress fracture or an acute injury generally not caused by inversion.

Fig. 15.6 Midmetatarsal fractures should be reduced to ensure that the metatarsal heads will be level and will bear equal weight when the fractures heal. The first two illustrations show the correct placement of a Kirschner wire so that the metatarsal head fragment is not elevated. Placement of a Kirschner wire as depicted in the latter two illustrations will cause elevation of the metatarsal head fragment. Complex fractures in the first metatarsal and occasionally in the lesser metatarsals may be fixed with 3.5-mm or 2.7-mm four-hole plates because Kirschner wires will not hold them in an anatomic position.

Fig. 15.7 Fractures in the metatarsophalangeal joints and in the proximal phalanges may be fixed with Kirschner wires. However, for fractures at the base of the first phalanx caused by avulsion of the tendons of the short flexor and the adductor muscles, better results are obtained with screw fixation. Anatomic restoration of the metatarsophalangeal joints is crucial for normal gait.

Fig. 15.6

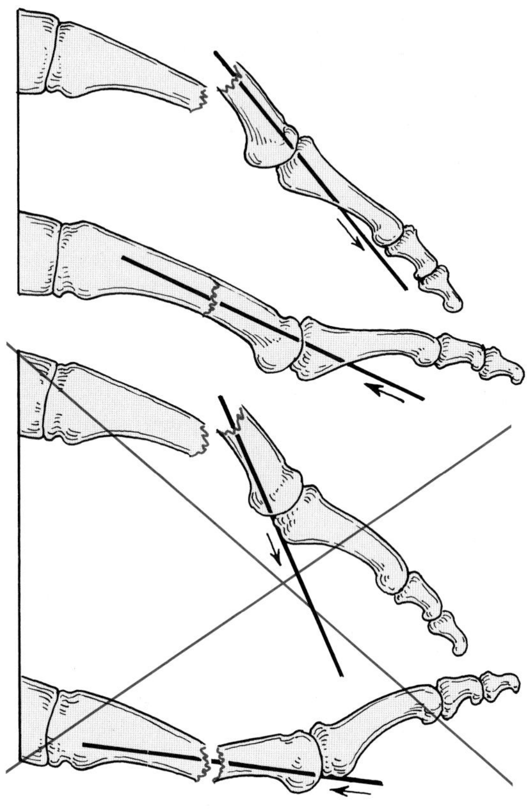

Fig. 15.7

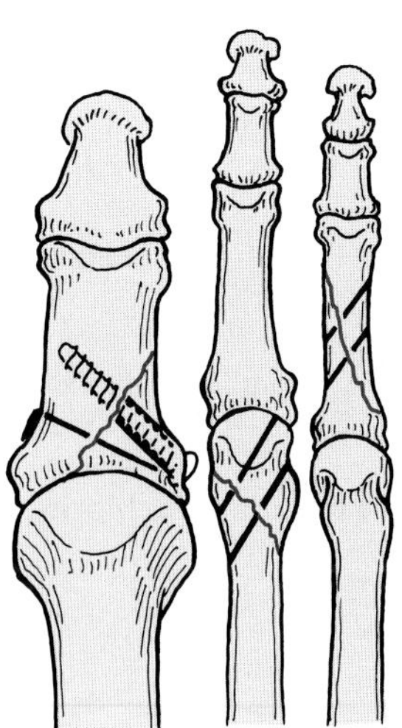

Avulsion fractures need not be fixed internally unless they are significantly displaced by 5 mm or more, but fractures at the metaphyseal/diaphyseal junction should be fixed even if they are only minimally displaced. They will heal very slowly, especially if they are stress fractures. Markedly displaced avulsion fractures in the metaphysis might on occasion need fixation by tension band or one or two small lag screws.

15.2.7 Metatarsophalangeal Joint Fractures

Both passive dorsiflexion and active plantar flexion at the metatarsophalangeal joints are very important to normal gait. Therefore, intra-articular fractures in this area should be fixed anatomically and motion should be initiated early. Since this can be difficult, it is fortunate that this type of fracture is rare.

The bones in the first metatarsophalangeal joint are large enough to allow open reduction and screw fixation. The occasional avulsion of the lateral base of a proximal phalanx, for example, can be put back in place with a small lag screw or tension band and early function can be restored (Fig. 15.7).

In lesser joints, the problem is rare and small fractures are best handled by Kirschner wire fixation and cast protection for about 3 weeks. Early motion should be started gently in the cast and activity increased as healing takes place. Attempts must be made to prevent major swelling both post-injury and postoperatively in all foot fractures. This is done by elevating the foot with active motion for 2 or 3 days postoperatively and thereafter by having the patient wear elastic hose and elevate the foot frequently, again with active mobilization.

A pneumatic venous foot pump is under evaluation for use in both postoperative and post-traumatic problems in the foot during the first 2 weeks postoperatively and might prove to reduce healing and rehabilitation time significantly.

References

Bèzes H, Massart P, Fourquet J-P (1984) Die Osteosynthese der Kalkaneusimpressionsfraktur. Unfallheilkunde 87:363

Büchler U, Fischer T (1987) Use of a minicondylar plate for metacarpal and phalangeal periarticular injuries. Clin Orthop 214:53

Hawkins LG (1970) Fractures of the neck of the talus. J Bone Joint Surg [Am] 52:991

Inman VT (1976) The joints of the ankle. Williams and Wilkins, Baltimore

Kavanaugh H, Brower TD, Mann RV (1978) The Jones fracture revisited. J Bone Joint Surg [Am] 60:776

Mann RA (ed) Surgery of the foot, 5th edn. Mosby, St Louis, p 279

16 THE SPINE

16.1 Introduction

The fundamental aim of fracture treatment in the limbs and the spine is the same: the restoration of normal anatomy and painfree function by anatomic reduction, optimal stabilization, atraumatic operative technique and early mobilization. A specific goal is the return of as much function as possible of the injured neural elements.

For some years now, high standards of fracture treatment have been achieved for fractures of the long bones, but similar results have only recently been obtained for spinal fractures. Operative stabilization of spinal injuries can bring about anatomic reduction, facilitate nursing and shorten the period of rehabilitation.

The ideal fixation system for the spine should provide enough stability to avoid the use of external support and allow early mobilization of the patient. Furthermore, it should only include the injured motion segments. Extension of instrumentation and/or fusions over uninjured segments should be avoided whenever possible.

The function of the spine is to provide support, allow motion and protect the neural elements. The biomechanical principles applied in the operative treatment of spinal lesions are basically the same as in fractures of the extremities. These include tension band fixation, compression, buttressing, etc., which can be applied both from the anterior and posterior aspects of the vertebral column. However, there are problems specifically related to the spine, such as the importance of the neurological lesions and the technical problems related to surgery.

It must be strongly emphasized that surgery of the spine is technically demanding. The techniques described in this chapter should only be undertaken by the experienced spinal surgeon.

Indications

The indications for operative stabilization in spinal injuries are as follows.

Absolute Indication

Progressive neurological deterioration in the presence of proven compression.

Relative Indications

- Irreducible fractures and dislocations, in particular those with neurological deficit.
- Open spinal injuries.
- Cessation of spontaneous recovery in incomplete neurological lesion at an early stage in the presence of proven compression.
- Polytrauma.

- Uncooperative (restless) patients at risk for neurological complications.
- Poor healing potential of the injury, e.g. pure discoligamentous lesions, odontoid fractures, etc.
- Unstable injuries.
- Deformities which may become clinically symptomatic.
- Facilitation of nursing, particularly in the elderly and in patients with uncontrollable pain.

Spinal Decompression

Anatomic reduction of the spinal fracture and/or dislocation is the most effective method of achieving neurological decompression in the majority of cases. Laminectomy must be condemned as an isolated procedure in the majority of cases. It may result not only in further neurological deterioration but also in progressive deformity. If laminectomy is performed, a stabilizing procedure must follow.

If compression of the neural elements persists after spinal reduction, the possibility of further surgical therapy and the timing thereof should be immediately considered.

16.2 Upper Cervical Spine

16.2.1 Stabilization

Atlanto-axial fusions may be indicated in certain cases of acute or chronic atlanto-axial instability. There are a number of approaches and surgical techniques to stabilize the C1–2 segment. Anterior transoral techniques carry well-known risks, particularly infection. Both the lateral and the combined anterior and posterior techniques require two approaches. For most lesions, we prefer the posterior approach.

16.2.1.1 Posterior Wiring Techniques

Standard Technique (after Gallie) (Fig. 16.1)

Principle

This technique provides a posterior stable construct for C1–2 instability particularly resistant to flexion forces.

Indications

- Fractures of the odontoid (dens) with anterior displacement.
- Rupture of the transverse ligament of C1.

Advantages

- Relatively easy technique.
- The graft firmly fixed between the two arches of C1 and C2.
- Aids in reduction of the anterior subluxation.

Disadvantages

- Sublaminar wiring technique.
- Cannot be used with associated fractures of the C1 arch.
- Is not suitable for posterior displacement of the atlas.

Surgical Technique

The patient is placed prone with the position of the head well controlled. Lateral image intensification is used to check position and reduction.

A midline incision extends from the occiput to C4. The soft tissues are cleared from the occiput, C1 and C2. Lateral dissection beyond 1.5 cm, particularly at C1, is avoided to prevent injury to the vertebral artery and venous plexus. The soft tissues are cleared circumferentially around the C1 arch in the midline to allow easy passage of the wire.

A 1.2-mm wire is fashioned into a loop with a hook configuration. The wire is passed from the inferior aspect of C1 anteriorly and cranially and looped over the superior surface of C1 (Fig. 16.1 a). The loop is carefully pulled backwards and distally sufficiently far to loop over the spinous process of C2 (Fig. 16.1 b). Unless the vertebrae are sufficiently reduced prior to insertion of the wire, there is a risk of damage to the spinal cord during this process. The arch of C1 and the lamina of C2 are decorticated by means of a high-speed burr.

A cortico-cancellous rectangular bone graft measuring 3 by 4 cm is removed from the posterior iliac crest. The graft is fashioned into an H configuration to fit snugly around the spinous process and over the lamina of C2. It is also notched laterally (Fig. 16.1 c).

The cancellous surface of the graft is shaped to conform with the slope of the arch of C1 and the lamina of C2 in order to provide maximal contact. The two free ends of the wire, which are laterally placed, are then brought across to the midline after the graft has been applied to the posterior surfaces of C1 and C2 (Fig. 16.1 d). The notches provide better fixation of the bone graft when tightening the wires. During the process of tightening the remaining reduction is achieved. Fragments of cancellous bone can then be packed around the bone graft between C1 and C2 (Fig. 16.1 e).

Fig. 16.1 Standard technique of C1–2 stabilization (Gallie).

a The 1.2-mm wire is fashioned into a loop with a hook configuration and then passed from the inferior aspect of C1 anteriorly and cranially and looped over the superior surface of C1.

b The loop is carefully pulled backwards and distally sufficiently far to loop over the spinous process of C2.

c A cortico-cancellous rectangular bone graft measuring 3 by 4 cm is fashioned into an H configuration to fit around the spinous process and over the lamina of C2. It is also notched laterally.

d The two free ends of the wire, which are laterally placed, are then brought across to the midline after the graft has been applied to the posterior surfaces of C1 and C2.

e Fragments of cancellous bone can be packed around the bone graft between C1 and C2.

Fig. 16.1

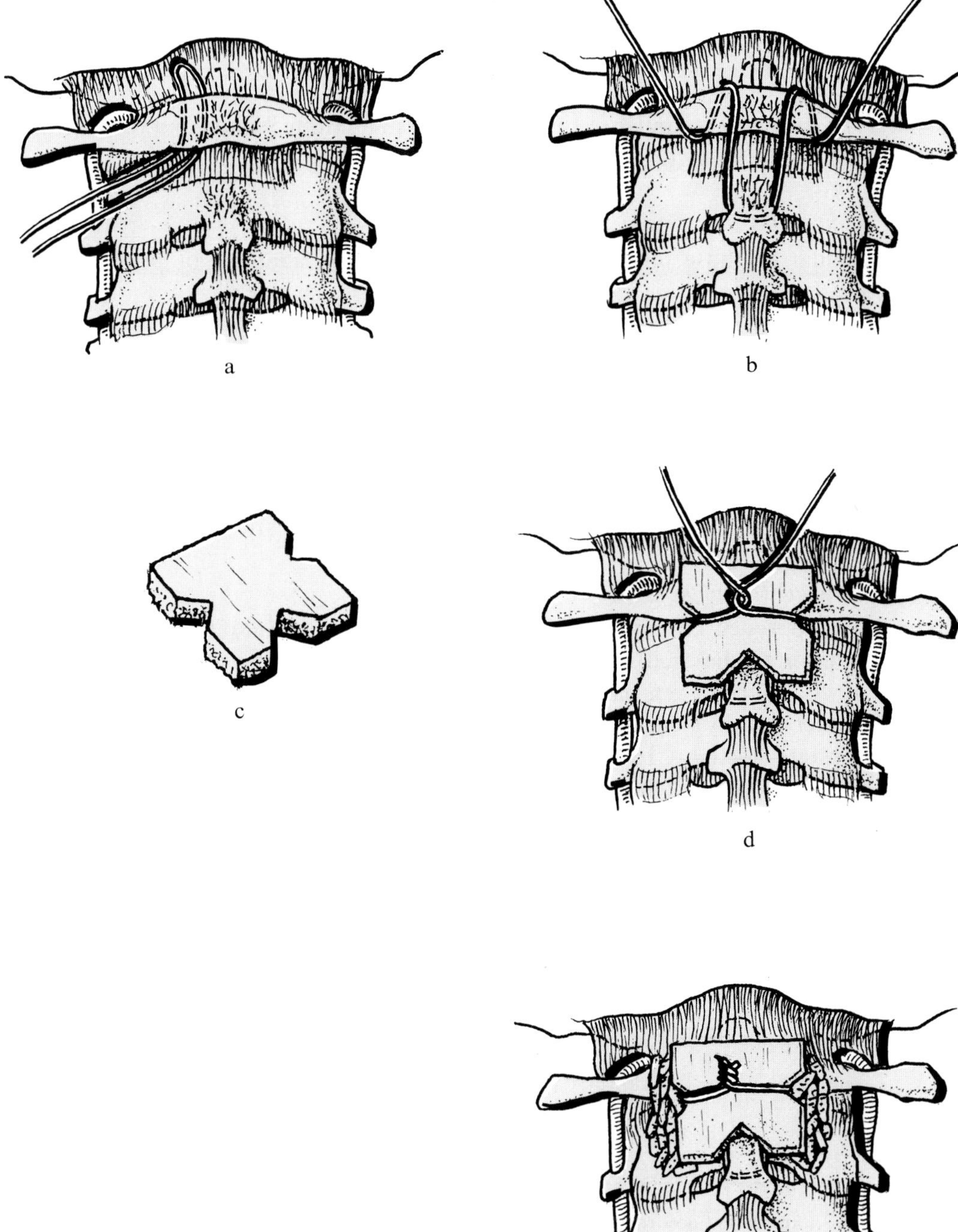

Postoperative Care

A firm collar preventing extension of the neck for a period of 6–10 weeks is recommended. It may be removed for daily care and, after 6 weeks, while resting.

Wedge Compression Technique (after Brooks and Jenkins) (Fig. 16.2)

Principle

The construct is similar to that used in the standard technique but provides more rotational and tensile strength.

Indications

Similar to those for the Gallie fusion, with the addition of posterior displacement of C1.

Advantage

– Biomechanically superior to the standard technique.

Disadvantages

– Requires the passage of sublaminar wires at two levels.
– Cannot be used for associated fractures of the C1 arch.

Surgical Technique

The approach is similar to that for the standard technique. In addition, the soft tissues anterior to the arch of C2 must be cleared, leaving the atlanto-axial membrane intact. A wire loop is then passed from the superior aspect of C1 around the arch of C1 and further distally beneath the lamina of C2 (Fig. 16.2a). A second wire is inserted on the opposite side (Fig. 16.2b). Two cortico-cancellous bone grafts, measuring approximately 1.5 by 3.5 cm, are taken from the posterior iliac crest. They are fashioned into a wedge with the cortical portion posterior. The wedges of bone are placed between the two vertebral arches after the undersurface of C1 and the superior surface of C2 have been decorticated by a high-speed burr (Fig. 16.2b). The double wires are then twisted to press the bone graft against the vertebral arches (Fig. 16.2c, d). One double wire provides the necessary stability, whereas four separate wires would just double the risk of neural injury.

Postoperative Care

The same as in the standard technique.

Fig. 16.2 C1–2 stabilization according to Brooks and Jenkins.

a A wire loop is passed from the superior aspect of C1 around the arch of C1 and further distally beneath the lamina of C2.

b A second wire is inserted on the opposite side. Two cortico-cancellous bone grafts measuring approximately 1.5 by 3.5 cm are fashioned into a wedge with the cortical portion posterior.

c After the two wedges of bone have been placed between the two vertebral arches and after the undersurface of C1 and the superior surface of C2 have been decorticated, the double wires are then twisted to press the bone graft against the vertebral arches.

d Lateral view.

Fig. 16.2

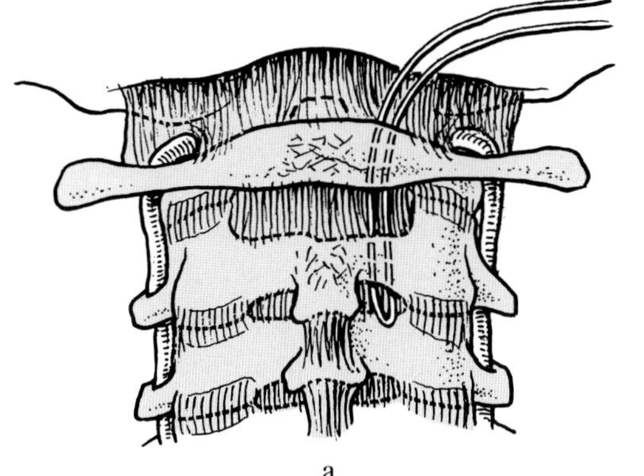

a

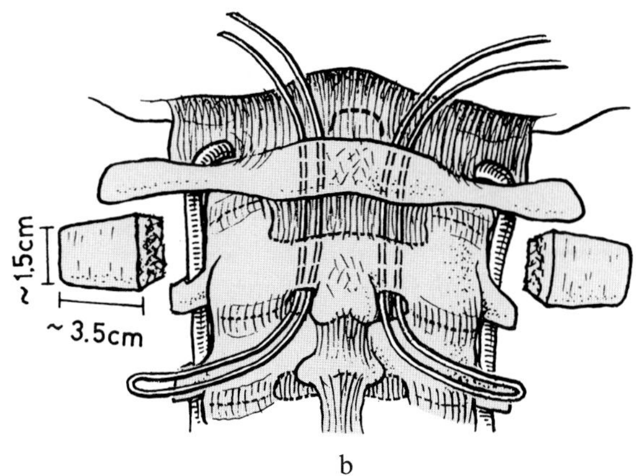

b

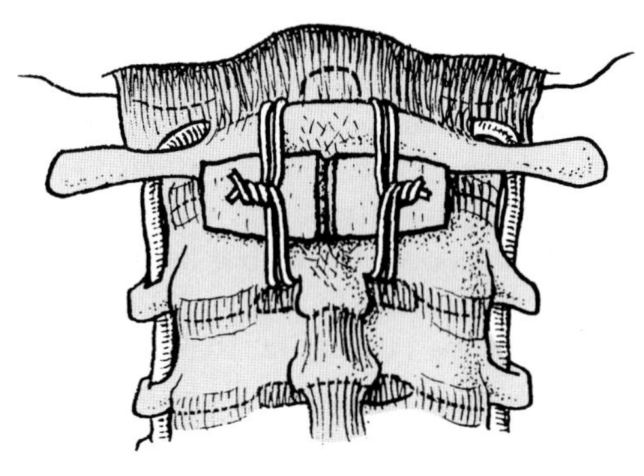

c

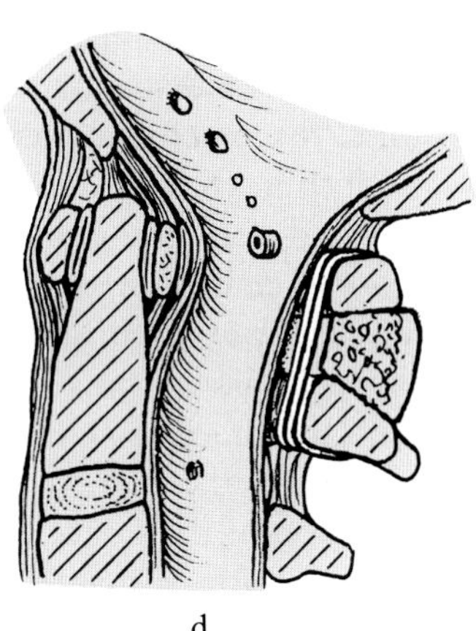

d

16.2.1.2 Transarticular Screw Fixation C1-2 (Fig. 16.3)

Indications

Acute and chronic atlanto-axial instability.

Advantages

- Biomechanically superior to wiring technique.
- Maintenance of reduction possible.
- Integrity of posterior arch of C1 is not necessary.

Disadvantage

- Technically demanding.

Surgical Technique

The patient lies in the prone position and the reduction of C1–2 is checked using lateral image intensifier control. The neck is flexed as much as possible to facilitate insertion of the screws, and the image intensifier is used to exclude redislocation.

A midline incision is performed from the occiput to the tip of the spinous process of C7. The arch of C1, the spinous processes, lamina and inferior articular processes of C2 and the lamina and articular masses of C3 are exposed subperiosteally. Persistent anterior dislocation of C1 or C2 may be reduced by pushing on the spinous process of C2 and/or by pulling gently on the posterior arch of C1, either with a Kocher clamp or with a sublaminar wire. Persistent posterior dislocation requires opposite forces.

A small dissector is used to expose the cranial surface of the lamina and isthmus of C2 by careful subperiosteal dissection up to the posterior capsule of the atlanto-axial joint (Fig. 16.3a). Medial to the isthmus the atlanto-axial membrane is visible. The laterally situated vertebral artery is not exposed. Using lateral image intensifier control, a long 2.5-mm drill is inserted in a strictly sagittal direction. The entry point of the drill is at the lower edge of the caudal articular process of C2 (Fig. 16.3a, b). The drill goes through the isthmus near to its posterior and medial surface. It then enters the lateral mass of the atlas close to its posterior-inferior edge (Fig. 16.3b). Anteriorly, the drill perforates the cortex of the lateral mass of C1. The screw length is measured and the direction of the screw canal is checked using the image intensifier. The screws are inserted after tapping with a 3.5-mm cortical tap (Fig. 16.3c). Proper caudocranial drilling may sometimes be difficult because the neck muscles and the upper torso prevent the correct

---

Fig. 16.3 Transarticular screw fixation of C1–2.

a The small dissector is used to expose the cranial surface of the lamina and isthmus of C2 by careful subperiosteal dissection up to the posterior capsule of the atlanto-axial joint.

b The entry point of the drill is at the lower edge of the caudal articular process of C2. The drill goes through the isthmus near to its posterior and medial surface. It then enters the lateral mass of the atlas.

c Measuring of the screw length and tapping of the screw hole with the 3.5-mm cortical tap.

d Following bilateral screw fixation, a posterior C1–2 fusion is performed and the graft is supplemented with a posterior wiring technique.

e Direct fusion of the atlanto-axial joints with insufficient stability of the posterior arch of C1: exposure of the atlanto-axial joint, removal of the cartilage of the posterior half of the facet joint, and packing of the resulting defect with cancellous bone.

Fig. 16.3

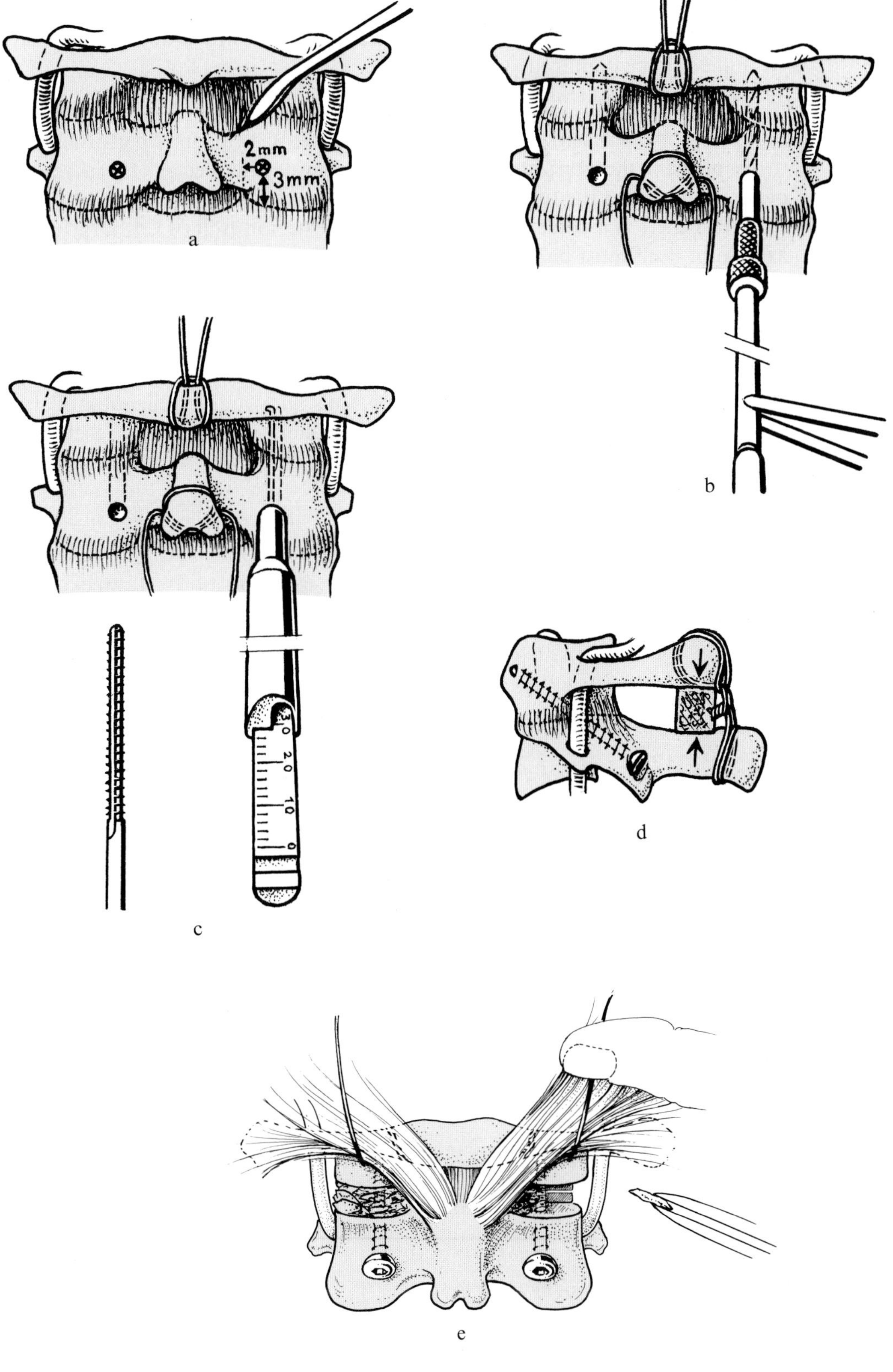

placement of the drill. Gently pulling the spinous process of C2 cranially with a towel clamp facilitates drilling.

Drilling in a horizontal direction must be avoided because:
- At the level of C2 the vertebral artery runs upward anteriorly to the C1–C2 joint and could be damaged.
- The screw could exit C2 anteriorly and not enter the atlas.

Following bilateral screw fixation, a posterior C1–C2 fusion is performed. It is preferable to supplement the graft with a posterior wiring technique, as this increases the stability of the fixation and the fusion rate (Fig. 16.3d).

When there is a defect or fracture of the posterior arch of C1, a fusion of the atlanto-axial joint itself must be performed. For visualization of the atlanto-axial joint, Kirschner wires are drilled into the posterior aspect of the lateral mass of the atlas. For this purpose, the greater occipital nerve is retracted cranially with a dissector. Once the Kirschner wires are in position and pulled cranially, the soft tissues containing the greater occipital nerve and its accompanying venous plexus can be retracted. The atlanto-axial joints are exposed by opening the posterior capsule, thus allowing visualization of the C1–C2 joint (Fig. 16.3e). The articular cartilage of the posterior half of the facet joint is removed with either a small chisel or a sharp curette, after which the joints are packed with cancellous bone and the screws are inserted.

Postoperative Care

Patients are immobilized in a firm collar for a period of 10–12 weeks but are allowed to remove the collar for daily care. After 6 weeks the collar can be discarded when resting. If additional posterior wiring has been used, a firm collar need only be worn for 3 weeks.

16.2.1.3 Anterior Screw Fixation of Odontoid (Dens) Fractures (Figs. 16.4–16.7)

Principle

Compression osteosynthesis by screw fixation (Fig. 16.4a, b).

Indication

The ideal indication is the transverse fracture of the neck of the odontoid process.

Figs. 16.4–16.7 Anterior screw fixation of odontoid (dens) fractures.

Fig. 16.4

a, b Compression osteosynthesis by screw fixation.

c Anterior screw fixation is contraindicated in oblique flexion fractures of the neck of the odontoid.

Fig. 16.5 Two image intensifiers are necessary to identify the odontoid process in the anteroposterior and lateral projections.

Fig. 16.4

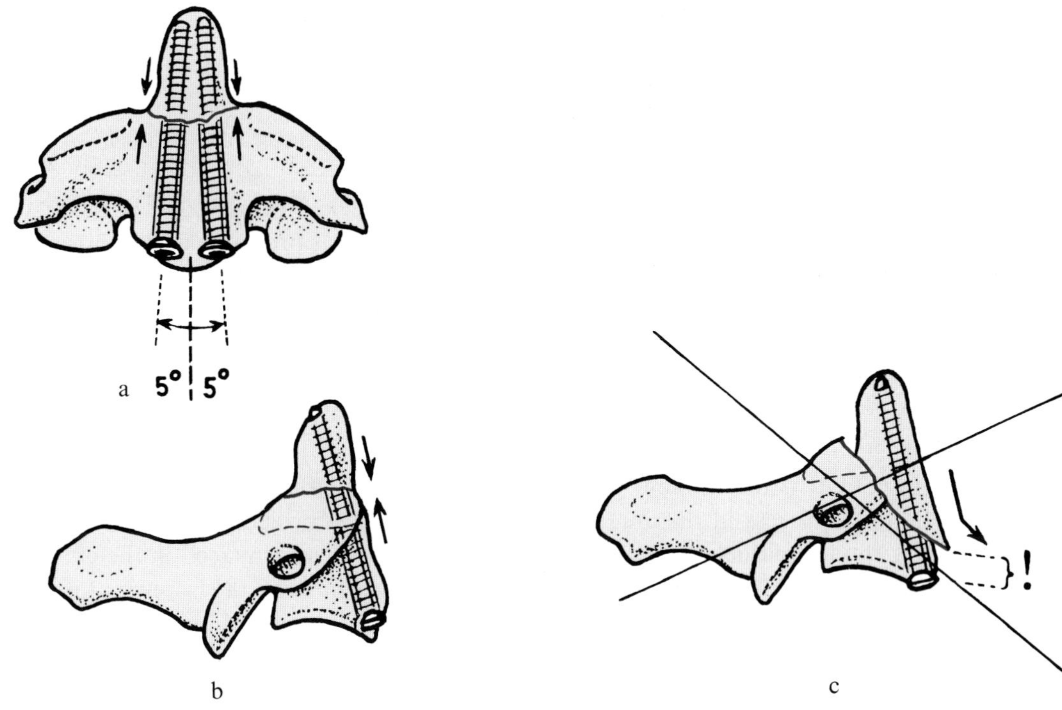

Fig. 16.5

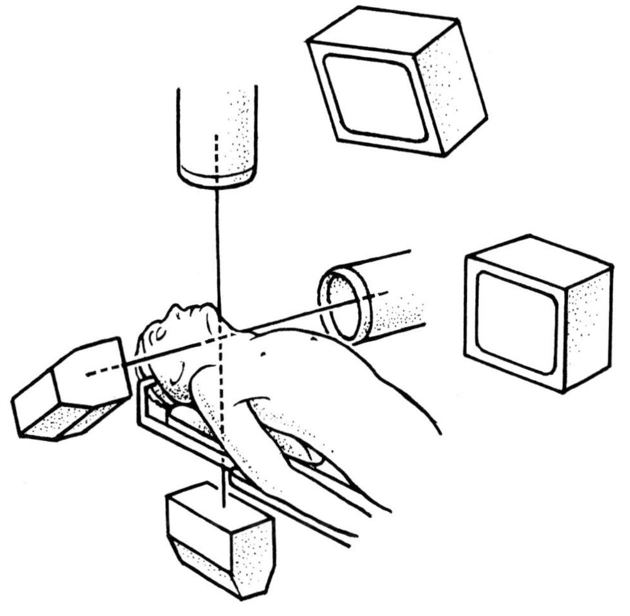

Advantages

- This procedure preserves the C1–C2 motion segment.
- Simple postoperative care and immobilization.
- Anterior approach less traumatic than posterior surgery.

Disadvantages

- Should not be used in the oblique flexion fractures of the neck of the odontoid (Fig. 16.4c).
- Technically difficult or impossible in short-necked patients, in patients with limited motion of the cervical spine and in patients with pronounced kyphosis of the upper thoracic spine.
- Requires high-resolution two-plane imaging (Fig. 16.5).
- Spinal stenosis is a contraindication because of the danger of cord injury associated with hyperextension of the neck.

Surgical Technique

The patient is in a supine position. Two image intensifiers are necessary to identify the odontoid process in the antero-posterior and lateral projections (Fig. 16.5). Without this help, the technique cannot not be carried out. The head is placed in the extended position to reduce the fracture and to facilitate the insertion of the screws. An anteromedian approach is used. The placement of the incision is determined by placing a long Kirschner wire along the side of the neck in the intended direction of the screw and viewing on the image intensifier.

The vertebral column is exposed anteriorly by blunt dissection and then exposed cranially until the inferior edge of the body of the second cervical vertebra is identified. Two Hohmann retractors are then inserted on either side of the odontoid (dens) to expose the body of the axis (Fig. 16.6a).

Standard Lag Screw Technique (Fig. 16.6b, c)

A long 2.5-mm drill is inserted into the anterior inferior edge of the C2 body. In the sagittal plane, the drill should be angled slightly posteriorly in order to exit at the posterior half of the tip of the odontoid (see Fig. 16.4b). Furthermore, in the frontal plane, the drill should be angled a few degrees towards the midline. A second drill is inserted in the same manner (Fig. 16.6b). One drill is removed and the entire hole in the distal fragment is overdrilled by a 3.5-mm drill (Fig. 16.6c). The depth of the hole to the tip of the odontoid is measured, tapped and the appropriate length 3.5-mm cortex screw is inserted. The same technique is used for the second screw.

Fig. 16.6 Exposure of the segment C2–3.

a Two Hohmann retractors are inserted, one on either side of the odontoid, to expose the body of the axis.

b A long 2.5-mm drill is inserted into the antero-inferior edge of the C2 body. In the sagittal plane the drill should be angled slightly posteriorly in order to exit at the posterior half of the tip of the odontoid (see Fig. 16.4b). In the frontal plane the drill should be angled a few degrees towards the midline. A second drill is inserted in the same manner.

c One drill is removed and the entire hole in the distal fragment is overdrilled using a 3.5-mm drill.

Fig. 16.6

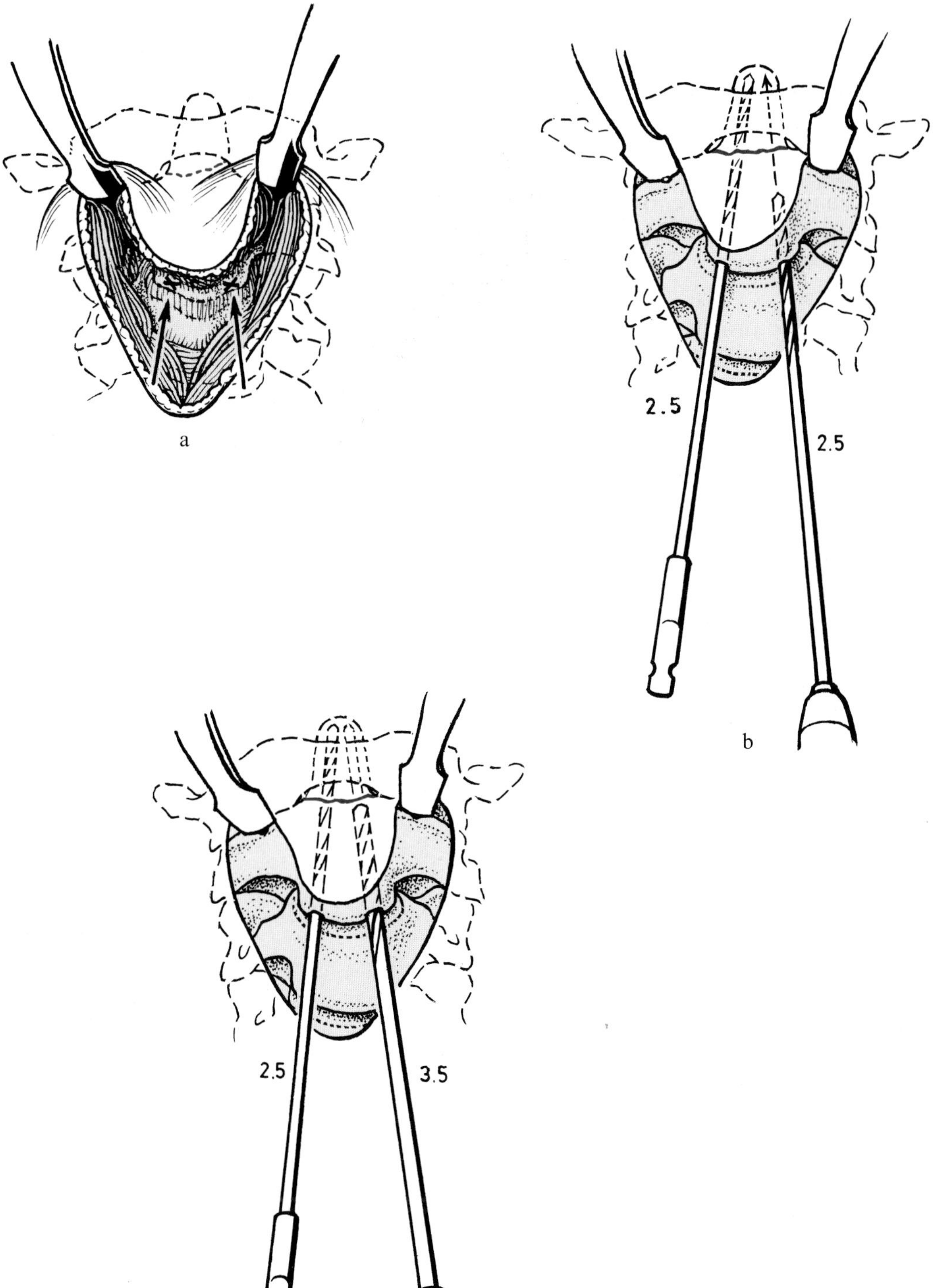

a

2.5

2.5

b

2.5

3.5

c

It is absolutely essential that tissue protectors are used when drilling and tapping, to avoid damaging vital structures. The oscillating attachment may also be used.

In patients of small stature, 2.7-mm screws are used with their appropriate drills and tap.

Cannulated Screw System (Fig. 16.7)

A hole is drilled with a long 3.5-mm drill at the antero-inferior edge of the vertebral body of C2 to a depth of 5 mm to facilitate later screw insertion (Fig. 16.7a). As previously described, two long 1.2-mm Kirschner wires, guided by a special sleeve, are inserted in the same direction. Each Kirschner wire is inserted until it penetrates the posterosuperior tip of the odontoid (Fig. 16.7b). The length of the screw is determined by measuring the protruding Kirschner wire. The appropriate length of self-tapping 3.5-mm cannulated cancellous bone screw is inserted with a cannulated screwdriver (Fig. 16.7c).

The progress of the screw *must* be observed with an image intensifier to ensure that the Kirschner wire does not migrate proximally into the foramen magnum.

Postoperative Care

The patient is treated with a firm collar for 6 weeks. The collar can be removed for daily care and when resting.

Fig. 16.7 Cannulated screw system technique.

a The entry point is made with a long 3.5-mm drill at the antero-inferior edge of the vertebral body of C2 to a depth of 5 mm to facilitate later screw insertion.

b Two long 1.2-mm Kirschner wires guided by a special sleeve are inserted until it penetrates the posterosuperior tip of the odontoid.

c The appropriate length of self-tapping 3.5-mm cannulated cancellous bone screw is inserted with a cannulated screwdriver.

Fig. 16.7

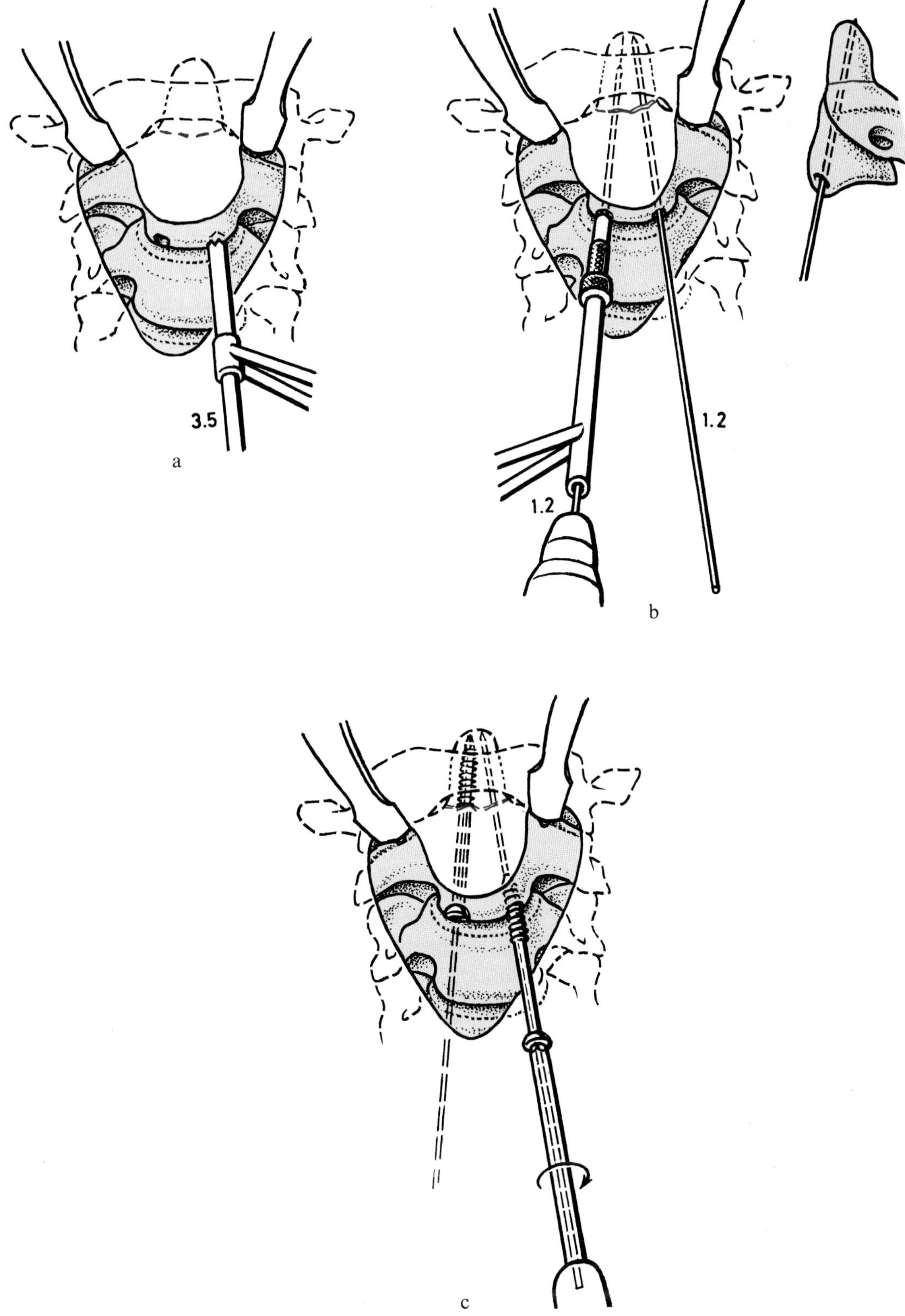

16.3 Lower Cervical Spine (C2-T1)

16.3.1 Posterior Techniques

16.3.1.1 Wiring Techniques

There are many wiring techniques for posterior fixation of the lower cervical spine. The most simple and least dangerous is interspinous wiring.

Interspinous Wiring (Fig. 16.8)

Principle

This technique applies the tension band principle.

Indications

Injuries of the posterior complex involving predominantly soft tissue with insignificant damage to the vertebral body.

Advantages

- Relatively easy.
- Safe.
- Large surface area for fusion.
- Short segment stabilization.

Disadvantages

- Wire breakage.
- Wire cut-out.
- Cannot be used in fractures of the vertebral arch including the spinous processes.

Surgical Technique

A midline posterior approach is used. It is essential to identify radiographically the levels to be fused. A hole is drilled on each side of the base of the spinous process of the upper vertebra of the injured segment (Fig. 16.8a). The entry point corresponds to the junction of the upper and middle portion of the process. A towel clip is placed in the holes, and with a gently rocking movement the holes are connected (Fig. 16.8b). A 1.2-mm wire is passed through the hole and then around the base of the inferior spinous process, leaving the interspinous soft tissue intact (Fig. 16.8c). The two ends of the wires are

---

Fig. 16.8 Interspinous wiring of the lower cervical spine.

a A hole is made on each side of the base of the spinous process of the upper vertebra of the injured segment, using a drill.

b The two tips of a towel clamp are placed in the holes, and with a gentle rocking movement the holes are connected.

c A 1.2-mm wire is passed through the hole and then around the base of the inferior spinous process, leaving the interspinous soft tissues intact.

d The two ends of the wire are tightened, curved around the inferior spinous process and twisted tight.

e The laminae are decorticated and cancellous bone graft is applied.

Fig. 16.8

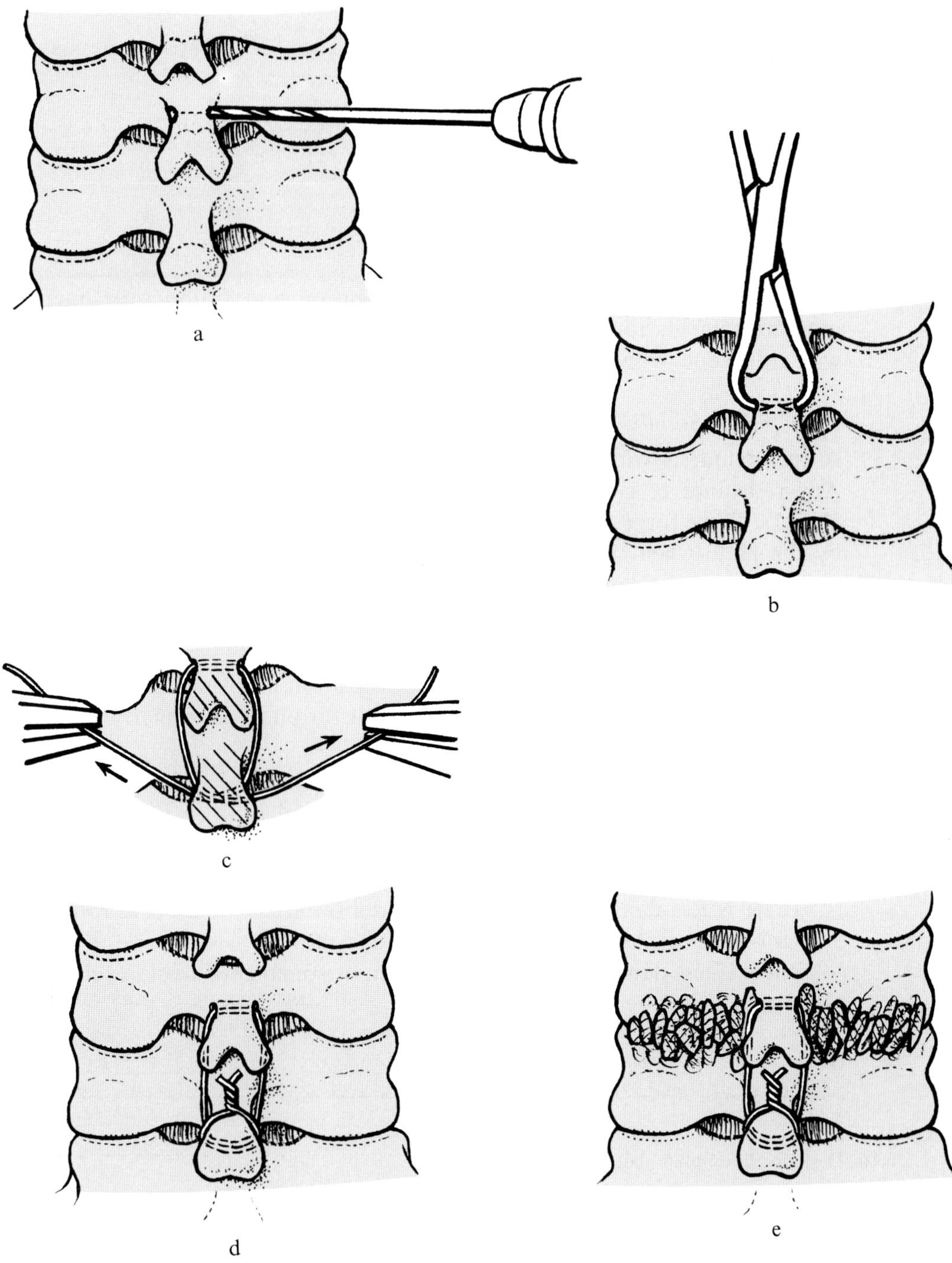

tightened. Lastly the wire ends are curved around the inferior spinous process and twisted tight (Fig. 16.8d). The laminae are decorticated with a high-speed burr, and cancellous bone graft is applied (Fig. 16.8e).

Postoperative Care

Similar to that for the posterior wiring techniques for the atlas and axis described above (Sect 16.2.1.1).

16.3.1.2 Plating Techniques

Hook Plates

Hook plates are used for posterior stabilization and fusion over one or two cervical motion segments (area of application: C2–C7). They are available in different lengths with either one or two holes (Fig. 16.9).

Principles of Stabilization

A spondylodesis with hook plates is a prestressed construct which is inherently stable. Any resistance to compression is due to the intervertebral joints and the interspinous H graft. These form a triangle in the horizontal plane. The compression force is provided by the plate when the screws are tightened. The spondylodesis is stable in all planes, since the resulting compression force lies within the triangle (Fig. 16.10).

Indications

- Discoligamentous instability due to subluxation or dislocation.
- Additional stabilization following anterior fusion in particularly unstable situations.
- Treatment of an anterior pseudarthrosis.

Advantages

- The primary stability achieved with the hook plate fixation is superior to that of interbody fusions and posterior cerclage wiring.
- There is less danger of injuring the vertebral artery or a nerve root than in posterior fusions using plates with screws inserted sagittally.
- There is less danger of injury to the dura or spinal cord than in sublaminar wiring.

Figs. 16.9–16.16 Posterior hook plate fixation.

Fig. 16.9 Hook plates are available in different lengths with either one or two holes.

Fig. 16.10 The spondylodesis is stable in all planes since the resulting compression force lies within the triangle formed by the facet joints and the interspinous graft.

Fig. 16.11 Positioning of the screws.

a The entry point for the screws lies 2–3 mm medially and cranially to the middle of the articular mass.

b Each screw diverges by 25° anterolaterally and runs parallel to the surface of the intervertebral joints.

c The inclination of the surface may be determined by inserting a fine dissector into the joint.

Fig. 16.9

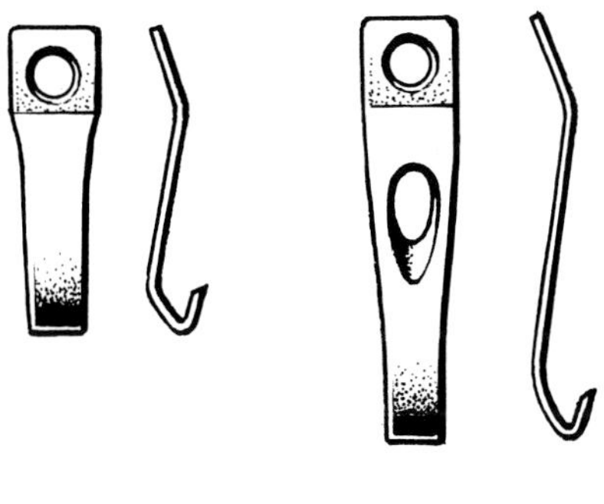

Fig. 16.10

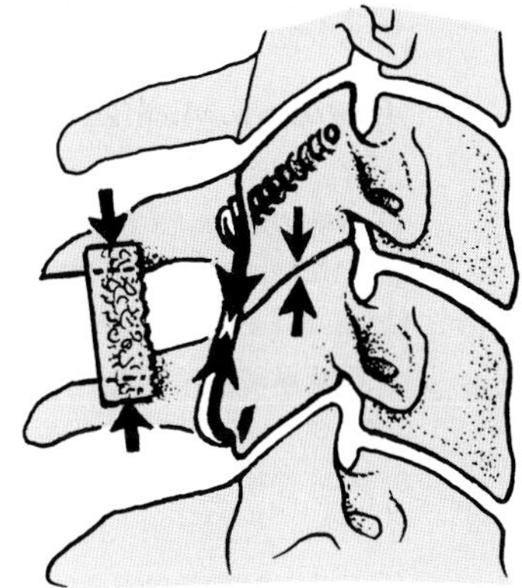

Fig 16.11

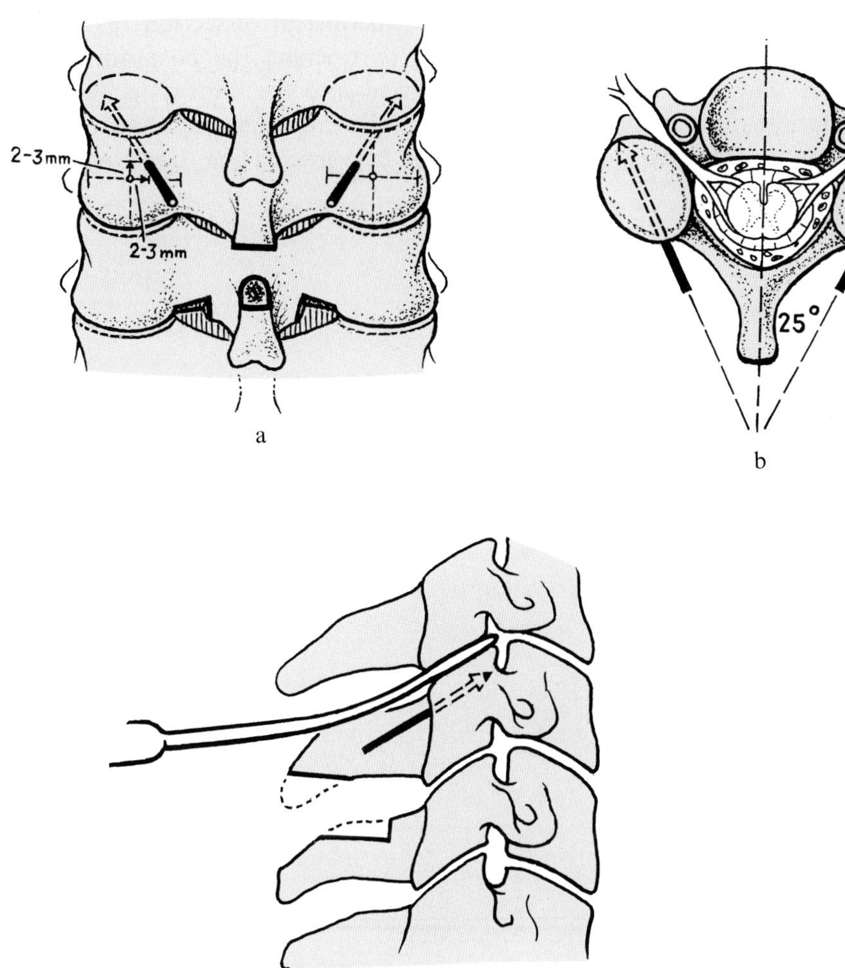

Disadvantage
Technically more demanding than wiring procedures.

Surgical Technique (Figs. 16.11–16.16)

Approach. Midline incision. Subperiosteal dissection of the posterior spinal elements.

Positioning of the screws. The entry point lies 2–3 mm medially and cranially to the middle of the articular masses (Fig. 16.11 a). Each screw diverges by 25° anterolaterally (Fig. 16.11 b) and runs parallel to the surface of the intervertebral joints. The inclination of the surfaces may be determined by inserting a fine dissector into the joints (Fig. 16.11 c). The screw canals are prepared using long 2.5-mm drills. The cortex of the articular processes on the far side is carefully perforated. The length of the drill hole is measured by the 3.5-mm depth gauge, and the canal is tapped only two-thirds of the distance. If a long spinous process hinders the preparation of the screw canals, it may be shortened.

Screws inserted into C2 must be directed 25° *toward the midline* and 25° cranially in order to avoid the vertebral artery and to pass through the isthmus of C2 into the subchondral bone of the upper articular surface (Fig. 16.12a, b). Perforation of the articular surface must be avoided.

The directions are determined by subperiosteal dissection of the soft tissues from the superior aspect of the isthmus and by opening the posterior capsule of the C1-2 joint. A thin dissector can then be inserted into the joint as a guide to determine the appropriate direction for screw insertion. The drill is inserted halfway between the upper and lower articular surfaces of C2 at a vertical line bisecting the articular mass (Fig. 16.12c).

Fig. 16.12 Screw fixation in C2.

a Direction of the screws in the horizontal plane. The screws are directed 25° towards the midline.

b In the sagittal plane the direction of the screws is 25° cranially.

c The drill is inserted halfway between the upper and lower articular surface of C2 at a vertical line bisecting the articular mass.

Fig. 16.12

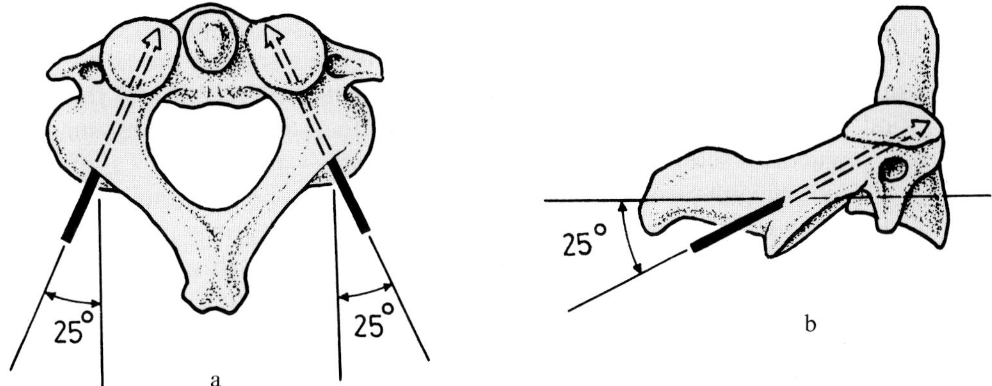

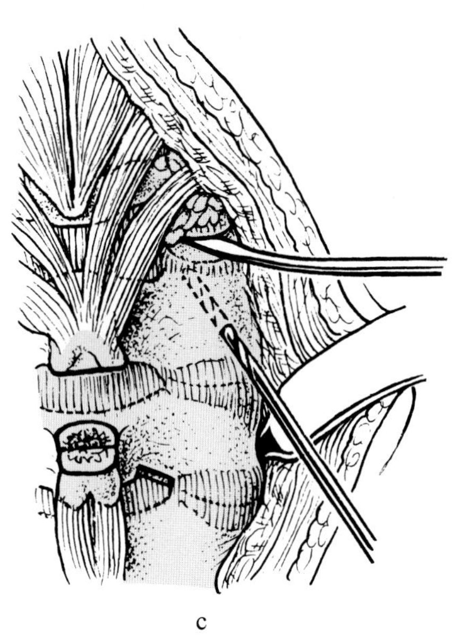

Hook and graft bed (Fig. 16.13). In order to prevent the hooks from sliding into the intervertebral joints, corresponding notches are cut into the lamina medial to the joints. The site of the H graft is prepared using an oscillating saw (Fig. 16.13). The lower notch must not be too deep in order to avoid a fracture of the spinous process.

Stabilizing one motion segment (Fig. 16.15). The plates are contoured by torque and bending to match the posterior aspect of the lamina as well as the articular mass (Fig. 16.14). A cortico-cancellous H graft is inserted between the spinous processes with the vertebrae in the neutral position. The contoured hook plates are placed into the prepared notches, and 3.5-mm cortex screws are inserted (Fig. 16.15a, b). In a very small articular mass, 2.7-mm cortex screws may be used.

Tightening the screws sandwiches the H graft. If a hook begins to lift out, the curvature of the hook should be increased. With two-hole plates, it is possible to secure the hook by inserting a short screw into the lower lamina, but this is rarely necessary. Finally, a cancellous bone graft is applied between the laminae and across the facet joints (Fig. 16.15a, b).

Stabilizing two motion segments (Fig. 16.16). With the long hook plates, two motion segments may be bridged (Fig. 16.16). The middle spinous process is removed. The upper screw canals, hook notches and graft bed are prepared and the plates appropriate in length are chosen and centered. They should be about 2 mm shorter to allow compression. The H graft is inserted, the plates applied and the upper screws inserted. They are tightened until some compression results. This is followed by drilling of the lower screw holes, parallel to the screws above. The drill is placed eccentrically through the upper part of the plate holes. First the lower screws are tightened, then the upper screws. With this technique compression is achieved in both motion segments.

Postoperative Care

A firm collar is worn for 6–8 weeks. It may be removed for daily care and, after 3 weeks, when resting.

Fig. 16.13 Hook and graft bed. In order to prevent the hooks from sliding into the intervertebral joints, corresponding notches are cut into the lamina medial to the joints. The site of the graft is prepared, using an oscillating saw.

Fig. 16.14 Contouring of the plates by torque and bending to match the posterior aspect of the lamina as well as the articular process.

Fig. 16.15 Stabilizing one motion segment. H-graft is inserted, the contoured hook plates are placed into the prepared notches, and 3.5-mm cortex screws are inserted:
a Lateral view.
b Posterior view.
Finally, the cancellous bone graft is applied between the laminae and across the facet joints.

Fig. 16.16 Stabilizing two motion segments. With the long hook plates two motion segments may be bridged. The middle spinous process is removed.

Fig. 16.13

Fig. 16.14

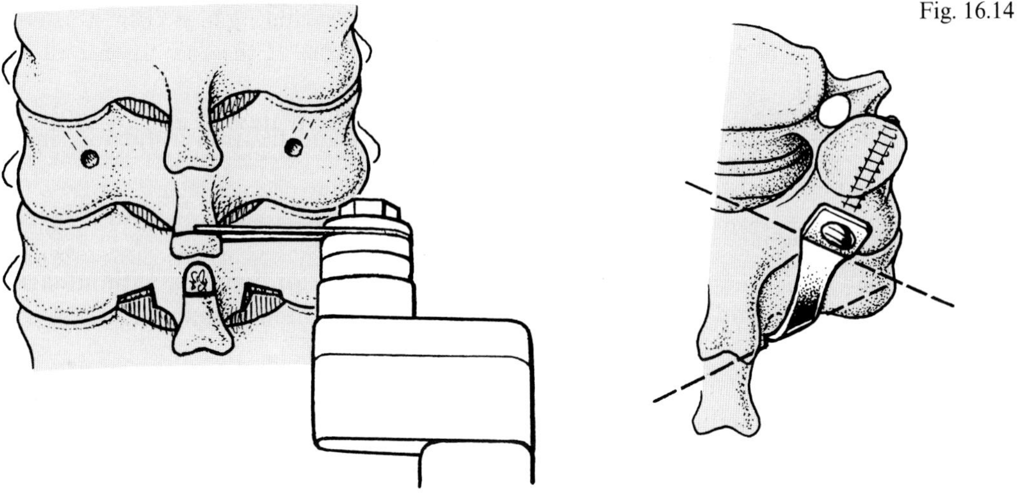

Fig. 16.15

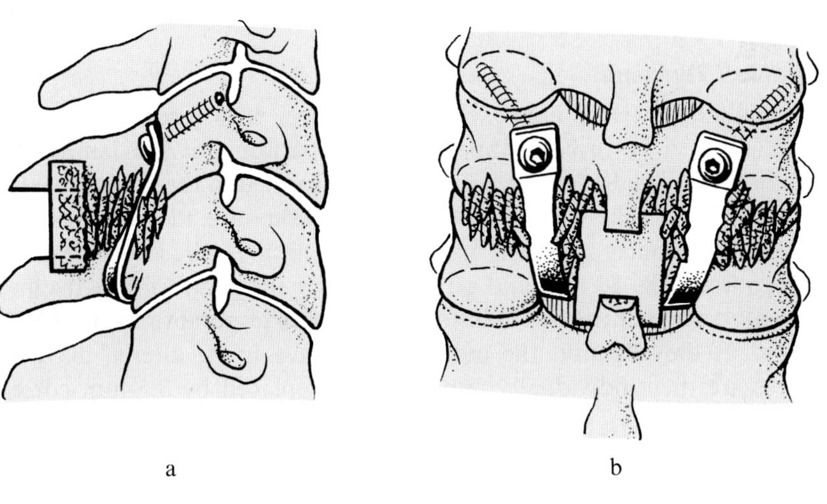

a

b

Fig.16.16

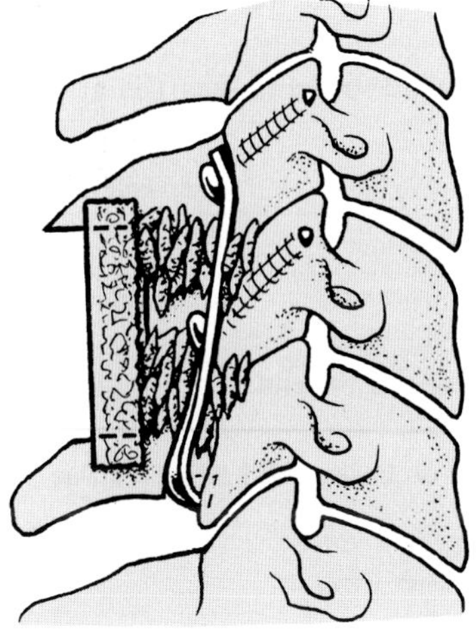

One-Third Tubular Plate Fixation (Fig. 16.17)

As an alternative to the one-third tubular plate, the 3.5-mm reconstruction plate may be used.

Principle

The posterior plating provides stable tension band fixation in flexion, increasing stability in rotation, and buttressing in extension.

Indication

Ligamentous and/or osseous lesions of the posterior complex without significant damage of the vertebral body. The lesions may be uni- or multisegmental.

Advantages

- Superior stability compared with wiring techniques.
- Can be used in the presence of laminar and spinous process fractures.
- Requires no special instrumentation.

Disadvantage

- Ideal screw placement may be compromised by the spacing of the holes.

Surgical Technique

A midline posterior approach is performed. It is essential to identify radiographically the levels to be fused. Subperiosteal preparation of the laminae and lateral masses is carried out. The Kirschner wires are then inserted in the lateral masses of the end vertebrae (Fig. 16.17a). The entry points and directions are the same as for the hook plates. A one-third tubular plate of appropriate length is chosen, hammered flat (Fig. 16.17b), contoured (Fig. 16.17c) and positioned over the protruding Kirschner wires (Fig. 16.17d) to check whether the end holes of the plate correspond to the entry points of the Kirschner wires. If they do not, the entry points have to be altered accordingly. The Kirschner wires are then individually removed and replaced by 3.5-mm cortex screws in the usual way (Fig. 16.17e). Care must be taken when perforating the anterior cortex of the lateral mass. If more than one motion segment is to be included, the end screws are not fully tightened, so that the plate can be adjusted and the remaining screws inserted. As the anatomic landmarks are hidden by the plate, check the entry point and direction of the drill in these holes with the image intensifier. The remaining screws are then introduced and all are tightened.

The laminae are decorticated and a cancellous bone graft is applied.

Fig. 16.17 Posterior plate fixation with the one-third tubular plate.

a Kirschner wires are inserted into the lateral masses of the end vertebra. The entry points and direction are the same as for the hook plate.

b The appropriate length of one-third tubular plate is chosen and hammered flat.

c The plate is contoured.

d The plate is positioned over the protruding Kirschner wires.

e The Kirschner wires are then individually removed and replaced by 3.5-mm cortex screws in the usual way.

Fig. 16.17

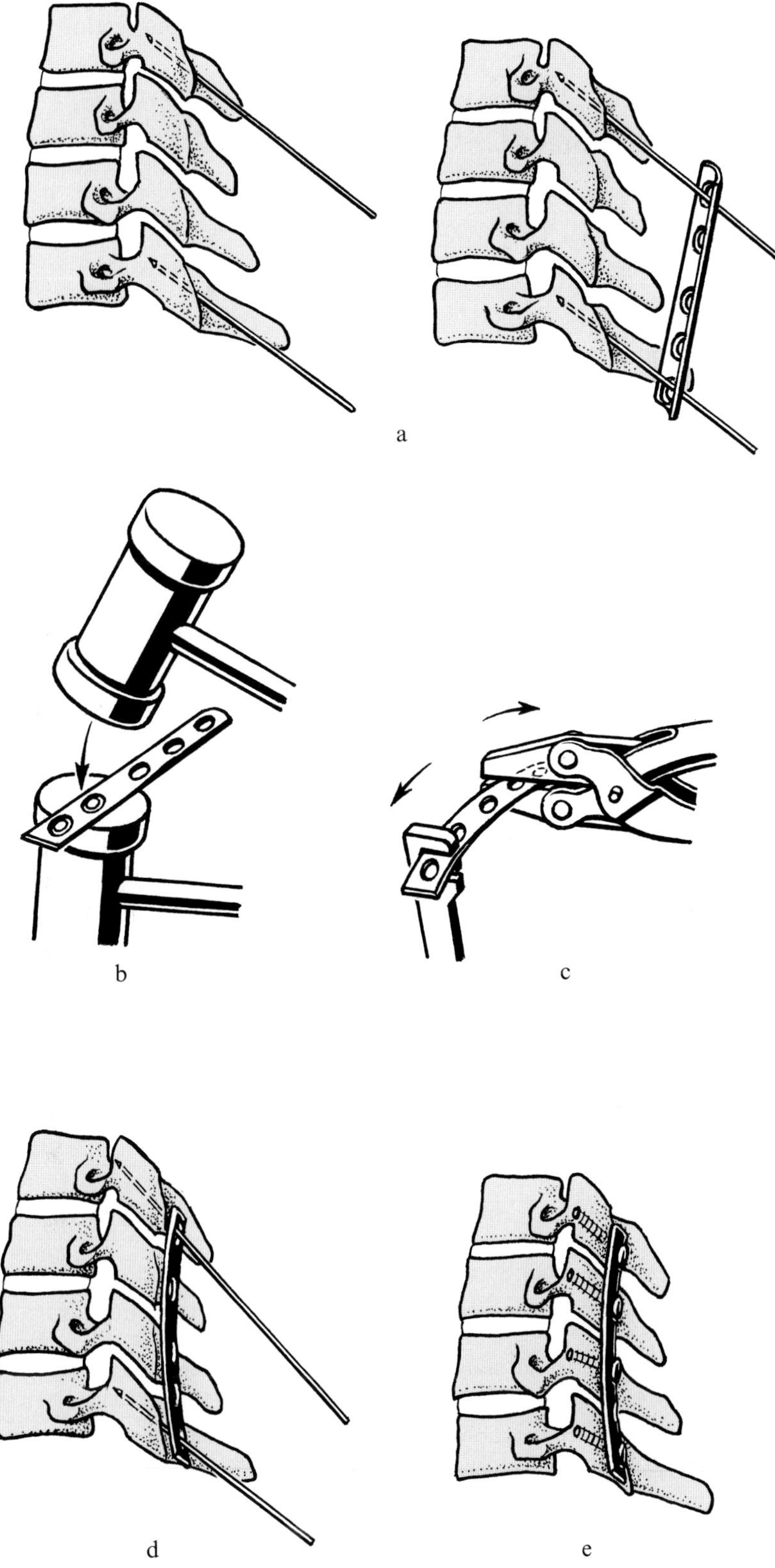

Postoperative Care

The patient wears a firm collar for 10–12 weeks. The collar can be removed for daily care, and after 6 weeks it need no longer be worn while resting.

16.3.2 Anterior Techniques

16.3.2.1 Plating

Principle

Anterior plate fixation is used to increase the stability of the anterior column following grafting techniques. The plate functions as a tension band in extension and as a buttress plate in flexion.

Indications

- To support the anterior column when instability persists, particularly in association with loss of height of the vertebral body following a severe wedge compression or burst fracture.
- Following partial or total vertebrectomy, for decompression of the spinal cord.

Standard H Plate (Figs. 16.18, 16.19)

Advantages

- Less instrumentation.
- More versatility regarding screw direction.
- Eccentric screw placement allows for compression of the graft.

Disadvantages

- The screws have to penetrate the posterior cortex of the vertebral body with potential risk to the spinal cord. (The oscillating attachment for the drill should be used.)
- Screw loosening with anterior migration can occur.
- No intrinsic stability of the fixation system (no fixed angle between screws and plate).

Figs. 16.18, 16.19 Anterior plating techniques: standard H plate.

Fig. 16.18 Preparation.

a The depth of the vertebral body is measured with the depth gauge through the intervertebral space after removal of the disc.

b The length of the protruding 2.5-mm drill is measured with a ruler.

c Ensure that the nut on the drill guide is tightly locked.

Fig. 16.19 Plate fixation.

a Using the preset special drill guide, the hole is drilled through the plate hole.

b The length is checked with the depth gauge.

c The anterior cortex of the vertebral body is tapped with the 3.5-mm tap.

Fig. 16.18

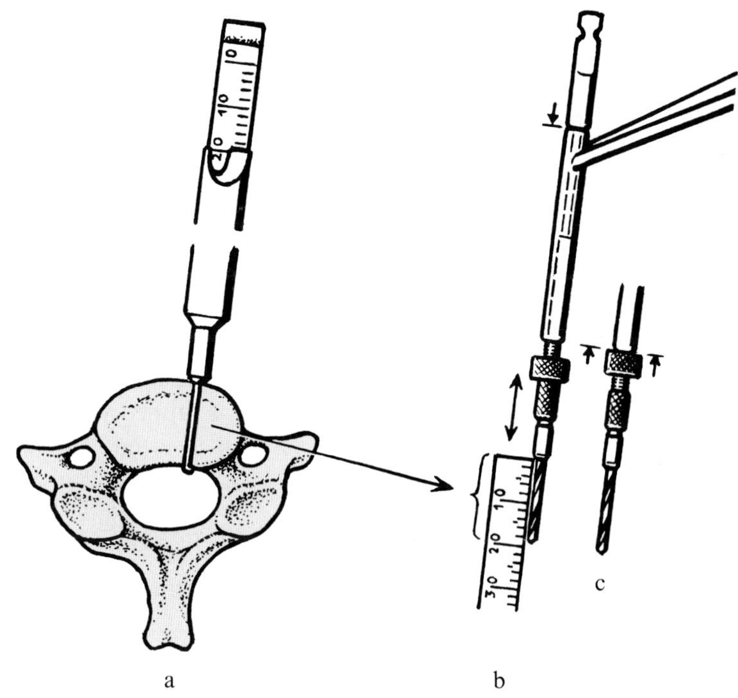

Fig. 16.19

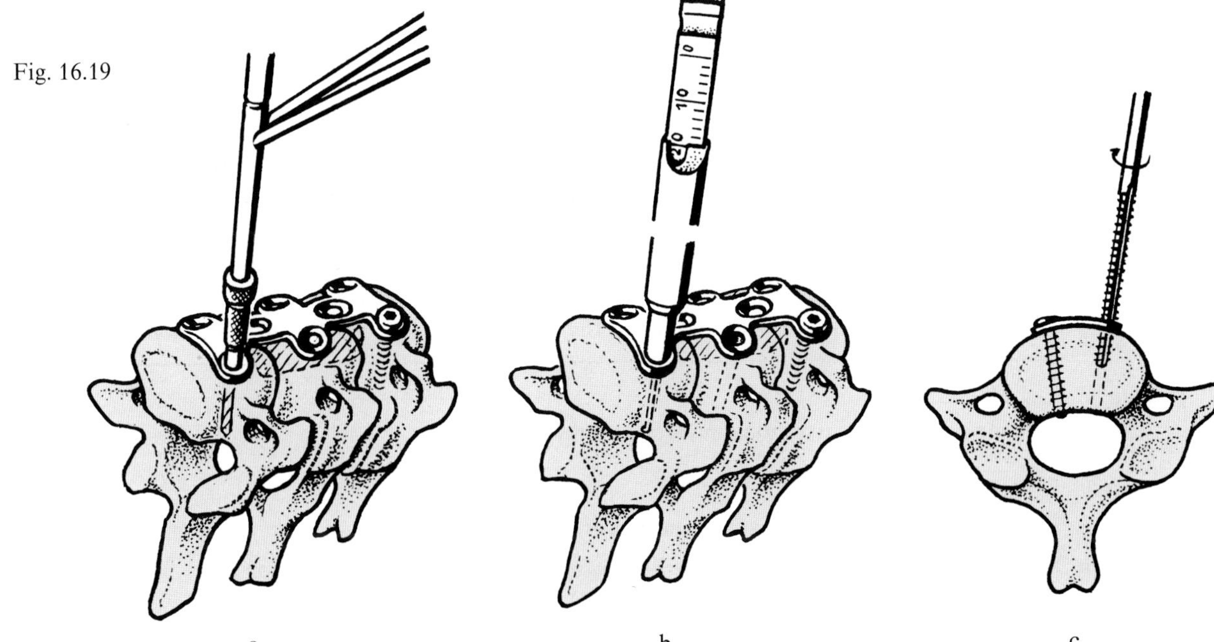

Surgical Technique

An anterior approach is used. It is essential to know the sagittal diameter of the vertebral body to prevent over-penetration of the posterior cortex with the drill.

In the majority of cases the disc at the site of injury has been removed prior to fusion, and at this stage, the depth of the vertebral body is measured with the depth gauge (Fig. 16.18a). The special drill guide with an inside diameter of 2.7 mm is set to the appropriate length and the length of the protruding 2.5-mm drill measured with a ruler (Fig. 16.18b). Ensure that the nut on the drill guide is tightly locked (Fig. 16.18c). Before drilling, a plate of suitable length is placed onto the anterior aspect of the vertebral bodies and held with a clamp. Using the preset special drill guide, the hole is drilled through the plate hole (Fig. 16.19a) and the length is checked with the depth gauge (Fig. 16.19b). If the posterior cortex has not been penetrated, then the special drill guide is adjusted to allow a further 1 mm of drilling. This is repeated if necessary and must be done with great care to prevent injury to the contents of the spinal canal.

The anterior cortex of the vertebral body is tapped with the 3.5-mm tap (Fig. 16.19c). The appropriate length 3.5-mm cortex screw is inserted. A similar procedure is performed with the other screw holes.

Postoperative Care

This is similar to the care described for the titanium locking screw-plate system below.

Titanium Locking Screw-Plate System (TLSP) (Figs. 16.20, 16.21)

Advantages

- The screws do not penetrate the posterior wall of the vertebral body.
- The locking of the screw head into the cylindrical holes provides intrinsic stability.
- Locking prevents migration of the screw anteriorly.

Disadvantage

The alignment of the screw holes in relation to the plate is fixed and can lead to difficulties in screw placement.

Principle

The expansion head of the screw is cylindrical with a rim stop and has a diameter of 4.5 mm. The screw head is cross-split just above the start of the thread (Fig. 16.20a, b) and can therefore be locked into the plate hole by means of a conical expansion

Figs. 16.20, 16.21 Anterior plating techniques: titanium locking screw-plate system.

Fig. 16.20 The system.

a The screw head is cross-split just above the start of the thread.

b It can therefore be locked into the plate hole by means of a conical expansion bolt.

Fig. 16.21 Surgical technique.

a The drill has a stop, which allows only 16 mm penetration into the vertebral body.

b The soft tissue protector is used when tapping the thread, and the tap also has a stop to prevent overpenetration.

c The two split leaves disengage when tightened, but remain on the screwdriver for ease of removal.

d When the small screw is driven in, it expands the head of the larger screw and locks it into the plate.

Fig. 16.20

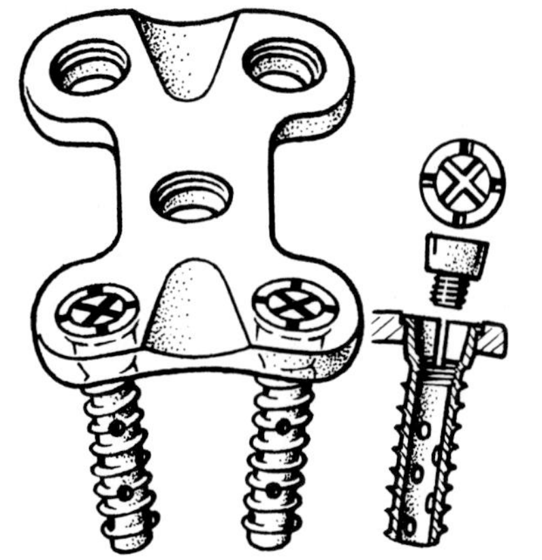

a b

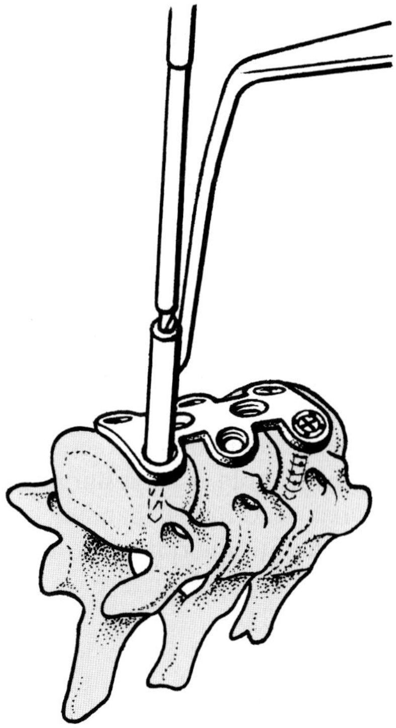

Fig. 16.21

a

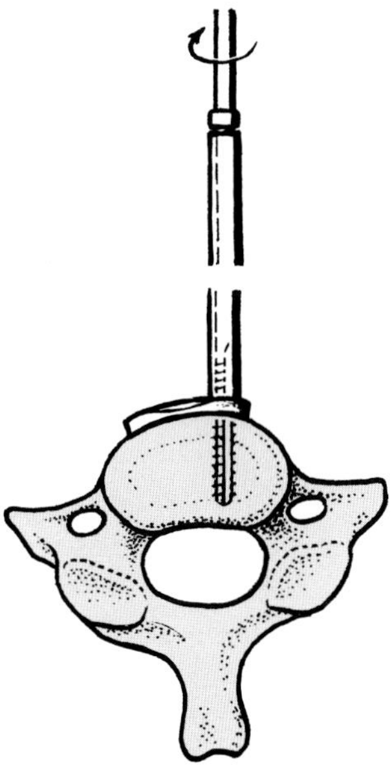

b

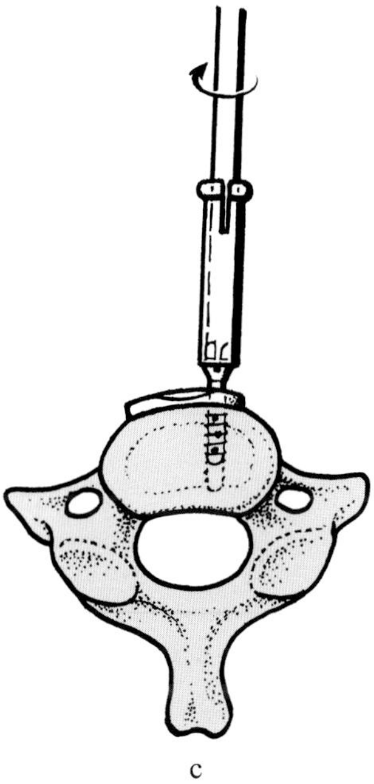

c 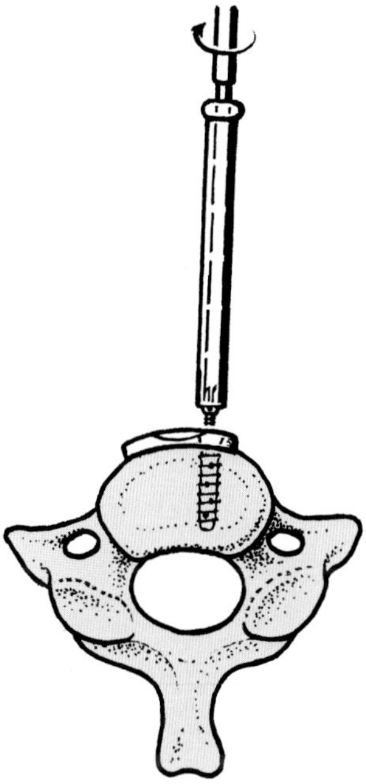 d

bolt (Fig. 16.20b). All screws are 14 mm long with a thread diameter of 4.0 mm. The diameter of the screw holes is 4.5 mm and the plate thickness 2.0 mm.

There is a wide range of plate sizes to allow application to the cervical and the upper thoracic spine. The titanium plasma spray coating of the screws gives a rough surface, increasing the area of contact. The screw is hollow to allow ingrowth of bone.

Surgical Technique

The spine is approached anteriorly through a transverse incision at the appropriate level. Since the discs are angled in the horizontal plane such that their direction changes from caudal to cranial as they extend from anterior to posterior, the plate size is selected to ensure that the screws penetrate the upper region of the vertebral bodies. This will prevent the screws from entering into the intervertebral disc above and below the level which requires fusion. Overriding of a normal disc by the plate must be avoided.

The plate is positioned and the first screw hole drilled with the aid of a special drill guide. The drill has a stop which allows only 16 mm penetration into the vertebral body (Fig. 16.21a). The soft tissue protector is used when tapping the thread, and the tap has also a stop to prevent overpenetration (Fig. 16.21b).

The screws are applied using the crosshead screw driver. The crosshead screwdriver is first inserted into the screw head and then a split sleeve is pushed over the screw head to hold it in position. A second split sleeve is necessary to prevent the cross-split screw head from expanding on insertion. The perforated hollow cylinder screw is screwed down until the rim of the screwhead is flush with the plate surface. The two split sleeves automatically disengage when tightened but remain on the screwdriver for ease of removal (Fig. 16.21c).

The plate is finally locked in place by the insertion of a small screw with a conical head. The small screw is held on the screwdriver by a split sleeve in the same way as the previously used screw. When the small screw is driven home it expands the head of the larger screw and locks it into the plate (Fig. 16.21d).

Postoperative Care

A collar is worn for 6 weeks but may be removed for daily care.

16.4 Thoracolumbar Spine

For stabilization of the thoracolumbar spine, anterior, posterior and combined techniques are used.

16.4.1 Anterior Technique: Fixation with the Large DCP (Fig. 16.23)

Principle

Anterior plate fixation is used to enhance stability of an anterior column following grafting techniques. The plate functions as a tension band in extension and as a buttress plate in flexion. From the practical point of view, it can be fixed to the front or the lateral aspect of the vertebral body without any relevant difference in stability.

Indications

- To support the anterior column when instability persists, particularly in association with loss of height of the vertebral body following a severe wedge compression or burst fracture.
- Following partial or total vertebrectomy for decompression of the spinal cord.

Advantages

- Short segment fixation.
- Relatively easy technique.

Disadvantages

- Loosening of the screws due to poor fixation in cancellous bone.
- Backing out of screws, especially if the plate is placed in the front of the vertebral body.
- No fixed angle between the screws and the plate.

Surgical Technique

A standard approach is made to expose the anterior vertebral column. The segmental vessels are ligated. Before applying a plate the anterior column is reconstructed with a tricortical iliac bone graft and supplemented with cancellous bone (Fig. 16.22a–c).

Anterior placement of the plate. After removal of the appropriate disc(s), the depth of the vertebra is measured with the depth gauge (see Fig. 16.22b). The special 3.2-mm drill guide is used to the appropriate length, and the length of the protruding drill measured with a ruler. The femoral plate thickness is 4 mm and is added to the measured depth (see H plate technique for cervical spine, Sect. 16.3.2.1). The broad DCP of appropriate length is applied to the anterior aspect of the vertebral body and fixed with 4.5-mm screws (Fig. 16.23a). If the bone is porotic, the 6.5-mm cancellous bone screws may be used, particularly in the end holes.

When considering anterior application of the plate the risk of grave complications inherent in this placement must be taken into account. Implant loosening, especially backing out of screws, may cause erosion of the esophagus, aorta or vena cava.

Lateral placement of the plate. An appropriate length broad DCP is placed on the lateral aspect of the vertebral body. The plate is applied using standard AO methods (Fig. 16.23b). The advantage of this technique is that one keeps away from the aorta and vena cava, especially should a screw become loose and back out.

Postoperative Care

The patient is mobilized with an appropriate thoracolumbar support for 12 weeks. The support may be removed for daily care and, after 6 weeks, when resting.

Fig. 16.22 Anterior fixation with the broad DCP in the thoracolumbar spine.

a The fragments of the fractured vertebral body are removed.

b The depth of the vertebral body is measured with the depth gauge, and the intervertebral defect is distracted with a bone distractor.

c The anterior column is reconstructed with one to three cortico-cancellous iliac bone grafts.

Fig. 16.23 Anterior or lateral placement of the plate.

a Application of the broad DCP of appropriate length to the anterior aspect of the vertebral body and fixation with 4.5-mm screws.

b Application of the plate, using standard AO techniques, to the lateral aspect of the spine.

Fig. 16.22

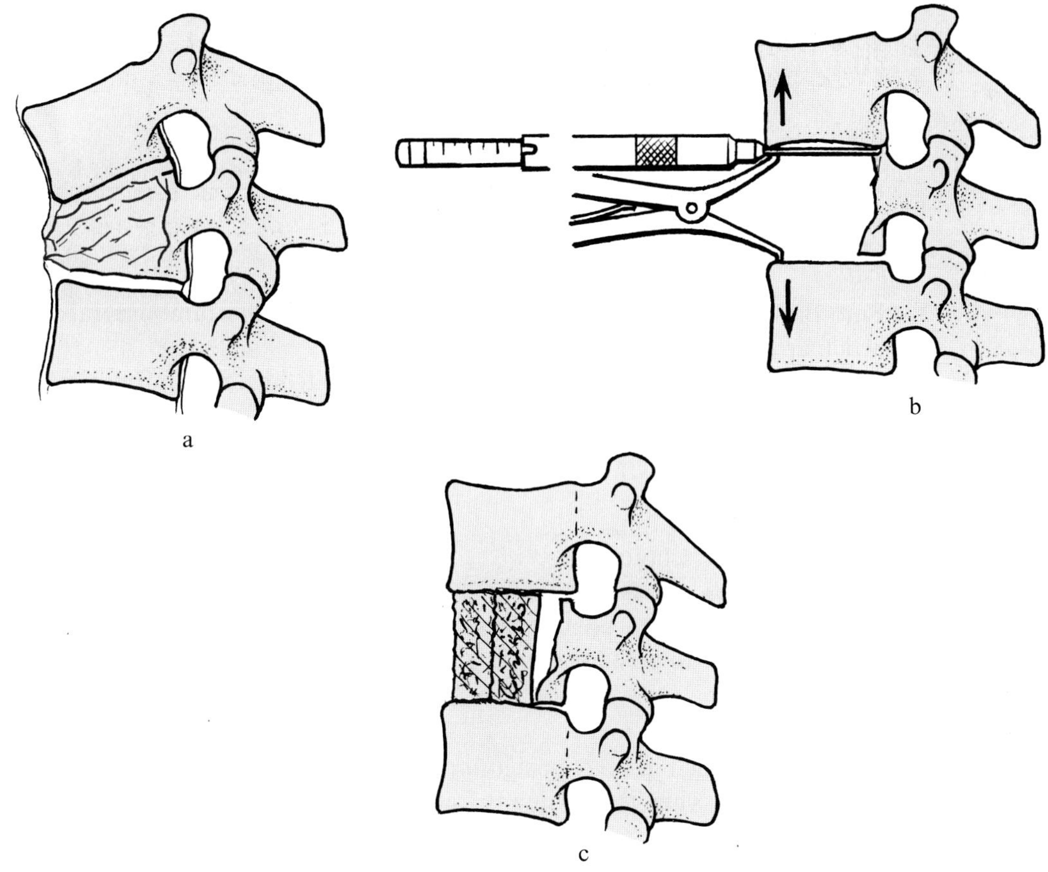

Fig. 16.23

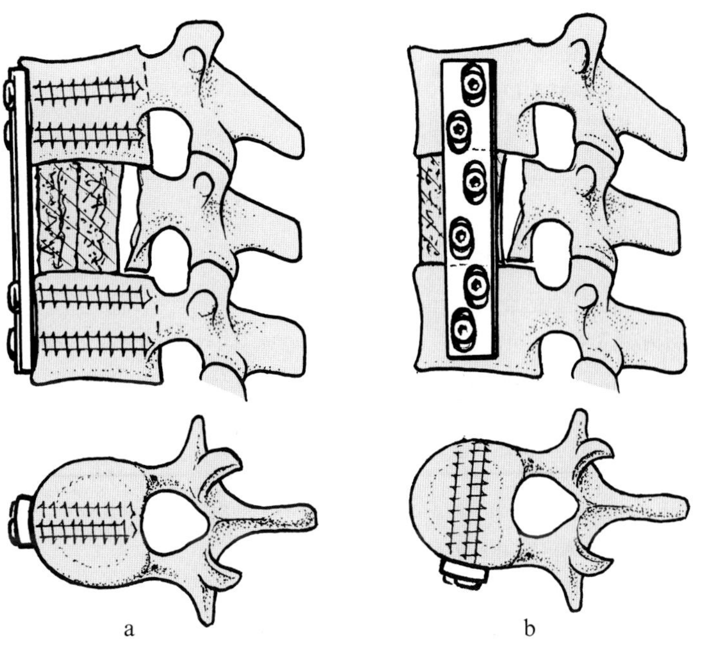

16.4.2 Posterior Techniques

16.4.2.1 Translaminar Screw Fixation (Figs. 16.24, 16.25)

Principle

Stabilization of a posterior fusion over one or two motion segments by transfixing the facet joints.

Indications

- Pure dislocations or subluxations from T12-L1 to the lumbosacral junction (minor articular process fractures can be ignored).
- Supplementary internal fixation of fractures treated by an interbody fusion or external fixation.

Advantages

- Short segment fixation.
- Relatively easy technique.
- No major inherent risk.
- The stability achieved is superior to that with other facet joint screw fixations (e.g. Boucher's) or with posterior wiring techniques.

Disadvantages

- Not recommended in severe osteoporosis.
- Not applicable when the lamina is fractured.

Surgical Techniques

Posterior midline approach. Exposure of the posterior vertebral elements including the bases of the transverse processes of the lower vertebra.

Using a special aiming device (Fig. 16.24a), the screw canals are prepared with a special long 3.2-mm drill. The two tips of the aiming device are placed onto the lamina and base of the transverse process respectively (Fig. 16.24b) so that the screw will pass through the spinous process, the inferior portion of the lamina, traverse the facet joint and exit near the base of the transverse process (Fig. 16.25a–c).

Figs. 16.24, 16.25 Translaminar screw fixation.

Fig. 16.24 Special aiming device for the screws.

a The device.

b Positioning of the aiming device. One tip of the device is placed upon the lower part of the lamina and the other upon the middle of the base of the transverse process.

Fig. 16.25 Surgical technique.

a The positioning of the translaminar screws seen from posterior.

b The screws seen in the horizontal plane.

c The screws seen from the side.

d The posterior vertebral elements, including the posterior half of the joints, are carefully decorticated and cancellous bone graft is applied.

Fig. 16.24

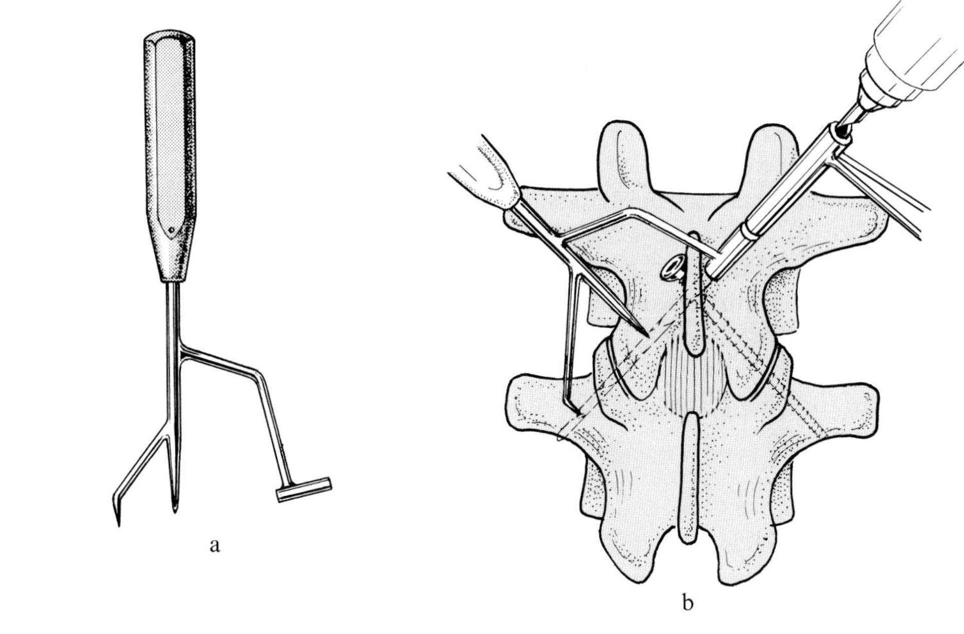

Fig. 16.25

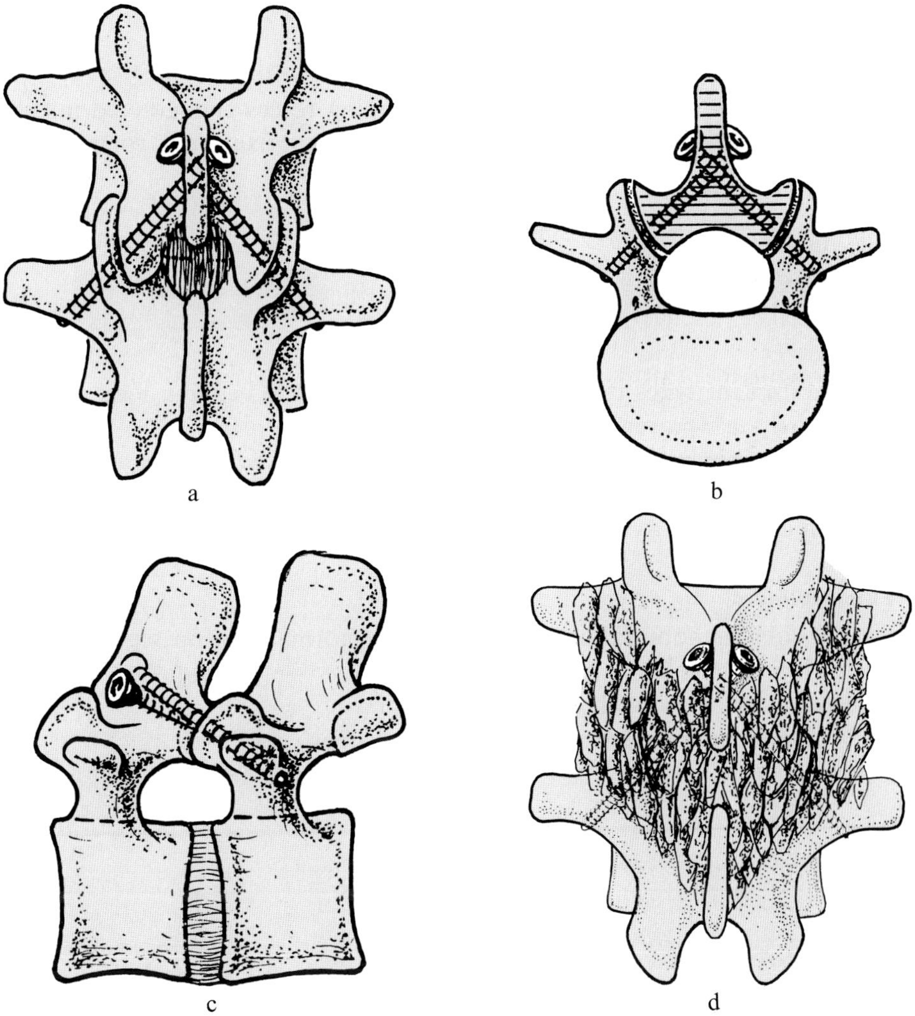

a

b

c

d

At the L5-S1 level, the screws are inserted into the lateral masses of the lamina, again using the special aiming device (Fig. 16.24). The length of each screw canal is measured, and the screw canals are tapped with the 4.5-mm tap. The tap needs only to traverse the facet joints. The proper 4.5-mm cortex screw is then inserted.

When preparing the first screw canal, one has to take into account that two screws are to be inserted. Therefore the first one should enter the spinous process and lamina slightly out of the ideal position either cranially or caudally in order to leave enough space for the second screw.

Given their diverging direction, the screws cannot be lagged. Translaminar screws function as threaded bolts which prevent motion in the respective segment but do not exert compression in the facet joints.

After insertion of the screws, the posterior vertebral elements including the posterior half of the joints are carefully decorticated and cancellous bone graft is applied (Fig. 16.25d).

Postoperative Care

The patient is mobilized when comfortable and wears a hyperextension brace for 10–12 weeks. The brace may be removed for daily care and during bedrest.

16.4.2.2 Locking Hook Spinal Rod System (Figs. 16.26, 16.27)

Principle

This implant is designed to resist high bending forces encountered in the injured spine. It is a distraction system which provides a four-point fixation to correct traumatic deformity.

Indications

Fractures of T3–T10.

Advantages

- The implant takes the axial compressive and the bending load and thus bridges the injured area, preventing dislocation.
- Both hooks are rigidly fixed to the rod for improved rotational stability.
- The upper hook design with the sliding cap provides higher posterior pull-out strength than other hook systems.

Disadvantages

- Requires immobilization of two or three normal motion segments above and below the injury.
- Hooks are placed within the spinal canal.
- Overdistraction of certain fractures may occur.

Figs. 16.26, 16.27 Locking hook spinal rod system.

Fig. 16.26 The implant.

Fig. 16.26

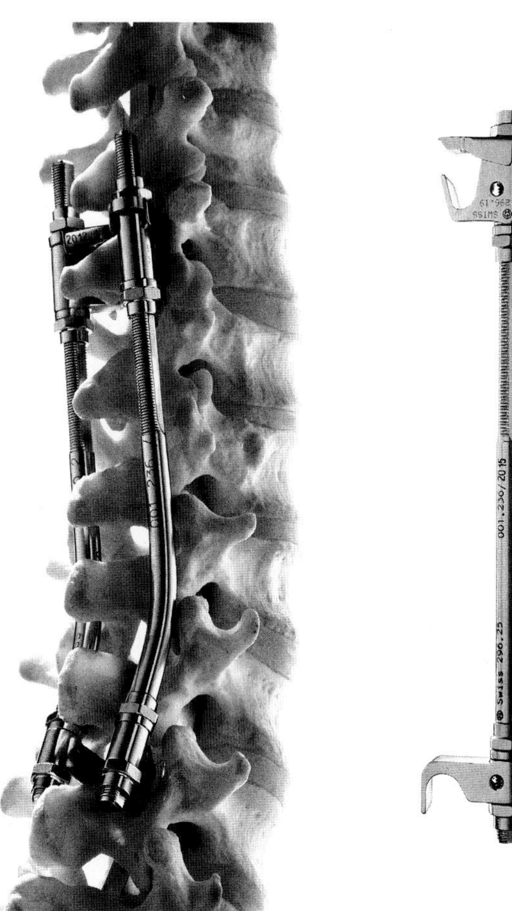

Description of the System

The implant consists of a rod, threaded at each end. The threaded portion is flattened on two sides (Fig. 16.26). At each end of the threaded sections, a hook is attached with its longitudinal position adjusted by means of nuts. The nuts contain a malleable collar which can be crimped to the flat surface of the rod to prevent loosening. The inferior hook is locked to a washer with a surface of radial grooves. The washer is keyed to the flat sides of the rod preventing rotation.

This provides rigid fixation in a variety of rotational positions. The upper hook has the same washer system as well as a sliding superior cover which can be advanced over the hook, locking the lamina.

Surgical Technique

The lower hook sites are prepared between the laminae of the first and second vertebra below the injury. A minimum amount of bone on the upper edge of the lamina and the medial border of the facet is removed to allow insertion of a trial lower hook. The lower border of the third lamina above the injury is removed to allow insertion of the trial upper hook into the spinal canal such that its upper surface is at the superior border of the lamina. In the thoracic spine, the rod does not usually require contouring, since the application of a straight rod usually results in correction of the deformity with an appropriate thoracic kyphosis remaining. The rod with the upper and lower hooks plus two locking washers and four nuts is inserted as a single assembly.

The lower hook is inserted first, through the narrow opening between the laminae (Fig. 16.27a). Using the hook holder on the upper hook, the angular deformity is corrected by downward pressure on the rod and hook (Fig. 16.27b).

The upper hook is inserted under the lamina by a hook holder, first at 90° to the rod to aid in final reduction and then progressively rotated to 30° to advance the hook up the rod and under the lamina. The sliding cover is then advanced over the lamina (Fig. 16.27c), locking it in place and the entire hook assembly is secured by tightening the nuts. The nut collars with the rod holder are tightened against the flat sides of the rod to prevent loosening of the nuts (Fig. 16.27d).

Insertion of this system corrects the deformity and restores most of the vertebral body height. Some distraction can be used to ensure solid fixation of the hooks to the posterior elements and to restore vertebral height. Sublaminar wires may be added to enhance stability in very unstable fractures.

Postoperative Care

No external immobilization is necessary. The patients are allowed to mobilize immediately.

Fig. 16.27 Surgical technique.

a The lower hook is inserted through the narrow opening between the lamina.

b Using the hook holder on the upper hook, the angular deformity is corrected by downward pressure on the rod and hook.

c The sliding cover is then advanced over the lamina and locked in place by tightening the nuts.

d The nut collars with the rod holder are tightened against the flat sides of the rod to prevent loosening of the nuts.

Fig. 16.27

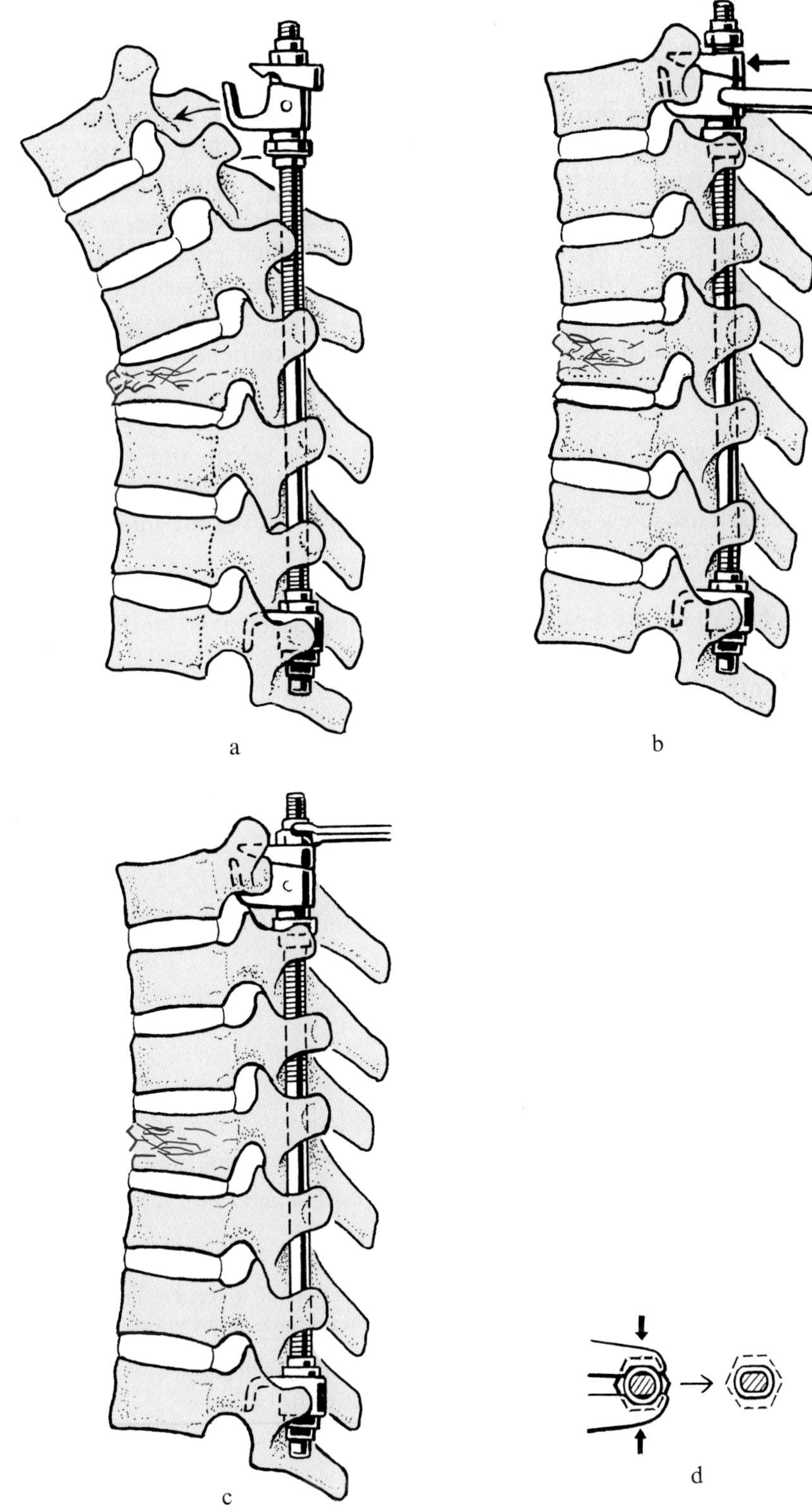

16.4.2.3 Pedicle Fixation

Determining the Position of Transpedicular Screws

Exact evaluation of the pedicles is an essential prerequisite for posterior plating and the application of fixator systems.

The pedicles are short conical tubes with an oval cross section. The objective is to insert the screws through the center of the pedicles, approximately parallel to the upper end plate or angled downward. The screws should converge toward the midline to a certain extent – up to 20% depending on the spinal level – in order to ensure that they do not penetrate the lateral wall of the vertebral body.

The long axis of the pedicle can be identified either by direct exposure or by image intensification. Although each method is reliable by itself, it is best to use a combination of the two. In addition, there are other aids for deciding screw position which are useful particularly when the anatomic landmarks are difficult to define due to distorted anatomic relationships.

Thoracic spine. The point of entry is just below the rim of the upper facet joint (Fig. 16.28a), 3 mm lateral to the center of the joint near the base of the transverse process. This screw should be angled 7–10° towards the midline (Fig. 10.28b) and 10–20° caudally (Fig. 16.28c).

Lumbar spine. At practically all levels the long axis of the pedicle pierces the lamina at the intersection of two lines: a vertical line tangential to the lateral border of the superior articular process, and a horizontal line bisecting the transverse process (Fig. 16.29a). Their point of intersection lies in the angle between the superior articular process and the base of the transverse process.

The screws should converge by 5° at the thoracolumbar junction (Fig. 16.29b) and by 10°–15° as one progresses from L2 to L5 (Fig. 16.29c).

Figs. 16.28–16.30 Determining the position of the transpedicular screws.

Fig. 16.28 Thoracic spine.

a The point of entry is just below the rim of the upper facet joint.

b, c The screw should be angled 7–10° towards the midline and 10–20° caudally.

Fig. 16.29 Lumbar spine.

a The entry point for the pedicle is at the intersection of a vertical line tangential to the lateral border of the superior articular process and a horizontal line bisecting the transverse process.

b The screws should converge by 5° at the thoracolumbar junction.

c The screws should converge by 10° at L2, increasing to 15° at L5.

Fig. 16.30 Sacrum.

a The entry point for the S1 pedicle is located at the intersection of a vertical line tangential to the lateral border of the S1 facet and a horizontal line tangential to its inferior border.

b The screws converge toward the midline.

c The screws aim toward the anterior corner of the promontorium.

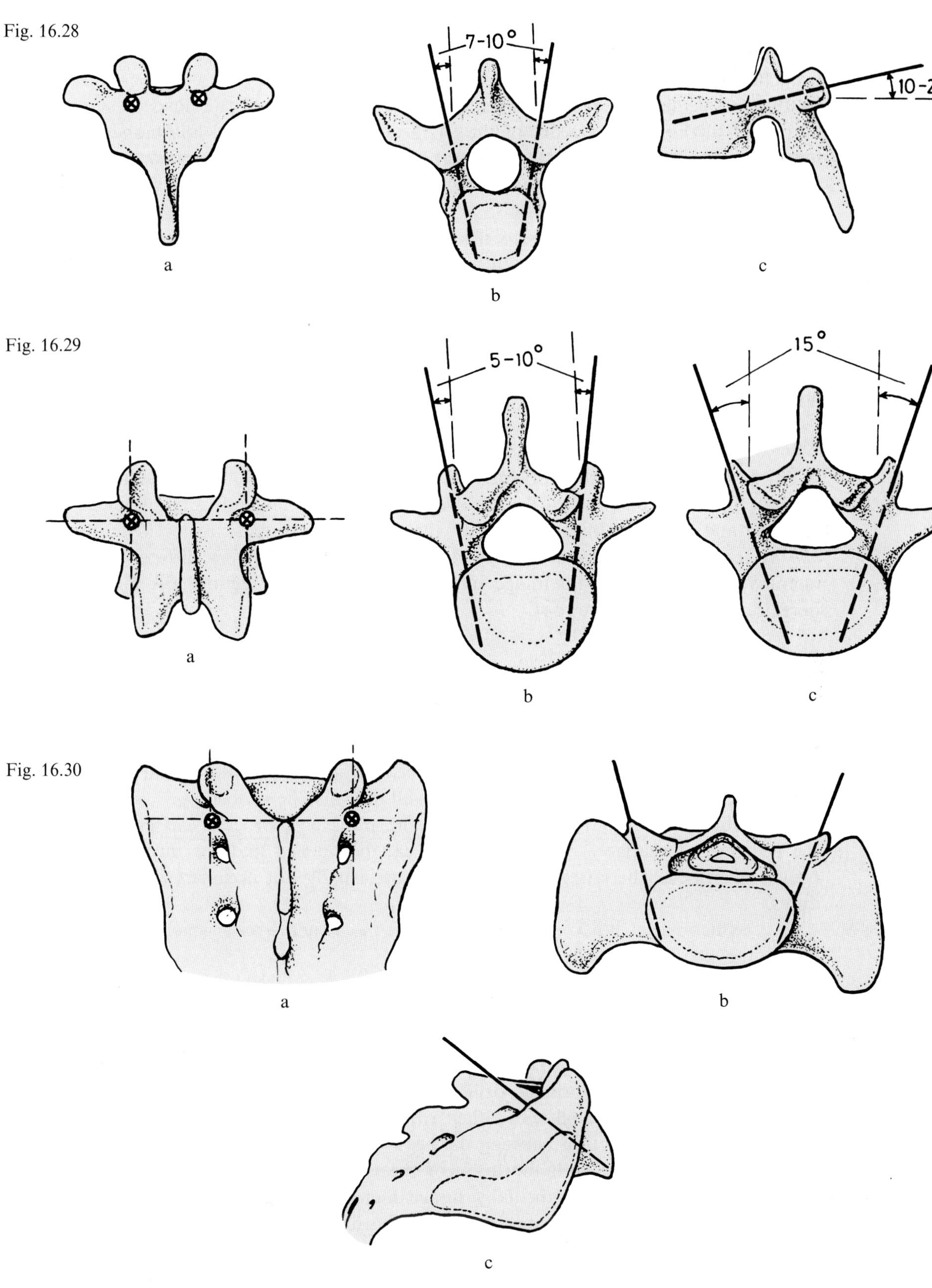

Fig. 16.28
a
7-10°
b
10-20°
c
Fig. 16.29
a
5-10°
b
15°
c
Fig. 16.30
a
b
c

Sacrum. Proper placement of screws in the sacrum is difficult because of its variable anatomy. The screws may be introduced at different points and in different directions, depending upon the instrumentation and the quality of the bone. The latter is important for achieving adequate purchase.

In general, the entry point is located at the intersection of two lines: a vertical line tangential to the lateral border of the S1 facet, and a horizontal line tangential to the inferior border of this facet (Fig. 16.30a). In most cases, the screws converge towards the midline (Fig. 16.30b) and aim towards the anterior corner of the promontorium (Fig. 16.30c).

An alternative possibility is to insert the screws more sagittally or parallel to the surface of the sacroiliac joint. The entry point shifts slightly medially as the screw direction diverges. Screws inserted parallel to the sacroiliac joint aim towards the anterior superior angle of the lateral mass of the sacrum.

When positioning screws in the sacrum so as to achieve optimal purchase, it is necessary to note the density of the bone – the subchondral bone is the strongest, whereas the lateral mass of the sacrum is often very osteoporotic, sometimes even hollow.

Radiographic Control of Screw Position

In any case, AP and lateral preoperative X-rays are indispensable. If there is any suggestion of anatomic variations, then CT scans are essential. They give information about pedicle diameter and direction. Intra-operatively, the use of image intensification is indispensable, too. It confirms the location and direction of the screws. In very difficult cases, intra-operative myelography with image intensification helps to identify the medial border in relationship to the nerve root.

Direct Visualization of the Pedicle

At the lumbar spine, the inferior and inferior lateral aspect of the pedicle can be exposed by dissecting subperiosteally from the base of the transverse process anteriorly. The soft tissues together with the spinal nerve and blood vessels are carefully retracted with a curved dissector. A small curved dissector is used to probe the lateral wall of the pedicle. If necessary, the inferior part of the medial wall may also be probed.

In addition, osteotomy of the base of the transverse process can help to identify the pedicle. Alternatively, the spinal canal can be opened and the medial wall of the pedicle identified. The latter two techniques are usually not necessary in routine procedures.

At the sacral level, it is very helpful to expose the S1 nerve root, which allows visualization of the lateral wall of the S1 canal.

Preparation of the Screw Canal

After identification of the entry point and the direction of the pedicle, the posterior cortex is perforated for approximately 5 mm using a 3.5-mm drill, preferably with the oscillating attachment. Continued drilling of the pedicle can be dangerous. A safer technique is to prepare the canal with either a thin awl or a small curette. This preparation is performed to the junction between the pedicle and vertebral body. The circumference of the canal is checked with the hook of the depth gauge to ensure that perforation has not occurred, particularly medially. Image intensification with the gauge or a Kirschner wire in place confirms the proper position. The depth gauge may be inserted into the cancellous bone of the vertebral body to about 80% of the AP body diameter. This length is then measured. Only the first few millimeters of the screw canal are tapped.

Notched Plates (Figs. 16.31, 16.32)

Principle

The plate functions as a splint when the vertebral body is not able to support axial load. If the anterior column is intact the plate functions as a posterior tension band.

Indications

- Fracture dislocations from T6 to S1.
- Supplementary stabilization to anterior interbody fusions.

Advantage

- Relatively easy to use.

Disadvantages

- A minimum of five vertebrae are bridged.
- In most cases, reduction of the fracture needs to be undertaken before application of the plate.

Surgical Technique

The fracture may be reduced with the aid of an image intensifier prior to surgery on the operating table.

Through a midline incision, the spinous processes, laminae, facet joints and transverse processes are exposed. If reduction of the spinal fracture has not been fully achieved, further manipulation to apply distraction can be undertaken using the Harrington outrigger inserted one level above and below the intended plated levels. A plate of appropriate length is placed over the posterior aspect of the spine and transverse processes and, if necessary, a bed is made to allow the plate to lie snugly on the bone. Initially the upper and lower screw canals are prepared. The pedicles are entered in the usual manner and Kirschner wires are inserted into each hole (Fig. 16.31 a).

The two plates are fitted into position over the Kirschner wires (Fig. 16.31 b). The appropriate length 4.5-mm cortex screws are inserted. The screws are tightened alternatively, allowing the spine to adapt to the plate.

Where possible, the remaining holes in the plates are then prepared and the screws inserted. A cancellous bone graft is placed over the decorticated laminae and transverse processes (Fig. 16.31 c).

Figs. 16.31, 16.32 Notched plates for the thoracolumbar spine.

Fig. 16.31 Surgical technique.

a The upper and lower screw canals are prepared, the pedicles are entered in the usual manner and Kirschner wires are inserted into each hole.

b The two plates are fitted into position over the Kirschner wires.

c A cancellous bone graft is placed over the decorticated lamina and transverse processes of the injured and the two adjacent vertebrae.

Fig. 16.31

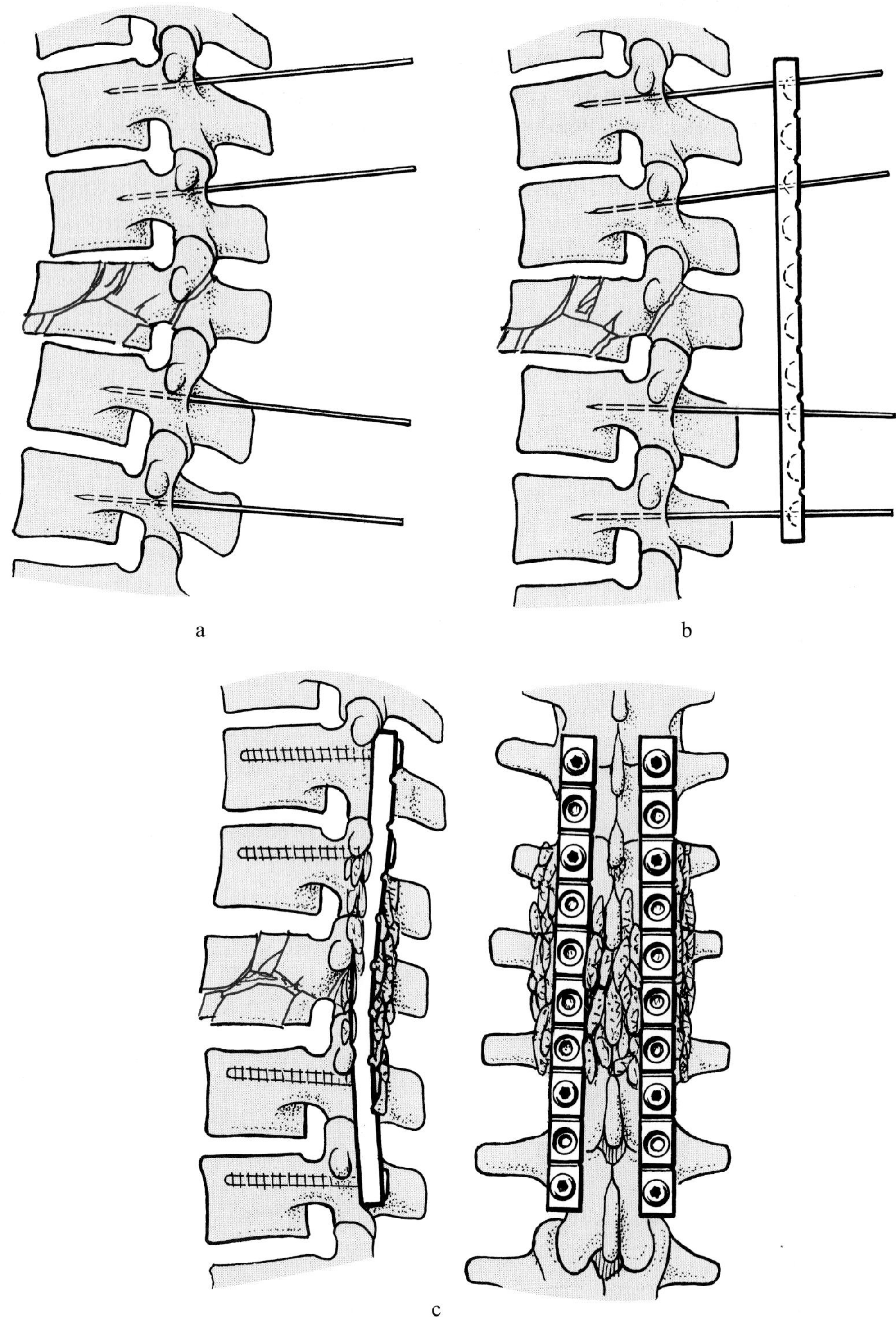

Correction of Kyphosis

If a kyphosis is present, the plates may be used for correction. They are not fully bent to match the deformity of the spine but are contoured to attain a normal curve.

Both plates are screwed to the two vertebrae below the fracture. The prominent upper portions of the plates are then manually approximated to the spine and the remaining screws inserted (Fig. 16.32a).

An alternative method of reduction is to contour the plate into the normal curve and then prepare the screw holes. Each screw is loosely inserted; then alternate ones are tightened from the apex of the deformity outwards so that the fracture is slowly reduced (Fig. 16.32b).

Postoperative Care

Early mobilization is allowed without external support.

The External Spinal Fixation System

The external spinal fixator system according to Magerl (1984) represents a fundamental step in spinal surgery in that it combines pedicle screw fixation with the advantages of a rod system, thus allowing the manipulation of the fixed spine area in all directions without introducing an additional instrument.

The external fixator is being increasingly used in the diagnostic work-up of chronic low back pain or multi-operated backs, where it acts as a temporary test fixation. In addition, the external fixator may be indicated in open fractures and spinal infections. In modern daily trauma surgery, however, the internal fixator system is now used more frequently, as the external spinal fixator is too inconvenient for the patient. Since the external fixator is no longer indicated in the standard treatment of spinal fractures, the technique for its application is not included in this chapter. Interested readers should refer to the relevant literature (Dick 1987; Magerl 1984).

Fig. 16.32 Correction of kyphosis.

a The prominent upper portions of the plates are manually approximated to the spine using a pusher and the remaining screws inserted.

b Each screw is loosely inserted, then alternate ones are tightened from the apex of the deformity outwards, so that the fracture is slowly reduced.

Fig. 16.32

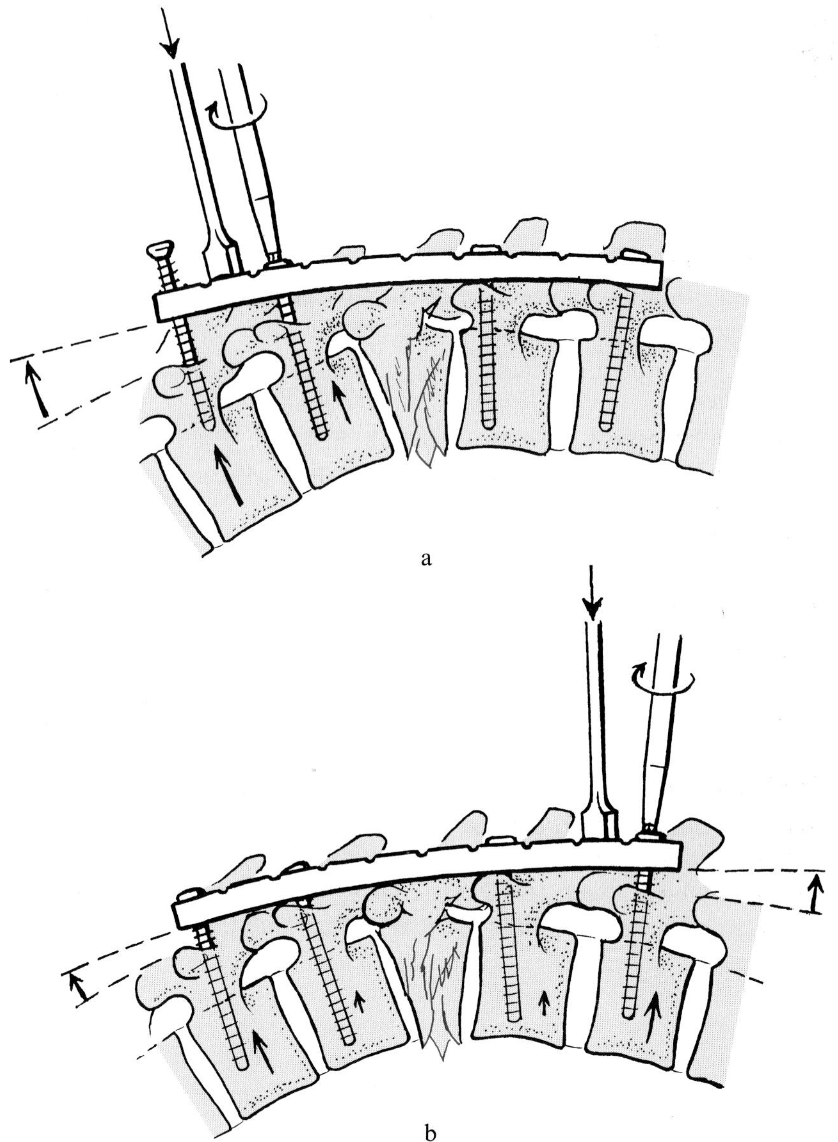

The Internal Spinal Fixation System (Figs. 16.33–16.41)

Principles

The internal fixator is a device which allows both stabilization and reduction without additional instrumentation. Long Schanz screws are inserted in the pedicles of the vertebral bodies and are connected to a threaded longitudinal rod by fully adjustable clamps. The implant acts as a tension band as well as a buttress system; it allows distraction as well as compression or fixation in a neutral position, each with or without kyphosis or lordosis prestress.

Indications

- Lower thoracic and lumbar spine fractures.
- Stabilization and correction of spinal segments in nontraumatic disorders of the spine (degenerative disease, tumors, deformities, infections, etc.).

Advantages

- A simple versatile system.
- Its use is independent of the fracture type.
- Short segment fixation.
- Schanz screws allow easy reduction.

Disadvantages

- It appears somewhat bulky.
- It should not be used in the upper thoracic spine (above T6) because the pedicles are too small.

Surgical Technique

Posterior midline approach. Subperiosteal dissection of the laminae laterally to the intervertebral joints. The entry points for the Schanz screws are determined carefully, as described above (Sect. 16.4.2). It is wise to use the bone nibbler to create a small flat area around the entry points in order to facilitate the further steps.

Figs. 16.33–16.41 Internal spinal fixation system.

Fig. 16.33 Surgical technique.

a Kirschner wires 2 mm in diameter are inserted into the pedicles to a depth of 3 cm.

b The first Kirschner wire is removed and a drill hole made with a 3.5-mm drill to a depth of 2 cm.

c The self-cutting Schanz screw is inserted by hand with the universal chuck to a depth of 4 cm (sacrum only 3 cm).

Fig. 16.34 Application of the threaded rods. The threaded rods of the internal fixator with loose clamps and clamp elements are applied, the rods lying medially to the screws. The flat sides of the rods are placed sagittally to facilitate the final crimping of the nut collars.

a Lateral view.

b Posterior view.

Fig. 16.33

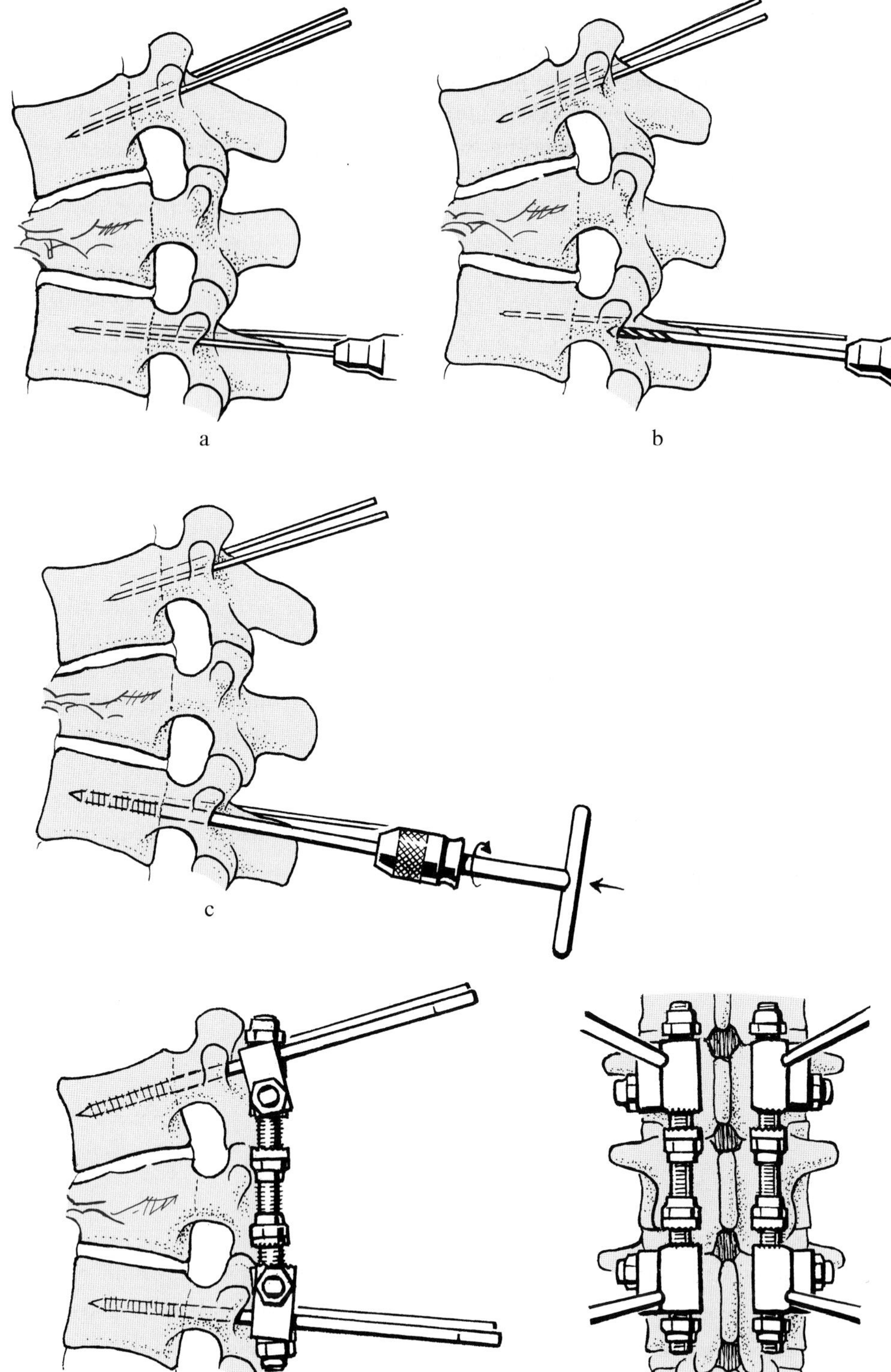

Fig. 16.34

Next, 2-mm Kirschner wires are inserted into the pedicles to a depth of 3 cm (Fig. 16.33a). Positioning of the Kirschner wires is checked using the image intensifier. In the lateral projection the level and the direction of the wires in relation to the endplate are determined. In the AP projection, the tips of the Kirschner wires should converge but not cross. The image intensifier in the anterior/posterior direction is repositioned for each Kirschner wire exactly parallel to the axis of the wire: thus the wire will be seen as a point, and its position in relation to the oval of the pedicle can be determined unequivocally.

When the Kirschner wires are correctly sited, they are replaced by the Schanz screws. The first Kirschner wire is removed and a drill hole made with a 3.5-mm drill to a depth of 2 cm (Fig. 16.33b). A depth gauge is used as a probe to ensure that the hole is surrounded by bone and penetration has not occurred. The self-cutting Schanz screw is easily inserted by hand with the universal chuck to a depth of 4 cm, except in of the sacrum, where more than 3 cm is unsafe (Fig. 16.33c). Lateral fluoroscopic control ensures that the anterior vertebral cortex is not perforated.

When all four Schanz screws are in place, the threaded rods of the internal fixator with loose clamps and clamp elements are applied, the rods lying medially to the screws (Fig. 16.34a, b). The flat sides of the rods are placed sagittally to enhance flexion stability and to facilitate the final crimping of the nut collars. The reduction technique depends on the type of fracture.

1. *Anterior vertebral body fracture with intact posterior wall*: The dorsal ends of the Schanz screws are manually approximated until the desired correction of the kyphosis has been attained. The clamp elements are allowed to slide freely towards each other during the maneuver by placing the distraction nuts away from the clamp elements (Fig. 16.35a). The center of rotation then lies at the posterior edge of the vertebral body. The appropriate nuts are tightened to fix the angle between the Schanz screws and the rods (Fig. 16.35b, c). The clamps are now distracted by adjusting the nuts on the rods. This distraction force relieves the pressure from the intervertebral disc (Fig. 16.35d) and completes the vertebral body reduction.

Fig. 16.35 Reduction technique for an anterior vertebral body fracture with intact posterior wall.

a The dorsal ends of the Schanz screws are manually approximated until the desired correction of the kyphosis has been attained. The clamp elements slide freely towards each other.

b The internal fixator with the laterally tightened nuts.

c The fixator with the new posteriorly tightened nuts.

d The clamps are now distracted by adjusting the nuts on the rods. The distraction completes the vertebral body reduction.

Fig. 16.35

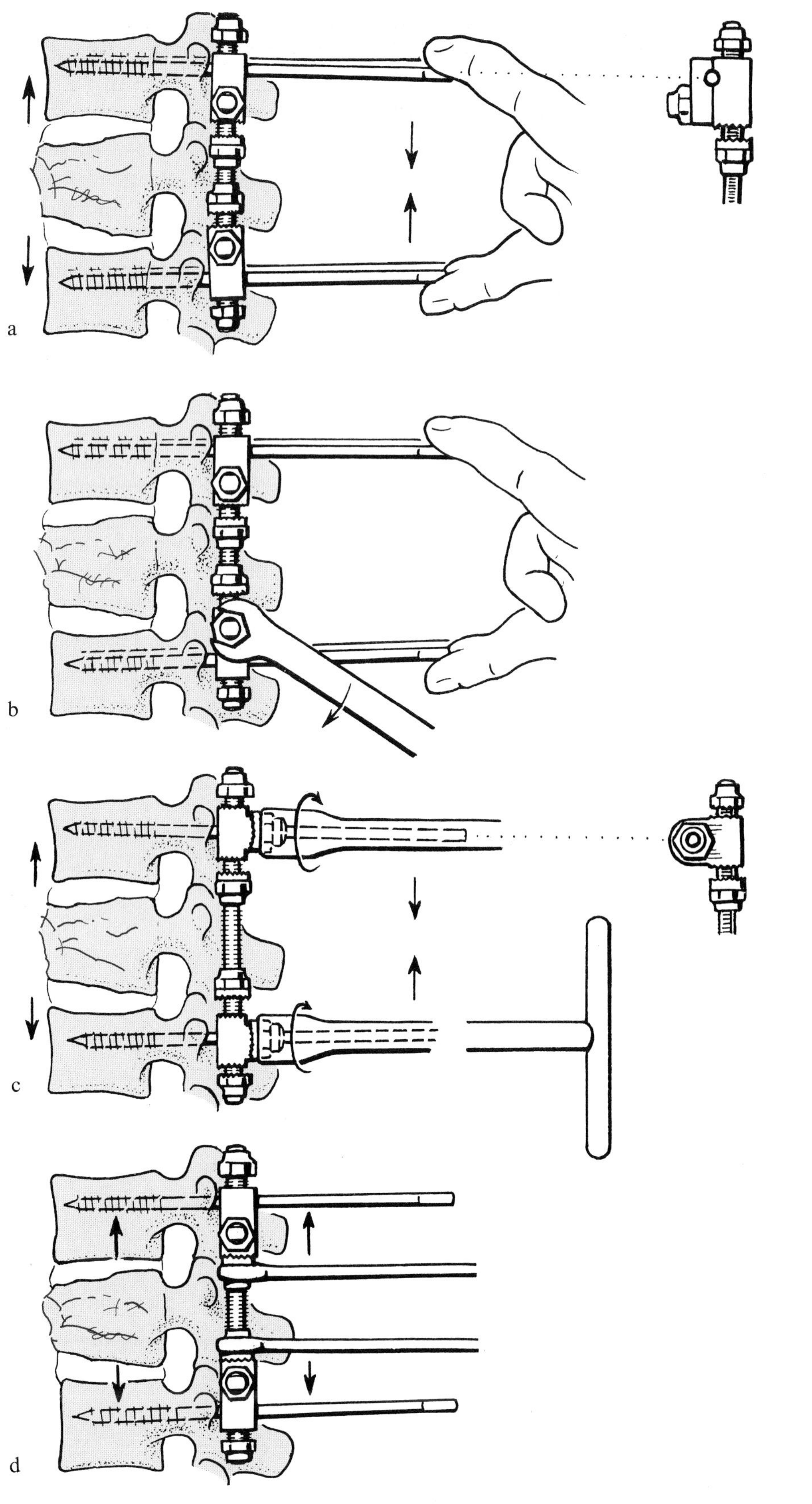

2. *Fracture types with fractured posterior wall*: In this form of fracture, there is a theoretical danger that posterior wall fragments might displace posteriorly into the canal during correction of the kyphosis when pressing together the ends of the Schanz screws. The posterior wall must be protected against compression. This can be achieved using the distraction nuts: prior to the reduction, a distance of 5 mm between the distraction nuts and the clamp elements for every 10° of attempted kyphosis correction (Fig. 16.36). When approximating the ends of the Schanz screws, the clamp elements will soon touch the distraction nuts and the center of rotation is transferred posteriorly to the level of the rods. The force now required to correct the kyphosis is much greater. Nuts are tightened to secure the correction. Distraction is now exerted to restore the original height of the vertebra.

3. *Posterior element fractures or disruption with distraction*: The implant acts as a pure tension band. Therefore, after reduction in the above-described manner with the clamp elements sliding freely, no distraction is carried out but slight compression is applied with the counternuts (Fig. 16.37).

4. *Complete disruption of the anterior and posterior elements with rotation*: The internal fixator acts as a neutralization device. The technique is similar to that described for type 3 above. All nuts and counternuts are firmly tightened and secured against spontaneous loosening by crimping the collar of the nuts into the flattening of the threads (Fig. 16.38a, b). The protruding ends of the Schanz screws are cut off as near as possible to the clamp elements, using the special bolt cutter (Fig. 16.39a, b).

Fig. 16.36 Fracture type with fractured posterior wall. The posterior wall must be protected against compression. This can be achieved using the distraction nuts: prior to the reduction, 5 mm is left between the distraction nuts and the clamp elements for every 10° of attempted correction of kyphosis.

Fig. 16.37 Slight compression is applied with the counternuts.

Fig. 16.38 Tightening the nuts.

a All nuts and counternuts are firmly tightened and secured against spontaneous loosening by crimping the collar of the nuts into the flattening of the threads.

b Detail view.

Fig. 16.39 Cutting the Schanz screws.

a The protruding ends of the Schanz screws are cut off as near as possible to the clamp elements, using the special bolt cutter.

b Detail view.

Fig. 16.36

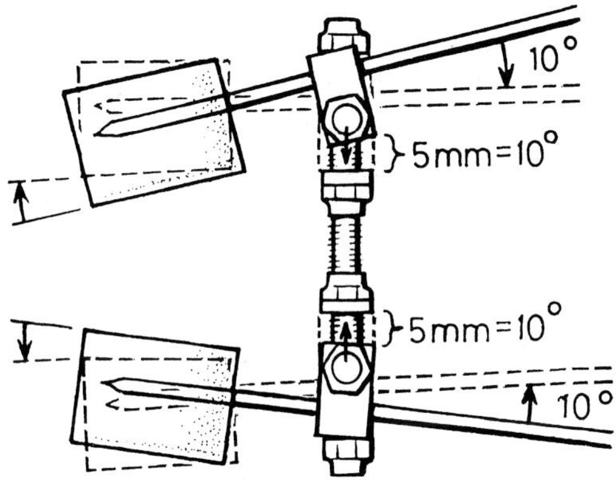

Fig. 16.37

Fig. 16.38

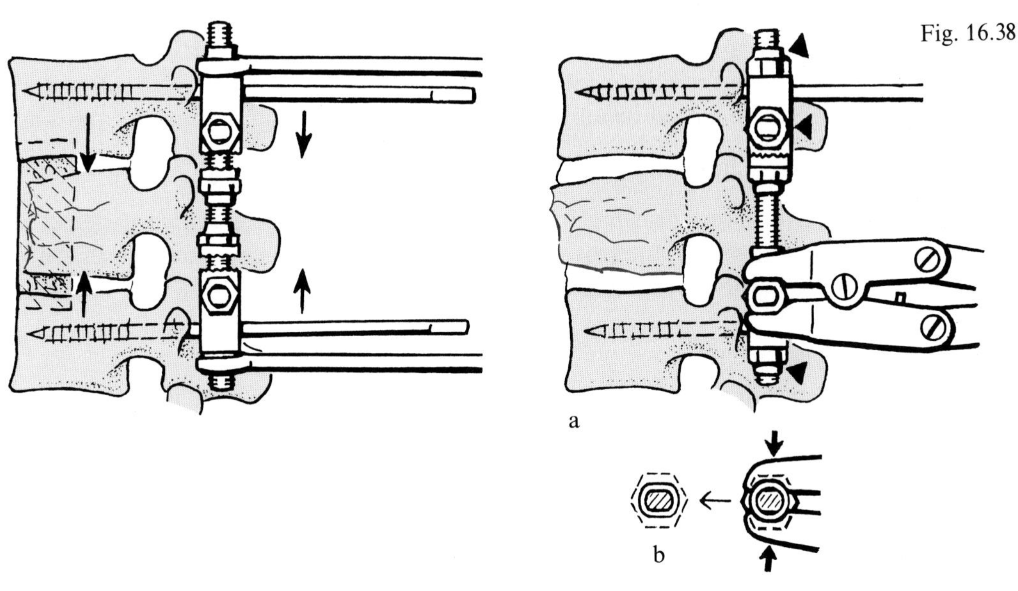

Fig. 16.39

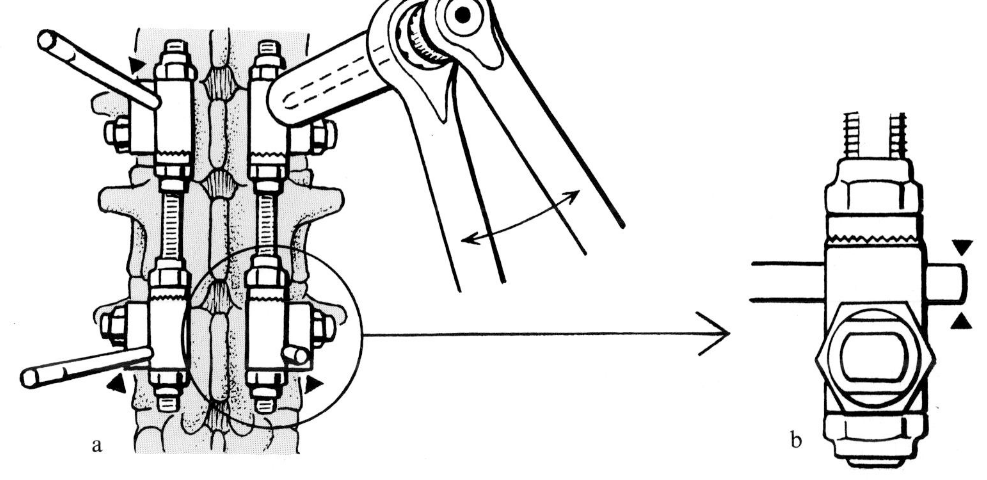

Additional Measures

1. In the majority of cases, reduction results in a large defect of bone stock in the vertebral body. It is an integral part of the fixator instrumentation to fill the anterior defects with autologous bone grafts. This is possible using the same posterior approach by the transpedicular bone grafting procedure described by Daniaux (1986): a channel of 6 mm diameter (Fig. 16.40a, b) is made into the pedicle of the fractured vertebra, the drill being directed slightly cranially towards the defect. As the entry point lies in line with the already inserted Schanz screws, it is situated lateral to the longitudinal rod and can be reached without impairment. The special funnel is then inserted into the drill hole (Fig. 16.40c) until the stop touches the bone: the tip then automatically reaches into the center of the vertebral body and protects the vertebral canal from unintended intrusion of bone graft particles through a fracture gap in the pedicle. Thus the transplanted bone is pushed anteriorly into the defect zone.

2. If the bony elements do not provide enough stability against lateral shear or rotation, a cross-linking device is added to the rods (Fig. 16.41).

3. If the patency of the spinal canal has not been restored and posterior wall fragments continue to protrude, hemilaminectomy and resection of one pedicle of the fractured vertebra is performed to reduce by impaction, or to extract, the posterior wall fragments: an alternative would be anterior decompression through a second approach.

4. Posterolateral fusion is indispensable.

5. Anterior bone grafting is necessary in the case of significant defect with mechanical impairment of the anterior column, since the incidence of fatigue fractures of the Schanz screws will otherwise increase.

Postoperative Care

Early mobilization is allowed, with an open frame type, three-point fixation brace to prevent excessive flexion or extension for 6–12 weeks postoperatively.

Fig. 16.40 Transpedicular cancellous bone grafting.

a The same posterior approach is used to identify the pedicle with a Kirschner wire.

b A channel of 6 mm diameter is made into the pedicle of the fractured vertebra, the drill being directed slightly cranially towards the defect.

c A special funnel is then inserted into the drill hole, and the cancellous bone is stuffed into the fractured vertebral body.

Fig. 16.41 Cross-linking device. If the bony elements do not provide enough stability against lateral shear or rotation, a cross-linking device is added to the rods.

Fig. 16.40

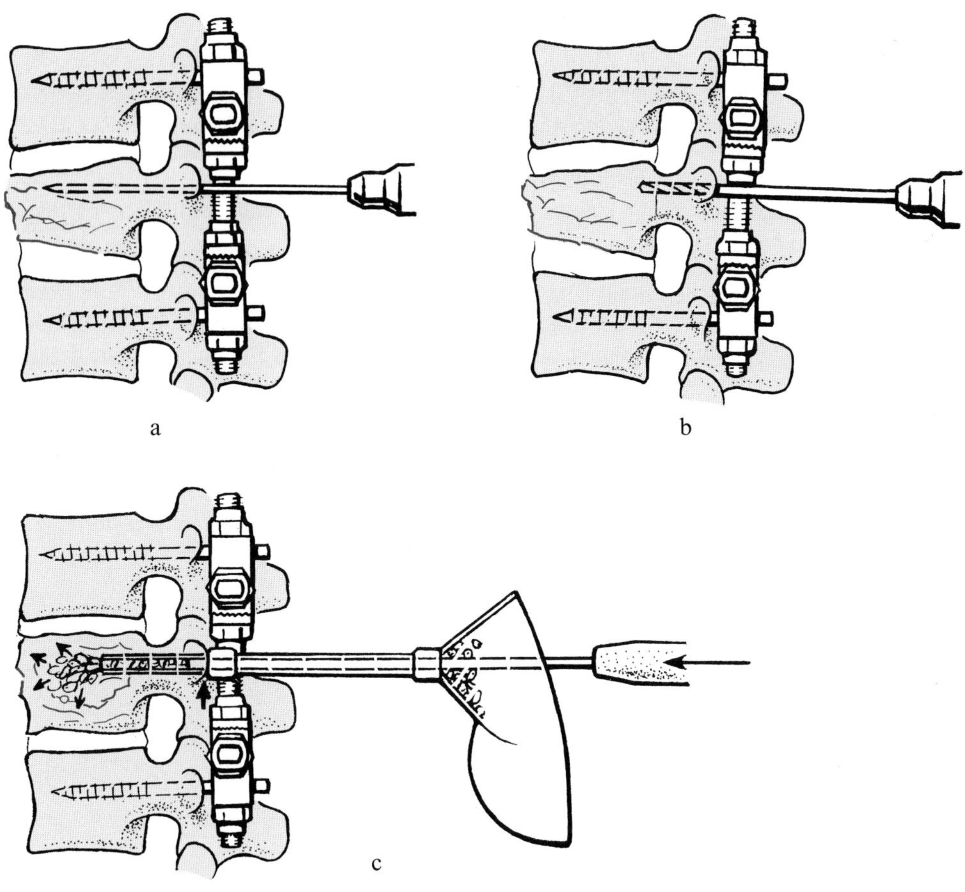

Fig. 16.41

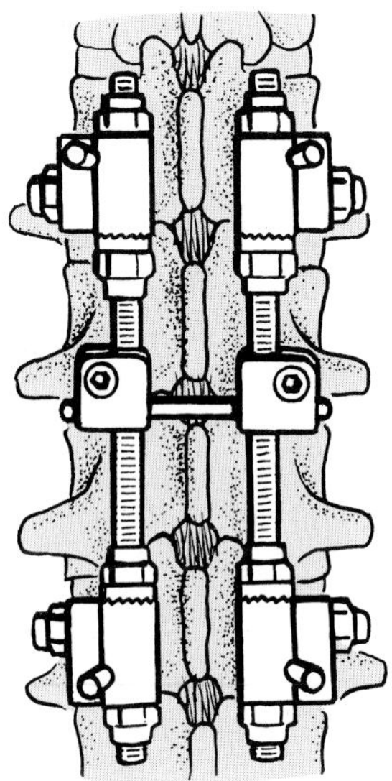

References

Aebi M, Mohler J, Zäch GA, Morscher E (1986) Indication, surgical technique and results of 100 surgically-treated fractures and fracture-dislocations of the cervical spine. Clin Orthop Rel Res 203:244–257

Aebi M, Etter C, Kehl T, Thalgott J (1987) The internal skeletal fixation system: a new treatment for thoracolumbar fractures and other spinal disorders. Clin Orthop Rel Res 227:30–43

Aebi M, Etter C, Coscia M (1989) Fractures of the odontoid process: treatment with anterior screw fixation. Spine 14:1065–1070

Böhler J (1982) Anterior stabilization for acute fractures and non-unions of the dens. J Bone Joint Surg [Am] 64:18–27

Daniaux H (1986) Transpedikuläre Reposition and Spongiosaplastik bei Wirbelkörperbrüchen der unteren Brust- und Lendenwirbelsäule. Unfallchirurg 89:197–213

Dick W (1987) The "fixateur interne" – a versatile implant for spine surgery. Spine 12:882–900

Dick W (1989) Internal fixation of thoracic and lumbar spine fractures. Huber, Bern

Grob D, Magerl F (1987) Operative Stabilisierung bei Frakturen von C1 und C2. Orthopäde 16:46–54

Magerl F (1984) Stabilization of the lower thoracic and lumbar spine with external skeletal fixation. Clin Orthop Rel Res 189:125–141

Magerl F (1985) The spine fixator. In: Weber BG, Magerl F (eds) The external fixator. AO/ASIF threaded rod system, spine fixator. Springer, Berlin Heidelberg New York

Morscher E, Sutter F, Jenny H, Olerud S (1986) Die vordere Verplattung der Halswirbelsäule mit dem Hohlschrauben-Plattensystem aus Titanium. Chirurg 57:702–707

17 COMPOUND FRACTURES

17.1 General Remarks

The management of an open fracture is a surgical emergency. Open fractures are often associated with additional injuries. The primary care and the priorities for the multiple trauma patient are considered elsewhere.

In any open injury, the aim is uncomplicated healing of the soft tissues and fracture to allow a return to normal function. In order to achieve this goal, the treatment must ensure that all remaining soft parts are well vascularized and free from contamination. The principles involved in achieving this aim are:

- Excision and removal of all dead tissue (to be repeated if necessary).
- The stabilization of the fracture by either an internal or, in the case of a more severe soft tissue injury, an external fixator or an unreamed nail.

Stable fixation allows more rapid restoration of the microcirculation of the soft tissues, which helps the bone to defend itself against infection.

17.2 Grading of Open Fractures

The grading system and the symbols used are explained in Chap. 1 together with the AO classification of fractures.

Open fractures are graded according to the degree of destruction of both the soft tissues and the bone. In fact, grading in these cases should not be restricted to the fracture but should be extended to include the three major constituents of the soft tissue cover: the integuments (I) [IC = closed fracture; IO = open fracture]; the muscles and tendons (MT); and the neurovascular system (NV).

17.2.1 First-Degree Open Fractures IO 1 (MT 1–4, NV 1–4)

In first-degree open fractures, the skin has been pierced from within by bone fragments. It must be stressed that the "first degree" is only applied when the surgeon is certain that the skin injury is from within. This may present as a small skin wound concealing associated major deep soft tissue injury, in particular damage to underlying muscle and neurovascular structures: IO 1 (MT 3–5, NV 3–4).

17.2.2 Second-Degree Open Fractures IO 2 (MT 1–5, NV 1–4)

In second-degree open fractures, the skin has been broken and crushed externally causing moderate damage to the skin, subcutaneous tissue and muscle. The severity of the fracture is variable.

17.2.3 Third-Degree Open Fractures IO 3 (MT 2–5, NV 2–5)

Third-degree open fractures are usually the result of high energy injuries with extensive damage to the skin, subcutaneous tissues, muscles and neurovascular structures. They are often associated with injuries to the nerves and vessels and are usually heavily infected. High-velocity gunshot wounds are included in this category. Amputation or near-amputation would be classified as IO 3 (MT 4, NV 5).

Use of these definitions will enable the surgeon to decide on the appropriate surgical procedure.

17.3 Management

First-degree injuries can be treated as closed fractures. With a second-degree injury, the initial treatment will differ from that of closed fractures but the postoperative care remains the same. Third-degree injuries are usually managed with external fixation or with unreamed nailing. As the standard methods of internal fixation are not appropriate, postoperative care will differ significantly.

17.3.1 Prevention of Further Contamination

Open fractures should always be considered as being contaminated with pathogenic organisms. Additional contamination with hospital bacteria between admission and operation must be prevented by strict asepsis. Therefore, a sterile field dressing should not be removed. Uncovered wounds should be treated immediately with an antibacterial solution and covered with a sterile dressing. Any further inspection of the wound must take place in an aseptic area (for example, in the operating room), with the surgeon wearing a sterile gown, mask and gloves. Photographs (e.g. Polaroids) of the wound required for planning and documentation purposes should be taken as early as possible. Gentle manipulation may be required to realign the limb, which is then placed in a radiotranslucent splint. The neurovascular status of the limb is regularly assessed. Radiographs of the fracture as well as of the joints above and below the fracture are then taken.

17.3.2 Excision of Dead Material and Devitalized Material

The wound must be cleared of any foreign material and all necrotic tissue. If excessive hemorrhage occurs, a tourniquet may be applied: this will allow a more detailed inspection but will also reduce the oxygen supply to the tissues. If the excision of dead tissue is carried out stepwise, a complete change of sterile equipment between the first and final stages is recommended. Copious irrigation of the wound with Ringer solution with or without antibiotics is mandatory.

17.3.2.1 Skin

Dead skin must be excised. If, for example in the lower leg, there is any doubt about the extent of the skin damage, it is advisable to initially excise as little skin as possible, knowing that the excision may have to be repeated within 48 h. The wound may be enlarged, if required, to inspect deeper tissues. Planning of this incision must take into consideration the method of bone stabilization and should not prejudice any later reconstructive plastic procedures. Fat should be removed from avascular skin in order to improve its potential for revascularization. In degloving injuries, skin should be defatted and applied as a free, full- or partial-thickness graft on well-vascularized wound ground – preferably muscle.

17.3.2.2 Fascia

The local fascia is incised to relieve or prevent increased pressure within the different compartments and to facilitate inspection of the muscle. Neighboring compartments to the fracture may be at risk and their decompression should also be considered.

17.3.2.3 Muscle

Dead muscle is a good culture medium and must be removed. The recognition of nonviable muscle can be difficult: it appears pale, lacks contractility and does not bleed when cut. Muscle of doubtful viability which is initially left, must be reassessed within the next few days.

Divided or ruptured tendons are not excised but rather are approximated with resorbable sutures.

17.3.2.4 Blood Vessels

Adequate blood supply to the limb must be preserved or restored as quickly as possible (6 h limit). While major veins should be repaired, small arteries and veins may usually be ligated. As it appears desirable to stabilize the bone before the vascular repair, it may be helpful to apply temporary vascular shunts. Next comes the rapid fixation of the bone, after which the definitive repair of the vessels may be performed. In the multiply injured patient with coagulation disorders, amputation is most often safer and quicker than difficult vascular repairs. In these cases, survival is more important than limb salvage.

17.3.2.5 Nerves

Divided nerves that can be identified should be approximated with one or two nonresorbable perineural sutures which can then be found for a later definitive reconstruction.

In a heavily contaminated wound, groping in the depths to find a nerve is not recommended as any formal nerve repair is preferably delayed.

17.3.2.6 Bone

Cortical bone devoid of soft tissue attachments should be removed unless:

1. It forms an integral part of an articular surface.
2. It comprises a major fragment needed for skeletal stability or preservation of limb. If the wound becomes infected, this fragment must be removed.

17.3.3 Stabilization of the Fracture

Stabilization of the fracture is essential to reduce dead space around the bone and to prevent any new soft tissue injury caused by moving fragments. Clinical and experimental work suggests that this will also reduce the likelihood of infection. Depending upon the severity of the soft tissue damage and the fracture pattern, different fixation techniques will be applied. It is essential, in bone stabilization, to avoid any additional damage to the already impaired blood supply by further dissection.

17.3.3.1 Moderate Soft Tissue Injuries

All first-degree and some selected second-degree open fractures may be treated using standard internal fixation techniques (screws, plates and the intramedullary nail).

The intramedullary nail, locked or unlocked, can be used for first-degree open fractures of the femur and the tibia, as well as for some second-degree injuries of the femur. For more severe injuries, especially in the tibia, the nail is not advocated. There is a certain tendency to apply unreamed nails. Even without reaming, however, the medullary blood supply will be damaged. Despite this, the short-term results of unreamed nailing look promising, and if the long-term results are also favorable this technique may offer a good alternative to external fixation. The surgical approach depends upon the size and location of the soft tissue wound; an enlargement of the original laceration or a separate incision may be necessary.

Internal fixation using screws and plates should be undertaken only if the following conditions apply:

- The plate can easily be covered with viable soft tissue.
- The plate may be applied in a biomechanically satisfactory position so that stable fixation can be achieved.
- Only minimal soft tissue dissection without stripping of bone fragments is required to apply the plate.
- Indirect reduction techniques are applied whenever possible without the use of retractors and bone forceps that encircle the bone.

17.3.3.2 Severe Soft Tissue Injuries

In the presence of severe soft tissue injuries, especially third-degree open fractures, stabilization should be carried out using external fixation (see Chap. 5). This provides the adequate stabilization of the fracture and the soft tissue lesion that is so essential in the initial management of severe injuries. In severely open articular fractures, lag screws may secure the anatomic alignment of the joint fragments and the external fixator – with or without bridging of the joint – prevents too much movement so that the soft tissues can heal. Very extensive lesions of the soft tissues, near- and complete amputation are often referred to as "fourth-degree open fractures." They are more precisely described by using – as appropriate – IO4 (MT4, NV5). The external fixator, if applied across a joint, should be removed as soon as the tissues have healed, usually in 2–3 weeks. Thereafter, further procedures may be considered. With regard to unreamed nailing, the remarks in Sect. 17.3.3.1 apply here as well.

17.3.3.3 Wound Closure

As a rule, open wounds are not to be closed, but cartilage as well as metal implants should be covered. To prevent drying out, the wound should be covered with sterile, paraffin-impregnated gauze or synthetic skin. Within days – when swelling has regressed – a secondary skin suture may be possible. Any tension must be avoided.

In degloving injuries and wounds with large flaps, healthy looking skin can be defatted and placed back as free split skin grafts. Large soft tissue losses, for example in the proximal tibia, may be covered by a gastrocnemius flap. Any more demanding procedures, such as rotational flaps or microvascular free flaps, should not be performed as emergencies.

17.3.3.4 Antibiotics

Antibiotics are compulsory for all open fractures. They are administered immediately upon admission. The selection of the drug and the duration of its use are controversial. The administration of antibiotics must not, however, preclude excising all devitalized tissue and stable fixation of bone.

The most frequent causes of infection in patients with open fractures are the following:

- Primary closure of wounds under tension.
- Incomplete and not repeated excision of poorly vascularized tissue.
- Inadequate hemostasis and insufficient wound drainage.
- Rough soft tissue handling during surgery.
- Failure to recognize a compartment syndrome.
- Wrong implant or poorly vascularized soft tissue cover.

17.3.3.5 Postoperative Treatment

The microcirculation of the soft tissues may be compromised by edema; elevation of the affected limb above the heart level is recommended except after an arterial repair or when a compartment syndrome is suspected. In the latter, pressure studies should be performed and passive motion as well as the neurovascular status must be observed closely.

Wounds left open must be kept moist by frequent or continuous irrigation with Ringer solution, fatty gauze dressings or artificial skin.

Gentle mobilization of the joints should begin as early as possible in the postoperative period. In articular fractures, continuous passive motion (CPM) appears advantageous.

Repeated inspection of the wound under operating room conditions is necessary at short intervals (24–48 h) until the surgeon is convinced that no avascular tissue remains.

At this stage, closure of the wound is permissible, providing it does not involve skin tension; larger defects may only require a muscle flap or a split skin graft. Where tendons, nerves, blood vessels or large bone areas are exposed, artificial skin can be used as a temporary dressing. As soon as possible (within 10 days) the definitive cover with either a soft tissue rotational flap or a microvascular free flap should be performed.

17.3.3.6 Subsequent Fracture Treatment

Once the soft tissues have healed, further thought may be given to the fracture per se. This particularly applies to those cases where the initial choice of fixation, for example external fixation, was a compromise because of the soft tissue injuries.

High-energy injuries and fractures with significant bony defects may require further cancellous bone graft. Fragment transport according to the Ilizarov technique may have to be considered (see Chap. 5).

The healing pattern of an open fracture rigidly stabilized with an external fixator may be slow. To accelerate healing, several possibilities are proposed: bone grafting, application of a brace, dynamization or destabilization and changing to another mode of external fixation or to internal fixation.

17.4 Conclusion

Four basic principles should be remembered in the management of open fractures:

- Excision of all nonviable tissue.
- Preservation of the blood supply to the bone and soft tissue.
- Stable fixation.
- Early active pain-free mobilization of muscles and joints.

References

Gustilo RB, Mendoza RM, Williams DN (1984) Problems in the management of type III (severe) open fractures; a new classification of type III open fractures. J Trauma 24:742–746

Matter P, Rittmann WW (1978) The open fracture. Huber, Bern

Patzakis MJ (1982) Management of open fractures. American Academy of Orthopaedic Surgeons, pp 62–64 (Instructional course lectures, vol 3)

Tscherne H, Gotzen L (1984) Fractures with soft tissue injuries. Springer, Berlin Heidelberg New York

18 FRACTURES IN CHILDREN

18.1 General Principles

The treatment of fractures in children is fundamentally different from that in adults, since only a few fractures require operative intervention (Fig. 18.1).

18.2 Diaphyseal Fractures

Closed treatment of diaphyseal fractures in children does not generally lead to dystrophy, joint stiffness or pseudarthrosis. These fractures heal rapidly, so the time available to achieve an acceptable reduction is much shorter than in the adult. Malunion can often result, but in many cases malunion can remodel itself by differential periosteal activity (shaft straightening) and asymmetric growth plate activity (axial realignment). The factors involved in initiating and controlling these remodelling activities are incompletely understood. In general, angulation in the plane of motion of the nearest joint will remodel itself. Torsional malunion can remodel itself if the fracture has occurred adjacent to a universal joint, especially at the proximal ends of the femur and of the humerus, whereas rotational malalignment of the tibia will not correct itself with growth. A second principle is that the nearer the child is to skeletal maturity, the less capacity (and time available) there is for remodeling. Some angular malunions, if of sufficient magnitude, can produce such asymmetric loading of the adjacent growth plate as to result in differential growth, causing an increase in the deformity.

18.2.1 Indications for Internal Fixation

Operative treatment of fractures in children should strongly be considered in:

1. Polytrauma including ipsilateral fractures.
2. Severe open fractures.
3. Patients with head injuries (or children with spastic cerebral palsy).
4. Femur fractures in adolescents.
5. Certain types of forearm fractures.
6. Certain types of physeal plate fracture (displaced intra-articular fractures).

18.2.2 Methods of Internal Fixation

The aim of internal fixation in children is to obtain an anatomic reduction and maintain that reduction using a minimum amount of metal. External immobilization can be used postoperatively without the risk of fracture disease.

External fixation is preferred in third-degree open fractures.

One-third tubular and 3.5-mm dynamic compression plates (DCPs and LC-DCPs) are used in the forearm, and DCPs or T plates in metaphyseal areas of the femur, tibia and humerus. Frequent use of the AO small fragment sets is mandatory! Closed intramedullary nailing may be used in femur fractures in adolescents. In proximal metaphyseal fractures of the tibia with valgus angulation, release of the pes anserinus from within the fracture gap may be needed to prevent progressive valgus deformity. Early removal of the metal is recommended after fracture healing. Anatomic reduction of shaft fractures has been said to increase the risk of overgrowth but this has never been scientifically substantiated.

18.3 Periarticular and Articular Fractures

18.3.1 General Principles/Classification

Articular and periarticular fractures in children are injuries which involve the physeal plate. The treatment and prognosis for physeal injuries depend on the pattern of the injury, i.e. whether the injury involves only the physeal plate, the physeal plate and the metaphysis, or the physeal plate and the epiphysis. The classification of physeal plate fractures is based on the pathoanatomy (pure separation, separation with a metaphyseal fragment, fracture of epiphysis) and gives guidance on treatment and prognosis (Fig. 18.2).

Type A (Salter-Harris I–II). The fracture line does not involve the germinal zone of the physeal plate. If a proper reduction is carried out, generally no growth disturbance is to be anticipated, but exceptions exist.

Type B (Salter-Harris III–IV). The fracture line crosses the epiphysis and the germinal zone of the physeal plate. An absolutely accurate reduction must be achieved, otherwise partial closure, with resulting eccentric growth disturbance, is to be anticipated. In addition, these injuries involve the articular surface and malunion can produce later joint degeneration.

Fig. 18.1 Relative surgical indications for fractures in children (after Weber). The diameter of each circle depicts the relative incidence of each fracture type and the shaded segment of each circle is proportional to the likelihood of surgical treatment being necessary.

Fig. 18.1

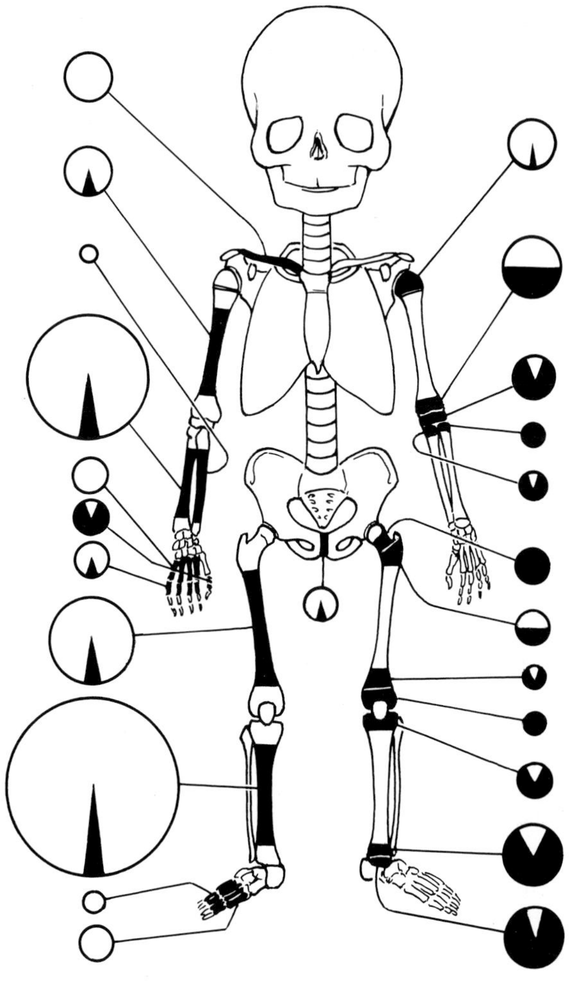

At the distal femur, ligamentous avulsion of an osteochondral block spanning the physis may occur: growth arrest is likely unless perfect reduction is achieved. Open abrasive injury of the periphery of the physis, resulting in destruction of the zone of Ranvier (Rang 1983), usually results in local growth arrest (Fig. 18.2).

Type C (Salter-Harris V). Compression of the physeal plate with impaction of epiphyseal bone into the metaphysis. There is severe damage to the growth area, and partial or complete closure of the epiphyseal plate, with consequent growth disturbance, is to be anticipated.

18.3.2 Indications for Internal Fixation

Displaced type B injuries are almost always treated operatively. These are the fractures that involve both the physeal plate and the articular surface. Usually, the pure physeal plate separations, with or without metaphyseal fragments (type A), are treated nonoperatively. However, multiple closed reduction maneuvers should be avoided, as damage to the germinal layer of the plate can ensue and premature closure of the plate may result. If a type A injury will not fully reduce with gentle reposition, then soft tissue interposition is usually responsible and surgical release is necessary.

Fig. 18.2 Classification of articular and periarticular fractures in children with involvement of the physeal plate; three main groups (M.E. Müller).

A The fracture passes through the junction of the zones of hypertrophy and provisional ossification. The fracture line does not involve the growth zones. Growth disturbance is unlikely (except at the proximal femur and proximal radius), even with incomplete reduction. Deformity in the plane of motion is likely to remodel itself as long as growth continues.

A1 (Salter-Harris type I) This is a pure shearing injury of the physeal plate and usually results from a rotational force.

A2 (Salter-Harris type II) This is partly a shear injury of the physis and partly a metaphyseal fracture (Thurston-Holland fragment). 70% of physeal injuries are type A2.

B The fracture line transverses all layers of the physis. If reduction is not anatomically perfect, growth disturbance is highly likely.

B1 (Salter-Harris type III) Partial physeal separation with an intra-articular epiphyseal fracture. Open reduction with screw fixation is strongly indicated. The screw must not penetrate the physeal plate.

B2 (Salter-Harris type IV) The fracture plane passes from the joint surface through all layers of the physis and through the metaphysis. As in type B1, screw fixation is strongly indicated using one screw in the epiphysis and one in the metaphysis, with neither crossing the growth plate.

B3 (M.E. Müller) An avulsion fracture of an insertion of a collateral ligament, taking with it a portion of the perichondrial ring (zone of Ranvier). Accurate reduction and fixation are required, but growth disturbance can still follow.

B4 (M. Rang) Open abrasive damage to the periphery of the physis, also injuring the zone of Ranvier. Partial closure is the usual sequel.

C (Salter-Harris type V) There is compression of the articular surface and impaction of epiphyseal bone into metaphyseal bone, with consequent disorganisation of part of the physeal cartilage. Partial growth arrest is to be expected and reconstructive procedures, such as those of Langenskiold and Osterman (1983), are necessary later.

C1, C2 Different degrees of impaction.

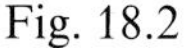
Fig. 18.2

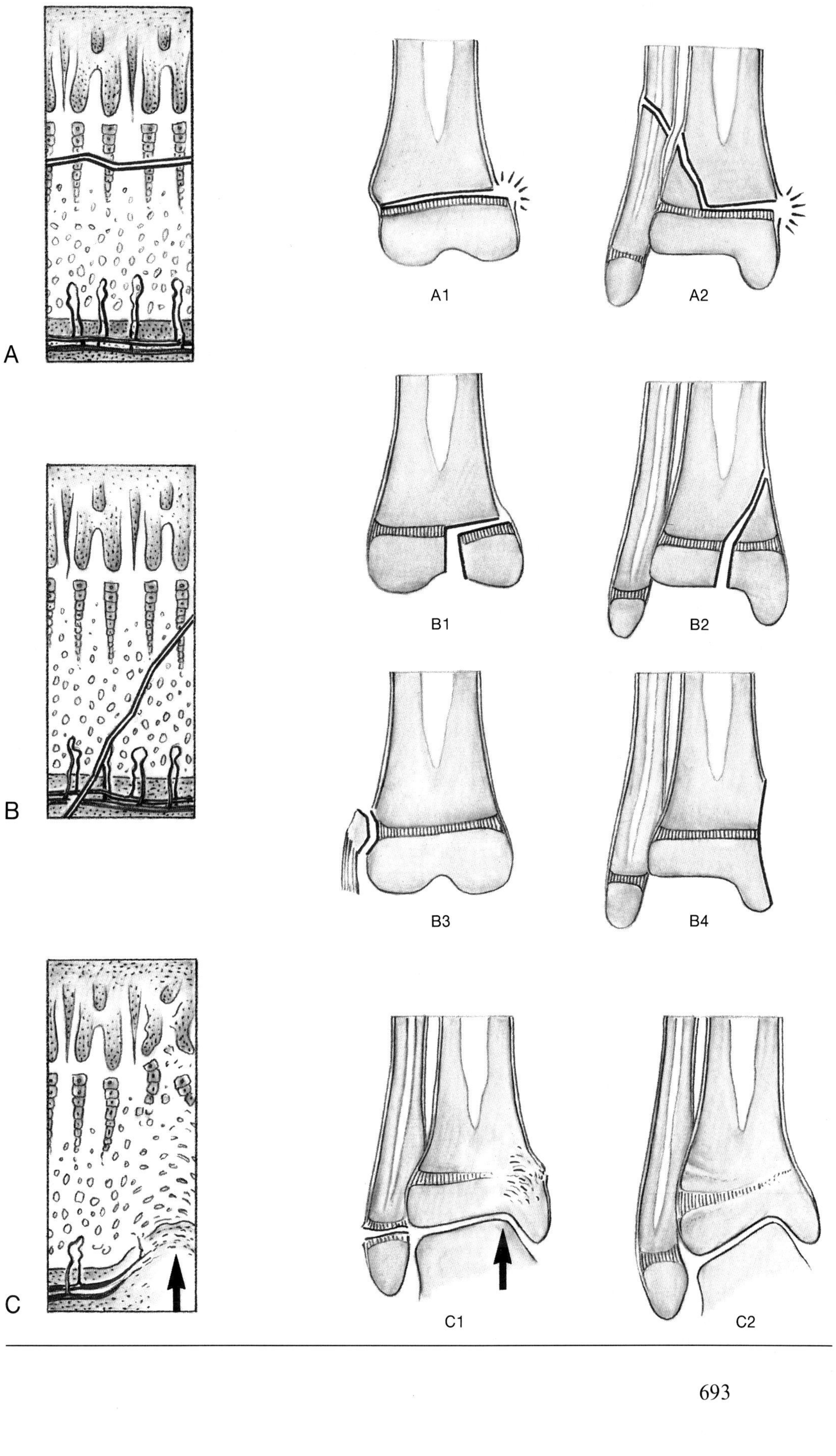

A1 A2

A

B1 B2

B3 B4

B

C1 C2

C

18.3.3 Methods of Internal Fixation

Kirschner wire fixation of epiphyseal and metaphyseal fragments is usually all that is necessary for internal fixation, as the hard cancellous bone in children affords excellent purchase for the wires. Physeal plates can, if necessary, be crossed with Kirschner wires, but never with interfragmentary screws unless growth is nearly complete. Kirschner wires can be used percutaneously to maintain a reduction that cannot be maintained by closed methods. Multiple drilling and insertion of several Kirschner wires at the same point is not recommended. Kirschner wires can be left protruding through the skin and removed at 2–3 weeks as the bone heals rapidly. Alternatively, interfragmentary cortex screws can be used parallel to the physeal plate. This method is recommended in severely displaced epiphyseal fractures (type B) as it produces a so-called waterproof reduction. The disadvantage of screw fixation is the necessity for a second operation to remove the metal. On the other hand, the drawback of using percutaneous wires is the increased risk of infection. When growth disturbance occurs, callus resection and interposition of fat, or cold-curing bone cement, may restore normal growth (Langenskiold and Osterman 1983).

18.4 Fractures of the Humerus

18.4.1 Proximal Humerus and Humeral Shaft

Most fractures of the proximal humerus and of the humeral shaft can be treated nonoperatively in a sling or occasionally in skeletal traction. The immobilization or traction is required usually for 2–3 weeks. Screw traction, rather than via a transolecranon pin, produces fewer complications (infection, early and late ulnar palsy, etc.) (Fig. 18.3). Occasionally, a proximal physeal plate separation has to be operated on because it cannot be reduced (e.g. due to interposition of the tendon of the long head of the biceps) or because a patient is close to skeletal maturity and the deformity is not expected to remodel itself (Fig. 18.4).

Fig. 18.3 Overhead traction via an olecranon screw is useful for proximal and supracondylar humeral fractures (Baumann: Worlock and Colton 1987).

Fig. 18.4 Proximal humeral epiphyseal separation. The usual metaphyseal displacement is into adduction and extension, so that the upper end of the distal fragment may even penetrate the anterior fibers of the deltoid muscle to come to lie subcutaneously. Irreducibility may be due to this muscular entrapment or to interposition of the tendon of the long head of the biceps.
Considerable degrees of displacement will remodel themselves at the proximal humerus, but gross deformity, especially in the older child, should be treated by open reduction and Kirschner wire transfixion.

Fig. 18.3

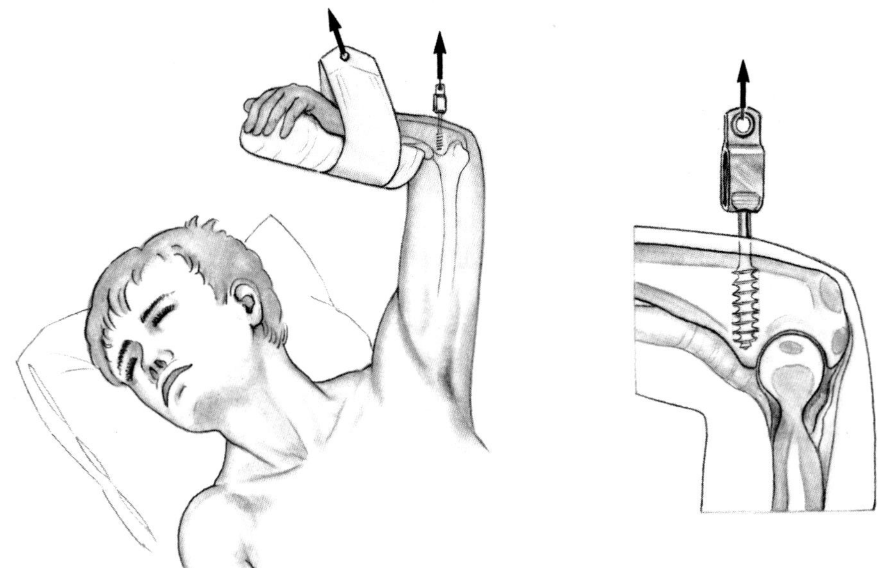

Fig. 18.4

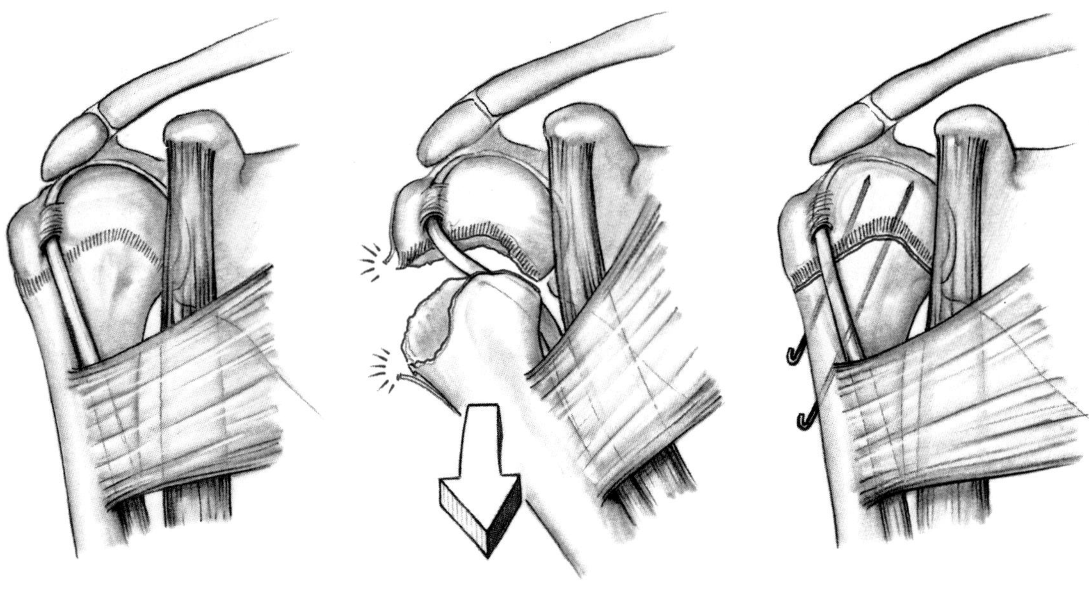

18.4.2 Distal Humerus

In all children's elbow fractures, comparative X-rays of both sides are necessary. Displaced supracondylar fractures of the humerus are almost always treated nonoperatively by reduction under general anesthesia, immobilization in a cast, or reduced and held with screw traction just distal to the olecranon. If stability of the reduced fracture can only be achieved in extreme flexion (with the attendant danger of muscle compartment ischemia), then either olecranon screw traction or percutaneous Kirschner wire fixation from the radial side is advisable, in order to maintain the reduction in a less flexed position (Fig. 18.5). Open reduction is indicated only if the fracture is irreducible or if it is associated with a vascular or nerve injury. For open reduction, the surgical approach can be lateral, bilateral or posterior, depending upon the nature and site of any associated neurovascular lesion. If cubitus varus is to be avoided, particular attention must be paid to the restoration of the correct angle (Baumann's angle) between the physeal plate of the lateral condyle and the long axis of the humerus. This angle must be approximately 70°–75° and should be comparable to the angle on the uninjured side (Fig. 18.6).

Fig. 18.5 Supracondylar fracture (if closed reduction fails). Stable fixation with two Kirschner wires left in place for 2–3 weeks.

Fig. 18.6 After reduction of a supracondylar fracture, the angle between the plane of the lateral condylar physis and the long axis of the humeral shaft (Baumann's angle) should equal that of the uninjured side, usually 70°–75°. Increase in this angle denotes varus malposition.

Fig. 18.5

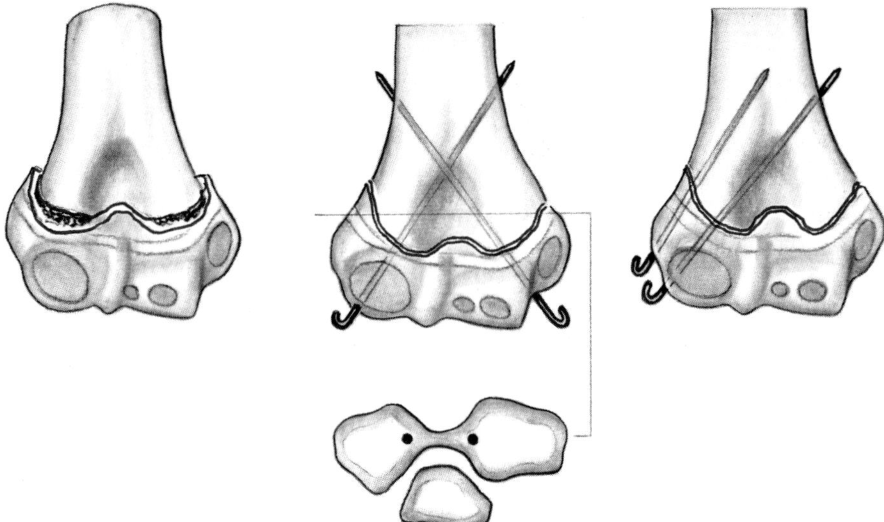

Fig. 18.6

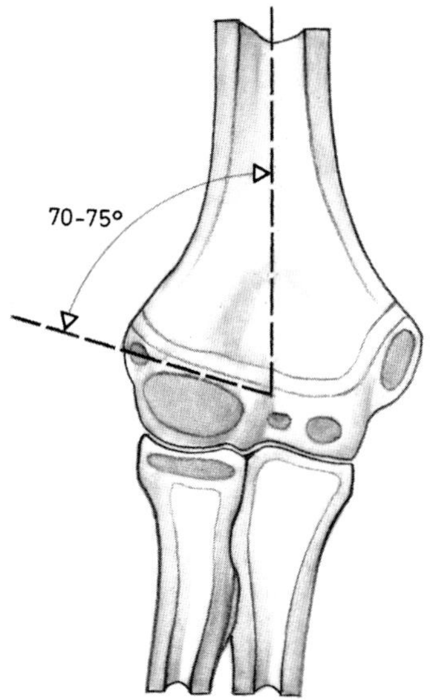

Displaced fractures of the lateral condyle are Salter-Harris type IV (B2) injuries. These intra-articular and epiphyseal fractures are usually treated by open reduction and Kirschner wire fixation for 2–3 weeks (Fig. 18.7). Cubitus varus can also result from capitellar overgrowth following this fracture, and cubitus valgus, with the danger of tardy ulnar palsy, may follow malreduction or non-union.

Fractures of the medial condyle of the Salter-Harris type IV also occur but are less common than lateral condylar injuries. The principles of their management are the same as for the lateral injury.

Very occasionally a Y-shaped intercondylar fracture can occur in a child. Effectively, this is analogous to the simultaneous occurrence of Salter-Harris type IV injuries of both medial and lateral condyles. Perfect realignment of the physeal plate is essential and may require compression screw fixation of the metaphyseal components combined with Kirschner wire stabilization of the epiphyseal, condylar mass. This fracture is often followed by growth disturbance and should only be treated by those surgeons with great experience of complex physeal trauma.

Fragments of the apophysis of the medial epicondyle which have become separated may become interposed in the joint, and although this fracture is not a true epiphyseal injury, it does carry the risk of non-union, irritation of the ulnar nerve and instability. Tension band fixation, or screw fixation in the older child, is advised in place of Kirschner wires alone (Fig. 18.8).

Fig. 18.7 Lateral condylar fracture separation at the distal humerus. Careful open reduction and fixation is indicated for this type B2 injury. Fixation is with Kirschner wires if the metaphyseal fragment is small (b), but with larger fragments, lag screw fixation totally within the metaphysis is preferable (c).

Fig. 18.8 Apophyseal injury at the distal humerus.

a, b Avulsion of the medial epicondylar apophysis fixed with Kirschner wires after open reduction.

c Alternative fixation with a figure-of-eight wire loop.

Fig. 18.7

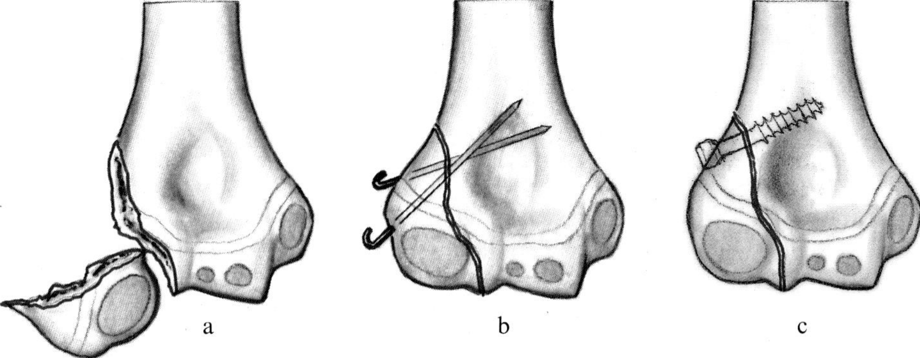

Fig. 18.8

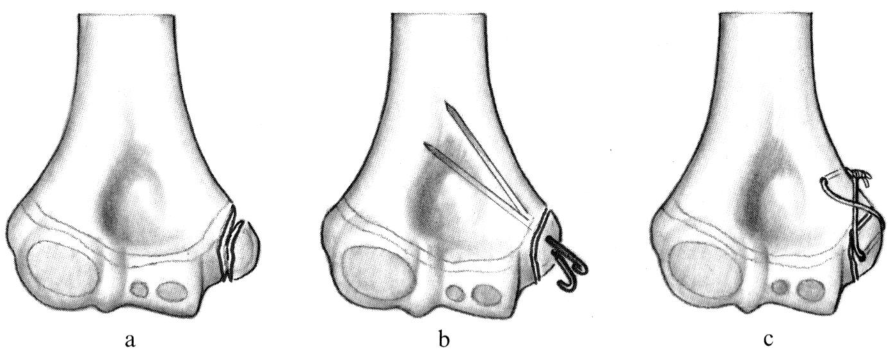

18.5 Fractures of the Forearm

18.5.1 Proximal Forearm, Radial Head and Neck

The epiphysis of the radial head is rarely fractured. If it is, then a Salter-Harris type IV (B2) injury has occurred and, if displaced, operative stabilization is mandatory if premature growth arrest is to be avoided.

Separation of the radial head, i.e., radial neck injury, may be a Salter-Harris type I (A1), type II (A2) or type IV (B2) injury, or a metaphyseal torus fracture (Fig. 18.9).

Because of the special vascular anatomy of the proximal radius (the proximal radial epiphysis has no soft tissue attachments and is totally covered by articular cartilage), a type A1 separation will virtually always result in physeal plate closure due to avascular necrosis of the epiphysis. On the other hand, a type A2 radial neck injury preserves those epiphyseal retinacular nutrient vessels associated with the metaphyseal fragment, and provided that the soft tissue attachments of this fragment are preserved, normal growth can continue. The distinction between the two types is paramount in planning treatment and predicting the outcome.

In general, in children under the age of about 8 years, radial head tilt (always into valgus) of up to 40° can be accepted, but above that age only 20° can be left unreduced.

One gentle closed manipulation is permitted, but failure to reduce to within the acceptable range is an indication for open reduction (Fig. 18.10).

Fixation is provided by means of a Kirschner wire (Fig. 18.11), supplemented by plaster fixation for 3 weeks.

Fig. 18.9 Fractures of the proximal radius. The proximal radial epiphysis receives its blood supply exclusively from the metaphyseal circulation via retinacular vessels passing in the periosteum of the neck and tightly bound to the perichondrium at the periphery of the growth plate. Certain patterns of separation of the radial head can imperil the epiphyseal vascularity and damage the germinal zone of the physis, resulting in growth arrest.

a Type B2 (Salter-Harris type IV) injury of the proximal radius is rare, but when displaced requires open reduction and internal fixation if growth arrest is to be avoided.

b, b′ Type A1 (Salter-Harris type I). Here, all the retinacular vessels are likely to be torn if displacement occurs. The head should be replaced and fixed with a Kirschner wire, but growth arrest is likely.

c Type A2 (Salter-Harris type II). In this injury, those metaphyseal vessels which are still associated with the metaphyseal bony fragment will continue to feed some of the retinacular vessels to the epiphysis. It is therefore of vital importance to distinguish between types A1 and A2. If open reduction is indicated in type A2, the soft tissue attachments to the metaphyseal fragment, which represent the sole remaining "life-line" to the epiphysis, must be preserved at all costs.

d Torus fracture of the proximal radial metaphysis, usually with valgus inclination.

Fig. 18.10 Fractures of the radial neck usually displace into valgus. A certain angulation is acceptable in children at different ages, from 20° in children over the age of 8 years to 40° in the very young. One gentle manipulative reduction maneuver is permissible, but if this fails, then open reduction will be required.

Fig. 18.11 Fixation of a fracture of the radial neck with a Kirschner wire. The wire should be removed at 2–3 weeks.

Fig. 18.9

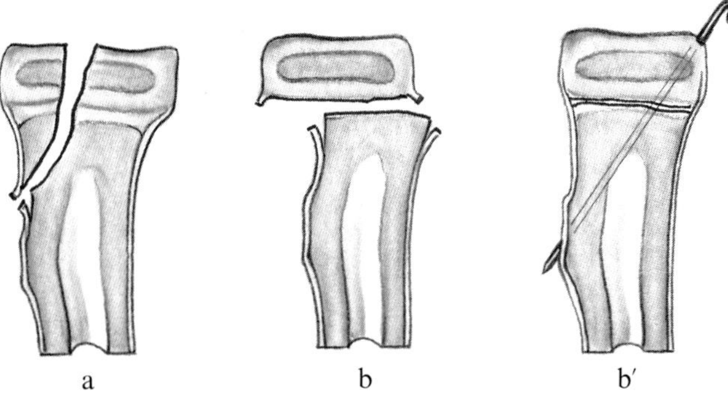

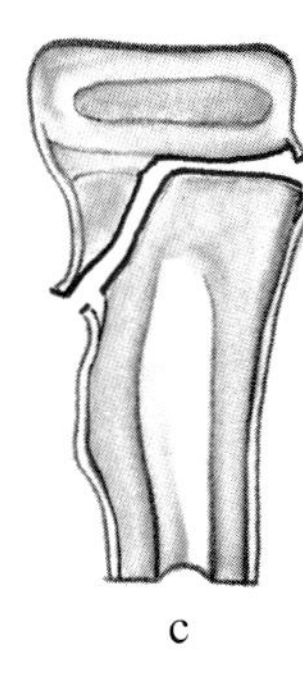

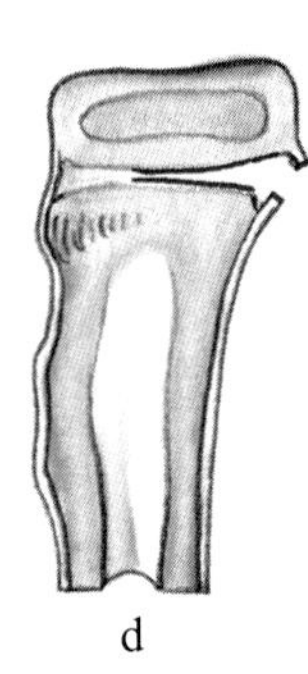

Fig. 18.10

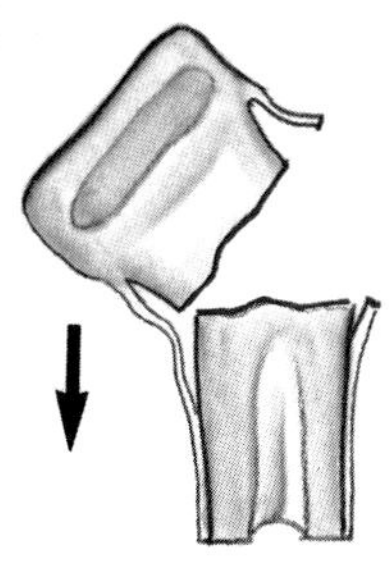

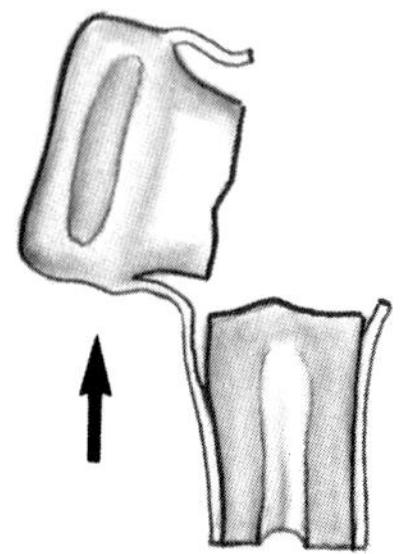

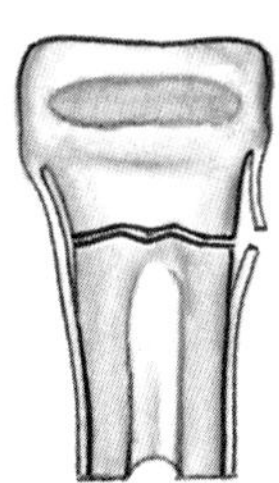

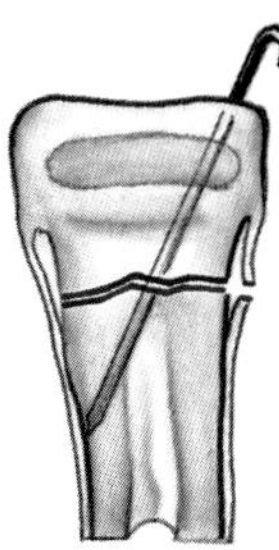

Fig. 18.11

18.5.2 Monteggia Fracture

In dealing with Monteggia fractures, if anatomic reduction of the ulna and radial head cannot be obtained or maintained, open reduction and internal fixation becomes necessary. Plate fixation of the ulnar fracture is recommended and leads to successful closed reduction of the radial head (Fig. 18.12). As the mechanism of this injury is one of hyperpronation of the forearm (Fig. 18.12a), the radial head is usually found to be stable in full supination, in which position the forearm should be immobilized for 3–4 weeks in a long-arm cast (Fig. 18.12b).

18.5.3 Shaft Fractures

Fractures of the forearm shaft in younger children can almost always be treated nonoperatively. The physiological bowing of the radius and ulna has to be restored to prevent limitation of pronation and supination. In the older child, poorly reduced forearm fractures are an indication for open reduction and plate fixation (Fig. 18.13). In general, displaced diaphyseal fractures of the forearm bones in children over 10 years of age should be managed as in the adult (Kay et al. 1986).

Fig. 18.12 The Monteggia fracture.

a This is a displaced fracture of the ulnar shaft with dislocation of the radial head, usually anteriorly or laterally (posterior displacement is rare in children). This injury is less common in children than in adults; it is usually caused by hyperpronation.

b If the ulnar fracture is unstable because it is oblique or multifragmentary, then open reduction and plating is necessary. If the position of the ulnar fracture is anatomic, the radial head will reduce if the forearm is placed in supination. Maintenance of this position with a cast for a short period is usually indicated.

Fig. 18.13 Diaphyseal fractures of the forearm bones in children are rarely fixed surgically under the age of about 10 years. Over this age, the indications for internal fixation are the same as in adults (Kay et al. 1986). The usual implants are 3.5-mm DCPs.

Fig. 18.12

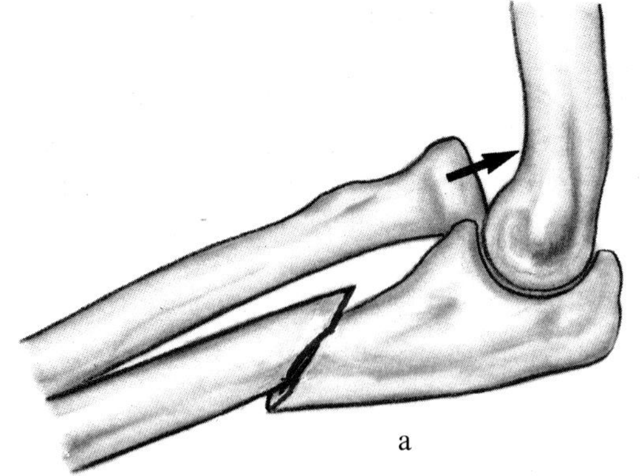

a

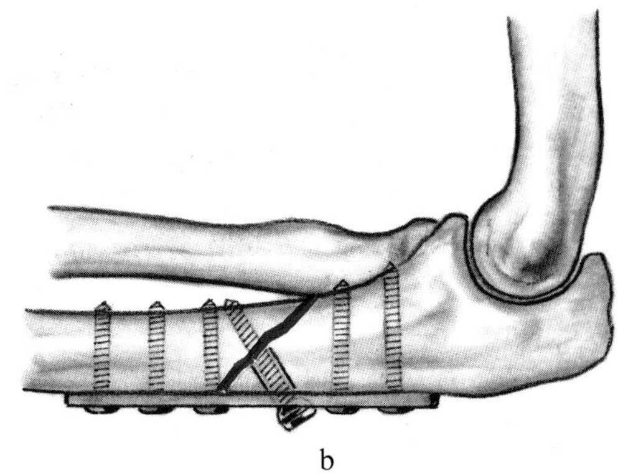

b

Fig. 18.13

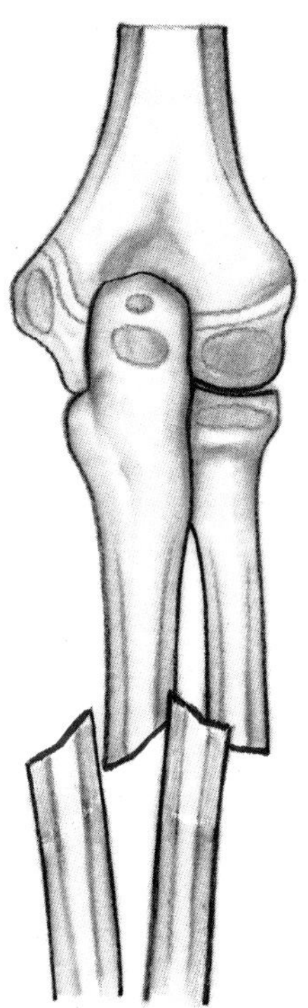

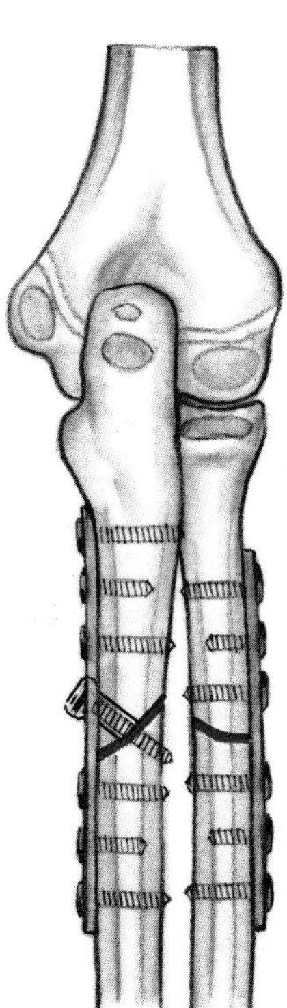

18.6 Fractures of the Femur

18.6.1 Proximal Femur

Fractures of the femoral neck, whether they be of the lateral type or of the medial subcapital shear type, comprise an absolute indication for open reduction and stable internal fixation.

Immediately after fracture, some of the retinacular vessels are usually intact. Displacement of the fragment leads to kinking of these vessels, which predisposes to thrombosis. Additionally, the hemarthrosis may lead to a joint tamponade, further threatening the epiphyseal vascularity, and therefore these fractures should be treated as surgical emergencies (Fig. 18.14).

Stable internal fixation is achieved by inserting one or more 6.5-mm diameter cancellous bone screws, taking care not to cross and thereby damage the physeal plate with the screw thread (Fig. 18.15). Nailing of these fractures is absolutely contraindicated. The cancellous bone is very hard, and in nailing, there is a great danger of driving the fragments apart and thereby tearing the retinacular vessels, which would also lead to avascular necrosis of the head.

18.6.1.1 The Technique of Open Reduction and Internal Fixation (ORIF)

The capsule is exposed in the space between the lesser glutei and tensor fasciae latae and opened at the acetabular side via a T-shaped capsulotomy. The fracture is exposed with the aid of three small retractors. One is inserted over the anterior pelvic rim, the second above the femoral neck and the third below it. Once reduced, the fracture is fixed temporarily with Kirschner wires and the reduction checked, particularly at the level of the calcar, by flexing and rotating the hip. Definitive fixation is then carried out with two 6.5-mm cancellous bone screws, again taking care not to pierce the physeal plate. The capsular incision is not fully closed, in order to avoid the danger of joint tamponade (Fig. 18.15).

The use of cannulated cancellous bone screws greatly facilitates this type of fixation.

Fig. 18.14 Intracapsular fractures of the femoral neck in children result in a joint tamponade which, because of the vascular anatomy of the proximal femoral epiphysis, will endanger any remaining blood supply to the femoral head. For this reason, closed reduction methods should never be used. Emergency arthrotomy and open reduction is always indicated.

Fig. 18.15 Transcervical femoral fracture in a child. Two large-diameter cancellous bone screws with 16-mm thread length are used, taking care not to penetrate the physeal plate. Cannulated screws may be used to good advantage. The capsular incision is not sutured, so as to permit drainage of the synovial joint space.

Fig. 18.14

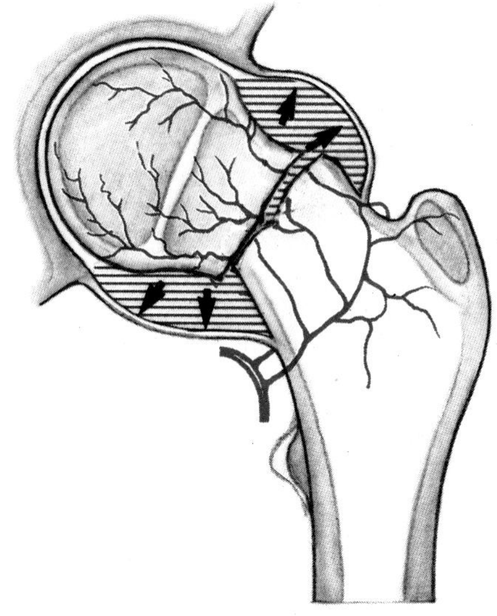

Fig. 18.15

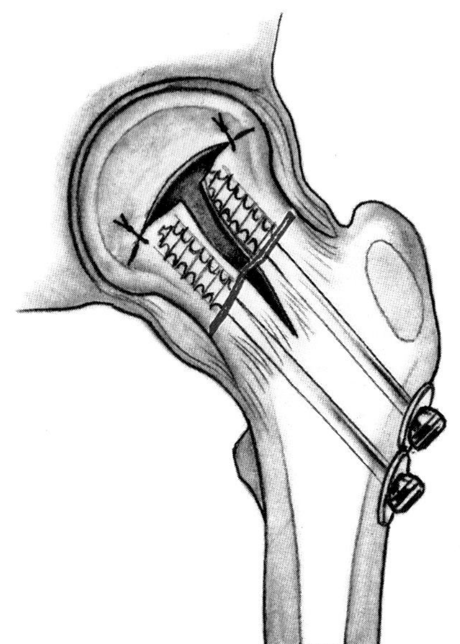

18.6.2 Femoral Shaft

Fractures of the femoral shaft are usually treated nonoperatively in skeletal traction on the Weber traction table with the hip and knee in 90° of flexion. The traction table allows radiologic control and correction of any rotational malalignment (Fig. 18.16). In adolescents, femoral diaphyseal fractures, particularly metaphyseal fractures, can be treated by internal fixation with plates or exceptionally with intramedullary nails.

18.6.3 Distal Femur

Distal femur fractures are mostly Salter-Harris type II (A2) separations of the epiphyseal plate with a metaphyseal fragment. They are difficult to reduce, and it is often difficult to maintain the reduction. If the fractures cannot be reduced, or can be reduced but not maintained, open reduction is needed and metaphyseal interfragmentary lag screw fixation is suggested (Fig. 18.17). Repeated closed reduction causes damage to the growth plate, and overlooked ligament avulsion fractures may explain the high frequency of growth disturbance at the distal femur.

Avulsion fractures of the lateral collateral ligament that span the plate should be treated by means of open reduction and internal fixation (ORIF) (Fig. 18.18).

Fig. 18.16 Fracture of the femoral shaft in skeletal traction on a Weber traction table. The knees and hips are flexed at 90°. The legs are abducted 20° as for an anteversion X-ray. The uninvolved limb is suspended in skin traction. The side with the fracture is placed in skeletal traction by means of a supracondylar threaded Steinmann pin inserted parallel to the knee joint and proximal to the growth plate. The fixed traction lifts the pelvis just clear of the mattress.

Fig. 18.17 Type A2 (Salter-Harris type II) injury of the distal femur. These should be fixed if displaced and unstable. A cortex lag screw compresses the metaphyseal fracture plane and must not transgress the physeal plate.

Fig. 18.18 Type B3 (M.E. Müller) injury. The fragment of ligamentous attachment must be anatomically reduced and fixed; small cancellous bone screws should be used if the bony segments are large enough, as Kirschner wires rarely succeed in closing the fracture gap.

Fig. 18.16

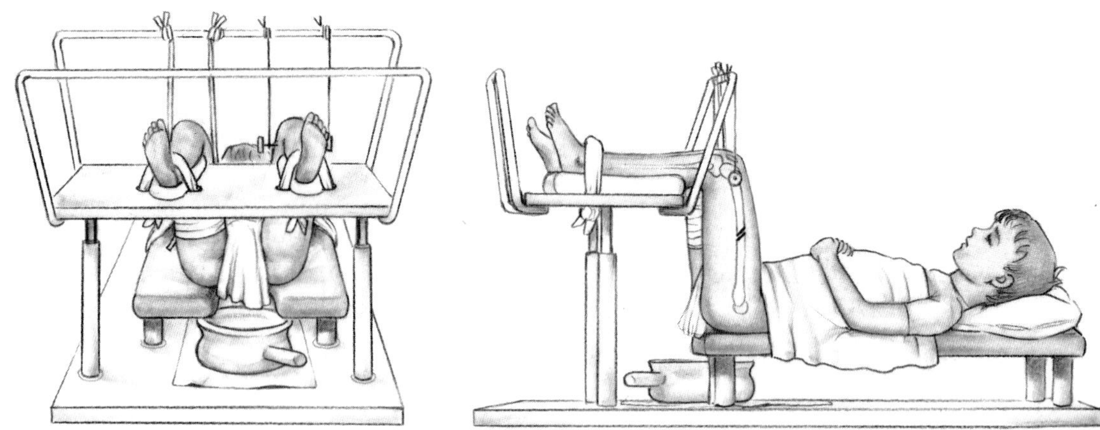

Fig. 18.17

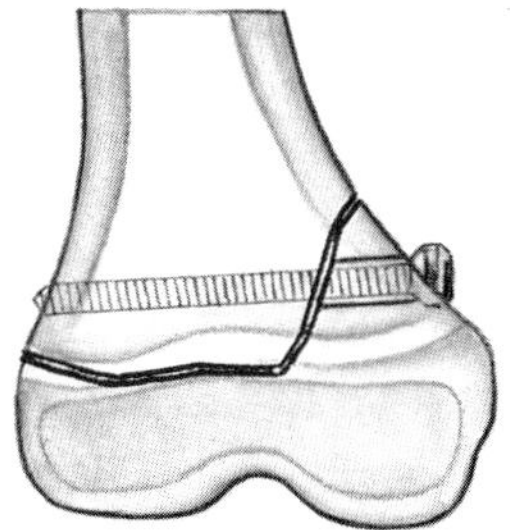

Fig. 18.18

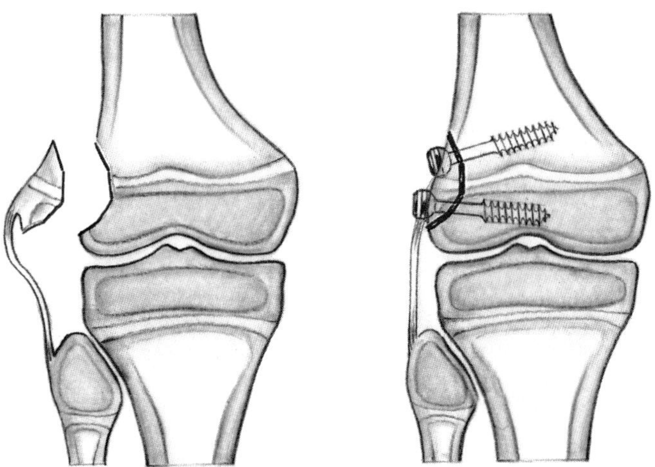

18.7 Fractures of the Tibia

A displaced avulsion fracture of the tibial tuberosity should be treated by means of ORIF. This usually occurs in an adolescent when the physeal plate is almost closed. Internal fixation is carried out with a tension band and/or interfragmentary cortex screws (Fig. 18.19). If the child is young, then a wiring technique which respects the growth zone of the apophysis of the tibial tuberosity is preferred (Fig. 18.20). Premature growth arrest at the tibial tuberosity can cause progressive genu recurvatum deformity.

A displaced avulsion fracture of the tibial intercondylar eminence can sometimes be treated closed and reduced by hyperextension. If reduction fails, there is a risk of permanent flexion deformity, and ORIF using a small cancellous bone screw is necessary. This screw should not pierce the proximal tibial physis (Fig. 18.21).

Fig. 18.19 Avulsions of the tibial tuberosity, usually in adolescents, require anatomic reduction and lag screw fixation.

a–d Various lag screw applications for specific fracture types.

Fig. 18.20 In the younger child, a wiring technique, respecting the growth plate, is used for tibial tuberosity detachments.

Fig. 18.21 Avulsion of the intercondylar eminence. Stabilize with a small cancellous bone screw, totally within the epiphysis.

Fig. 18.19

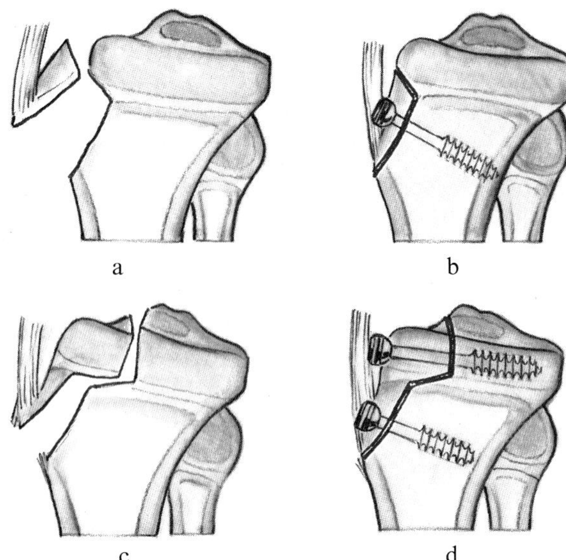

Fig. 18.20

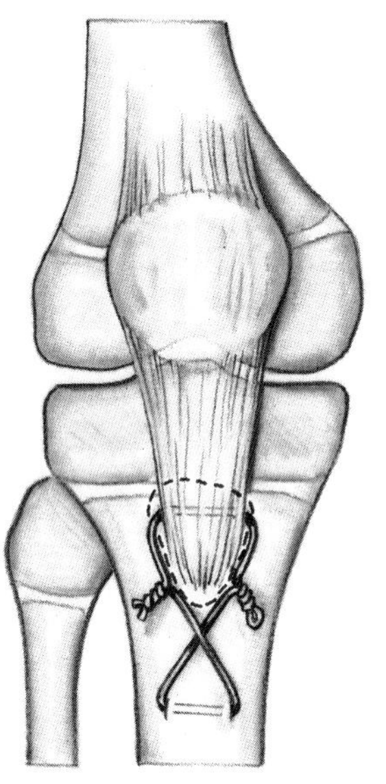

Fig. 18.21

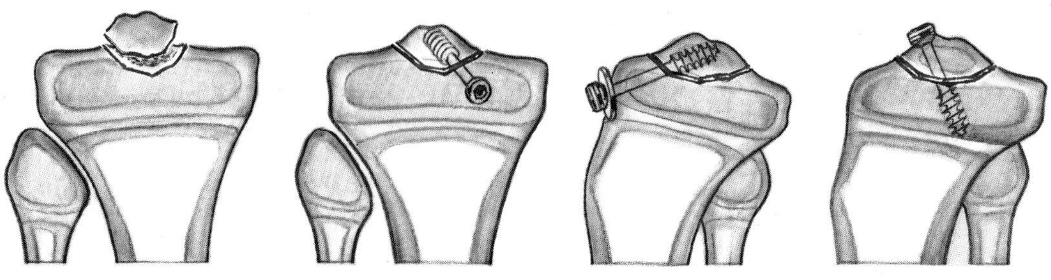

18.8 Distal Tibial Growth-Plate Fractures

Open reduction with internal fixation is indicated when the fracture line crosses the epiphysis, physeal plate and/or metaphysis and remains displaced. Remaining articular incongruity is also an indication for surgery. For these fractures we prefer interfragmentary cortex lag screw fixation, rather than simple Kirschner wire fixation to achieve a perfect anatomic reduction of the physeal lesion (Figs. 18.22–18.25).

The triplane fracture is unique to the ankle. This is a complex injury involving the distal tibial epiphysis, physeal plate and metaphysis. The most frequent variety consists of a vertical sagittal fracture through the epiphysis, a horizontal shear injury of the physeal plate and a vertical coronal fracture plane separating a posterior metaphyseal fragment (Fig. 18.26a). This pattern, if displaced, will usually require ORIF to reconstruct the articular surface (Fig. 18.26b) (Tinnemans and Severijnen 1975).

Displaced talus fractures in children should also be treated using interfragmentary lag screw fixation.

18.9 Other Fractures

Displaced patella and olecranon fractures should be treated as in adults.

Fig. 18.22 Type A2 (Salter-Harris type II) fracture separation of the distal tibial epiphysis, the result of an abduction force. Irreducibility, due to medial periosteal interposition, or marked instability after manipulative reduction are indications for open reduction and fixation with an intrametaphyseal 3.5-mm cortex lag screw.

Fig. 18.23 Type B1 (Salter-Harris type III) medial malleolar separation. Anatomic reduction and fixation with one or two intra-epiphyseal small cancellous bone screws is usually indicated.

Fig. 18.24 Type B2 (or B1) (Salter-Harris type IV and III) avulsion injuries of the anterior tibial tuberosity (Tillaux-Chaput) occur in adolescence, just before natural physeal closure. Anatomic reduction of the joint surface is essential, followed by fixation with one or more small cancellous bone screws. At this stage of skeletal maturity, the usual physeal considerations are less important.

Fig. 18.25 Type B2 (Salter-Harris type IV) medial injury. The precise realignment of the joint surface and the physis are vitally important. Fixation by lag screws utilizes cortex screws in the metaphysis and cancellous bone screws in the epiphysis. The physis must not be transgressed if normal, longitudinal growth is to be preserved.

Fig. 18.26 The classical two-part triplane injury (Marmor). This occurs usually at that stage of skeletal maturity when spontaneous fusion of the distal tibial physis has just started anteromedially. The fused portion of the medial malleolus (its anterior half) remains attached to the tibial shaft, whereas the unfused portion separates, together with a posterior metaphyseal fragment. The resultant complex fracture surfaces lie in three planes: sagittal, horizontal and coronal. In order to restore the joint surface, fixation with lag screws is essential.

Fig. 18.22

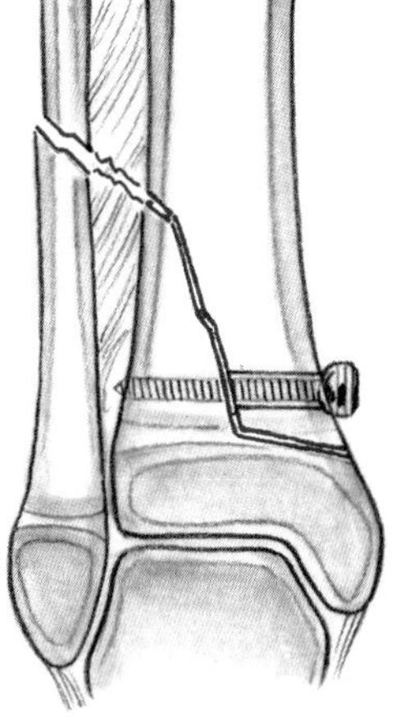

Fig. 18.23

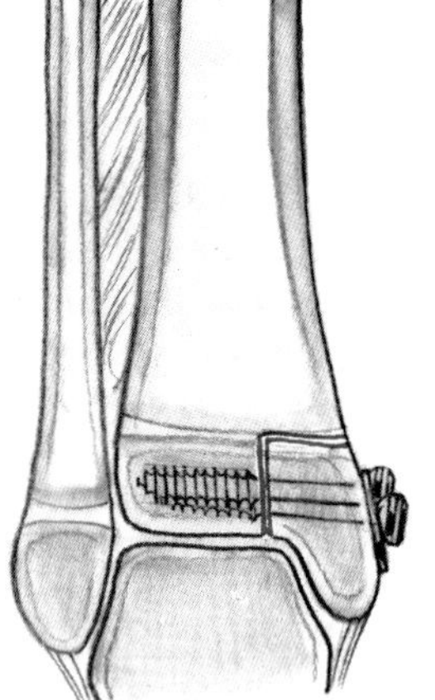

Fig. 18.24

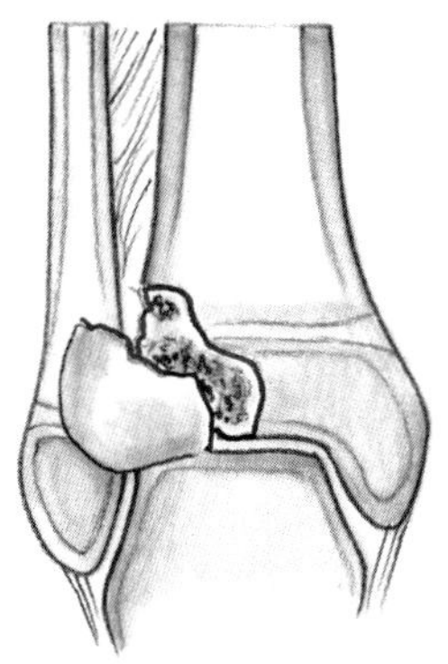

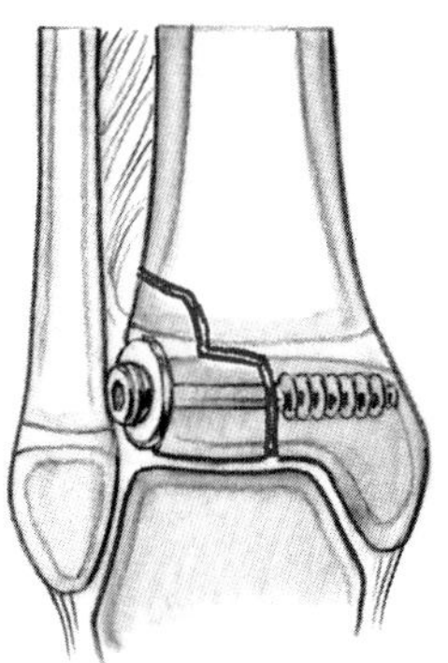

Fig. 18.25

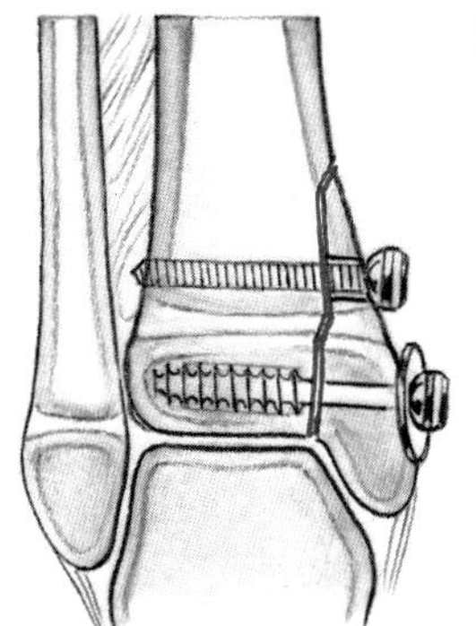

Fig. 18.26

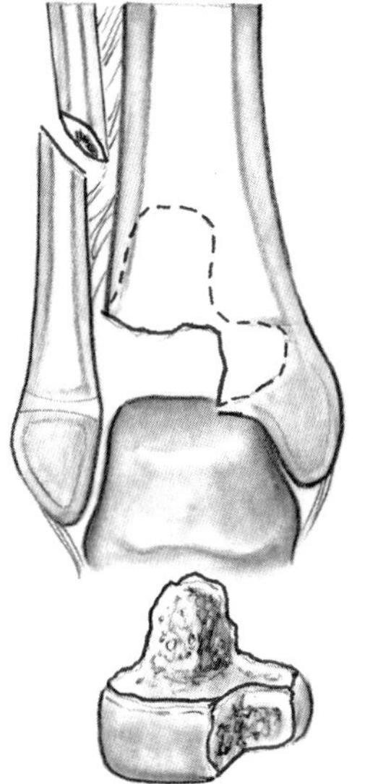

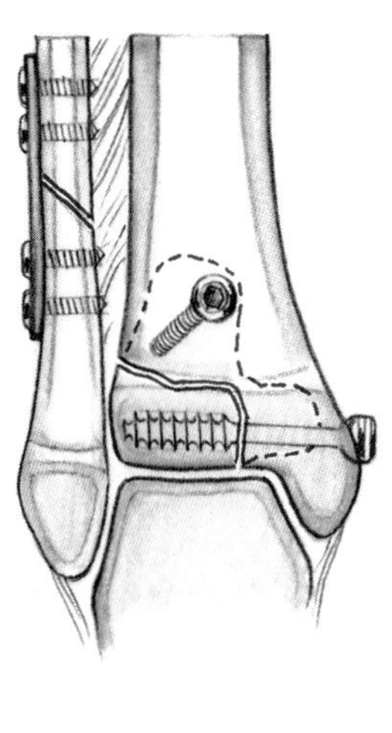

References

Brouwer KJ (1981) Torsional deformities after fractures of the femoral shaft in childhood. Acta Orthop Scand 52 [Suppl 195]

Broudy AS, Jupiter J, May JW Jr (1979) Management of supracondylar fracture with brachial artery thrombosis in a child: case report and literature review. J Trauma 19 (7): 540–543

Kay S, Smith C, Oppenheim WL (1986) Both-bone midshaft forearm fractures in children. J Pediatr Orthop 6: 306–310

Langenskiold A, Osterman K (1983) Surgical elimination of posttraumatic partial fusion of the growth plate. In: Houghton G, Thompson G (eds) Problematic musculoskeletal injuries in children. Butterworth, London

Rang M (1983) Children's fractures, 2nd edn. Lippincott, Philadelphia, p 24

Tinnemans JGM, Severijnen RSVM (1975) The triplane fracture of the distal tibial epiphysis in children. Injury 12: 393–396

Weber BG (1977) Fibrous interposition causing valgus deformity after fracture of the upper tibial metaphysis in children. J Bone Joint Surg [Br] 59: 290–292

Weber BG, Brunner C, Freuler F (1980) Treatment of fractures in children and adolescents. Springer, Berlin Heidelberg New York

Worlock PH, Colton CL (1987) Severely displaced supracondylar fractures of the humerus in children. J Pediatr Orthop 7: 49–53

19 PSEUDARTHROSES

19.1 Definitions

19.1.1 Delayed Union

In 4–6 months, most fractures will unite or at least show progressive healing on serial X-rays. If a fracture has not healed by that time, it is considered to be a delayed union. Even if the initial internal fixation had rendered the fracture lines well adapted and hardly visible, these fracture lines will become progressively wider and some cloudy, poorly delineated "irritation callus" may be present. Resorption areas around the internal fixation devices will show evidence of loosening and irritation.

19.1.2 Non-Union

There is an arrest of the bony fracture repair process with formation of fibrous or cartilaginous interposition tissue between the main fragments, and the fracture has remained ununited for 6–8 months. There are two basic patterns of non-unions (Fig. 19.1): the reactive, hypertrophic, vascular non-union; and the nonreactive, atrophic or even avascular non-union.

19.1.2.1 Reactive Non-Union

Over 90% of non-unions which result from conservative fracture treatment and a smaller percentage which follow operative treatment are of the reactive, hypertrophic or vascular type (Fig. 19.1 a). Radiologically they are characterized by the florid bone reaction which is responsible for flaring and sclerosis at the bony ends. This reaction leads to the so-called elephant's foot non-union. Somewhat less reactive tissue at the bony end is present in the so-called horse's hoof non-union (Fig. 19.1 a″). The radiologically evident sclerosis does not represent dead bone but rather excessive appositional bone formation with an excellent blood supply. This has very important therapeutic implications. Once absolutely immobilized, the interposed cartilage or connective tissue rapidly mineralizes and changes into bone. Therefore the ends of such a hypertrophic non-union need not be resected unless realignment becomes necessary, and bone grafting is usually unnecessary. Once immobilized, with either an intermedullary nail or a compression plate, preferably using one or two interfragmentary screws, these non-unions begin to ossify within a few weeks.

19.1.2.2 Nonreactive, Atrophic, More or Less Avascular Non-Union (Fig. 19.1 b)

Radiologically these non-unions are characterized by the absence of callus and the presence of interposition tissue at the bony ends. From a prognostic as well as from a therapeutic point of view, they can be equated with the so-called oligotrophic vascular non-unions of Weber and Cech (1976) characterized by the lack of callus. These oligotrophic and atrophic non-unions require stable internal fixation and, in addition, extensive decortication and cancellous bone grafting. With the increase in the number of internal fixations leading to partial devascularization of bony ends and free fragments, there has been a similar increase in the incidence of these atrophic non-unions.

19.1.3 Pseudarthrosis

For many surgeons, the designation pseudarthrosis is synonymous with non-union. Correctly used it means a non-union which develops a neoarthrosis with a synovial lining and sometimes with joint fluid in the cleft or cavity. This is called a synovial pseudarthrosis. Clinically there is false motion and radiologically a wide gap can be seen. The vascularity of the bony ends will have the same characteristics as described for non-union in Sect. 19.1.2. A technetium-99m bone scan will usually show a cold cleft between hot ends. Operative intervention is the only reliable method for obtaining union of a synovial pseudarthrosis.

An important subdivision of delayed unions, non-unions and pseudarthroses relates to infection. We therefore classify the three prevailing conditions as noninfected, previously infected and infected. Evidence of previous or manifest infection will influence the therapeutic planning.

Another important aspect related to therapeutic planning is whether the non-unions have their bony ends in contact or whether there is a bony defect. Bony defects of a few centimeters may be bridged by cancellous bone autotransplants. Major defects, whether noninfected, previously infected or manifestly infected, are best treated with fragment transport according to the principles of Ilizarov (Ilizarov et al. 1972) (see Chap. 5).

Fig. 19.1 The two types of noninfected non-union.

a The reactive hypertrophic, well-vascularized type. (a′) elephant's foot type (rich in callus), (a″) horse's hoof type (minimal callus), (a‴) oligotrophic (without callus).

b Nonreactive atrophic type, between poorly vascularized or dead bone fragments. (b′) partially necrotic fragment, (b″) necrotic fragment, (b‴) defect, (b⁗) atrophic type.

Fig. 19.1

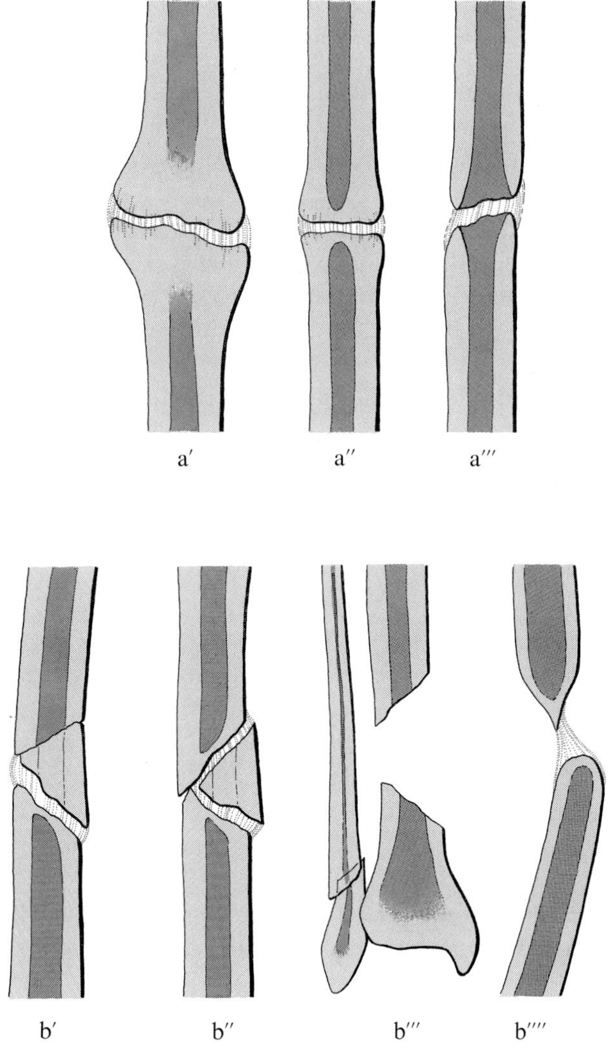

19.2 Etiology of Delayed Unions, Non-Unions and Pseudarthroses

Delayed union, and subsequent non-union and pseudarthrosis result from the following:

- Excess motion due to: inadequate immobilization.
- Gap between fragments due to: soft tissue interposition; distraction by traction or hardware; malposition, over-riding or displacement of fragments; and loss of bone substance.
- Loss of blood supply due to: damage to nutrient vessels; excessive stripping or injury to periosteum and muscle; free fragments; severe comminution; and avascularity due to hardware or poor operative technique.
- Infection due to: bone death (sequestrum); osteolysis (gap); and loosening of implants (motion).
- Other reasons include: old age; nutrition; steroids; anticoagulants; radiation; and burns. All of these predispose to but do not cause non-union.

19.3 Objectives of Non-Union Therapy

1. If possible to *correct deformity* i.e. angulation, rotation, sideward displacement and length.
2. To *mobilize adjacent stiff joints*, especially in metaphyseal and epiphyseal non-unions. This is accomplished by arthrotomy and arthrolysis, and release of ligamentous, capsular and muscle contracture.
3. To *obtain union* of the fracture in a reasonable time, and with as few operative procedures as possible.
4. In infected non-unions, in addition to number 3, to *eradicate infection*. This may require several operations to gain union first and then remove the infection, or vice versa.

19.4 Rationale of Non-Union Therapy

19.4.1 Nonoperative Rationale

19.4.1.1 Immobilization

In delayed unions, immobilization with a cast or brace and non-weight-bearing may induce a vascular non-union to unite. Fibular osteotomy with weight-bearing in a cast may often succeed in uniting a tibial non-union; however, the result is very often shortening and varus deformity. Therfore, we suggest leaving the fibula undisturbed in open treatment of a tibial non-union. If weight-bearing casts or braces succeed in healing a femoral non-union, the result is frequently a malunion and permanent impairment of the knee.

19.4.1.2 Electrical Stimulation

In various forms, electrical stimulation is said to induce union in 60%–80% of non-unions, but these methods:

- Do not usually succeed: with gaps of more than 1 cm; in avascular and synovial pseudarthroses; where motion at the fracture is difficult to control (i.e. proximal femur or humerus); and in metaphyseal non-unions.
- Do not correct malposition or shortening.
- Often require long plaster, non-weight-bearing immobilization causing atrophy of bone and soft tissue, stiffness of joints and loss of function.

19.4.2 Operative Rationale

Correct the causative factors by:

- Decreasing motion using stable reduction and fixation with strong (tension band) plates and well-seated screws under compression (lag screws), intramedullary nails, or external fixators when indicated.
- Closing the gap using: compression between fragments; cortico-cancellous bone grafts (Fig. 19.2); or fragment transport according to Ilizarov's principles.
- Encouraging revascularization: by shingling (Figs. 19.3, 19.4) and cancellous bone grafts – these can induce an avascular non-union to heal and sometimes even an infected one too; by early exercise and function (facilitated by stable fixation), thus decreasing muscle atrophy, fibrosis and joint stiffness; or by microsurgical composite free flaps (bone and soft tissues) and vascular repair.

Fig. 19.2 To obtain bone from the inner table of the anterior wing of the ilium. Make your incision 1–2 cm either medial or lateral to the iliac crest. Reflect the skin and keep it retracted with two small Hohmann retractors.

a Use a gouge to obtain corticocancellous strips 6–10 cm long from the inner table. Cut these strips into smaller pieces 5–6 mm wide and 15 mm long.

b If you need only cancellous bone, use a broad osteotome. Lift up a large flap of pure cortical bone parasacrally which you hinge inferiorly. At the end allow it to fall back into place. Once exposed, the cancellous bone is removed using a chisel with a U-shaped profile. The parasacral part of the ilium provides the richest source of cancellous bone.

c The greater trochanter provides good quality cancellous bone. The cortical window should be carefully closed.

Fig. 19.2

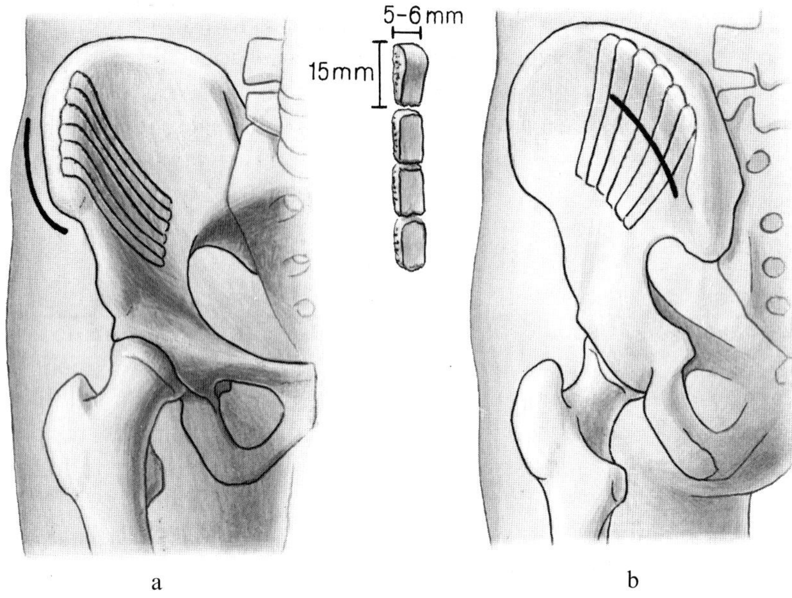

a b

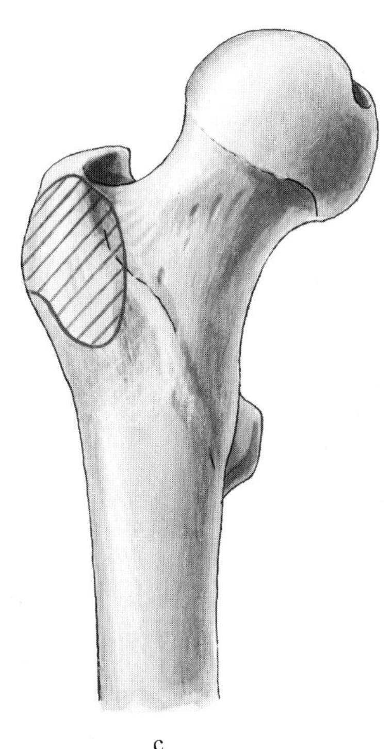

c

19.5 Principles of the Operative Treatment

The classification of delayed unions, non-unions and pseudarthroses is used as a basis for treatment. It should be stressed at the outset that prevention is better than treatment! Every area of avascular or necrotic diaphyseal bone can be the cause of a delayed union or non-union if it is greater than 1 cm. Therefore it should be obvious to every surgeon who diagnoses such an area at operation that a cancellous bone graft should be added.

19.5.1 Noninfected

A delayed union should be anticipated at 3 months and treated aggressively by gaining stability and if necessary bone grafting. If well aligned, treatment may be by non-weight-bearing brace or cast immobilization, or by open reduction and internal fixation (ORIF).

If there has been previous internal fixation with plates and lag screws which shows loosening and/or widening of fracture gaps, then changing or adding a lag screw, tightening the loose screws, adding a bone graft and shingling (Figs. 19.3, 19.4) may all give rise to rapid union. Removing a loose tibial or femoral plate and replacing it with a reamed intramedullary nail is usually a successful alternative method of treatment in vascular delayed unions.

If a diaphyseal non-union is present and is vascular (elephant's foot, or horse's hoof type callus), then merely stabilizing the fracture, avoiding a resection of the non-union tissue or fracture ends and without using either a bone graft or a cast, will induce rapid healing. Only if there is malalignment must the ends be fashioned prior to stable internal fixation. Shingling or decortication is performed to induce rapid healing. If there is poor blood supply and minimal callus (oligotrophic towards atrophic non-union) a cancellous bone graft is mandatory!

If there is an avascular diaphyseal nonreactive non-union, then shingling and a bone graft are added to restart the healing process, plus of course, a stable internal fixation device as above. When the bone is osteoporotic and the screws do not hold, methyl methacrylate cement can be injected from a syringe into the loose screw holes, the screws reinserted and the cement allowed to harden. The screws are then terminally tightened. (Fig. 19.8b).

Note: No cement should be injected into screw holes adjacent to or in the fracture, or be allowed to remain around the bone!

Fig. 19.3 The decortication of Judet (shingling) as also described by Phemister.

a Carry the incision down to the bone. Expose the bone by chiseling off small flakes, taking care that these flakes retain their soft tissue attachment and thus their blood supply.

b The decortication should extend one-half to three-quarters of the way round the bone and about 5 cm proximal and distal of the non-union. This sheet of mobile, living cortical flakes of bone usually rapidly consolidates with the formation of a strong fixation callus regardless of whether one is treating a non-infected or an infected pseudarthrosis.

Fig. 19.4

a In treating oligotrophic or atrophic pseudarthroses, both fragments are decorticated.

b In this way pockets are created for the bone graft between the bone and its soft tissue cover. One should also decorticate whenever a corrective osteotomy is made through a fracture callus.

Fig. 19.3

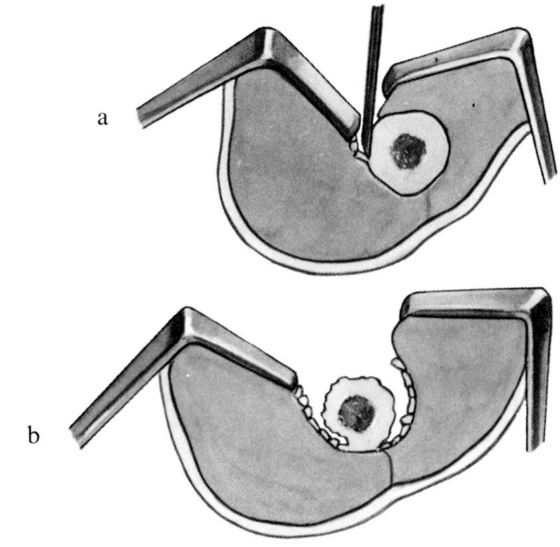

Fig. 19.4

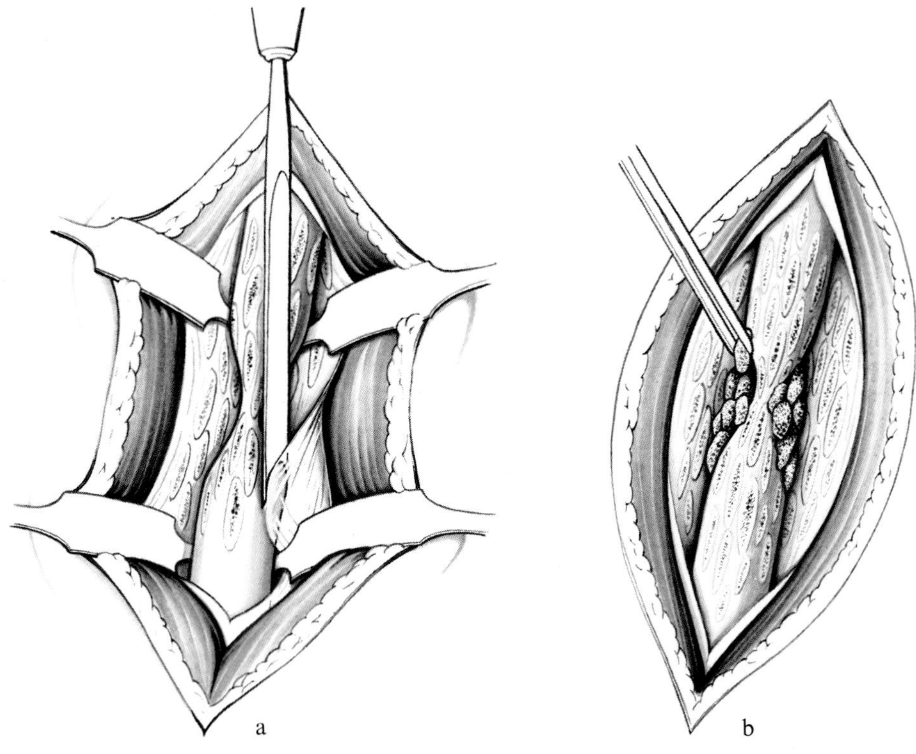

If there is a large diaphyseal defect caused by lengthening, or by loss of bone stock from, for example, an open fracture, then external fixators, a bridge plate, or a locked intramedullary nail can all be used for stabilization. Depending on the length of the gap, a good alternative bridging method is a cortico-cancellous or vascularized composite bone graft (i.e. fibular). With normal mobility of the foot, lengthening of up to 2 cm can be carried out using the compressor/distractor during the internal fixation procedure. If more than 2 cm gradual lengthening is required, the Ilizarov technique using the AO tubular fixator is recommended (see Chap. 5).

The same principles of bone grafting are applied to synovial pseudarthroses depending on the presence or absence of vascular bone ends and callus. In addition, the bone ends are fashioned and shingled, the pseudarthrosis tissue resected, the medullary canals opened and the fracture reduced to correct alignment. Stable internal fixation is added to complete the procedure.

In metaphyseal non-unions the following procedure is suggested:

- Mobilize stiff joints (either at initial operation or as a separate procedure): open joint, capsulotomy, or capsulectomy; resect hypertrophic synovium and lyse adhesions; remove loose fragments and bodies; release adjacent muscles, ligamentous and joint contractures; and gently manipulate joints until "free".
- Align articular surfaces and fix temporarily with Kirschner wires: stabilize with one or preferably more interfragmentary lag screws, or if a defect is present, use position screws to fix the articular metaphyseal fragments, filling in defects with autologous cancellous bone.
- Stably fix the reconstructed metaphyseal fragment to the shaft with a blade plate, T, L, or buttress plate. Use axial compression for stability, if possible; use at least two (preferably three) points of fixation to gain purchase on the porotic metaphyseal fragment. Cancellous bone grafting is necessary when there is a large gap or avascular bone; occasionally use external fixators with pin-adjusting clamps if the metaphyseal fragment is very small. (Temporary overbridging of the joint may be considered if necessary.) Cement in screw or blade holes may occasionally be necessary in porotic bone.
- Start early active motion of adjacent joints by prompt removal of temporary external splints, physiotherapy and continuous passive and active mobilization (hinged cast braces may occasionally be necessary for added protection).

19.5.2 Infected

In the treatment of infected nondraining non-unions, the following procedure is recommended:

Quiescent (dry, nondraining for at least 3 months): use short-term antibiotic prophylaxis; excise dead bone and scarred, nonvascularized soft tissues and remove loose hardware; shingle; correct alignment; perform cancellous bone grafting in hypotrophic or avascular types; stabilize using plates or medullary nails or by external fixators; mobilize adjacent joints by physiotherapy, active and continuous passive motion.

Active (nondraining but with abscess and fever). A two-stage procedure is recommended – the first stage consisting in thorough debridement. Excise and debride, irrigate well; drain using open treatment or closed suction irrigation; antibiotic beads may be useful; stabilize with external fixators; use parenteral antibiotics pre-, intra- and postoperatively; and continue treatment as in infected draining non-unions. The second stage

– after 10–20 days if wound healing proceeds normally – consists in shingling and application of a cancellous bone autotransplant.

In the treatment of infected draining non-unions, the following procedure is recommended:

A two- or three-stage procedure is recommended. The first stage may consist in by-pass bone grafting i.e. fibula protibia, posteromedial femur or humerus grafting. Stabilization usually makes use of external fixators. Exceptionally, plate fixation after thorough debridement may be considered.

When the by-pass has become solid (after several months) radical debridement of sinuses, dead soft tissue, abscess cavity, dead infected bone and removal of loose hardware – if not done at first salvage procedure – should be carried out. Drainage may be by open irrigation or closed suction irrigation; use antibiotics pre-, intra- and for short periods postoperatively. In a third stage, an additional cancellous bone graft, muscle or skin pedicle flap, or vascularized free transplant will be considered. Postoperatively, mobilization of stiff joints with CPM and by active mobilization should be instituted. External fixators will be left in place until union. Partial weight-bearing until union should be with hinged casts or braces when necessary.

19.6 Preoperative Planning (see also Chap. 2)

In the operative treatment of non-unions, there are no emergencies except in sepsis. Therefore, there is time for careful and thorough preoperative planning, which is essential to a successful outcome.

The history will raise and answer many questions. Was the fracture open or closed? High or low velocity? Was there infection or allergy to antibiotics or medication? What operative procedures were performed and were there complications? Were implants used and removed? Were there skin grafts or muscle transfers? What other injuries or fractures were sustained? Will residual disability of other injured parts affect the prospective non-union treatment?

The physical examination will determine deformity, motion at the fracture, the site of pain, stiffness of adjacent joints, atrophy, the status of the skin and scars, nerve or vascular damage, limb shortening, etc.

A review of previous X-rays is important to the understanding of the etiology of the non-union. A review of the original accident X-rays will frequently show fragments that have since healed in malposition.

Implants and instruments should be carefully considered and planned as primary devices or for secondary back-up if the primary device should fail. Special instruments or devices should be ordered well in advance so that at the time of operation all possible methods of fixation are available. The operating room personnel and nurses should be consulted early to ensure that various implants and instruments are indeed available. In addition, the availability of sterile tourniquets, special traction tables, lights, image intensification, X-ray control, etc. should be checked preoperatively and the position of the patient planned.

Other diagnostic tests and procedures which may be considered include: arthroscopy, which may be necessary to ascertain the articular damage in a metaphyseal articular non-union; sinograms or sinus methylene blue injections preoperatively, which give information as to the depth and direction; preoperative cultures of sinuses, tissue biopsies and abscess aspiration, which will help to isolate the offending organisms in infected non-unions, and determine their sensitivity; AP and lateral arteriograms, which should be done in cases of open fractures with scarring or where there has been complex previous surgery, when circulation is questionable or vascularized tissue transfers are contemplated – ultrasonic and Doppler studies sometimes obviate the need for arteriograms; bone scans, which are of value in synovial pseudarthroses; gallium scans, which are useful in determining infection; EMG, nerve conduction tests and careful neurological examination preoperatively, which are useful in determining the status and degree of nerve damage, and may aid or preclude the need for nerve exploration and repair at the time of non-union surgery.

Consultations with specialists from other areas preoperatively will frequently aid in avoiding complications and postoperative litigation. This means consulting specialists from the fields of anesthesia, plastic surgery and the blood bank, for example, as well as the infectious disease team to assess correct antibiotic therapy in infected cases. In noninfected cases, prophylactic antibiotics (usually cephalosporins) are used preoperatively, intraoperatively and postoperatively for a maximum of 36 h to prevent infection in these multiply operated limbs.

Fig. 19.5

a Pseudarthroses of the clavicle are stabilized with a six- to seven-hole 3.5-mm DCP or a 3.5-mm reconstruction plate.

b Quite often it is necessary to resect the ends of the non-union and to insert an intercalary bone graft. In treating these pseudarthroses, an attempt must be made to re-establish the normal length of the clavicle. The DCP can be precisely contoured when inserted from the front. This placement of the plate takes advantage of the relatively flat surface of the clavicle.

c Here a 3.5-mm reconstruction plate and lag screw are used to regain clavicle shape and length plus an additional cancellous bone graft.

Fig. 19.6

a In treating the humerus a broad eight- or nine-hole 4.5-mm DCP must be used. The screws must grip at least eight cortices on each side of the pseudarthrosis. The plate is usually applied to the lateral cortex. We use the broad plate, not because it is more rigid, but because its holes are staggered.

b The non-unions and pseudarthroses of the humerus are often of the nonreactive, atrophic type. This type of non-union appears more often in the humerus than anywhere else. Where the fracture goes on to form a nonreactive non-union, it is often associated with an exceptional degree of osteoporosis. We feel that in order to obtain rapid consolidation it is necessary to decorticate as well as to bone graft the non-union. The decortication should be done only on the side of the bone where the screws do not gain purchase. Where screws do not hold, methyl methacrylate cement may be used but care should be taken not to allow any of the cement to enter the non-union or go outside of the confines of the bone.

Note: In the treatment of a non-union of the humerus associated with stiff elbow the plate should usually be placed on the dorsal aspect to effect a tension band fixation. Where the fixation has not been perfect, the arm should be immobilized in a double-plaster splint or lightweight cast brace for 4–6 weeks to protect the internal fixation and prevent the screws from being pulled out.

Fig. 19.7

a For non-unions of the radius or ulna in large men, we use a seven-hole or longer tension band narrow 4.5-mm DCP. Note the positioning of the seven-hole plate on the ulna which is at right angles to the previous screw holes. For both bones, in women and small men we prefer an eight-hole or longer 3.5-mm DCP.

b Two hypertrophic non-unions of the radius and ulna are stabilized here by a plate and one interfragmentary screw. The length of both bones should be carefully maintained to obtain a normal distal radioulnar joint.

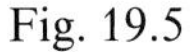

Fig. 19.5

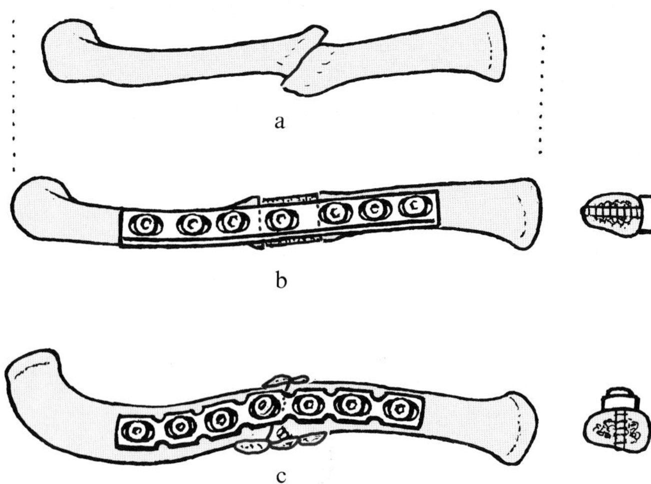

Fig. 19.6

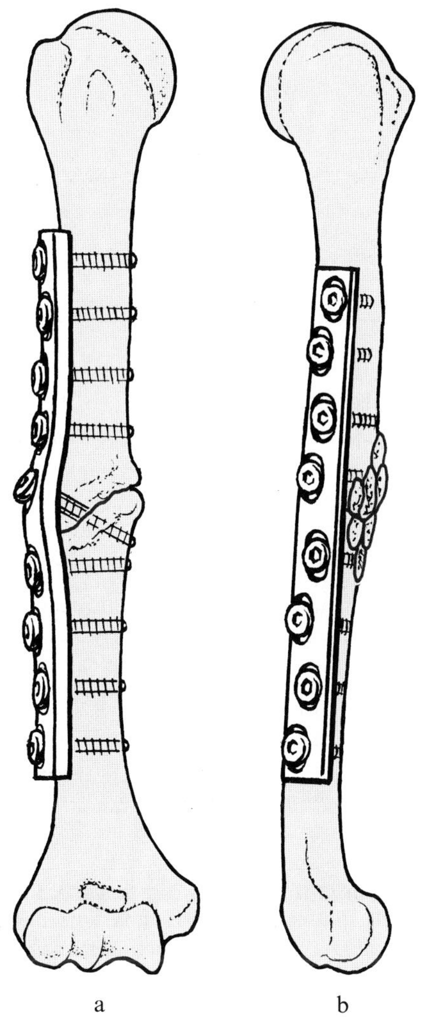

a b

Fig. 19.7

a b

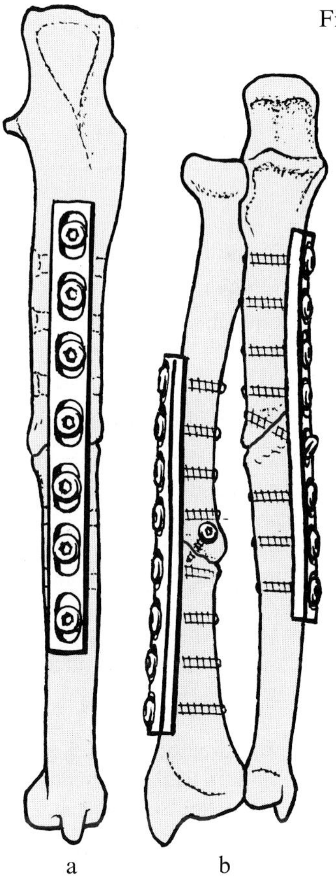

19.7 Operative Techniques to Achieve Union

The numerous and specific techniques utilized in the treatment of delayed unions, non-unions and pseudarthroses are illustrated in Figs. 19.5–19.40 and explained in the legends.

Fig. 19.8

a Non-unions through the surgical neck of the humerus fixed with a T plate.

b If the bone is severely osteoporotic and screws do not hold, then consider using cortex screws and cement.

Fig. 19.9

a An oblique supracondylar pseudarthrosis of the humerus. Note the lag screw across the pseudarthrosis.

b This Y-shaped supracondylar pseudarthrosis is fixed with a one-third tubular plate medially. This medial plate should be applied on the crest, and the lateral plate placed posteriorly. A 3.5-mm reconstruction plate may be used to good advantage. Note also the bone graft. The ulnar nerve may have to be transposed anteriorly because of the medial implant. A transverse lag screw (or position screw) is used to fix the intercondylar fracture.

Fig. 19.10 This transverse supracondylar non-union was stabilized with a spoon plate posteriorly. The tip of the olecranon was resected to avoid impingement on the plate in the olecranon fossa and was used as a bone graft.

Fig. 19.11 A non-union of the proximal ulna (Monteggia fracture with butterfly fragment). A 3.5-mm reconstruction plate is used posteriorly with a lag screw into the butterfly. The proximal intramedullary screw gains better hold on the osteoporotic proximal fragment. A bone graft is used around the non-union. Note the screw hole of the compressor/distractor, which indicates its use to good advantage.

Fig. 19.12

a, b Note the use of the small T plate in the treatment of the metaphyseal pseudarthrosis of the proximal phalanx. A bone graft is added in the defect. A good alternative is the finger condylar plate.

Fig. 19.8

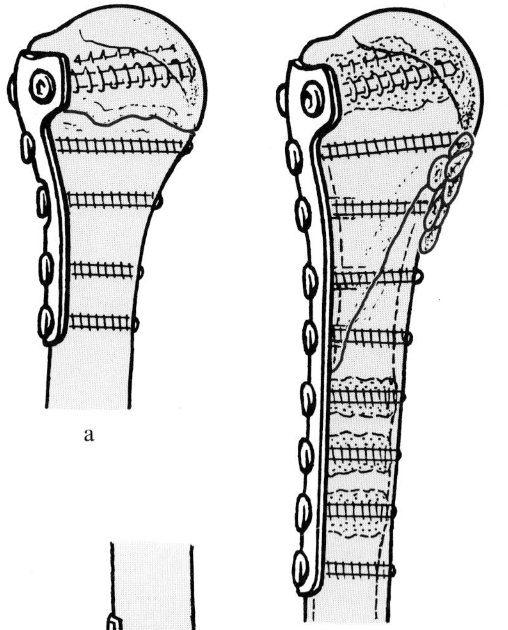

a

b

Fig. 19.9

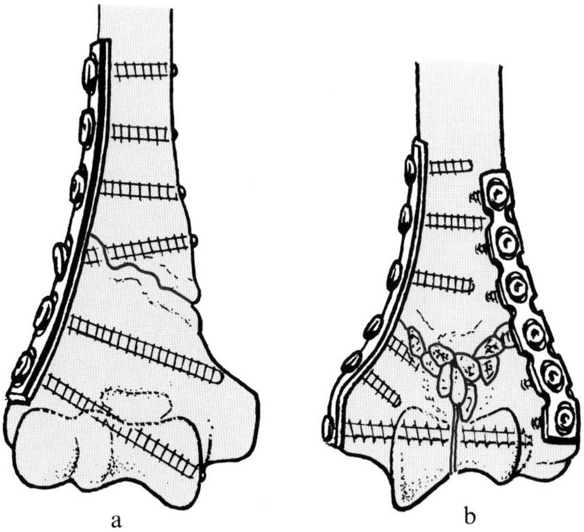

a

b

Fig. 19.10

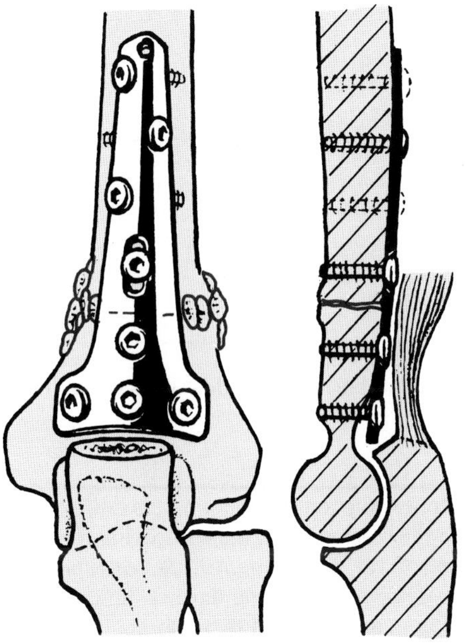

Fig. 19.11

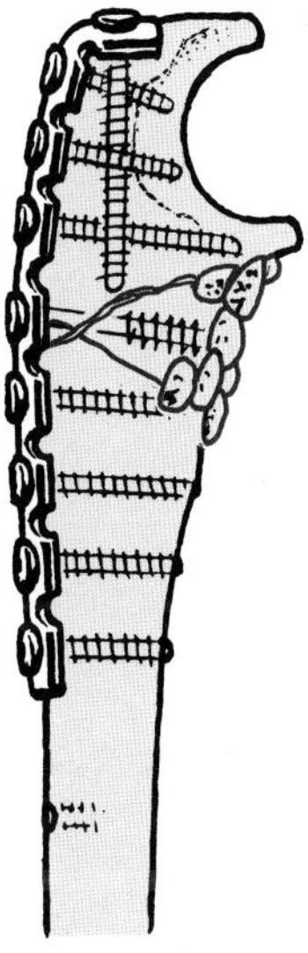

Fig. 19.12

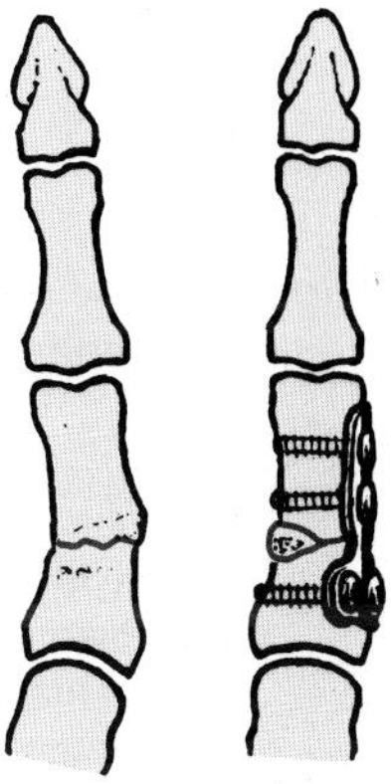

a

b

Fig. 19.13 The non-unions of the middle third of the femur (and tibia) are the ideal indications for intramedullary nailing.

Figs. 19.14, 19.15 The interlocking universal nail is used under the following conditions: where axial or rotational stability is difficult to achieve with standard nailing; where the fracture is in the subtrochanteric or supracondylar region of the femur (Fig. 19.14) or similar areas of the tibia (Fig. 19.15); or where leg length is to be maintained. Reaming does not have to be as aggressive as with standard nailing, since the interlocking screws give stability to the fracture rather than the contact produced by reaming.

Fig. 19.16 Broaching the sealed medullary canal with the 6-mm thick hand reamer.

Fig. 19.13 Fig. 19.14 Fig. 19.15 Fig. 19.16

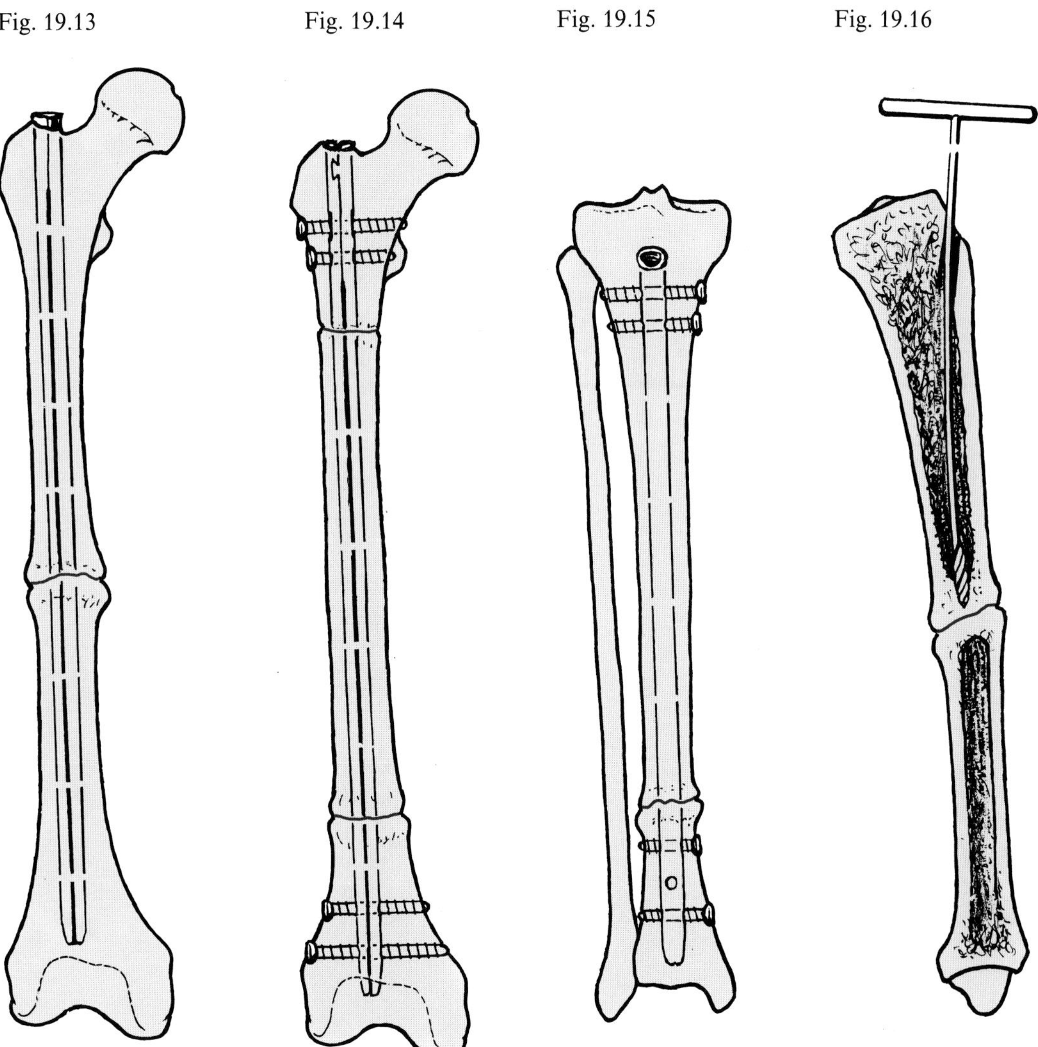

Fig. 19.17 The tension band plate is always placed on the tension or convex side of the deformity.

a In the more common varus deformity, the plate, almost always a narrow 4.5-mm DCP, is placed on the convex or lateral side.

b The valgus deformity is less common. Here the plate is applied on the medial side. If the fibula is longer, no osteotomy is required. If the fibula has healed with shortening or deformity, it must be osteotomized prior to the correction of the tibia.

c In a posterior bowing of the tibia (recurvatum), the plate is placed on the posterior aspect.

Note: In all of the above mid-tibial non-unions, an intramedullary nail is an excellent alternative to plating when deformity can be corrected.

Fig. 19.18 The use of the tension device to correct a significant varus deformity of the tibia. The plate is first fixed with four screws, usually to the distal fragment. The tension device is then fixed to the proximal fragment with a long cortex screw which is then gradually tightened. With the development of increasingly higher tension on the lateral side, the varus deformity is gradually corrected and the lateral portion of the non-union comes under quite marked axial compression. A fibular osteotomy becomes necessary only if there is a considerable deformity of the fibula.

Fig. 19.19 This model illustrates how correction of the varus of the tibia (a) results in overall lengthening of the bone (b) despite the shortening which takes place as a result of axial compression.

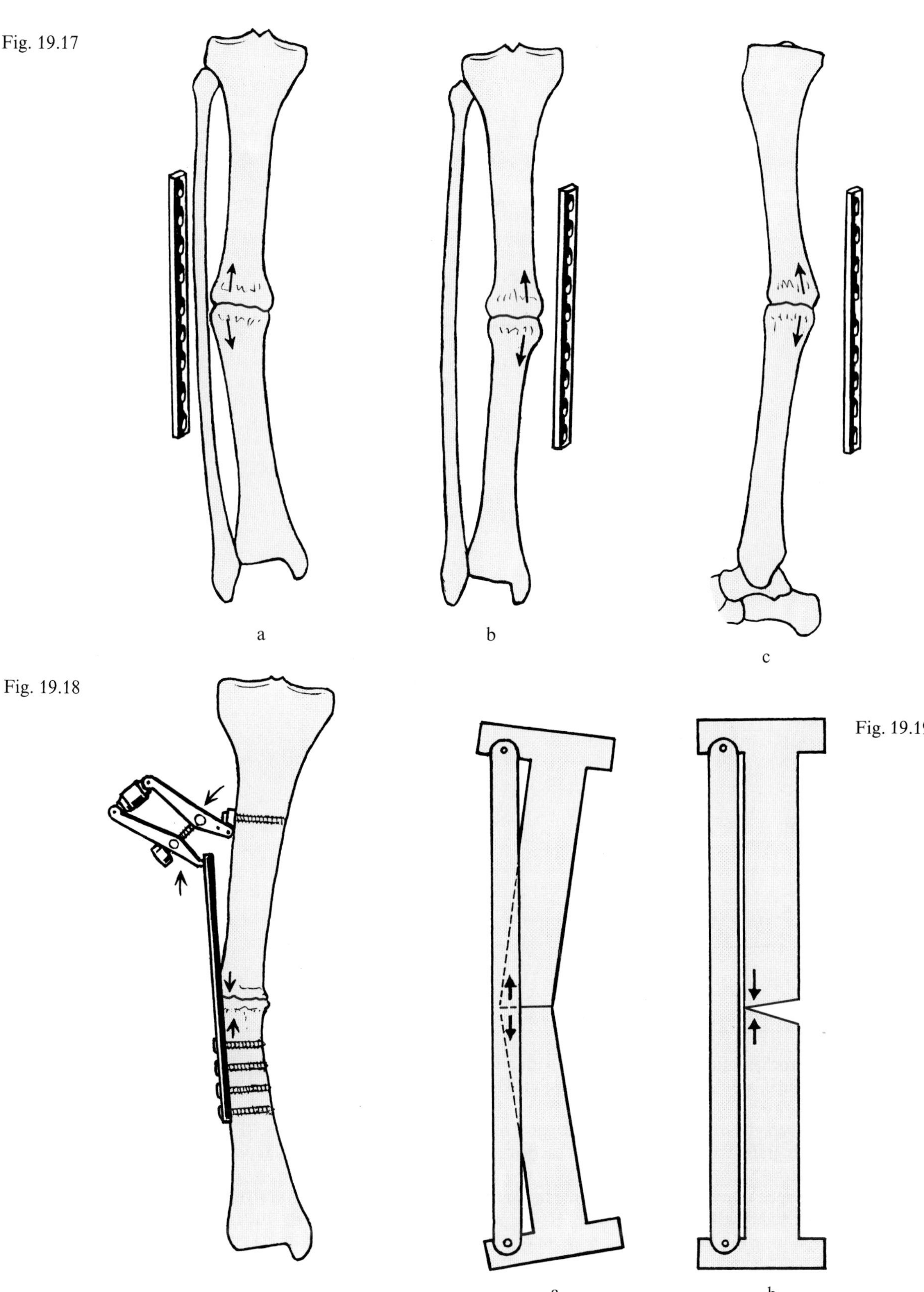
Fig. 19.17
a
b
c
Fig. 19.18
Fig. 19.19
a
b

Fig. 19.20 Subtrochanteric non-union treated with a dynamic condylar screw, an interfragmentary lag screw across the plate, a bone graft and compression. The condylar blade plate can also be used (see Fig. 19.32).

Fig. 19.21 Supracondylar pseudarthroses are good indications for condylar plates. If a defect is present medially, this is grafted and decortication is carried out. A lag screw is added when possible.

Fig. 19.22 Y-shaped intercondylar and supracondylar non-union stabilized with a dynamic condylar screw, a bone graft and axial compression.

Fig. 19.23 A failed supracondylar non-union in osteoporotic bone treated previously with a dynamic condylar screw salvaged with a condylar buttress plate. The large hole left by the condylar screw is filled with a bone graft or cement, as are the other screw holes that do not provide a sufficient hold. A bone graft is added.

Fig. 19.20

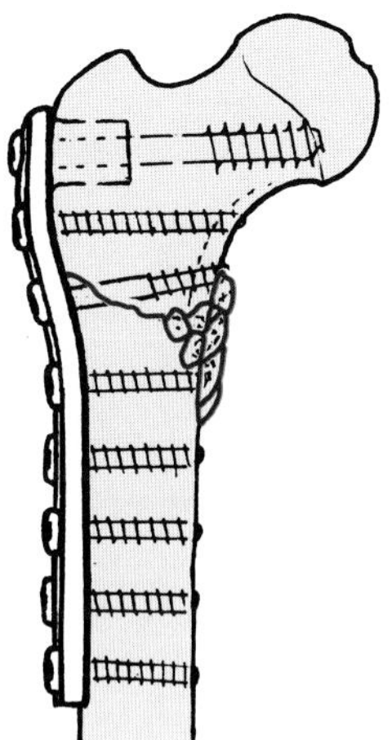

Fig. 19.21

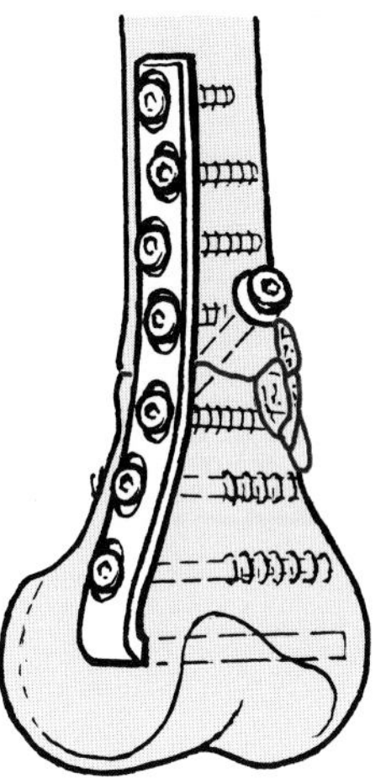

Fig. 19.22

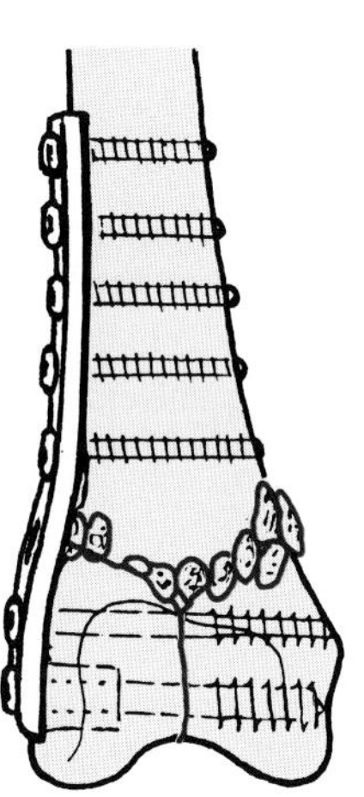

Fig. 19.23

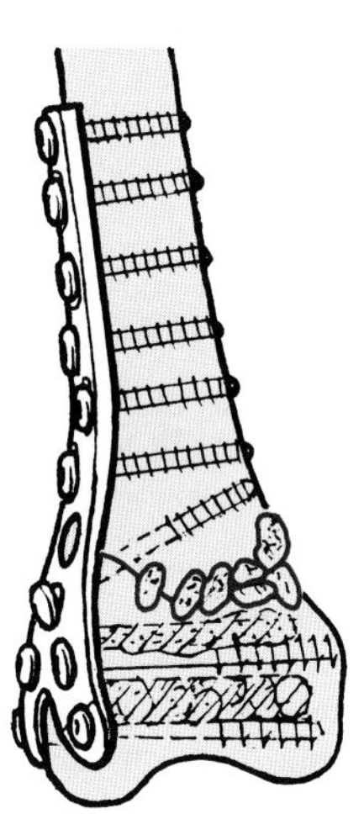

Fig. 19.24 A double pseudarthrosis – one on either side of the knee joint.

a If the joint is destroyed, we recommend two long compression plates at right angles to one another. These not only stabilize the pseudarthroses but enable us at the same time to carry out an arthrodesis of the knee joint in a physiological position.

b Here the arthrodesis of the knee is performed with a long universal intramedullary nail with interlocking screws above and below. This is especially used after failed total knee arthroplasty where there is loss of bone, infection and poor skin.

Fig. 19.25 A pseudarthrosis of the proximal tibia stabilized with a T plate or L plate laterally and a semi-tubular plate anteriorly.

Fig. 19.26 In pseudarthrosis of the medial malleolus, it is difficult to achieve any interfragmental compression with a lag screw because of the severe osteoporosis. We therefore insert a graft into a slot cut at right angles to the pseudarthrosis. We occasionally excise the medial malleolus if the fragment is small and below the tibial plafond.

For lateral malleolar type B non-unions, a third-tubular or 3.5-mm DCP is contoured and applied after a plate-independent lag screw has been inserted. Rotation of the fibula must be carefully controlled. A bone graft may be needed to regain length. A distal intramedullary screw may help to gain purchase in porotic bone.

Fig. 19.27 Previously infected pseudarthroses with a broad area of contact between the ends.

a In a pseudarthrosis of the tibia with varus deformity and a broad area of contact between the ends, fixation and axial alignment is achieved with a long 9- to 12-hole plate applied on the lateral side. Screws are inserted first proximally and second distally, leaving the pseudarthroses and the surrounding tissue undisturbed; in oligotrophic non-unions, decortication and cancellous bone graft will be added.

b Whenever there is a small defect which increases the risk of a flare-up of sepsis, it may be better to and fix the pseudarthrosis by external fixation and perform a tibiofibular synostosis. Note that the fibular osteotomy is carried out distally and never at the level of the pseudarthrosis. A cancellous bone graft fills the defects created by curettage, shingling and synostosis. A double-tube, one-plane or a two-plane, unilateral fixator may be indicated in such cases (V frame).

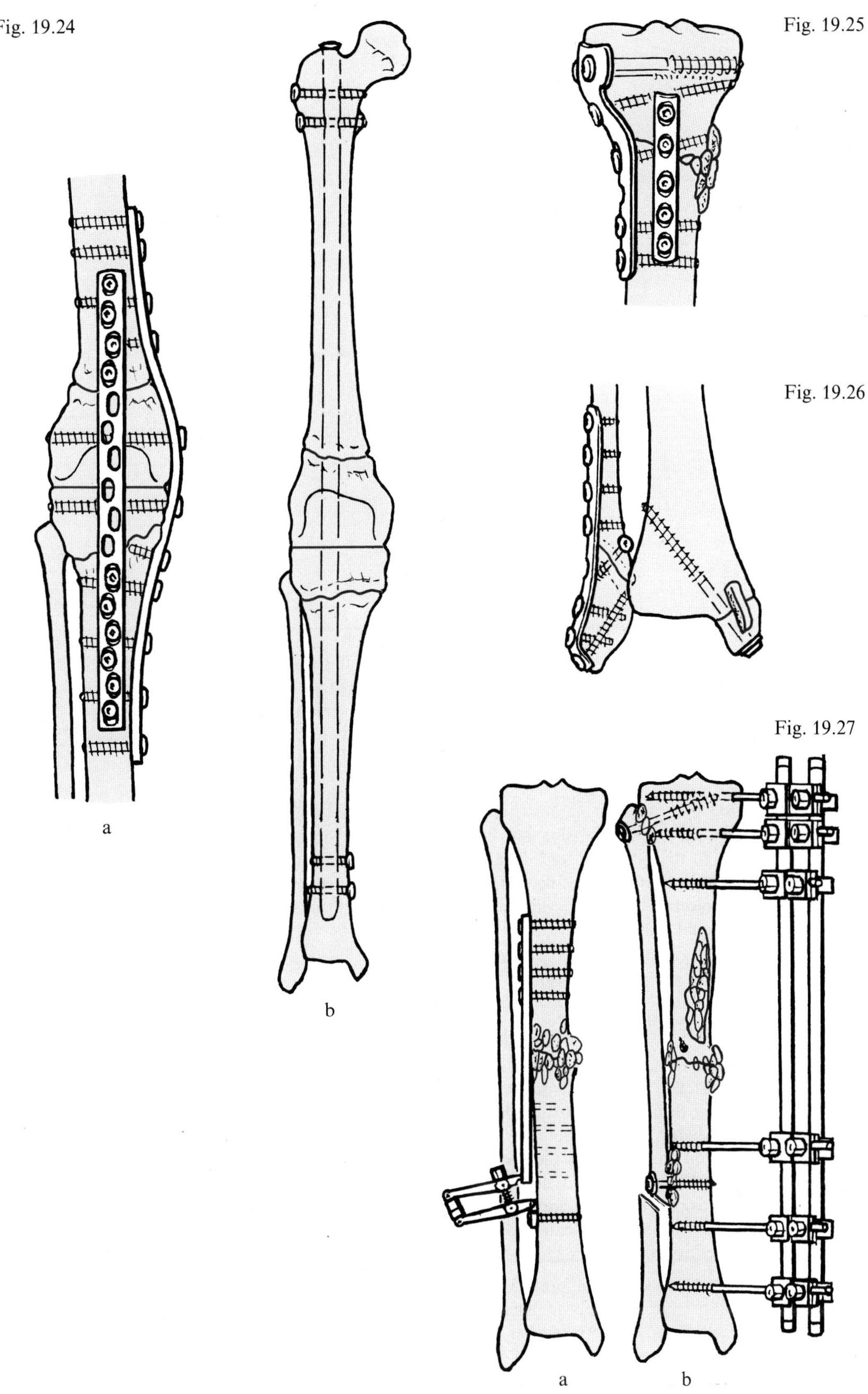

Fig. 19.24

Fig. 19.25

Fig. 19.26

Fig. 19.27

Fig. 19.28 Pseudarthroses with bone loss. In the humerus it suffices to carry out extensive decortication, a bone graft and stabilization with the modular external fixator. The Schanz screws in the two fragments are inserted at an angle close to 90° to avoid any risk to the radial nerve. A subsequent tension band plating would become necessary if the pseudarthrosis were to persist. Plating in conjunction with cancellous autotransplant as a primary procedure may also be considered.

Fig. 19.29

a Large defects in the ulna are bridged with a 3.5-mm DCP or 3.5-mm reconstruction plate which is fixed to the proximal and distal fragment while the hand is maintained in full supination. The trough alongside the plate is filled with small corticocancellous bone fragments. Subsequently the arm must be protected in plaster, since a single plate in the presence of a large defect does not provide enough rotational stability.

b Alternatively a vascularized fibular graft or Ilizarov type of corticotomy and AO external fixator could be used.

Fig. 19.30 Pseudarthrosis of the femur with bone loss.

a An AO-Ilizarov procedure is carried out with resection of the infected bone ends and a corticotomy just distal to the lesser trochanter, using a 4.5-mm Schanz screw double-bar construction. The transport segment distal to the corticotomy is moved distally 0.20 mm four to five times a day until it obliterates the pseudarthrosis defect. To prevent a varus tendency from developing, the second tube is used as a tension band because the threaded bar used for transport offers very little axial stability. Additionally the proximal head and neck fragments may be lengthened proximally at the corticotomy site using the proximal transport nut after loosening the tube nuts of the proximal fragment until normal femoral length is achieved. A cancellous bone graft is added at the distal pseudarthrosis site if union is slow or does not occur.

b A vascularized fibular graft may be used instead of the above with a double-tube external fixator for stability and an additional cancellous iliac graft after gradual lengthening with the external fixator. A cancellous bone graft after lengthening with the double-bar external fixator may be used to fill a smaller defect instead of the fibular graft. The external fixator may be removed in favor of a long special lengthening plate at that time, or later if necessary, or a locked intramedullary rod may be substituted.

Fig. 19.28

Fig. 19.29

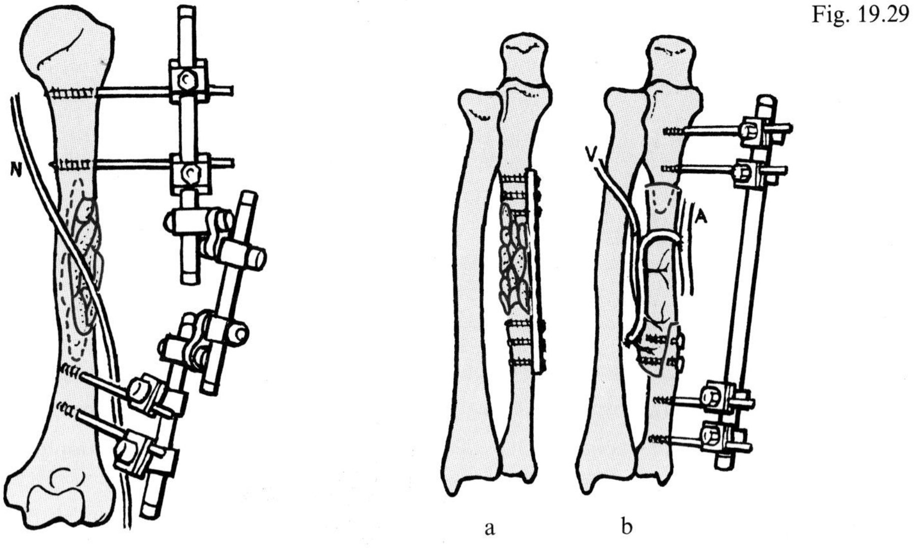

Fig. 19.30

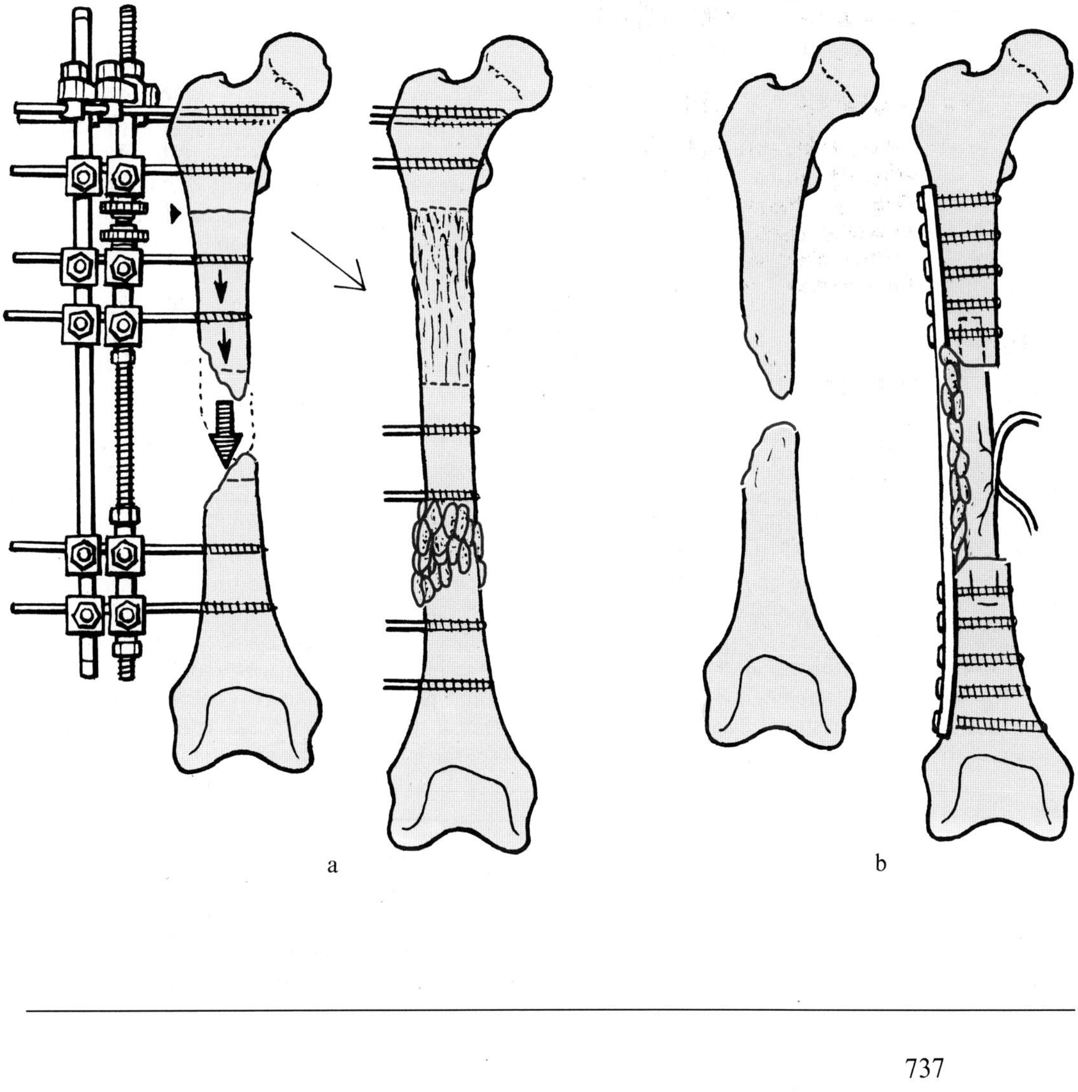

a

b

Fig. 19.31 Using the intramedullary nail in a hypertrophic pseudarthrosis of the femur.

a Note the large resorption cavity in which the distal end of the nail moves about.

b If the nail has good purchase above, stability can be obtained by simply advancing a longer and wider nail a further 2–3 cm through the distal end of the resorption cavity.

c Alternatively, if previously infected, the medullary canal may be reamed to debride it, and the non-union stabilized by interlocking nailing. Normally, however, we recommend removal of the nail, debridement of the medullary cavity by over-reaming, and stabilization with a double-tube external fixator. The local sinus and infected soft tissues are debrided and the wound left open. Antibiotic beads may be added. A carefully controlled closed suction irrigation system could also be used for about 1 week if the wound is closed. Secondarily, after 3–4 weeks a pure cancellous bone graft is inserted into the debrided bony defect following removal of antibiotic beads.

Fig. 19.32 Subtrochanteric pseudarthrosis.

a, b We strongly recommend the use of a condylar plate or DCS with axial compression as a means of achieving stability. This must be combined with posteromedial bone grafting. A fistula will persist till the plate is removed. In a number of months, however, the pseudarthrosis will be sufficiently consolidated to permit removal of the implant. Then debridement and probably some additional cancellous bone grafting will follow. If healing of the lateral cortex appears doubtful, an external fixator may be applied for a few weeks as a safeguard against refracture.

Fig. 19.33

a In the middle of the shaft, it is possible to use the two-tube external fixator as a means of stabilization. Note the additional medial bone graft.

b Weber's wave plate is a very good alternative. It has three basic aims or potentials:

1. It allows for ingrowth of vessels into the cancellous bone onlay graft beneath the plate.
2. It reduces the danger of fatigue fracture of the plate by distributing bending stresses over a long sector of the plate, thus avoiding local stress concentrations.
3. If the lateral cortex is preserved or reconstructed, the wave plate can act as a very efficient tension band of the lateral cortex so that the support by the medial cortex, normally required in plating, particularly of the femur, is substituted by the lateral cortex.

Fig.19.34 A pseudarthrosis of the distal femur can be stabilized by means of a double-frame external fixator. This is accomplished by inserting two Steinmann pins above and two below the pseudarthroses. These are then prestressed against each other in such a way that the pseudarthrosis is brought under axial compression. As seen from (a) the front, and (b) the lateral side.

Fig. 19.35

a An infected pseudarthrosis of the distal femur with a stiff knee joint can at times be salvaged by grafting laterally and then immobilizing the leg in a cast in up to 60° of valgus through the pseudarthrosis to permit the formation of a lateral bony bridge.

b 6–7 weeks later, the deformity can be corrected manually and casted. The lateral bony bridge then acts as a tension band and the corrective force results in a strong axial compressive force which will aid in the rapid consolidation of the pseudarthrosis.

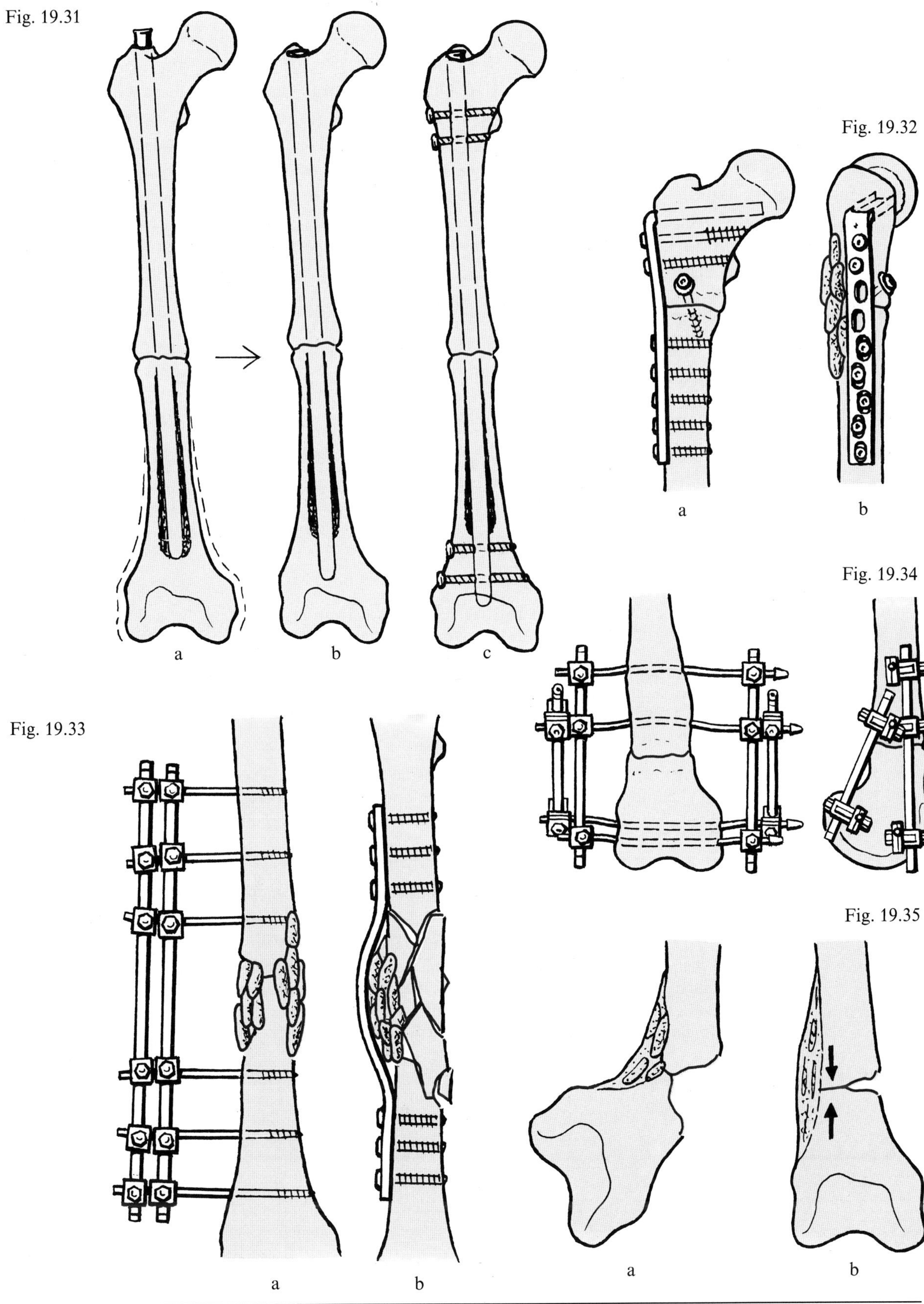

Fig. 19.31
a
b
c
Fig. 19.32
a
b
Fig. 19.34
Fig. 19.33
Fig. 19.35
a
b
a
b

19.8 Postoperative Treatment

Non-unions of the lower extremities are mobilized as soon as possible postoperatively by supervised exercises and/or a CPM machine even as early as in the recovery room. Partial weight-bearing with crutches or a walker is prescribed until there is evidence of a bony bridge on serial X-rays. This really means 10–20 kg of weight-bearing taught to the patient by a physiotherapist using a scale or a special beeping shoe device to facilitate compliance by the patient. When sufficient bony bridging is evident on X-rays, a gradually progressive, weekly increase in weight-bearing is allowed. Active motion exercises should be supervised carefully by a physiotherapist until maximum joint motion is achieved. Hinged casts or cast braces are added postoperatively, either to support unstable joints, weak limbs and bone until strength returns or to prevent noncompliant patients from loosening or breaking their internal fixation.

In the upper extremity, early active supervised exercises and/or a CPM machine follow immediately after surgery, or when splints are removed a few days later to allow traumatized soft tissues to rest. A sling is most often used to support and protect the arm postoperatively but does not prevent active movements. Pushing, pulling or lifting are not allowed until union takes place. Hinged braces are prescribed when necessary to prevent stress on the internal fixation, or to support ligamentous repair.

Fig. 19.36

a If the intramedullary nail provides a reasonable degree of fixation, just carry out a decortication and a cancellous bone graft through an anterolateral or posterolateral approach, depending upon the preoperative arteriogram and the vascularity that is present. If instability exists, revise the intramedullary nailing. Ream further and insert a larger size nail or an interlocking nail.

b Alternatively, remove the nail and stabilize with a two-plane, unilateral external fixator and do a fibula pro tibia synostosis.

Fig. 19.37 This synostosis was carried out in the presence of an intact fibula. There is some bone contact and a medial fistula. The approach is lateral. The tibia and fibula are decorticated and an extensive bone graft is carried out. A V-shaped external fixator is added for medial support.

Fig. 19.38 Tibiofibular synostosis in the presence of infection and bone loss.

a Carry out a bone graft as far proximally as possible, but take care not to damage the anterior tibial artery and peroneal nerve. In addition, carry out a graft distally to secure union above and below. A cancellous graft may be added at the defect after thorough debridement.

b This is another method of achieving a fibula protibia synostosis. The fibula is plated to achieve alignment, length and stability. Screws may be used superiorly after the superior tibiofibular joint has been eradicated and bone grafted, and distally a fibular osteotomy with the excision of 1–2 cm of fibula is performed and the distal fibula fixed to the tibia with a lag screw and a bone graft.

Fig. 19.39 Pseudarthrosis of both the tibia and fibula at the same level with poor contact between the fragments: first immobilize the pseudarthrosis by means of four or six Schanz screws and a double-tube external fixator. As soon as the infection has abated, carry out a decortication and cancellous bone graft through a posterolateral approach. Late debridement of the infected area may be necessary to eradicate infection. If so, a final cancellous bone graft is used to fill the defect.

Fig. 19.40 The "AO-Ilizarov" technique is certainly an excellent means of bridging large defects in the tibia by performing a proximal or distal metaphyseal corticotomy, and moving the central segment with overlying living soft tissues to close the defect, not only in the bone but in the soft tissues as well. A preliminary debridement of the infected bone ends is performed. A tibiofibular synostosis, as illustrated, may not always be necessary.

Fig. 19.36

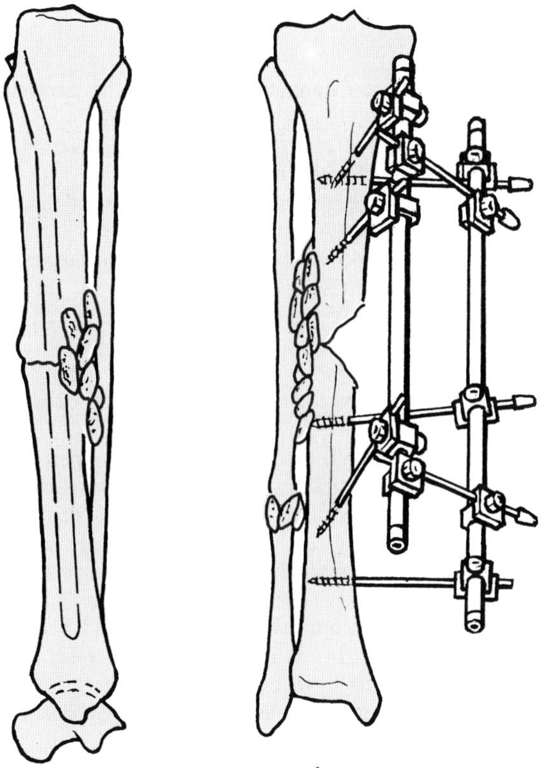

a

b

Fig. 19.37

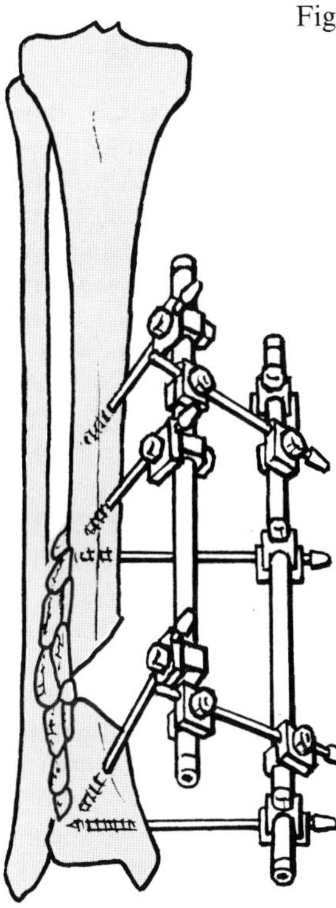

Fig. 19.38

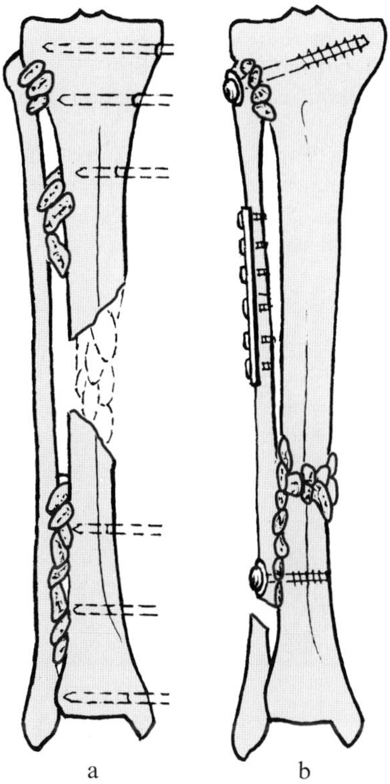

a

b

Fig. 19.39

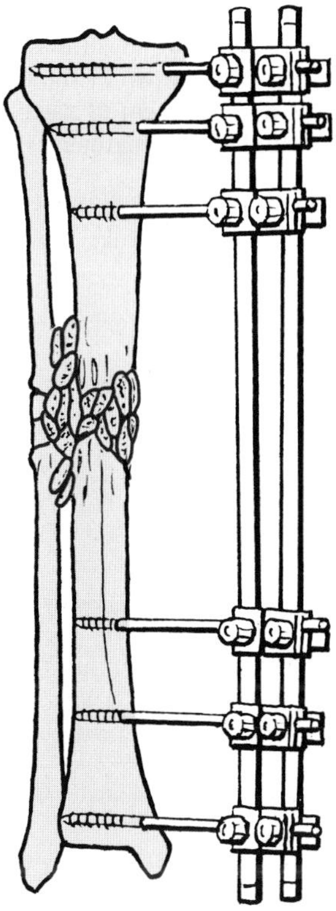

Fig. 19.40

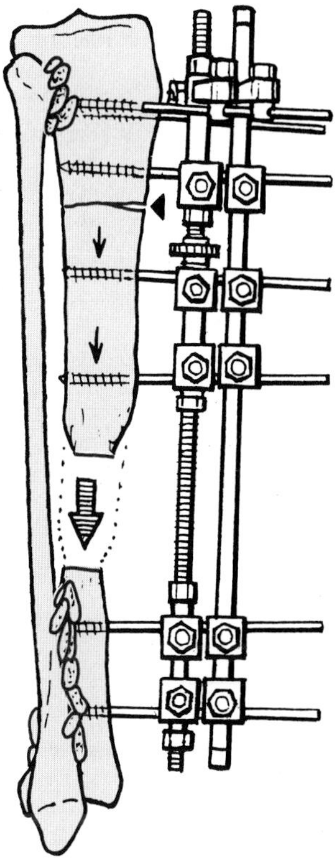

References

Anderson LD, Boyd HB, Johnston DS (1965) Changing concepts in the treatment of non-union. Clin Orthop 43:37

Bassett CAL, Mitchell SN, Gaston SR (1981) Treatment of ununited tibial diaphyseal fractures with pulsing electromagnetic fields. J Bone Joint Surg [Am] 63:511–523

Brighton CT, Pollack SR (1985) Treatment of recalcitrant non-union with a capacitively coupled electric field. A preliminary report. J Bone Joint Surg [Am] 67:577–585

Eggers GWN, Shindler TO, Pomerat CM (1949) The influence of the contact compression factor on osteogenesis in surgical fractures. J Bone Joint Surg [Am] 31:693

Friedrich B, Klaue P (1977) Mechanical stability and post-traumatic osteitis: an experimental evaluation of the relation between infection of bone and internal fixation. Injury 9:23

Ilizarov GA, Kaplunov AG, Degtarev VE, Ledaiev VI (1972) Treatment of pseudarthroses and ununited fractures complicated by purulent infection, by the method of compression-distraction osteosynthesis. Ortop Travmatol Protez 33:10–14

Judet J, Judet R (1961) L'ostéogénèse et les retards de consolidation et les pseudoarthroses des os longs. 8e Congrès SICOT, New York 1960. Imprimeries des Sciences, Bruxelles

Kempf I, Grosse A, Lafforgue D (1978) L'apport du verrouillage dans l'enclouage centro-médullaire des os longs. Rev Chir Orthop 64:635–651

Meyer S, Weiland AJ, Willenegger H (1975) The treatment of infected non-union of fractures of long bones. J Bone Joint Surg [Am] 57:836

Müller ME (1965) Treatment of nonunions by compression. Clin Orthop 43:83–92

Müller ME (1979) Reconstructive bone surgery. In: Müller ME, Allgöwer M, Schneider R, Willenegger H (eds) Manual of internal fixation, 2nd edn. Springer, Berlin Heidelberg New York, pp 333–395

Müller J, Schenk RK, Willenegger H (1968) Experimentelle Untersuchungen über die Entstehung reaktiver Pseudoarthrosen am Hunderadius. Helv Chir Act 35:301

Papineau LJ, Alfageme A, Dalcourt JP, Pilon L (1979) Ostéomyélite chronique: excision et greffe de spongieux à l'air libre après mises à plat extensives. Int Orthop 3:165

Perren SM, Cordey J (1980) The concepts of interfragmentary strains. In: Uhthoff HF (ed) Current concepts of internal fixation of fractures. Springer, Berlin Heidelberg New York

Phemister DB (1947) Treatment of un-united fractures by onlay bone grafts without screw or other fixation and without breaking down of the fibrous union. J Bone Joint Surg 29:946

Rosen H (1979) Compression treatment of pseudarthroses. Clin Orthop 138:154–166

Weber BG, Brunner C (1981) The treatment of nonunions without electrical stimulation. Clin Orthop 161:24–32

Weber BG, Cech O (1976) Pseudarthrosis. Pathophysiology, biomechanics, therapy, results. Huber, Bern

Weiland AJ, Moore JR, Daniel RK (1983) Vascularized bone autografts: experience with 41 cases. Clin Orthop 174:87

20 INFECTIONS

20.1 Prophylaxis of Infection

Since the work of Jack Burke (1961), it has been clearly established that true prophylaxis in surgical patients means preoperative administration of the prophylactic agent in such a way that all tissues encountered during surgery will have a therapeutic level of the agent present. This clearly means that true prophylaxis can only be applied in elective surgery or – with regard to fractures – when deciding to operate on a closed fracture.

Open fractures are unanticipated wounds. Preventative medicine, and thus true prophylaxis, is therefore not possible. Administering antibiotics at the earliest possible moment may, however, still be helpful in preventing contamination from developing into overt infection in open fractures.

20.1.1 Indication for Antibiotic Prophylaxis

Antibiotic prophylaxis does have its hazards: it may induce a feeling of false security and therefore negligence in asepsis. This was particularly obvious in the kind of prophylaxis, once commonly practised, which consisted in starting antibiotics after operation and continuing this treatment over days and weeks. Ample evidence has accumulated that this policy very often eliminated relatively harmless germs of the gut and induced antibiotic resistance in dangerous bacteria, particularly in various staphylococci.

With today's knowledge, antibiotic prophylaxis has proven to be successful. However, careful handling of tissues and strict asepsis in combination with the elimination of dead tissue remain the best means of preventing infection.

Postlethwait (1977) classified wounds into four types: clean, clean contaminated, contaminated and dirty. In surgery of the locomotor system, most of the wounds will be surgically inflicted and therefore clean or – if dealing with open fractures brought to the hospital shortly after the accident – clean contaminated. An additional category exists for this kind of surgery: the wound with overt infection, particularly of the bones involved. There we talk of "osteitis". ("Osteomyelitis" is very often loosely used, but this term should be reserved for hematogenous infection of bones!)

Simple closed fractures which are treated by open reduction and internal fixation represent clean wounds. Usually there is no indication for prophylactic antibiotics, but there are some exceptions. Very difficult reconstructions requiring massive implants are likely to reduce local resistance to infection. Therefore, when dealing with a very difficult fracture problem such as an acetabular fracture or a pilon fracture, antibiotic prophylaxis appears indicated. The same holds true for fractures requiring reintervention. In cases with overt infection (draining sinuses), the term "antibiotic prophylaxis" does not apply, but preoperative bacteriologic examination is crucial to establish a clear antibiogram. Even then, antibiotics will only supplement sound surgical debridement with removal of dead tissue and particularly dead bone.

20.1.2 Selection of Antibacterial Agents

It must be stressed that in every hospital there should be a very strict antibiotic policy including the selection of antibiotics. Nowadays, most hospital centers use second- or third-generation cephalosporins. As the available agents change rapidly, no very specific advice can be given here. Preoperative application – normally intravenously at the beginning of anesthesia – is the most important principle to be observed.

Effective prophylaxis requires adequate dosage. This will vary according to the pharmacokinetics of the chosen agent. Antibiotics with long-lasting effective blood levels are required. Shorter-acting agents will have to be repeated during the first 24 h, but antibiotic prophylaxis should not exceed 24 to 36 h. We aim for "one-shot" antibiotic prophylaxis. At the time of writing, ceftriaxone seems to fulfill these criteria.

20.2 Postoperative Hematoma

After 12–18 h, a hematoma becomes an excellent culture medium for bacteria. In this connection, different bacteriological investigations have shown that up to 20% of residual postoperative hematomas are contaminated. Therefore they should be evacuated as soon as possible. This basic principle should be rigorously adhered to.

The evacuation must be performed under strict aseptic conditions in the operating area. The operative wound has to be sufficiently reopened so that the whole hematoma, including clots, can be removed and washed out with saline or Ringer solution. In some cases, as in the lower leg, where the hematoma may be located at a distance from the operative wound, a separate incision is recommended.

After removal of the hematoma, a new suction drain has to be inserted followed by primary wound closure. To avoid transmission of skin organism, the tube must be inserted from inside out prior to the wound closure.

Exceptionally, a small liquid subcutaneous hematoma can be aspirated by puncture. In such cases, the needle must always be inserted through a previous stab incision in order to avoid the implantation of skin particles.

20.3 Infection

In spite of optimal aseptic conditions and adequate preoperative, operative and postoperative management (see Chap. 6), occasional postoperative wound infection cannot be completely avoided. However, in the majority of cases, its evolution into a neglected chronic stage infection can be avoided by means of early diagnosis and immediate radical surgery.

For *early diagnosis*, an experienced surgeon should make the clinical assessment, as the course of a postoperative wound infection is very variable. The first signs of infection (swelling, redness, pain, fever, elevated leucocyte counts) can appear days, weeks or even months after internal fixation representing early, delayed or late manifestation, the clinical signs of which can be either acute or subacute. Exploratory punctures are not always reliable; a negative bacteriologic result does not necessarily exclude the presence of a fresh infection.

Immediate, aggressive surgery is the treatment of choice – following the old-established principle of *ubi pus, ibi evacua* that has to be respected in all fields of surgery. The procedure consists in adequate reopening of the operative wound and debridement of the infected tissue, careful removal of all remaining hematoma and excision of necrotic tissue, particularly subcutaneous fat, fascia and muscles. After such a thorough debridement, stable implants are to be left in place (tighten screws) and an irrigation drain is set up. Stably fixed bone should not be removed in this first phase, even if the vascularity of one or other of the parts seems to be decreased. Only loose fragments should be removed. In contrast, loosened implants must be removed, because they encourage the spread of infection, especially in bone. In such cases, stability should then be achieved by other means, preferably by external fixation. Further debridement may be necessary a few days later. Revascularization of fragment ends may occur.

The main purposes of irrigation-drainage are mechanical cleansing and the combating of retention. It makes "economical" wound opening possible, avoiding retention and preserving already existing vascular contacts between soft tissues and bone.

Irrigation-drainage is carried out with Ringer solution. Previously we used additional topical antibiotics such as neomycin, bacitracin and polymyxin, but these have been progressively abandoned due to bacterial resistance. Initially the irrigation-drainage should be performed continuously and maintained until the clinical signs of infection have disappeared and symptoms of retention are no longer present. In general it takes only a few days, but occasionally it may require more than 10 days.

A special problem is whether the debridement should be followed by closing the wound or leaving it open, with closed or open irrigation-drainage. The principal disadvantage of wound closure is the risk of retention and recurrence of infection. Closure may be justified only in cases with a freshly infected hematoma without bone involvement or after reliable debridement. In most cases, open wound treatment should be considered as standard procedure, regardless of whether the wound is partially closed by some stitches for adaption. Usually we try to use vital soft tissues to protect bone, plates, tendons, nerves, vessels and joint capsules.

This very active management of postoperative wound infection after osteosynthesis is justified on the grounds of the following advantages:

- Early containment of the infection.
- High rate of spontaneous reossification without additional bone grafting.
- High percentage of full functional repair.
- Very low rate of invalidity.

To illustrate these facts, a long-term study (5–29 years follow-up) of 40 infected shaft fractures may be mentioned (Willenegger and Roth). In all 40 cases, primary internal fixation was performed. Observation of clinical signs, early diagnosis and immediate surgical treatment of wound infection took place in one and the same clinic (Willenegger). In all 40 cases there was bone involvement.

Fracture type, treatment. Of the 40 fractures, 29 were closed and 11 open. There were 26 internal fixations of the tibia, 10 of the femur, three of the forearm and one of the humerus. Twenty-two cases were treated using plates and screws and 18 by intramedullary nailing.

Results in bone. In 31 patients (75%!) spontaneous bone healing was observed without bone grafting and without restabilization. In nine cases (25%) the infection developed into a chronic stage and left an osteitic focus which necessitated excision and cancellous bone grafting. In four of these cases restabilization was not required because the bone was already consolidated; in five there was an infected non-union which needed additional restabilization by exchange of implants. No recurrent infection was observed in the 40 cases.

Functional results. Full functional restoration was obtained in 33 of the 40 patients. In two cases, an irrelevant disability persisted (−15° supination in forearm, −5° dorsiflexion in foot). Thirty-five patients recovered full working capacity, while in five patients the working capacity was reduced by between 5% and 30%.

Results as good as these cannot be expected in the neglected chronic stages of postoperative wound infection. Such infections are combined with non-union and require focus elimination, bone grafting and restabilization (see Chap. 19). The repair problems involved in the case of large bone defects are especially difficult, requiring extensive bone grafting, transfer of microvascular composite grafts or fragment transport according to the method of Ilizarov.

References

Boyd RJ, Burke JF, Colton T (1973) A double-blind clinical trial of prophylactic antibiotics in hip fracture. J Bone Joint Surg [Am] 55:1251–1254

Burke JF (1961) The effective period of preventive antibiotic action in experimental incisions and dermal lesions. Surgery 50:161–168

Carlsson AS, Lidgren L, Lindberg L (1977) Prophylactic antibiotics. Acta Orthop Scand 48:405–409

Cushing RD (1977) Antibiotics in trauma. Surg Clin North Am 57:165–177

De Piro JT, Bowden TA, Hooks VH (1984) Prophylactic parenteral cephalosporins in surgery. JAMA 252:3277–3282

Geroulanos S, Lüthy R, Turina M, Largiadèr F, Senning A (1985) Antibiotikaprophylaxe in der Chirurgie. Helv Chir Acta 52:149–158

Guglielmo BJ, Hohn DC, Koo PJ, Hunt TK, Sweet RL, Conte JE (1983) Antibiotic prophylaxis in surgical procedures. A critical analysis of the literature. Arch Surg 118:943–955

Hell K (1988) Half-life of antibiotics – an important factor in surgical single-dose prophylaxis. In: Hell K, Hobsley M (eds) Antibiotic prophylaxis in surgery. International Society of Surgery, Reinach, Switzerland

Hill C, Flamant R, Mazas F, Evrand J (1985) Prophylactic cefazolin vs placebo in total hip replacement. Lancet I:795–797

Hirschmann JV (1987) Controversies in antimicrobial prophylaxis. Chemioterapia 6:202–207

Kaiser AB (1986) Antimicrobial prophylaxis in surgery. N Engl J Med 315:1129–1138

Peters G (1987) Perioperative Antibiotikaprophylaxe in der Chirurgie. Dtsch Med Wochenschr 112:644–646

Postlethwait RW (1977) Infection. In: Sabiston DC (ed) Textbook of surgery. Saunders, Philadelphia

Roth B, Müller J, Willenegger H (1985) Intraoperative Wundspülung mit einem neuartigen lokalen Antiseptikum. Helv Chir Acta 52:61–65

Willenegger H, Roth B (1986) Behandlungstaktik und Spätergebnisse bei Frühinfarkt nach Osteosynthese. Unfallchirurgie 12:241–246

SUBJECT INDEX

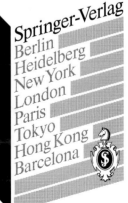

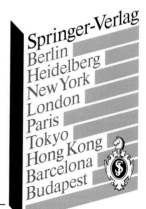